In Silico Strategies for Prospective Drug Repositionings

In Silico Strategies for Prospective Drug Repositionings

Editors

Lucreția Udrescu
Ludovic Kurunczi
Paul Bogdan
Mihai Udrescu

MDPI • Basel • Beijing • Wuhan • Barcelona • Belgrade • Manchester • Tokyo • Cluj • Tianjin

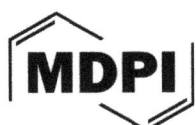

Editors
Lucreția Udrescu
Department I-Drug Analysis
"Victor Babeș" University
of Medicine and Pharmacy
Timișoara
Romania

Ludovic Kurunczi
Department I-Physical
Chemistry
"Victor Babeș" University of
Medicine and Pharmacy
Timișoara
Romania

Paul Bogdan
Ming Hsieh Department of
Electrical and Computer
Engineering
University of
Southern California
Los Angeles
United States

Mihai Udrescu
Department of Computer and
Information Technology
Politehnica University
of Timisoara
Timișoara
Romania

Editorial Office
MDPI
St. Alban-Anlage 66
4052 Basel, Switzerland

This is a reprint of articles from the Special Issue published online in the open access journal *Pharmaceutics* (ISSN 1999-4923) (available at: www.mdpi.com/journal/pharmaceutics/special_issues/drug_reposition).

For citation purposes, cite each article independently as indicated on the article page online and as indicated below:

LastName, A.A.; LastName, B.B.; LastName, C.C. Article Title. *Journal Name* **Year**, *Volume Number*, Page Range.

ISBN 978-3-0365-6134-9 (Hbk)
ISBN 978-3-0365-6133-2 (PDF)

© 2023 by the authors. Articles in this book are Open Access and distributed under the Creative Commons Attribution (CC BY) license, which allows users to download, copy and build upon published articles, as long as the author and publisher are properly credited, which ensures maximum dissemination and a wider impact of our publications.

The book as a whole is distributed by MDPI under the terms and conditions of the Creative Commons license CC BY-NC-ND.

Contents

About the Editors . . . . **vii**

Preface to "In Silico Strategies for Prospective Drug Repositionings" . . . . **ix**

Raul Pérez-Moraga, Jaume Forés-Martos, Beatriz Suay-García, Jean-Louis Duval, Antonio Falcó and Joan Climent
A COVID-19 Drug Repurposing Strategy through Quantitative Homological Similarities Using a Topological Data Analysis-Based Framework
Reprinted from: *Pharmaceutics* **2021**, *13*, 488, doi:10.3390/pharmaceutics13040488 . . . . **1**

Dan-Yang Liu, Jia-Chen Liu, Shuang Liang, Xiang-He Meng, Jonathan Greenbaum and Hong-Mei Xiao et al.
Drug Repurposing for COVID-19 Treatment by Integrating Network Pharmacology and Transcriptomics
Reprinted from: *Pharmaceutics* **2021**, *13*, 545, doi:10.3390/pharmaceutics13040545 . . . . **19**

Linda Brunotte, Shuyu Zheng, Angeles Mecate-Zambrano, Jing Tang, Stephan Ludwig and Ursula Rescher et al.
Combination Therapy with Fluoxetine and the Nucleoside Analog GS-441524 Exerts Synergistic Antiviral Effects against Different SARS-CoV-2 Variants In Vitro
Reprinted from: *Pharmaceutics* **2021**, *13*, 1400, doi:10.3390/pharmaceutics13091400 . . . . **35**

Speranta Avram, Miruna Silvia Stan, Ana Maria Udrea, Cătălin Buiu, Anca Andreea Boboc and Maria Mernea
3D-ALMOND-QSAR Models to Predict the Antidepressant Effect of Some Natural Compounds
Reprinted from: *Pharmaceutics* **2021**, *13*, 1449, doi:10.3390/pharmaceutics13091449 . . . . **49**

Yong Xiang, Kenneth Chi-Yin Wong and Hon-Cheong So
Exploring Drugs and Vaccines Associated with Altered Risks and Severity of COVID-19: A UK Biobank Cohort Study of All ATC Level-4 Drug Categories Reveals Repositioning Opportunities
Reprinted from: *Pharmaceutics* **2021**, *13*, 1514, doi:10.3390/pharmaceutics13091514 . . . . **69**

Priyanka Ramesh, Woong-Hee Shin and Shanthi Veerappapillai
Discovery of a Potent Candidate for RET-Specific Non-Small-Cell Lung Cancer—A Combined In Silico and In Vitro Strategy
Reprinted from: *Pharmaceutics* **2021**, *13*, 1775, doi:10.3390/pharmaceutics13111775 . . . . **95**

Stefania Olla, Maristella Steri, Alessia Formato, Michael B. Whalen, Silvia Corbisiero and Cristina Agresti
Combining Human Genetics of Multiple Sclerosis with Oxidative Stress Phenotype for Drug Repositioning
Reprinted from: *Pharmaceutics* **2021**, *13*, 2064, doi:10.3390/pharmaceutics13122064 . . . . **113**

Vlad Groza, Mihai Udrescu, Alexandru Bozdog and Lucreția Udrescu
Drug Repurposing Using Modularity Clustering in Drug-Drug Similarity Networks Based on Drug–Gene Interactions
Reprinted from: *Pharmaceutics* **2021**, *13*, 2117, doi:10.3390/pharmaceutics13122117 . . . . **127**

Muthu Kumar Thirunavukkarasu, Utid Suriya, Thanyada Rungrotmongkol and Ramanathan Karuppasamy
In Silico Screening of Available Drugs Targeting Non-Small Cell Lung Cancer Targets: A Drug Repurposing Approach
Reprinted from: *Pharmaceutics* **2021**, *14*, 59, doi:10.3390/pharmaceutics14010059 155

Albert Li, Jhih-Yu Chen, Chia-Lang Hsu, Yen-Jen Oyang, Hsuan-Cheng Huang and Hsueh-Fen Juan
A Single-Cell Network-Based Drug Repositioning Strategy for Post-COVID-19 Pulmonary Fibrosis
Reprinted from: *Pharmaceutics* **2022**, *14*, 971, doi:10.3390/pharmaceutics14050971 173

Utid Suriya, Panupong Mahalapbutr and Thanyada Rungrotmongkol
Integration of In Silico Strategies for Drug Repositioning towards P38 Mitogen-Activated Protein Kinase (MAPK) at the Allosteric Site
Reprinted from: *Pharmaceutics* **2022**, *14*, 1461, doi:10.3390/pharmaceutics14071461 187

Débora Chaves Cajazeiro, Paula Pereira Marques Toledo, Natália Ferreira de Sousa, Marcus Tullius Scotti and Juliana Quero Reimão
Drug Repurposing Based on Protozoan Proteome: In Vitro Evaluation of In Silico Screened Compounds against *Toxoplasma gondii*
Reprinted from: *Pharmaceutics* **2022**, *14*, 1634, doi:10.3390/pharmaceutics14081634 201

Verena Schöning and Felix Hammann
Drug-Disease Severity and Target-Disease Severity Interaction Networks in COVID-19 Patients
Reprinted from: *Pharmaceutics* **2022**, *14*, 1828, doi:10.3390/pharmaceutics14091828 217

Viktor A. Zouboulis, Konstantin C. Zouboulis and Christos C. Zouboulis
Hidradenitis Suppurativa and Comorbid Disorder Biomarkers, Druggable Genes, New Drugs and Drug Repurposing—A Molecular Meta-Analysis
Reprinted from: *Pharmaceutics* **2021**, *14*, 44, doi:10.3390/pharmaceutics14010044 233

Trang T. T. Truong, Bruna Panizzutti, Jee Hyun Kim and Ken Walder
Repurposing Drugs via Network Analysis: Opportunities for Psychiatric Disorders
Reprinted from: *Pharmaceutics* **2022**, *14*, 1464, doi:10.3390/pharmaceutics14071464 255

About the Editors

Lucreția Udrescu

Lucreția Udrescu is a specialist pharmacist and Professor in the Department I–Drug Analysis and Environmental Chemistry, Hygiene, and Nutrition at the Faculty of Pharmacy, the Victor Babeș University of Medicine and Pharmacy Timișoara, Romania. She received her Ph.D. in Chemistry from the Romanian Academy in 2015. Her research interests are computational drug repositioning, drug interactions (clinical evaluation and prediction), the internet of medical things applied in pharmacovigilance, and biopharmaceutical drug profile optimization using cyclodextrins.

Ludovic Kurunczi

Ludovic Kurunczi is a retired Professor from the Faculty of Pharmacy of the Victor Babeș University of Medicine and Pharmacy Timișoara, Romania. Before 1989, he was a researcher at the Institute of Chemistry Timișoara, Romania, and a member of a research team running a multi-year technological project that directed the production of two insecticides from the laboratory level to the resultant industrial unit (during this period, he coauthored 10 Romanian patents). Since 1990, he has been a professor of Physical Chemistry, Methodology of Scientific Research, and Drug Design at the Faculty of Pharmacy. In his career, he addressed the following research domains: the chemistry of the organophosphorus compounds, computational chemistry (molecular modeling, quantum chemistry), Quantitative Structure Activity (Property) Relationships (QSA(P)R), cheminformatics (similarity search, Discriminant Analysis–DA, Principal Component Analysis–PCA, Partial Least Squares–PLS), protein structure handling, molecular docking, virtual screening. His publications include five books, 14 chapters, and 120 research articles with over 1260 citations. Over the years, he participated in more than 15 research projects. He is the supervisor of 9 doctoral theses (one in progress) coordinated at the Department of Computational Chemistry, "Coriolan Drăgulescu", Institute of Chemistry Timișoara of the Romanian Academy.

Paul Bogdan

Paul Bogdan is the Jack Munushian Early Career Chair and associate professor (with tenure) in the Ming Hsieh Department of Electrical and Computer Engineering at University of Southern California. His work has been recognized with a number of distinctions, including the 2012 A.G. Jordan Award from the Electrical and Computer Engineering Department, Carnegie Mellon University for outstanding Ph.D. thesis and service, the 2012 Best Paper Award from the Networks-on-Chip Symposium (NOCS), the 2012 D.O. Pederson Best Paper Award from IEEE Transactions on Computer-Aided Design of Integrated Circuits and Systems, the 2012 Best Paper Award from the International Conference on Hardware/Software Codesign and System Synthesis (CODES+ISSS), the 2013 Best Paper Award from the 18th Asia and South Pacific Design Automation Conference. His main areas of interest are network science, complex systems, synthetic and system biology, systems pharmacology, neuroscience, cyber–physical systems, fractal modeling and control of biological systems, machine learning, artificial intelligence, and design methodologies for large scale heterogeneous many core systems.

Mihai Udrescu

Mihai Udrescu is a Professor of Computer Engineering in the Department of Computer and Information Technology at the Politehnica University of Timisoara, Romania. Between September 2019 and February 2020, he was a Fulbright Visiting Scholar in the Electrical and Computer Engineering department at Carnegie Mellon University. He received his Ph.D. in Computer Engineering from the Politehnica University of Timisoara in 2006. Mihai Udrescu's present research concentrates on developing machine learning techniques and emerging (quantum) computing methods for analyzing complex biological, technological, and social systems.

Preface to "In Silico Strategies for Prospective Drug Repositionings"

Drug design means planning a new chemical structure that purposely interacts with the biological targets known as being relevant for a given medical condition. The discovery of new drugs is one of the pharmaceutical research's most exciting and challenging tasks. Unfortunately, the conventional drug discovery procedure is chronophagous and cumbersome. However, over time, the successfully developed medicines—acting as planned on the intended targets—are also proven to work on other targets as efficient therapies for other diseases. Medicines have a proven proclivity to having multiple functions; a well-known example is Aspirin, initially used as an analgesic but later uncovered as an antiplatelet drug at low doses.

In this context, the process of systematically finding new functions for approved drugs—often called drug repositioning—becomes a valuable strategy in drug discovery. The literature also mentions similar terms: repurposing, reprofiling, redirecting, rediscovery, retasking, rescuing, recycling, redirection, therapeutic switching, etc. [1]. The common denominator of all these taxonomic variants is identifying a new indication for an existing drug. Nevertheless, there are significant differences in the characterizations of the repurposed entity—from "old drugs" [2] to "drug candidates from academic institutions and public sector laboratories not yet fully pursued" [3], "drugs that have previously passed safety testing for human use", or "drugs that have advanced to the clinical trial stage of development but have failed or stalled at that stage" [4].

Pursuing drug repurposing has obvious financial reasons. In 2004, Ashburn and Thor [5] argued that a solution for the pharma industry—facing high costs for launching new drugs—is to focus on drug repositioning. Indeed, in a 2020 June FDA virtual conference [6], participants estimated the costs for a repurposed drug to reach the market to be USD 500 thousand (for a development period of 1–3 years), in contrast to over USD 1.5 billion for a new drug (for a development period of 12–19 years). Such significant cost reductions mean drug repurposing is also suitable for identifying existing drugs as efficient in rare diseases with low economic incentives. Drug repositioning's massive potential to impact healthcare practices is further emphasized by the growth of this subject in the scientific literature. Thus, the number of papers containing the terms "drug" and "repurposing" has grown exponentially between 2005 and 2019 [7] (790 documents accumulated in 2019, according to Scopus).

Twenty years ago, pharmacists and medical doctors relied on fortuity to reposition medicines. The reason is that the drug-target search space is enormous, and exploring it requires vast human and material resources. Nevertheless, efficiently benefiting from serendipity requires that opportunity (drugs' apparent propensity for multiple functions) meets preparation (systematic, practical methods). The recent progress in machine learning, complex systems, and big data computational analysis provides systematic methods for drug repositioning. Such approaches successfully prune the drug-repositioning search space, providing valuable hints to experimental biologists and biochemists. As such, computational repositioning was recently employed as a valuable tool for identifying potential therapies for COVID-19.

Following this new and exciting trend, our Special Issue's scope was to collect papers introducing innovative computational methods to identify potential candidates for drug repositioning. The papers in this Special Issue introduce a wide array of in-silico strategies, such as complex network analysis, big data, machine learning, molecular docking, molecular dynamics simulation, and QSAR; these strategies target diverse diseases and medical conditions: COVID-19 and post-COVID-19 pulmonary fibrosis, non-small lung cancer, multiple sclerosis, toxoplasmosis, psychiatric disorders, or skin conditions such as Hidradenitis Suppurativa.

The editors are grateful to *Pharmaceutics* for allowing us to host this highly interdisciplinary, distinctive Special Issue. Our special thanks go to Candice Zhuo, the Assistant Editor, who strongly supported this project and facilitated our communication with the Editorial Office at *Pharmaceutics*. We also appreciate the work of all Assistant Editors involved in this Special Issue.

References:

[1] Langedijk, J. Continuous innovation in the drug life cycle. Ph.D. Thesis, Utrecht University, Utrecht, Netherlands, 2016 19 december (ISBN: 978-94-6233-489-2)

[2] Avram, S., Curpan, R., Halip, L., Bora, A., Oprea, T.I. Off-patent drug repositioning. Journal of Chemical Information and Modeling 2020, 60(12):5746-5753.

[3] Allarakhia, M. Open-source approaches for the repurposing of existing or failed candidate drugs: learning from and applying the lessons across diseases. Drug Design, Development and Therapy 2013, 7, 753-766.

[4] Pharmaceutical Companies Repurposing Drugs to Accelerate Growth.

[5] Ashburn, T.T., Thor, K.B. Drug Repositioning: Identifying and Developing New Uses for Existing Drugs. Nature Reviews Drug Discovery 2004, 3(8):673-683.

[6] FDA Drug Topics: CURE ID: Capturing Clinicians Experiences Repurposing Drugs to Inform Future Studies in the Era of COVID-19.

[7] Maria Shkrob and Jabe Wilson. Drug Repurposing Could Open the Door to New Therapies. Technology Networks. September 4, 2020.

Lucreția Udrescu, Ludovic Kurunczi, Paul Bogdan, and Mihai Udrescu
Editors

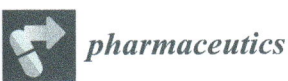

Article

A COVID-19 Drug Repurposing Strategy through Quantitative Homological Similarities Using a Topological Data Analysis-Based Framework

Raul Pérez-Moraga [1,2,†], Jaume Forés-Martos [1,2,3,†], Beatriz Suay-García [1,2], Jean-Louis Duval [4], Antonio Falcó [1,2,*] and Joan Climent [1,5,*]

1. ESI International Chair@CEU-UCH, Universidad Cardenal Herrera-CEU, CEU Universities, San Bartolomé 55, Alfara del Patriarca, 46115 Valencia, Spain; raulcl1994@gmail.com (R.P.-M.); fores.martos.jaume@gmail.com (J.F.-M.); beatriz.suay@uchceu.es (B.S.-G.)
2. Departamento de Matemáticas, Física y Ciencias Tecnológicas, Universidad Cardenal Herrera-CEU, CEU Universities, San Bartolomé 55, Alfara del Patriarca, 46115 Valencia, Spain
3. Biomedical Research Networking Center of Mental Health (CIBERSAM), 28029 Madrid, Spain
4. ESI Group, 3bis rue Saarinen, 94528 Rungis, France; Jean-Louis.Duval@esi-group.com
5. Departamento de Producción y Sanidad Animal, Salud Pública Veterinaria y Ciencia y Tecnología de los Alimentos, Universidad Cardenal Herrera-CEU, CEU Universities, C/Tirant lo Blanc 7, Alfara del Patriarca, 46115 Valencia, Spain
* Correspondence: afalco@uchceu.es (A.F.); joan.climentbataller@uchceu.es (J.C.)
† These authors have contributed equally to this work.

Abstract: Since its emergence in March 2020, the SARS-CoV-2 global pandemic has produced more than 116 million cases and 2.5 million deaths worldwide. Despite the enormous efforts carried out by the scientific community, no effective treatments have been developed to date. We applied a novel computational pipeline aimed to accelerate the process of identifying drug repurposing candidates which allows us to compare three-dimensional protein structures. Its use in conjunction with two in silico validation strategies (molecular docking and transcriptomic analyses) allowed us to identify a set of potential drug repurposing candidates targeting three viral proteins (3CL viral protease, NSP15 endoribonuclease, and NSP12 RNA-dependent RNA polymerase), which included rutin, dexamethasone, and vemurafenib. This is the first time that a topological data analysis (TDA)-based strategy has been used to compare a massive number of protein structures with the final objective of performing drug repurposing to treat SARS-CoV-2 infection.

Keywords: COVID-19; drug repurposing; topological data analysis; persistent Betti function

1. Introduction

On 11 March 2020, the World Health Organization (WHO) declared the Coronavirus Disease 2019 (COVID-19) outbreak, produced by the novel SARS-CoV-2 virus, a global pandemic [1]. To date, three previously approved antiviral drugs and one antimalarial medication (remdesevir, iopinavir, interferon-1, and hydroxychloroquine) have been tested for efficacy against SARS-CoV-2 infection by the WHO SOLIDARITY consortium in a large multicentric study. The results of the trial suggested that these treatments had little or no effect in a set of clinical outcomes which included overall mortality, time to initiation of mechanical ventilation, and duration of hospital stay [2].

With the third wave ongoing in many countries, herd immunity a distant prospect, and new strains challenging the existing vaccines, it is still a pressing need to find adequate treatments for the disease. De novo drug development and testing, including preclinical research and clinical trials, is a slow process that could take more than 12 years [3,4]. However, the current sanitary emergency makes it imperative to shorten this time frame. Therefore, sustained efforts to identify potential candidates for drug repurposing are necessary.

In the context of COVID-19, Kumar and co-workers compiled sets of genes linked to the disorder and studied their distribution in the human interactome [5]. They first identified the interactome subnetworks' hub genes in which the disease-related genes were placed. Then, they queried the drug–gene interaction database to identify Food and Drug Administration (FDA)-approved drugs that had the hub genes as their target (i.e., chloroquine, lenalidomide, pentoxifylline) [6,7]. Zhou and collaborators compiled a list of human proteins that physically interact with four previous human coronaviruses (SARS-CoV, MERS-CoV, HCoV-229E, and HCoV-NL63) and used network proximity measures to prioritize 16 potential anti-human coronavirus repurposable drugs including melatonin, mercaptopurine, and sirolimus [8]. Drug repurposing studies using virtual screening procedures based on molecular docking have also been reported. To cite an example, Kerestsu et al. used a protease inhibitors database (MEROSP) and the geometric structure of the 3C-Like virus protease (3CLpro) to identify 15 potential inhibitors using the surflex-Dock software [9].

Here, we present a general-purpose drug repositioning workflow and its application to the specific case of COVID-19. Our procedure is based on recent developments in the field of topological data analysis (TDA) and its use in the study of biological geometric structures [10]. In particular, our method relies on the idea that drugs that are known to target a specific protein would likely target other proteins that present high degrees of topological similarities with the initial protein. Therefore, the accumulated knowledge of drug–protein interactions available in public repositories such as DrugBank in combination with the information about protein three-dimensional structures found in the Protein Data Bank (PDB) can be used to predict new potential drug protein targets based on the computation of protein–protein topological similarities. Figure 1 contains a brief summary of the general methodology.

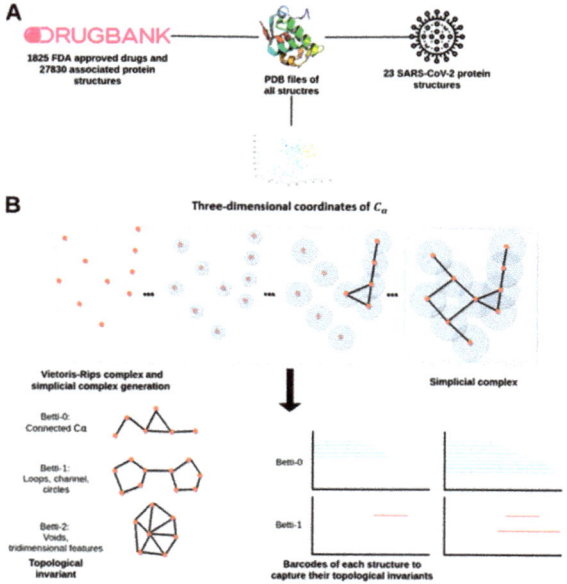

Figure 1. *Cont.*

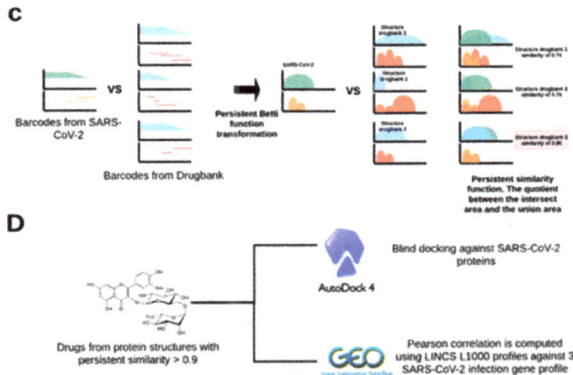

Figure 1. Bioinformatic work-flow used. (**A**) Data preprocessing and acquisition (**B**) Topological data analysis phase, Vietoris–Rips complexes at scale ε are computed to generate the barcodes. Each ε-associated Betti number captures a unique topological feature of the protein. (**C**) To compare barcodes of viral proteins against structures with known drugs, it is necessary to transform barcodes into comparable curves using persistent Betti functions (PBFs). (**D**) Candidate drugs from proteins with a mean persistent similarity score above 0.9 were validated by a dual in silico strategy. We used AutoDock 4 to analyze the capacity of the drug to bind against viral proteins. Transcriptomics analysis was performed to test the capacity of the candidate drugs to revert the transcriptomics effect induced by the COVID-19.

2. Results

2.1. Drugs, Protein Targets, and PDB Structures Included in This Study

DrugBank queries yielded 1825 drugs approved by the American Food and Drug Administration (FDA). The identified drugs had 1821 known unique protein targets, for which 27,839 three-dimensional structures were available in the protein databank. The first three persistent Betti functions (PBFs, see Section 4.2) were successfully calculated for 25,800 of the 27,839 structures, whereas computational limitations prevented us from estimating the remaining 1622 structures' PBFs. We also retrieved multiple protein structures from SARS-CoV-2 that were available in PDB, including the Spike protein receptor binding domain, the RNA-dependent RNA polymerase (NSP12), the endoribonuclease (NSP15), the ADP ribose phosphatase (NSP3), the RNA binding protein (NSP9), the 3C-like protease, and the NSP 8 and 7. In total, we calculated the PBFs of 23 viral protein structures. Table 1 shows the complete information regarding the included SARS-CoV-2 protein structures.

2.2. TDA Results, Viral Proteins Showing Mean Persistent Similarities above 0.9 with Structures Targeted by Known FDA-Approved Drugs

We compared 23 PDB structures derived from SARS-CoV-2 with 25,800 structures belonging to proteins that are known targets of FDA-approved drugs through the computation of 593,400 persistent similarity measures. We selected a stringent threshold of 0.9 for the mean of the persistent similarity measures (see Section 4.2) in order to call two protein structures similar. Three viral structures, the 3CL protease (6M2Q), the RNA-dependent RNA polymerase (6M71), and the NSP15 endoribonuclease (6W01), presented a mean of the persistent similarity measures with values higher than the selected threshold with proteins known to be targeted by approved drugs. The 3CL protease was found to be associated with 284 PDB structures (Supplementary Table S1), most of them classified as Aldo/Keto reductases and protein kinases, which were targeted by 55 different pharmacological compounds (Supplementary Table S2). The RNA-dependent RNA polymerase was found to be significantly associated with 361 PDB structures (Supplementary Table S3), which in many cases belonged to the protein kinase and flavin-containing oxidoreductase families, and that were found to be targeted by 204 unique drugs (Supplementary Table S4). Finally, the viral NSP15 endoribonuclease presented topological similarity values higher than 0.9 with 13 PDB structures (Supplementary Table S5), where the most abundant group was the poly(Adp-RIbose) Polymerase Catalytic Domain. These structures were targeted by 45 drugs (Supplementary Table S6).

Table 1. Protein Data Bank (PDB) structures of SARS-CoV-2 proteins analyzed in the study. Entry ID (column 1) encodes the PDB identifyers of the analyzed protein structures, Structure Title (column 2) provides the protein structure description, Macromolecular Name (column 3) is the protein short name and Chain ID (column 4) are the studied chains.

Entry ID	Structure Title	Macromolecule Name	Chain ID
6LVN	2019-nCoV HR2 Domain	Spike protein S2	A, B, C, D
6YI3	The N-terminal RNA-binding domain of the SARS-CoV-2 nucleocapsid phosphoprotein	Nucleoprotein	A
6M3M	SARS-CoV-2 nucleocapsid protein N-terminal RNA binding domain	SARS-CoV-2 nucleocapsid protein	A, B, C, D
6VYO	RNA binding domain of nucleocapsid phosphoprotein from SARS coronavirus 2	Nucleoprotein	A, B, C, D
6WJI	C-terminal Dimerization Domain of Nucleocapsid Phosphoprotein from SARS-CoV-2	SARS-CoV-2 nucleocapsid protein	A, B, C, D, E, F
6LXT	Structure of post fusion core of 2019-nCoV S2 subunit	Spike protein S2	A, B, C, D, E, F
6VSB	Prefusion 2019-nCoV spike glycoprotein with a single receptor-binding domain up	SARS-CoV-2 spike glycoprotein	A, B, C
6VYB	SARS-CoV-2 spike ectodomain structure (open state)	Spike glycoprotein	A, B, C
6W41	Crystal structure of SARS-CoV-2 receptor binding domain in complex with human antibody CR3022	CR3022 Fab heavy chain	H
		CR3022 Fab light chain	L
		Spike protein S1	C
6YLA	Crystal structure of the SARS-CoV-2 receptor binding domain in complex with CR3022 Fab	Spike glycoprotein	A, E
		Heavy Chain	B, H
		Light chain	C, L
6M0J	Crystal structure of SARS-CoV-2 spike receptor-binding domain bound with ACE2	Angiotensin converting enzyme 2	A
		Spike receptor binding domain	E
6M17	2019-nCoV RBD/ACE2-B0AT1 complex	Sodium-dependent neutral amino acid transporter B(0)AT1	A, C
		Angiotensin converting enzyme 2	B, D
		SARS-coV-2 Receptor Binding Domain	E, F
6M2Q	SARS-CoV-2 3CL protease (3CL pro) apo structure (space group C21)	SARS-CoV-2 3CL protease	A
6W4B	Crystal structure of Nsp9 RNA binding protein of SARS CoV-2	Non-structural protein 9	A, B
6W9Q	Peptide-bound SARS-CoV-2 Nsp9 RNA replicase	3C-like proteinase peptide, Nonstructural protein 9 fusion	A
6VXS	Crystal Structure of ADP ribose phosphatase of NSP3 from SARS CoV-2	Non-structural protein 3	A, B
6W9C	Crystal structure of papain-like protease of SARS CoV-2	Papain-like proteinase	A, B, C
6WCF	Crystal Structure of ADP ribose phosphatase of NSP3 from SARS-CoV-2 in complex with MES	Non-structural protein 3	A
6WEN	Crystal Structure of ADP ribose phosphatase of NSP3 from SARS-CoV-2 in the apo form	Non-structural protein 3	A
6WIQ	Crystal structure of the co-factor complex of NSP7 and the C-terminal domain of NSP8 from SARS CoV-2	SARS-CoV-2 NSP7	A
		SARS-CoV-2 NSP8	B
6M71	SARS-Cov-2 RNA-dependent RNA polymerase in complex with cofactors	SARS-Cov-2 NSP 12	A
		SARS-Cov-2 NSP 8	C
		SARS-Cov-2 NSP 7	B, D
6W01	1.9 A Crystal Structure of NSP15 Endoribonuclease from SARS CoV-2 in the Complex with a Citrate	Uridylate-specific endoribonuclease	A, B
6VWW	Crystal Structure of NSP15 Endoribonuclease from SARS CoV-2	Uridylate-specific endoribonuclease	A, B

Drugs known to target proteins presenting a mean of the persistent similarity measures larger than 0.9 with the SARS-CoV-2 structures were subjected to blind docking with the viral proteins. Blind docking was carried out using the complete viral protein and drug structure information preprocessed as detailed in Section 4, which included polar hydrogen addition. A set of potential repurposable candidates was then selected based on the topological similarity criteria (a mean of the persistent similarity measures), the correlations between the transcriptomic profiles observed in patients infected by SARS-CoV-2 and those generated by treating cell lines with the candidate drugs, and the blind docking analyses results. Therefore, the selected candidates are known to target proteins with large topological similarities with a specific viral protein, present high affinities with the viral structures, and have the capacity to partially revert the transcriptomic effects induced by the viral infection. Figure 2 provides a schematic overview of the narrowing-down process followed to identify the final 16 drug candidates. Furthermore, the full description of the candidates can be consulted in Table 2.

We identified six repurposable candidates to target the 3CL viral protease (6M2Q). Cholic acid, an amphipathic sterol, presented the strongest binding energies (BE = -15.06 kcal/mol), and was found to negatively correlate with transcriptomic dataset 2 (DS2 r = -0.11). Rutin (BE = -14.52 kcal/mol, DS2 r = -0.184 DS3 r = -0.1), a flavonoid-3-o-glycoside with known antioxidant and cytoprotective activity, was also selected [11,12]. Two non-steroidal anti-inflammatory drugs, indomethacin (BE = -13.31 kcal/mol, DS2 r = -0.12) and sulindac (BE = -13.14 kcal/mol, DS2 r = -0.12), were also identified. Whereas indomethacin presents antipyretic and analgesic properties [13], sulindac is used to treat conditions that involve chronic inflammation, such as arthritis [14]. Finally, sulfisoxazole (BE = -11.59 kcal/mol DS2 r = -0.13), a sulfanilamide used as a broad-spectrum antibiotic, and dasatinib (BE = -10.94 kcal/mol DS2 r = -0.15), a tyrosine kinase inhibitor indicated for the treatment of chronic myeloid leukaemia [15], were also identified as drugs with the potential of targeting the viral 3CL protease.

Five compounds were found to be candidates to target the SARS-CoV-2 NSP15 endoribonuclease (6W01), which included two corticosteroids, dexamethasone (BE = -11.42 kcal/mol, DS2 r = -0.15) and spironolactone (BE = -10.99 kcal/mol, DS1 r = -0.12 and DS2 r = -0.1), which are indicated for the treatment of allergies and asthma and resistant hypertension, respectively [14,16,17]; phenolphthalein (BE = -11.15 kcal/mol, DS1 r = -0.13), a compound historically used as a laxative [18]; mifepristone (BE = -10.04 kcal/mol, DS1 r = -0.13, DS2 r = -0.14), a synthetic steroid progesterone antagonist drug that is indicated for Cushing's syndrome and is also used as an emergency contraceptive pill [19,20]; and, finally, carbamazepine (BE = -9.66 kcal/mol, DS2 r = -0.15), a pharmacologically active molecule related to the group of tricyclic antidepressants, mainly used as anticonvulsant [14,21].

Lastly, the analysis of the NSP12 RNA-dependent RNA polymerase (6M71) yielded multiple antineoplastic drugs as possible repurposing candidates: vemurafenib (BE = -8.09 kcal/mol DS2 r = -0.16), a BRAF inhibitor [22,23]; sorafenib (BE = -7.34 kcal/mol DS1 r = -0.11, DS2 r = -0.15), a multitarget protein kinase inhibitor [24]; levonorgestrel (BE = $-7,21$ kcal/mol, DS2 r = -0.14), a synthetic progestogen used as a first-line oral emergency contractive pill [14]; the opioid antagonist naloxone (BE = -7.07 kcal/mol, DS2 r = -0.11); and raloxifene (BE = -7.05 kcal/mol, DS1 r = -0.13 and DS2 r = -0.17), a selective estrogen receptor modulator mainly used to treat osteoporosis in postmenopausal women and avoid bone loss [25]. Supplementary File 2 shows the interacting residues between the three viral proteins and the 16 drugs identified as potential repurposing candidates.

2.3. Transcriptomic Data Analysis Results

Differential gene expression analyses were carried out with the three identified datasets including samples infected with SARS-CoV-2 and uninfected controls, and were followed by Gene Set Enrichment Analysis (GSEA) and LINCS L1000 analysis. GSEA analyses allow the identification of coordinated changes in the expression of genes belonging to specific biological processes and pathways in case samples compared to controls. GSEA results are reported using the Normalized Enrichment Score (NES) and the p-value adjusted by multiple comparisons (p-adj). LINCS L1000 analyses aim to find drugs capable of reverting the transcriptomic effects produced by SARS-CoV-2 infection. Differential gene expression analysis of DS1 yielded 451 deregulated genes (DEGs), of which 213 were found to be upregulated and 238 were downregulated in SARS-CoV-2 infected samples compared to controls. The top upregulated genes were derived from the virus open reading frames. Gene Set Enrichment Analysis (GSEA) showed that pathways linked to the immune response were heavily upregulated in SARSCoV-2-infected samples. Instances of such pathways included immune response mediated by circulating immunoglobulin (p-adj = 1.8×10^{-25}), B-cell mediated immunity, (p-adj = 3.2×10^{-22}), and adaptive immune response (p-adj = 2.0×10^{-20}). The FDA-approved drugs showing the strongest negative correlation in LINCS L1000 analysis were niclosamide, bisacodyl, and perhexiline (r = $-0.21, -0.19, -0.18$, respectively). GSEA analysis of the transcriptomic signatures produced by these medications suggested that they induce significant gene expression changes in pathways linked to interleukin signaling and NF-kB activation. Genes included in the set of potential 105 therapeutics for SARS were also found to be upregulated in the bisacodyl signature (NES = 1.61, p-adj = 2.19×10^{-2}). The JAK-STAT complex and the TCF-dependent signaling pathways were found to be downregulated in the perhexiline and niclosamide signatures, respectively.

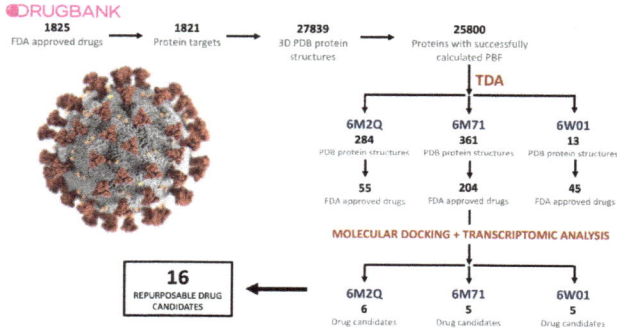

Figure 2. Schematization of the narrowing-down process followed to identify the final 16 drug candidates.

A total of 8380 DEGs were identified in the DS2 analysis. A total of 4606 genes were found to be upregulated, and 3774 were found to be downregulated in SARS CoV-2 infected samples compared to uninfected controls. Upregulated genes were enriched in components of the humoral immune response, epidermis development, keratinization, and B-cell-mediated immunity (p-adj = $1.1 \times 10^{-20}, 8.2 \times 10^{-20}, 1.3 \times 10^{-18}, 2.5 \times 10^{-10}$, respectively), among others. The top negatively correlated drugs included instances of several different compound families, such as anti-inflammatories (phenylbutazone, r = -0.21), antidiabetics (troglitazone, r = -0.20), antimalarials (chloroquine, r = -0.20), and other compounds such as nicotine (r = -0.17). Treatment with phenylbutazone was found to upregulate the gene expression of genes included in the interleukin-12 and 17 signaling pathways. In contrast, interleukin-4 and 13 signaling-related genes tended to be downregulated by chloroquine treatment (NES = -1.45, p-adj = 4.30×10^{-2}). Genes involved in the viral mRNA translation and the ISG15 antiviral mechanism were also upregulated in the gene expression profiles induced by treatment with chloroquine, phenylbutazone, and troglitazone. In addition, the SARS-CoV infection pathway was found to be upregulated in samples treated by chloroquine and troglitazone. ADORA2B-mediated anti-inflammatory cytokine production-related genes were downregulated by the treatment of the three top negatively correlated drugs.

DS3 presented the lowest yield in terms of differentially expressed genes. A total of 188 genes were found to be upregulated to controls, whereas 31 genes were found to be downregulated in infected samples compared to controls. Twenty-nine biological processes were found to be significantly upregulated and were mainly linked to mechanisms aimed to fight the viral infection and immune system-related processes including, defense response to virus (p-adj = 7.2×10^{-13}), myeloid leukocyte-mediated immunity (p-adj = 8.8×10^{-15}), regulation of cytokine production (p-adj = 1.5×10^{-8}), and response to interferon-gamma (p-adj = 1.9×10^{-8}), among others. Chloroquine was found to be the top negatively correlated drug (r = -0.11), followed by others such as pazopanib, spectinomycin, and troglitazone (r = -0.11, -0.11, -0.10, respectively). The correlations observed in this dataset tended to be weaker than those computed for DS1 and DS2. GSEA analyses of the drug signatures showed that troglitazone increased the expression of genes classified as potential therapeutics for SARS (NES = 1.46, p-adj = 4.65×10^{-2}), in addition to antiviral pathways such as the ISG15 and IFN-stimulated antiviral mechanisms. Spectinomycin was found to reduce the expression of interferon-gamma signaling 135 and interleukin 2, 3, and 5 pathway-related genes, whereas pazopanib was found to upregulate viral-related pathways such as viral mRNA translation influenza and SARS-CoV-2 infection. Supplementary File 1 includes the complete differential gene expression and enrichment analysis results for transcriptomic datasets 1, 2, and 3, whereas Supplementary File 2 contains the full LINCS L1000 analysis information.

Table 2. Drug repurposing candidates based on the topological, trascriptomic, and docking criteria. PC: Pearson correlation. LE: Lowest energy conformation in the cluster. Candidates with a PC of <−0.1 may revert the transcriptomic effects of SARS-CoV-2 infection. The maximum number of the AutoDock cluster is 150. Drug ID (colum 2) encodes the DrugBank ID of the corresponding drug (column 1).

Drug Name	Drug ID	PC DS1 (GSE150316)	PC DS2 (CRA002390)	PC DS3 (GSE147507)	AutoDock LE (kcal/mol)	AutoDock Cluster
\multicolumn{7}{c}{6M2Q (SARS-CoV-2 3CL Protease)}						
CholicAcid	DB02659	−0.09	−0.11	−0.08	−15.06	74
Rutin	DB01698	−0.07	−0.18	−0.1	−14.52	149
Indomethacin	DB00328	−0.07	−0.12	−0.05	−13.31	146
Sulindac	DB00605	−0.07	−0.12	−0.07	−13.14	73
Sulfisoxazole	DB00263	−0.05	−0.13	−0.09	−11.59	77
Dasatinib	DB01254	−0.04	−0.15	−0.09	−10.94	43
\multicolumn{7}{c}{6W01 (NSP15 Endoribonuclease)}						
Dexamethasone	DB01234	−0.07	−0.15	−0.08	−11.42	49
Phenolphthalein	DB04824	−0.13	−0.1	−0.04	−11.15	101
Spironolactone	DB00421	−0.12	−0.1	−0.09	−10.99	110
Mifepristone	DB00834	−0.13	−0.14	−0.06	−10.04	28
Carbamazepine	DB00564	−0.08	−0.14	−0.07	−9.66	86
\multicolumn{7}{c}{6M71 (NSP12 RNA-dependent RNA polymerase)}						
Vemurafenib	DB08881	−0.09	−0.16	−0.08	−8.09	13
Sorafenib	DB00398	−0.11	−0.15	−0.05	−7.34	30
Levonorgestrel	DB00367	−0.08	−0.14	−0.08	−7.21	89
Naloxone	DB01183	−0.06	−0.12	−0.09	−7.07	69
Raloxifene	DB00481	−0.13	−0.17	−0.07	−7.05	6

2.4. GSEA Analysis of the Repurposing Candidates

We determined the transcriptomic impact of the treatment with the selected candidates on two sets of biological processes linked to COVID-19, viral infections, and immune-related pathways by performing Gene Set Enrichment Analysis (GSEA) of their gene expression signatures derived from LINCS L1000. The transcriptomic profiles generated by cholic acid, rutin, sulfafurazole, and sulindac treatment (candidates to target the 3CL protease) were found to be enriched in the ISG15 antiviral mechanism. Furthermore, genes related to interleukin-1 and 12 signaling tended to be upregulated in rutin's signature, in addition to genes belonging to the potential therapeutics for SARS gene set (NES = 1.51, p-adj = 3.85×10^{-2}) whereas WNT ligand biogenesis and trafficking (NES) genes were found to be downregulated by rutin treatment (NES = -1.99, p-adj = 2.12×10^{-3}) (Supplementary Table S7). RNA-dependent RNA polymerase drug candidates, levonorgestrel and raloxifene, were found to be enriched in pathways related to antiviral processes such as ISG15 antiviral mechanism (levonorgestrel, NES = 2.08, p-adj = 9.95×10^{-4}; raloxifene, NES = 2.06, p-adj = 8.13×10^{-4}) and antiviral mechanism by IFN-stimulated genes (levonorgestrel, NES = 1.95, p-adj = 1.22 × 10^{-3}; raloxifene, NES = 1.94, p-adj = 1.12 × 10^{-3}). In addition, interferon alpha/beta signaling was observed to be depleted in raloxifene-treated cells (NES = −1.52, p-adj = 4.59 × 10^{-2}) (Supplementary Table S8). Finally, in the case of NSP15 endoribonuclease candidate drugs, dexamethasone produced gene expression signatures upregulated in pathways associated with viral infection response, such as ISG15 antiviral mechanism (NES = 1.82, p-adj = 3.17 × 10^{-3}) and the antiviral mechanism by IFN-stimulated genes (NES = 1.59, p-adj = 1.20 × 10^{-2}). This pathway was also found to be upregulated in the gene expression profiles of carbamazepine and mifepristone. Finally, interleukin-7 signaling (NES = −1.64, p-adj = 3.47 × 10^{-2}) and interferon alpha/beta signaling (NES = −1.68, p-adj = 5.48 × 10^{-3}) were downregulated by dexamethasone treatment (Supplementary Table S9). Figure 3 shows a dot plot representation of the GSEA analysis results.

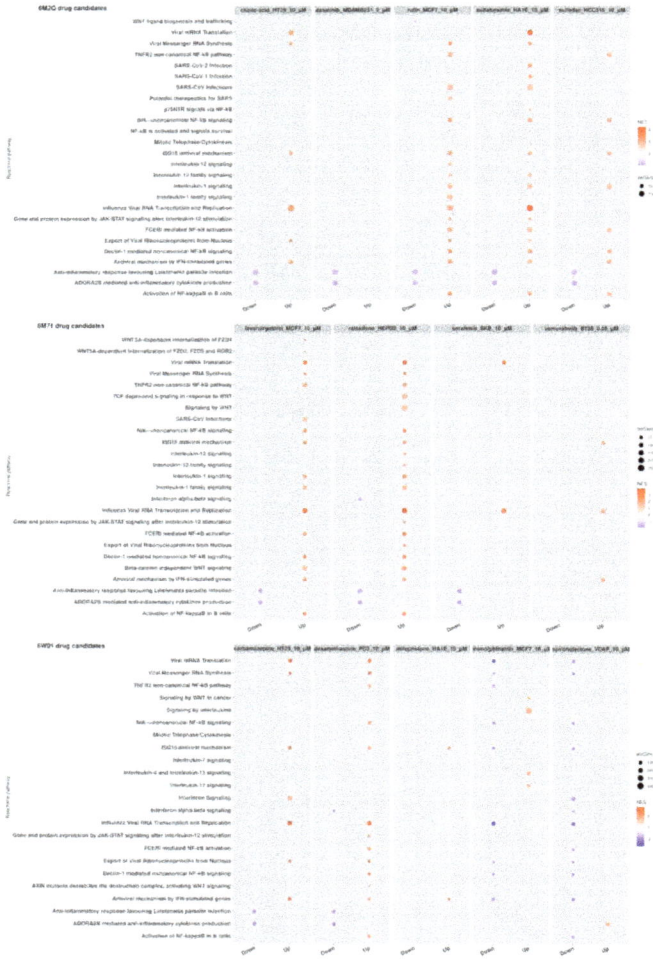

Figure 3. Gene Set Enrichment Analysis (GSEA) results for candidate drugs for 6M2Q, 6M71, and 6W01 SARS-CoV-2 structures with the expression signature yields from correlation analyses from DS2. Reactome pathways related to the immune system and viral infections. Only drugs with at least one pathway with an adjusted *p*-value < 0.05 are displayed. The GSEA table with the results is available in Supplementary Tables S7–S9.

3. Discussion

On December 31st, 2019, the World Health Organization (WHO) was officially notified about several cases of pneumonia in Wuhan City, China, caused by COVID-19, a disease with no effective treatment nor a specific vaccine at that time, which history and quest for a cure is a daily struggle and is constantly being rewritten. As specific antiviral treatments are still under development and the vaccination campaign has faced difficulties derived from unmet forecasts in the process of production and distribution, drug repurposing strategies suggesting the use of FDA-approved drugs continue to be a valuable option to find candidate drugs for the effective treatment of COVID-19 in a short timeframe.

Here, we report a novel TDA-based strategy for drug repurposing in combination with current methodologies of molecular docking, differential expression analysis of SARS-CoV-2 infected cells, and correlation with FDA-approved drugs transcriptomic profiles. Our results indicate that the proposed TDA-based formalism is a promising tool to address biological problems from a dual perspective. First, from a structural biology perspective, we used the Vietoris–Rips complex to compute the PBF encoding the shape of each protein structure. Next, to measure the degree of similarity between proteins we introduced the persistent similarity measure (PSM, see Section 4.2). This allowed us to classify proteins based solely on the C atomic coordinates. TDA-based methods have been previously proposed as a method to study the topological invariants of the three-dimensional structure of biomolecules. Several studies have employed this framework to classify protein structures using only the three-dimensional coordinates of the atoms from crystallographically resolved proteins. For instance, Xia and collaborators performed TDA-based methods on three-dimensional biomolecular structures to study their structural characteristics, flexibility prediction, and folding properties [10]. Hence, they defined the molecular topological fingerprints (MFTs) to extract the topological information from protein structures using the so-called persistent Betti numbers [26]. K. Dey and colleagues proposed another topology-based method to generate protein signatures to create a fast domain classifier using a support vector machine [27]. Interestingly, our mean persistence similarity metric was able to achieve results comparable to those obtained by the state-of-the-art structural alignment method, DALI [28], and presented a high predictive power clustering protein in terms of external classifications.

Molecular docking simulation is a rapid screening method to test compound binding activity. Additionally, transcriptomic data represent a rich alternative resource for inferring non-obvious relationships between drugs and genes. Previous in silico molecular docking studies have highlighted the potential of repurposed drugs for the treatment of COVID-19 [29–35]. However, here we used in silico molecular docking combined with transcriptomic small molecule treatment data from LINCS L1000 to determine which FDA-approved drugs may reverse the effects of SARS-CoV-2 infection. The gene expression profiles in response to the identified drugs support the docking results and offer a plausible perspective for the pathways associated with protein responses to drugs binding to SARS-CoV-2 proteins. To our knowledge, this is the first time that an application of barcode-based similarity measures has been used for the analysis of large datasets of PDB structures.

The generation of PBF depends upon the previous construction of Vietoris–Rips complexes, which have a computational store cost that scales exponentially with the number of points defining a particular structure. Moreover, in the worst case, the standard algorithm to compute the barcodes has cubic complexity in the number of simplices. Although our analyses were carried out in a cluster with 32 cores and up to 500 GB of RAM, the computational cost of the barcode generation of the excluded 1622 genes exceeded the available amount of RAM or required an exponential amount of runtime.

Among all of the SARS-Cov-2 proteins analyzed (n = 23, Table 1), only three showed a persistent similarity score above 0.9 against other protein structures targeted with known drugs. Interestingly, these proteins are key components in coronavirus replication and structural assembly: the Viral 3CL protease (6M2Q), a chymotrypsin-like protease that is essential for the production of non-structural proteins [36]; the nsp12 RNA-dependent

RNA polymerase (6M71), the main component of coronavirus replication and transcription machinery, and because of that an excellent target for new therapeutics [37]; and the nsp15 endoribonuclease (6W01), a protein with a poorly defined role in SARS-CoV-2 infection, but which has been described to be linked to pRB downregulation affecting host cell cycle division and coronavirus infection in other coronaviruses (SARS-CoV), and with a role as an antagonist of host dsRNA sensors during coronavirus infection in macrophages to evade innate immune system defenses [38,39]. Hence, in this study, we selected three proteins from the SARS-CoV-2 coronavirus as the best candidates to find repurposed drugs to combat the disease.

Our differential expression analyses revealed that troglitazone, niclosamide, and chloroquine, among multiple candidates, were the top negatively correlated drugs that may revert the effects of SARS-CoV-2 infection to the cell transcriptome. Moreover, chloroquine is already under study in several clinical trials, although recent results reported by the WHO SOLIDARITY study stated that chloroquine has no significant effect on hospitalized COVID-19 patients, in terms of the overall mortality level [2]. Niclosamide is also being evaluated under a Phase 2 clinical trial [40]. In addition, the antiviral activity of the niclosamide has been demonstrated against SARS-CoV in in vitro studies [41] and recent investigations against SARS-CoV-2 [42], and also previously against other MERS coronaviruses [43].

To date, no therapeutic agents have been proven to be effective against SARS-CoV-2. Several treatments have been reported under investigation specifically to treat COVID-19 as the result of drug repurposing strategies [44,45] and, as this draft is being written, up to 700 research papers have already been published. The number of clinical trials using repurposed drugs such as hydroxychloroquine, remdesivir, and lopinavir/ritonavir, among others, alone or in combination, is also exponentially growing, although in most cases unfortunately the results are not as good as initially expected [46–48]. Recently, a new treatment, plitidepsin, has been reported as the most potent antiviral drug against the coronavirus [49].

Our more promising candidates arise from the combination of molecular docking and transcriptomic results, and the cornerstone of our work, the TDA-based formalism. Among the 16 compounds related to the three SARS-CoV-2 proteins analyzed, nine have been described as possible candidates in other repurposing studies and five of these have already shown antiviral activity or have already been described as possible COVID-19 treatments (Supplementary Table S10), although preclinical studies will be required to determine their efficacy. In this direction, 3 of the 16 compounds are being evaluated under different clinical trials (indomethacin ($n = 2$), dexamethasone ($n = 40$), and spironolactone ($n = 4$)).

Rutin and indomethacin were amongst the notable compounds selected from 3CL main protease. In addition, they have been proven as good candidates in other studies. Rutin is a polyphenolic flavonoid that has shown a wide range of pharmacological applications due to its significant antioxidant properties [50]. Our results from GSEA analyses revealed that rutin might act in early stages of SARS-CoV-2 infection by activating the interferon-induced ISG15 pathway. ISG15 is an interferon-induced protein that has been implicated as a central player in the host antiviral response, and is the key element for the innate immune response against viral infection [51]. Furthermore, ISG15 modulates the immune system stimulating the IFN-gamma production by NK cells that lead to the promotion of early viral response [52]. Although the result of the possible interaction between rutin and 3CL protease has been reported by other studies using an in silico approach [53], our results provide a transcriptomic dimension to the possible effect of rutin during infection with SARS-CoV-2. Moreover, to our knowledge this is the first time the natural compound rutin has been related with the antiviral activity induced by the protein ISG15.

Dexamethasone, a corticosteroid used in a wide range of conditions for its anti-inflammatory and immunosuppressive effects, could be one of the most promising repurposed drugs chosen to treat COVID-19 disease, based on some results that prove a decrease in the incidence of death versus the usual care group among patients receiving invasive mechanical ventilation [54]. This compound was chosen because of its immunosuppressant properties to treat the cytokine storm induced by the immune response to coronavirus infection in late stages of the disease. Nonetheless, our results indicated that dexamethasone could also be a good candidate to target nsp15 endoribonuclease, although some repurposed works also suggested it as the target of the main protease [55]. These data could support the idea of administering corticosteroids, not just at the advanced infection stage, but also at the beginning. However, a recent study tested multiple pharmacological compounds derived from the steroids in vitro and demonstrated that dexamethasone has no antiviral activity against SARS-CoV-2 [56]. Nevertheless, we also found other corticosteroids that could interact with nsp15 protein, such as mifepristone, which suppressed viral growth conferring more than 95% of cell survival rate after viral infection and drug administration in vitro [56].

Lastly, the RNA-dependent RNA polymerase nsp12 of SARS-CoV-2 is a protein that performs essential functions in the coronavirus life cycle with no host cell homolog. This is an advantage for antiviral drug development, reducing the risk of affecting any protein present in human cells, as has been proven by many drug repurposing studies directed against nsp12 RdRP [57–60]. Vemurafenib, sorafenib, and raloxifene may be potential candidates against nsp12 RdRP. Vemurafenib can disturb the cellular Raf/MEK/ERK signaling cascade via binding in the ATP-binding site of BRAF(V600E) kinase and inhibiting its function [61], whereas sorafenib is another kinase inhibitor that targets VEGFR, PDGFR, and RAF kinases [62]. Interestingly, SARS-CoV-1 uses Raf/MEK/ERK signaling pathways to promote its replication via various mechanisms, indicating that this signaling cascade is a critical therapeutic target for host-directed SARS-CoV-2 antivirals [63–65].

4. Materials and Methods

4.1. Data Acquisition

DrugBank queries were carried out to retrieve the information regarding drugs with known protein targets [66]. In short, the DrugBank database version 5.1.5 (https://go.drugbank.com/releases/5-1-5, accessed on 21 March 2020) was downloaded in XML format, and the dbparser package and custom R scripts were employed to extract the relevant information [67]. We only selected drugs approved by the American Food and Drug Administration (FDA) and retrieved the names and UniProt identifiers of their protein targets. Then, UniProt IDs were mapped to their respective Protein Data Bank (PDB) structures using the Retrieve/ID mapping tool available at UniProt. All of the PDB structures targeted by FDA-approved drugs were downloaded in PDB format and stored for downstream analysis. Protein Data Bank queries were also performed to identify the three-dimensional structures of SARS-CoV-2 proteins.

4.2. A Topological Data Analysis Based Formalism to Compare, at Quantitative Level, the Homological Similarities of Pairwise Three-Dimensional Molecules Considered as Surfaces

In this paper, we used an adapted a TDA-based strategy which combines concepts and results from Algebraic Topology to compare three-dimensional protein structures [68–70]. More precisely, we considered the shape of the protein structure as a surface for which we only know a sample of points that are given by the coordinates of its C_α. Using this information, we construct a set of simplicial complexes associated to that protein. This set is composed by three classes of geometrical objects: isolated points, non-intersecting segments connecting these points, and non-intersecting triangles composed using non-intersecting segments. To quantify the above geometrical information, we associate a non-negative continuous function to each of the three components of a simplicial complex. The first function, denoted by f_0, represents the structure of the position of the individual points, the second function f_1, corresponds to the non-intersecting segments and finally, the third function f_2 correspond to the triangles. These three functions are called the persistent Betti Functions (PBFs) and allow us to characterize the representation of a protein's tertiary structure.

Therefore, we computed the persistent Betti functions using PDB structures from DrugBank. To compare the shape of both structures, one given by the PBF $\{f_i\}_{i=0}^{i=2}$ of each structure from DrugBank, against the PBF of *SARS-CoV-2* proteins $\{f_i^{SARS-Cov-2}\}_{i=0}^{i=2}$ we construct the persistent similarity measure (PSM), which is defined as

$$PSM_i = \frac{\int \min\left(f_i(x), f_i^{SARS-Cov-2}(x)\right)dx}{\int \max\left(f_i(x), f_i^{SARS-Cov-2}(x)\right)dx} \text{ for } i = 0, 1, 2. \quad (1)$$

Then, we calculate the mean of the persistent similarity measures:

$$\overline{PSM} = \frac{1}{3}(PSM_0 + PSM_1 + PSM_2) \quad (2)$$

for each protein comparison. A $\overline{PSM} \geq 0.9$ threshold value was established, considering those drugs whose target protein had a value of 0.9 or higher for their mean persistent similarity measure with a *SARS-CoV-2* protein as drug repurposing candidates.

4.3. Data Preprocessing and Persistent Similarity Measures Computation

All protein structures in PDB format were loaded into the R environment using the bio3d package [71]. Then, the coarse-grain representation of each structure was generated by selecting only the three-dimensional atomic coordinates of the alpha-carbons of the amino acids [26]. Two main reasons compelled us to work with this reduced representation. First, the construction of simplicial complexes scales exponentially with the number of initial points present in the point cloud. Therefore, structures defined by a very large number of points are not computationally tractable even in state-of-the-art computers. Second, all-atom models present a high degree of detail that could mask the general structure of the protein. Barcodes were constructed using the R package of TDAstats [72]. TDAstats makes use internally of the Ripser C++ library [73], an optimized fast software package for simplicial complexes and barcodes construction.

4.4. Protein–Ligand Binding with AutoDock 4.2

Ligand preparation was carried out as follows: First, the FDA-approved drugs in SDF format were retrieved from DrugBank. A custom R script and Open Babel v.3.0.0 were used to transform SDF into the mol2 format [74–77]. Following, the MGLTools v.1.5.7 toolkit was employed to add the polar hydrogens and protonation at pH 7.4. Then, mol2 drug structures were converted into PDBQT format, and their stereochemical properties were computed using AutoDock 4.2 [78]. A virtual screening library was then constructed using the preprocessed drug structures. Drugs containing atoms different from those included in the following list (H, C, N, O, F, Mg, P, S, Cl, Ca, Mn, Fe, Zn, Br, I) were discarded from the subsequent analyses because AutoDock does not include the values of their atomic force fields and is, therefore, unable to perform molecular docking using them. Polar hydrogens were also added to the SARS-CoV-2 protein PDB structures which were also transformed to the PDBQT format. Docking was carried out using AutoDock 4.2 [78], a molecular docking software package developed by the Scripps Research Institute. A grid box spanning the whole protein structure was set to perform blind docking. AutoDock was configured following the manual recommendations [79]. We increased the parameter ga_runs from 10 to 150 to improve the accuracy of the results.

4.5. Differential Gene Expression Analyses of SARS-CoV-2 Infected Human Samples and Cell Lines and Uninfected Controls

We carried out searches for transcriptomic datasets of patients and human-derived cell lines including samples infected with SARS-CoV-2 and uninfected controls. At the time the searches were carried out, three datasets were identified. Dataset 1 (DS1) was found in the gene expression omnibus (GEO) under ID GSE150316 [80]. This includes formalin-fixed paraffin-embedded samples from multiple tissues (i.e., lung, jejunum, heart) derived from SARS-CoV-2-infected individuals and uninfected controls obtained in autopsies. We restricted our analysis to lung samples. Twenty-one samples (16 cases and five controls) were selected for downstream analysis.

Dataset 2 (DS2) gathers samples derived from bronchoalveolar lavage fluids (BALF) of SARS-CoV-2 infected patients (four samples derived from two patients with two technical replicates) and three healthy controls [81]. Samples derived from infected patients were stored at the National Genomics Data Center under accession number CRA002390, whereas control samples were downloaded from the NCBI SRA database and were available under the identifiers SRR10571724, SRR10571730, and SRR10571732. Sequence alignment using the human reference genome hGR38 and count extraction were carried out using the Rsubread package [82].

Finally, the third dataset (DS3) was available in GEO under accession ID GSE147507 [83]. It presented a complex design including both primary cell lines derived from the human lung epithelium and transformed lung alveolar which were either mock treated or infected with different viruses including the influenza A virus (IAV), the respiratory syncytial virus (RSV), and SARS-CoV-2, in addition to samples derived from infected ferrets and two technical replicates of a lung sample derived from a SARS-CoV-2-infected human patient. We restricted our analysis to the cell lines NHBE, A549, and Calu-3, which were either infected with SARS-CoV-2 or were mock treated. The infected human lung samples and the healthy lung biopsies were also included. Overall, 28 samples were analyzed in this dataset.

For each dataset, differential gene expression analysis between SARS-CoV-2 infected samples and uninfected controls was carried out using the DESeq2 package [84].

4.6. Identification of LINCS 1000 Signatures Negatively Correlated with the SARS-CoV-2 Differential Gene Expression Profiles

LINCS L1000 contains an extensive collection of gene expression profiles generated using thousands of perturbagens (i.e., small molecules, ligands, micro-environments, CRISPR gene over-expression, and knockdown perturbations) and different cell lines, doses, and exposure times [85]. In particular, LINCS L1000 Level 5 data includes differential gene expression signatures computed by comparing three technical replicates of the same perturbation to appropriate controls. Level 5 LINCS L1000 phases I (GSE92742) and II (GSE70138) datasets were downloaded from GEO. Signatures involving FDA-approved drugs were identified with the help of the information contained in file *repurposing_drugs_20180907.txt* and *repurposing_samples_20180907.txt* available at the LINCS L1000 repurposing hub [85] (see Supplementary Materials). Drugbank and LINCS 1000 data were merged based on Pubchem compound identifiers. Then, the subset of signatures corresponding to FDA approved medications with 435 known Pubchem identifiers were selected. Overall, we obtained 52,144 expression signatures generated using 1313 approved drugs. To identify drugs with the potential of reverting the differential expression profiles generated by SARS-CoV-2 infection, we computed Pearson's correlations between each expression signature derived from LINCS L1000 and the differential expression profiles from DS1, DS2, and DS3, and picked those drugs exhibiting the most negative correlations.

4.7. Gene Set Enrichment Analysis (GSEA)

Dysregulated biological processes were identified for each transcriptomic dataset using the pre-ranked Gene Set Enrichment Analysis (GSEA) implementation of the fgsea package [86]. The C5 molecular signatures collection, which contains gene sets derived from the three branches of Gene Ontology (GO), was used as a source of functional information. GO terms including more than 500 or less than 15 genes were filtered out. GSEA analyses were also performed for those LINCS L1000 level 5 expression signatures negatively correlated with the differential gene expression profiles generated by the SARS-CoV-2 infection to determine their effect in specific pathways and biological processes. Reactome (version 73) was used as a source of pathway information and analyses were carried out using the clusterProfiler R-package (https://www.rdocumentation.

org/packages/clusterProfiler/versions/3.0.4, accessed on 21 March 2020) [87]. Biological processes and pathways presenting false discovery rate (FDR) adjusted p-values were called to be significantly deregulated.

5. Conclusions

In conclusion, our strategy of quantitative homological similarities using TDA-based formalism would allow researchers and clinicians to select optimal candidates from drug repurposing to achieve the desired target, not only regarding the SARS-CoV-2 coronavirus, but also any new viruses that may appear in the future, by choosing the best targets among all virus proteins. In this specific case, targeting nsp15 endonuclease and nsp12 RNA polymerase, in addition to other promising drug targets of the 3CL main protease, could support the development of a cocktail of anti-coronavirus treatments that could also be potentially used for the discovery of broad-spectrum antivirals. In particular, we identified 16 potential repurposable drug candidates including cholic acid, rutin, indomethacin, sulindac, sulfisoxazole, dasatinib, dexamethasone, phenolphthalein, spironolactone, mifepristone, carbamazepine, vemurafenib, sorafenib, levonorgestrel, naloxone, and raloxifene. Furthermore, by choosing a precision multidrug treatment, we could rescue any specific drug failure or avoid any future drug resistance due to possible acquired mutations in any of the proteins as a consequence of continuous virus replication and spreading, because the virus will be attacked from different fronts. Nevertheless, our results based on multidrug combinations should be validated in both in vitro and in vivo experiments, not just to prove the effectiveness of the treatment, but also to select the best combination against SARS-CoV-2 infection and consequent disease symptoms.

Supplementary Materials: The following are available online at https://www.mdpi.com/article/10.3390/pharmaceutics13040488/s1, File S1: Differential gene expression and GSEA analyses results for the three transcriptomic datasets, File S2: INCS L1000 analyses results for the three transcriptomic datasets, File S3: Supplementary tables. File S4: interacting residues between the viral proteins and the drugs identified as potential repurposing candidates. File S5: repurposing_drugs_20180907. File S6: repurposing_samples_20180907. Table S1: Proteins targeted by Drugbank FDA-approved medications showing average persistent similarity measures higher than 0.9 with 6M2Q, Table S2: Transcriptomic and molecular docking analyses results for drugs with the potential of targeting the SARS-CoV-2 3CL protease in apo conformation (6M2Q), Table S3: Proteins targeted by Drugbank FDA-approved medications showing average persistent similarity measures higher than 0.9 with 6M71, Table S4: Transcriptomic and molecular docking analyses results for drugs with the potential of target-ing the SARS-CoV-2 RNA dependent RNA polymerase (6M71), Table S5: Proteins targeted by Drugbank FDA-approved medications showing average persistent similarity measures higher than 0.9 with 6W01, Table S6: Transcriptomic and molecular docking analyses results for drugs with the potential of targeting the SARS-CoV-2 NSP15 Endoribonuclease (6W01), Table S7: GSEA results for top drugs targeting the 3CL protease (6M2Q), Table S8: GSEA results for top drugs tar-geting the RNA-dependent RNA polymerase (NSP12)(6M71), Table S9: GSEA results for top drugs targeting the SP15 Endoribonuclease (6W01), Table S10: Previous research analyzing the effects of our candidate drugs in SARS-CoV-2 infection.

Author Contributions: Conceptualization, A.F. and J.C.; methodology, A.F., R.P.-M. and J.F.-M.; software, A.F., R.P.-M. and J.F.-M.; validation, A.F., R.P.-M. and J.F.-M.; formal analysis, J.F.-M. and R.P.-M.; investigation, J.F.-M., R.P.-M. and J.C.; resources, A.F. and R.P.-M.; data curation, J.F.-M. and R.P.-M.; writing—original draft preparation, A.F., R.P.-M., J.F.-M. and J.C.; writing—review and editing, B.S.-G., J.F.-M. and A.F.; visualization, A.F., J.F.-M., B.S.-G. and J.C.; supervision, A.F., J.-L.D. and J.C.; project administration, A.F. and J.-L.D.; funding acquisition, A.F. and J.-L.D. All authors have read and agreed to the published version of the manuscript.

Funding: This work is partially supported by grants FONDOS SUPERA COVID-19, 2020–2021 and Funda-ción BBVA a equipos de investigación científica SARS-CoV-2 y COVID-19, IA4COVID19 2020-2022.

Data Availability Statement: All data used in this work was obtained from the following public repositories: Drug Bank (https://go.drugbank.com/ (accessed on 21 March 2020)), Gene Expression

Omnibus (https://www.ncbi.nlm.nih.gov/geo/ (accessed on 21 March 2020)), Protein Data Bank (https://www.rcsb.org/ (accessed on 21 March 2020)), and the Genome Sequence Archive (https://bigd.big.ac.cn/gsa/browse/CRA002390 (accessed on 21 March 2020)).

Conflicts of Interest: The authors declare no conflict of interest.

References

1. Al-Mandhari, A.; Samhouri, D.; Abubakar, A.; Brennan, R. Coronavirus Disease 2019 outbreak: Preparedness and readiness of countries in the Eastern Mediterranean Region. *East. Mediterr. Health J.* **2020**, *26*, 136–137. [CrossRef]
2. WHO Solidarity Trial Consortium; Faust, S.; Horby, P.; Lim, W.S.; Emberson, J.; Mafaham, M.; Bell, J.; Linsell, L.; Staplin, N.; Brightling, C.; et al. Repurposed Antiviral Drugs for Covid-19—Interim WHO Solidarity Trial Results. *N. Eng. J. Med.* **2020**, NEJMoa2023184. [CrossRef]
3. Mohs, R.C.; Greig, N.H. Drug discovery and development: Role of basic biological research. *Alzheimers Dement.* **2017**, *3*, 651–657. [CrossRef]
4. DiMasi, J.A.; Feldman, L.; Seckler, A.; Wilson, A. Trends in risks associated with new drug development: Success rates for investigational drugs. *Clin. Pharmacol. Ther.* **2010**, *87*, 272–277. [CrossRef] [PubMed]
5. Kumar, S. Covid-19: A drug repurposing and biomarker identification by using comprehensive gene-disease associations through protein-protein interaction network analysis. *Preprints* **2020**. [CrossRef]
6. Griffith, M.; Griffith, O.L.; Coffman, A.C.; Weible, J.V.; McMichael, J.F.; Spies, N.C.; Koval, J.; Das, I.; Callaway, M.B.; Eldred, J.M.; et al. DGIdb: Mining the druggable genome. *Nat. Methods* **2013**, *10*, 1209–1210. [CrossRef]
7. Freshour, S.L.; Kiwala, S.; Cotto, K.C.; Coffman, A.C.; McMichael, J.F.; Song, J.J.; Griffith, M.; Griffith, O.L.; Wagner, A.H. Integration of the drug-gene interaction database (dgidb) with open crowdsource efforts. *Nucleic Acids Res.* **2021**, *49*, D1144–D1151. [CrossRef]
8. Zhou, Y.; Hou, Y.; Shen, J.; Huang, Y.; Martin, W.; Cheng, F. Network-based drug repurposing for novel coronavirus 2019-nCoV/SARS-CoV-2. *Cell Discov.* **2020**, *6*, 14. [CrossRef] [PubMed]
9. Keretsu, S.; Bhujbal, S.P.; Cho, S.J. Rational approach toward COVID-19 main protease inhibitors via molecular docking, molecular dynamics simulation and free energy calculation. *Sci. Rep.* **2020**, *10*, 17716. [CrossRef]
10. Xia, K.; Wei, G.W. Persistent homology analysis of protein structure, flexibility, and folding. *Int. J. Numer. Methods Biomed. Eng.* **2014**, *30*, 814–844. [CrossRef] [PubMed]
11. Javed, H.; Khan, M.M.; Ahmad, A.; Vaibhav, K.; Ahmad, M.E.; Khan, A.; Ashafaq, M.; Islam, F.; Siddiqui, M.S.; Safhi, M.M.; et al. Rutin prevents cognitive impairments by ameliorating oxidative stress and neuroinflammation in rat model of sporadic dementia of Alzheimer type. *Neuroscience* **2012**, *210*, 340–352. [CrossRef] [PubMed]
12. Richetti, S.K.; Blank, M.; Capiotti, K.M.; Piato, A.L.; Bogo, M.R.; Vianna, M.R.; Bonan, C.D. Quercetin and rutin prevent scopolamine-induced memory impairment in zebrafish. *Behav. Brain Res.* **2011**, *217*, 10–15. [CrossRef] [PubMed]
13. Lucas, S. The Pharmacology of Indomethacin. *Headache* **2016**, *56*, 436–446. [CrossRef] [PubMed]
14. Munjal, A.; Wadhwa, R. *Sulindac*; [Updated 2020 November 27] in StatPearls [Internet]; StatPearls Publishing: Treasure Island, FL, USA, January 2021. Available online: https://www.ncbi.nlm.nih.gov/books/NBK556107/ (accessed on 1 April 2021).
15. Keskin, D.; Sadri, S.; Eskazan, A.E. Dasatinib for the treatment of chronic myeloid leukemia: Patient selection and special considerations. *Drug Des. Dev. Ther.* **2016**, *10*, 3355–3361. [CrossRef]
16. Shefrin, A.E.; Goldman, R.D. Use of dexamethasone and prednisone in acute asthma exacerbations in pediatric patients. *Can. Fam. Physician* **2009**, *55*, 704–706. [PubMed]
17. Nakano, S.; Kobayashi, N.; Yoshida, K.; Ohno, T.; Matsuoka, H. Cardioprotective mechanisms of spironolactone associated with the angiotensin-converting enzyme/epidermal growth factor receptor/extracellular signal-regulated kinases, nad(p)h oxidase/lectin-like oxidized low-density lipoprotein receptor-1, and rho-kinase pathways in aldosterone/salt-induced hypertensive rats. *Hypertens. Res.* **2005**, *28*, 925–936. [CrossRef]
18. National Center for Biotechnology Information. "PubChem Compound Summary for CID 4764, Phenolphthalein" PubChem. Available online: https://pubchem.ncbi.nlm.nih.gov/compound/Phenolphthalein (accessed on 1 April 2021).
19. Díaz-Castro, F.; Monsalves-Álvarez, M.; Rojo, L.E.; del Campo, A.; Troncoso, R. Mifepristone for treatment of metabolic syndrome: Beyond cushing's syndrome. *Front. Pharmacol.* **2020**, *11*, 429. [CrossRef]
20. Silvestre, L.; Dubois, C.; Renault, M.; Rezvani, Y. Voluntary interruption of pregnancy with mifepristone (ru 486) and a prostaglandin analogue. *N. Eng. J. Med.* **1990**, *322*, 645–648. [CrossRef]
21. Al-Quliti, K.W. Update on neuropathic pain treatment for trigeminal neuralgia. The pharmacological and surgical options. *Neurosciences* **2015**, *20*, 107–114. [CrossRef]
22. National Center for Biotechnology Information. "PubChem Compound Summary for CID 42611257, Vemurafenib" PubChem. Available online: https://pubchem.ncbi.nlm.nih.gov/compound/Vemurafenib (accessed on 1 April 2021).
23. Sosman, J.A.; Kim, K.B.; Schuchter, L.; Gonzalez, R.; Pavlick, A.C.; Weber, J.S.; McArthur, G.A.; Hutson, T.E.; Moschos, S.J.; Flaherty, K.T.; et al. Survival in BRAF V600-mutant advanced melanoma treated with vemurafenib. *N. Engl. J. Med.* **2012**, *366*, 707–714. [CrossRef]

24. Liu, L.; Cao, Y.; Chen, C.; Zhang, X.; McNabola, A.; Wilkie, D.; Wilhelm, S.; Lynch, M.; Carter, C. Sorafenib blocks the RAF/MEK/ERK pathway, inhibits tumor angiogenesis, and induces tumor cell apoptosis in hepatocellular carcinoma model PLC/PRF/5. *Cancer Res.* **2006**, *66*, 11851–11858. [CrossRef] [PubMed]
25. National Center for Biotechnology Information. "PubChem Compound Summary for CID 5035, Raloxifene" PubChem. Available online: https://pubchem.ncbi.nlm.nih.gov/compound/Raloxifene (accessed on 1 April 2021).
26. Cang, Z.; Mu, L.; Wu, K.; Opron, K.; Xia, K.; Wei, G.W. A topological approach for protein classification. *Mol. Based Math. Biol.* **2015**, *3*, 140–162. [CrossRef]
27. Dey, T.K.; Mandal, S. Protein classification with improved topological data analysis. *DROPS* **2018**, *113*, 6:1–6:13. [CrossRef]
28. Holm, L. Dali and the persistence of protein shape. *Protein Sci.* **2020**, *29*, 128–140. [CrossRef] [PubMed]
29. Baby, K.; Maity, S.; Mehta, C.H.; Suresh, A.; Nayak, U.Y.; Nayak, Y. Targeting SARS-CoV-2 RNA- dependent RNA polymerase: An in silico drug repurposing for COVID-19. *F1000Res* **2020**, *9*, 1166. [CrossRef]
30. Acharya, A.; Agarwal, R.; Baker, M.B.; Baudry, J.; Bhowmik, D.; Boehm, S.; Byler, K.G.; Chen, S.Y.; Coates, L.; Cooper, C.J.; et al. Supercomputer-Based Ensemble Docking Drug Discovery Pipeline with Application to Covid-19. *J. Chem. Inf. Model.* **2020**, *60*, 5832–5852. [CrossRef] [PubMed]
31. Marak, B.N.; Dowarah, J.; Khiangte, L.; Singh, V.P. Step toward repurposing drug discovery for COVID- 19 therapeutics through in silico approach. *Drug Dev. Res.* **2020**. [CrossRef]
32. Trezza, A.; Iovinelli, D.; Santucci, A.; Prischi, F.; Spiga, O. An integrated drug repurposing strategy for the rapid identification of potential SARS-CoV-2 viral inhibitors. *Sci. Rep.* **2020**, *10*, 13866. [CrossRef]
33. Jia, Z.; Song, X.; Shi, J.; Wang, W.; He, K. Transcriptome-based drug repositioning for coronavirus disease 2019 (COVID-19). *Pathog. Dis.* **2020**, *78*, ftaa036. [CrossRef]
34. Kumar, Y.; Singh, H.; Patel, C.N. In silico prediction of potential inhibitors for the main protease of SARS-CoV-2 using molecular docking and dynamics simulation based drug-repurposing. *J. Infect. Public Health* **2020**, *13*, 1210–1223. [CrossRef]
35. Elmezayen, A.D.; Al-Obaidi, A.; Sahin, A.T.; Yelekci, K. Drug repurposing for coronavirus (COVID-19): In silico screening of known drugs against coronavirus 3CL hydrolase and protease enzymes. *J. Biomol. Struct. Dyn.* **2020**, 1–13. [CrossRef] [PubMed]
36. Kneller, D.W.; Phillips, G.; O'Neill, H.M.; Jedrzejczak, R.; Stols, L.; Langan, P.; Joachimiak, A.; Coates, L.; Kovalevsky, A. Structural plasticity of SARS-CoV-2 3CL Mpro active site cavity revealed by room temperature X-ray crystallography. *Nat. Commun.* **2020**, *11*, 3202. [CrossRef] [PubMed]
37. Gao, Y.; Yan, L.; Huang, Y.; Liu, F.; Zhao, Y.; Cao, L.; Wang, T.; Sun, Q.; Ming, Z.; Zhang, L.; et al. Structure of the RNA-dependent RNA polymerase from COVID-19 virus. *Science* **2020**, *368*, 779–782. [CrossRef] [PubMed]
38. Bhardwaj, K.; Liu, P.; Leibowitz, J.L.; Kao, C.C. The coronavirus endoribonuclease Nsp15 interacts with retinoblastoma tumor suppressor protein. *J. Virol.* **2020**, *86*, 4294–4304. [CrossRef] [PubMed]
39. Deng, X.; Hackbart, M.; Mettelman, R.C.; O'Brien, A.; Mielech, A.M.; Yi, G.; Kao, C.C.; Baker, S.C. Coronavirus nonstructural protein 15 mediates evasion of dsRNA sensors and limits apoptosis in macrophages. *Proc. Natl. Acad. Sci. USA* **2017**, *114*, E4251–E4260. [CrossRef] [PubMed]
40. Niclosamide in COVID-19; Identifier: Nct04542434. 29 February 2000. Available online: https://clinicaltrials.gov/ct2/show/NCT04542434 (accessed on 1 April 2021).
41. Jeon, S.; Ko, M.; Lee, J.; Choi, I.; Byun, S.Y.; Park, S.; Shum, D.; Kim, S. Identification of Antiviral Drug Candidates against SARS-CoV-2 from FDA-Approved Drugs. *Antimicrob. Agents Chemother.* **2020**, *64*, e00819-20. [CrossRef]
42. Wu, C.J.; Jan, J.T.; Chen, C.M.; Hsieh, H.P.; Hwang, D.R.; Liu, H.W.; Liu, C.Y.; Huang, H.W.; Chen, S.C.; Hong, C.F.; et al. Inhibition of severe acute respiratory syndrome coronavirus replication by niclosamide. *Antimicrob. Agents Chemother.* **2004**, *48*, 2693–2696. [CrossRef]
43. Gassen, N.C.; Niemeyer, D.; Muth, D.; Corman, V.M.; Martinelli, S.; Gassen, A.; Hafner, K.; Papies, J.; Mösbauer, K.; Zellner, A.; et al. Skp2 attenuates autophagy through beclin1- ubiquitination and its inhibition reduces mers-coronavirus infection. *Nat. Commun.* **2019**, *10*, 5770. [CrossRef]
44. Wang, X.; Guan, Y. COVID-19 drug repurposing: A review of computational screening methods, clinical trials, and protein interaction assays. *Med. Res. Rev.* **2021**, *41*, 5–28. [CrossRef]
45. Riva, L.; Yuan, S.; Yin, X.; Martin-Sancho, L.; Matsunaga, N.; Pache, L.; Burgstaller-Muehlbacher, S.; de Jesus, P.D.; Teriete, P.; Hull, M.V. Discovery of SARS-CoV-2 antiviral drugs through large-scale compound repurposing. *Nature* **2020**, *586*, 113–119. [CrossRef]
46. Beigel, J.H.; Tomashek, K.M.; Dodd, L.E.; Mehta, A.K.; Zingman, B.S.; Kalil, A.C.; Hohmann, E.; Chu, H.Y.; Luetkemeyer, A.; Kline, S.; et al. Remdesivir for the Treatment of Covid-19—Final Report. *N. Engl. J. Med.* **2020**, *383*, 1813–1826. [CrossRef] [PubMed]
47. Wang, Y.; Zhang, D.; Du, G.; Du, R.; Zhao, J.; Jin, Y.; Fu, S.; Gao, L.; Cheng, Z.; Lu, Q.; et al. Remdesivir in adults with severe COVID-19: A randomised, double-blind, placebo-controlled, multicentre trial. *Lancet* **2020**, *395*, 1569–1578. [CrossRef]
48. Cao, B.; Wang, Y.; Wen, D.; Liang, W.; Ou, C.; He, J.; Liu, L.; Shan, H.; Lei, C.; David, S.C.; et al. A Trial of Lopinavir-Ritonavir in Adults Hospitalized with Severe Covid-19. *N. Engl. J. Med.* **2020**, *382*, 1787–1799. [CrossRef]
49. White, K.M.; Rosales, R.; Yildiz, S.; Kehrer, T.; Miorin, L.; Moreno, E.; Jangra, S.; Uccellini, M.B.; Rathnasinghe, R.; Coughlan, L.; et al. Plitidepsin has potent preclinical efficacy against SARS-CoV-2 by targeting the host protein eEF1A. *Science* **2021**, *371*, 926–931. [CrossRef]
50. Sharma, S.; Ali, A.; Ali, J.; Sahni, J.K.; Baboota, S. Rutin: Therapeutic potential and recent advances in drug delivery. *Expert Opin. Investig. Drugs* **2013**, *22*, 1063–1079. [CrossRef]

51. Perng, Y.C.; Lenschow, D.J. ISG15 in antiviral immunity and beyond. *Nat. Rev. Microbiol.* **2018**, *16*, 423–439. [CrossRef] [PubMed]
52. Kang, S.; Brown, H.M.; Hwang, S. Direct Antiviral Mechanisms of Interferon-Gamma. *Immune Netw.* **2018**, *18*, e33. [CrossRef]
53. Hu, X.; Cai, X.; Song, X.; Li, C.; Zhao, J.; Luo, W.; Zhang, Q.; Ekumi, I.O.; He, Z. Possible SARS-coronavirus 2 inhibitor revealed by simulated molecular docking to viral main protease and host toll-like receptor. *Future Virol.* **2020**, *15*, 359–368. [CrossRef]
54. RECOVERY Collaborative Group; Beigel, J.H.; Tomashek, K.M.; Dodd, L.E.; Mehta, A.K.; Zingman, B.S.; Kalil, A.C.; Hohmann, E.; Chu, H.Y.; Luetkemeyer, A.; et al. Dexamethasone in hospitalized patients with covid-19—Preliminary report. *N. Engl. J. Med.* **2020**, NEJMoa2021436. [CrossRef]
55. Sarkar, I.; Sen, A. In silico screening predicts common cold drug Dextromethorphan along with Prednisolone and Dexamethasone can be effective against novel Coronavirus disease (COVID-19). *J. Biomol. Struct. Dyn.* **2020**, 1–5. [CrossRef]
56. Matsuyama, S.; Kawase, M.; Nao, N.; Shirato, K.; Ujike, M.; Kamitani, W.; Shimojima, M.; Fukushi, S. The inhaled steroid ciclesonide blocks sars-cov-2 rna replication by targeting the viral replication- transcription complex in cultured cells. *J. Virol.* **2020**, *95*, e01648-20. [CrossRef] [PubMed]
57. Ribaudo, G.; Ongaro, A.; Oselladore, E.; Zagotto, G.; Memo, M.; Gianoncelli, A. A computational approach to drug repurposing against SARS-CoV-2 RNA dependent RNA polymerase (RdRp). *J. Biomol. Struct. Dyn.* **2020**, 1–8. [CrossRef]
58. Parvez, M.S.A.; Karim, M.A.; Hasan, M.; Jaman, J.; Karim, Z.; Tahsin, T.; Hasan, N.; Hosen, M.J. Prediction of potential inhibitors for RNA-dependent RNA polymerase of SARS-CoV-2 using comprehensive drug repurposing and molecular docking approach. *Int. J. Biol. Macromol.* **2020**, *163*, 1787–1797. [CrossRef]
59. Ahmad, J.; Ikram, S.; Ahmad, F.; Rehman, I.U.; Mushtaq, M. SARS-CoV-2 RNA Dependent RNA polymerase (RdRp)—A drug repurposing study. *Heliyon* **2020**, *6*, e04502. [CrossRef] [PubMed]
60. Pokhrel, R.; Chapagain, P.; Siltberg-Liberles, J. Potential RNA-dependent RNA polymerase inhibitors as prospective therapeutics against SARS-CoV-2. *J. Med. Microbiol.* **2020**, *69*, 864–873. [CrossRef] [PubMed]
61. Pleschka, S.; Wolff, T.; Ehrhardt, C.; Hobom, G.; Planz, O.; Rapp, U.R.; Ludwig, S. Influenza virus propagation is impaired by inhibition of the Raf/MEK/ERK signalling cascade. *Nat. Cell Biol.* **2001**, *3*, 301–305. [CrossRef] [PubMed]
62. Adnane, L.; Trail, P.A.; Taylor, I.; Wilhelm, S.M. Sorafenib (BAY 43-9006, Nexavar), a dual-action inhibitor that targets RAF/MEK/ERK pathway in tumor cells and tyrosine kinases VEGFR/PDGFR in tumor vasculature. *Methods Enzymol.* **2006**, *407*, 597–612. [CrossRef]
63. Pleschka, S. RNA viruses and the mitogenic Raf/MEK/ERK signal transduction cascade. *Biol. Chem.* **2008**, *389*, 1273–1282. [CrossRef]
64. Cai, Y.; Liu, Y.; Zhang, X. Suppression of coronavirus replication by inhibition of the MEK signaling pathway. *J. Virol.* **2007**, *81*, 446–456. [CrossRef]
65. Ghasemnejad-Berenji, M.; Pashapour, S. SARS-CoV-2 and the Possible Role of Raf/MEK/ERK Pathway in Viral Survival: Is This a Potential Therapeutic Strategy for COVID-19? *Pharmacology* **2021**, *106*, 119–122. [CrossRef]
66. Wishart, D.S. Drugbank: A comprehensive resource for in silico drug discovery and exploration. *Nucleic Acids Res.* **2006**, *34*, D668–D672. [CrossRef] [PubMed]
67. Ali, M.; Ezzat, A. DrugBank Database XML Parser. Dainanahan, R Package Version 1.2.0. 2020. Available online: https://CRAN.R-project.org/package=dbparser (accessed on 21 March 2020).
68. Munkres, J. *Elements of Algebraic Topology*; Perseus Publishing: Cambridge, MA, USA, 1984.
69. Robins, V. Towards computing homology from finite approximations. *Topol. Proc.* **1999**, *24*, 503–532.
70. Pérez-Moraga, R.; Forés-Martors, J.; Suay-García, B.; Duval, J.L.; Falcó, A.; Climent, J. A COVID-19 Drug Repurposing Strategy Through Quantitative Homological Similarities by using a Topological Data Analysis Based Formalism. *Preprints* **2020**, 2020120281. [CrossRef]
71. Grant, B.J.; Rodrigues, A.P.C.; ElSawy, K.M.; McCammon, J.A.; Caves, L.S.D. Bio3d: An R package for the comparative analysis of protein structures. *Bioinformatics* **2006**, *22*, 2695–2696. [CrossRef] [PubMed]
72. Wadhwa, R.R.; Williamson, D.F.; Dhawan, A.; Scott, J.G. Tdastats: R pipeline for computing persistent homology in topological data analysis. *J. Open Source Softw.* **2018**, *3*, 860. [CrossRef] [PubMed]
73. Bauer, U. Ripser: Efficient computation of Vietoris-Rips persistence barcodes. *arXiv* **2019**, arXiv:1908.02518.
74. Jain, B.J.; Lappe, M. Joining softassign and dynamic programming for the contact map overlap problem. *BIRD* **2007**, *4414*, 410–423. [CrossRef]
75. Lancia, G.; Carr, R.; Walenz, B.; Istrail, S. 101 optimal pdb structure alignments: A branch-and-cut algorithm for the maximum contact map overlap problem. In Proceedings of the Fifth Annual International Conference on Computational Biology, Montreal, QC, Canada, 22–25 April 2001; pp. 193–202. [CrossRef]
76. Fox, N.K.; Brenner, S.E.; Chandonia, J.M. SCOPe: Structural Classification of Proteins–extended, integrating SCOP and ASTRAL data and classification of new structures. *Nucleic Acids Res.* **2014**, *42*, D304–D309. [CrossRef]
77. O'Boyle, N.M.; Banck, M.; James, C.A.; Morley, C.; Vandermeersch, T.; Hutchison, G.R. Open Babel: An open chemical toolbox. *J. Cheminform.* **2011**, *3*, 33. [CrossRef]
78. Morris, G.M.; Huey, R.; Lindstrom, W.; Sanner, M.F.; Belew, R.K.; Goodsell, D.S.; Olson, A. AutoDock4 and AutoDockTools4: Automated docking with selective receptor flexibility. *J. Comput. Chem.* **2009**, *30*, 2785–2791. [CrossRef]
79. Forli, S.; Huey, R.; Pique, M.; Sanner, M.; Goodsell, D.; Olson, A. Computational protein-ligand docking and virtual drug screening with the autodock suite. *Nat. Protoc.* **2016**, *11*, 905–919. [CrossRef]

80. Desai, N.; Neyaz, A.; Szabolcs, A.; Shih, A.R.; Chen, J.H.; Thapar, V.; Nieman, L.T.; Solovyov, A.; Mehta, A.; Lieb, D.J.; et al. Temporal and spatial heterogeneity of host response to sars-cov-2 pulmonary infection. *Nat. Commun.* **2020**, *11*, 6319. [CrossRef]
81. Xiong, Y.; Liu, Y.; Cao, L.; Wang, D.; Guo, M.; Jiang, A.; Guo, D.; Hu, W.; Yang, J.; Tang, Z.; et al. Transcriptomic characteristics of bronchoalveolar lavage fluid and peripheral blood mononuclear cells in covid-19 patients. *Emerg. Microbes Infect.* **2020**, *9*, 761–770. [CrossRef] [PubMed]
82. Liao, Y.; Smyth, G.K.; Shi, W. The R package rsubread is easier, faster, cheaper and better for alignment and quantification of rna sequencing reads. *Nucleic Acids Res.* **2019**, *47*, e47. [CrossRef] [PubMed]
83. Blanco-Melo, D.; Nilsson-Payant, B.E.; Liu, W.C.; Møller, R.; Panis, M.; Sachs, D.; Albrecht, R.A.; tenOever, B.R.; Uhl, S.; Hoagland, D.; et al. Imbalanced host response to sars-cov-2 drives development of covid-19. *Cell* **2020**, *181*, 1036–1045. [CrossRef] [PubMed]
84. Love, M.I.; Huber, W.; Anders, S. Moderated estimation of fold change and dispersion for RNA-seq data with DESeq2. *Genome Biol.* **2014**, *15*, 550. [CrossRef] [PubMed]
85. Subramanian, A.; Narayan, R.; Corsello, S.M.; Peck, D.D.; Natoli, T.E.; Lu, X.; Gould, J.; Davis, J.F.; Tubelli, A.A.; Asiedu, J.K.; et al. A Next Generation Connectivity Map: L1000 Platform and the First 1,000,000 Profiles. *Cell* **2017**, *171*, 1437–1452. [CrossRef]
86. Korotkevich, G.; Sukhov, V.; Sergushichev, A. Fast gene set enrichment analysis. *bioRxiv* **2019**. [CrossRef]
87. Yu, G.; Wang, L.G.; Han, Y.; He, Q.Y. ClusterProfiler: An R package for comparing biological themes among gene clusters. *OMICS* **2012**, *16*, 284–287. [CrossRef] [PubMed]

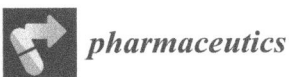

Article

Drug Repurposing for COVID-19 Treatment by Integrating Network Pharmacology and Transcriptomics

Dan-Yang Liu [1], Jia-Chen Liu [2], Shuang Liang [2], Xiang-He Meng [2], Jonathan Greenbaum [3], Hong-Mei Xiao [2], Li-Jun Tan [1,*] and Hong-Wen Deng [1,2,3,*]

1. Laboratory of Molecular and Statistical Genetics, College of Life Sciences, Hunan Normal University, Changsha 410081, China; danyang.liu@foxmail.com
2. Center for System Biology, Data Sciences, and Reproductive Health, School of Basic Medical Science, Central South University, Changsha 410013, China; ljch1999@csu.edu.cn (J.-C.L.); 196501012@csu.edu.cn (S.L.); xhmeng2020@csu.edu.cn (X.-H.M.); hmxiao@csu.edu.cn (H.-M.X.)
3. Tulane Center of Biomedical Informatics and Genomics, Deming Department of Medicine, Tulane University School of Medicine, New Orleans, LA 70112, USA; jgreenb8@tulane.edu
* Correspondence: ljtan@hunnu.edu.cn (L.-J.T.); hdeng2@tulane.edu (H.-W.D.)

Citation: Liu, D.-Y.; Liu, J.-C.; Liang, S.; Meng, X.-H.; Greenbaum, J.; Xiao, H.-M.; Tan, L.-J.; Deng, H.-W. Drug Repurposing for COVID-19 Treatment by Integrating Network Pharmacology and Transcriptomics. *Pharmaceutics* **2021**, *13*, 545. https://doi.org/10.3390/pharmaceutics13040545

Academic Editors: Lucreția Udrescu, Ludovic Kurunczi, Paul Bogdan and Mihai Udrescu

Received: 10 February 2021
Accepted: 26 March 2021
Published: 14 April 2021

Publisher's Note: MDPI stays neutral with regard to jurisdictional claims in published maps and institutional affiliations.

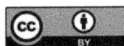

Copyright: © 2021 by the authors. Licensee MDPI, Basel, Switzerland. This article is an open access article distributed under the terms and conditions of the Creative Commons Attribution (CC BY) license (https://creativecommons.org/licenses/by/4.0/).

Abstract: Since coronavirus disease 2019 (COVID-19) is a serious new worldwide public health crisis with significant morbidity and mortality, effective therapeutic treatments are urgently needed. Drug repurposing is an efficient and cost-effective strategy with minimum risk for identifying novel potential treatment options by repositioning therapies that were previously approved for other clinical outcomes. Here, we used an integrated network-based pharmacologic and transcriptomic approach to screen drug candidates novel for COVID-19 treatment. Network-based proximity scores were calculated to identify the drug–disease pharmacological effect between drug–target relationship modules and COVID-19 related genes. Gene set enrichment analysis (GSEA) was then performed to determine whether drug candidates influence the expression of COVID-19 related genes and examine the sensitivity of the repurposing drug treatment to peripheral immune cell types. Moreover, we used the complementary exposure model to recommend potential synergistic drug combinations. We identified 18 individual drug candidates including nicardipine, orantinib, tipifarnib and promethazine which have not previously been proposed as possible treatments for COVID-19. Additionally, 30 synergistic drug pairs were ultimately recommended including fostamatinib plus tretinoin and orantinib plus valproic acid. Differential expression genes of most repurposing drugs were enriched significantly in B cells. The findings may potentially accelerate the discovery and establishment of an effective therapeutic treatment plan for COVID-19 patients.

Keywords: SARS-CoV-2; COVID-19; drug repurposing; network-based pharmacology

1. Introduction

The severe acute respiratory syndrome coronavirus 2 (SARS-CoV-2) caused the coronavirus disease 2019 (COVID-19) and triggered the largest pandemic since 1918 [1], which was responsible for >100 million cases and >2 million deaths reported globally [2]. However, there are no specific antiviral drugs for SARS-CoV-2 infection so far, for the reduction of morbidity and mortality of COVID-19, active symptomatic support was urgently needed [3].

According to recent reports [4–6], the majority of COVID-19 patients are currently given antiviral and antibiotic treatments or combination therapy including oseltamivir, ribavirin, lopinavir, ritonavir, and moxifloxacin. Additionally, several drugs are under clinical trials to verify their safety and efficacy for COVID-19 treatment, such as favipiravir, remdesivir, and hydroxychloroquine [7]. However, existing therapeutic options for the treatment of COVID-19 remain controversial. For example, remdesivir is an FDA Emergency Use Authorization (not FDA-approval) viral RNA polymerase inhibitor which has been widely used in COVID-19 patients [8], however, a recent randomized clinical trial demonstrated there was no significant beneficial effect [9]. Similarly, the COVID-19 WHO SOLIDARITY trial showed that other proposed treatments such as hydroxychloroquine, lopinavir, and interferon regimens appeared to have little or no effect on hospitalized COVID-19 patients [10]. Therefore, there is an urgent necessity to develop novel potential candidates for COVID-19 treatment.

Traditional drug development is a time-consuming and costly process that frequently takes 10–15 years and costs about 2–3 billion dollars from initial lab-scale experiments through the three phases of clinical trials and final approval for clinical usage [11]. Drug repurposing, as an effective and rapid drug discovery strategy from existing drugs [11,12], is considered the most practical approach as a rapid response to the emergent pandemic since the candidate treatments have already previously been tested for their safety [13]. The availability of the genomic sequence of SARS-CoV-2 has rapidly accelerated the development of clinical perspectives and recommendations. For example, David E. Gordon et al. identified 332 SARS-CoV-2 human protein-protein interactions and 69 drug candidates including 29 FDA-approved drugs, 12 clinical trial drugs, and 28 drugs at a preclinical stage [14]. Additionally, gene set enrichment analysis (GSEA) can be applied to identify underlying pathological processes using gene expression of COVID-19 patients, which can retrieve efficient drugs from patient-derived gene expression data using drug–target gene sets [15]. Therefore, the application of GSEA for drug targets based on drug–transcriptome-responses datasets and disease-associated gene sets can serve as an excellent screening tool for diseases that lack a safe and reliable cellular model for in vitro screening, such as COVID-19 [16].

This study uses an integrated network-based pharmacologic and transcriptomic approach to screen drug candidates for COVID-19 treatment. Network-based pharmacology is an effective and holistic tool to identify drug treatments, where the drug effects are provided by the distance between drugs and disease in the interactome [17]. Additionally, several databases containing genome-wide expression profiles of human cell lines treated with bioactive compounds have been developed for drug discovery [18]. Transcriptional profiling studies have successfully identified potential therapies for diseases such as breast cancer [19], diabetes [20], and Parkinson's [21]. Using a network-based pharmacology approach combined with the transcriptional profiling databases, we detected 18 single drug candidates (e.g., dexamethasone, chloroquine, and tretinoin) and 30 synergistic drug combinations as potential therapies for COVID-19.

2. Materials and Methods

We screened novel drug combinations for COVID-19 by integrated network-based pharmacology and transcriptome analysis based on the following steps: (1) collection of COVID-19 related genes; (2) collection of target-available drugs and construction of drug–target modules; (3) calculation of network-based proximity between drug–target modules and COVID-19 related genes; (4) filtering drugs based on gene set enrichment analysis (GSEA); (5) network-based prediction of drug combinations (Figure 1). These steps will be detailed in the following.

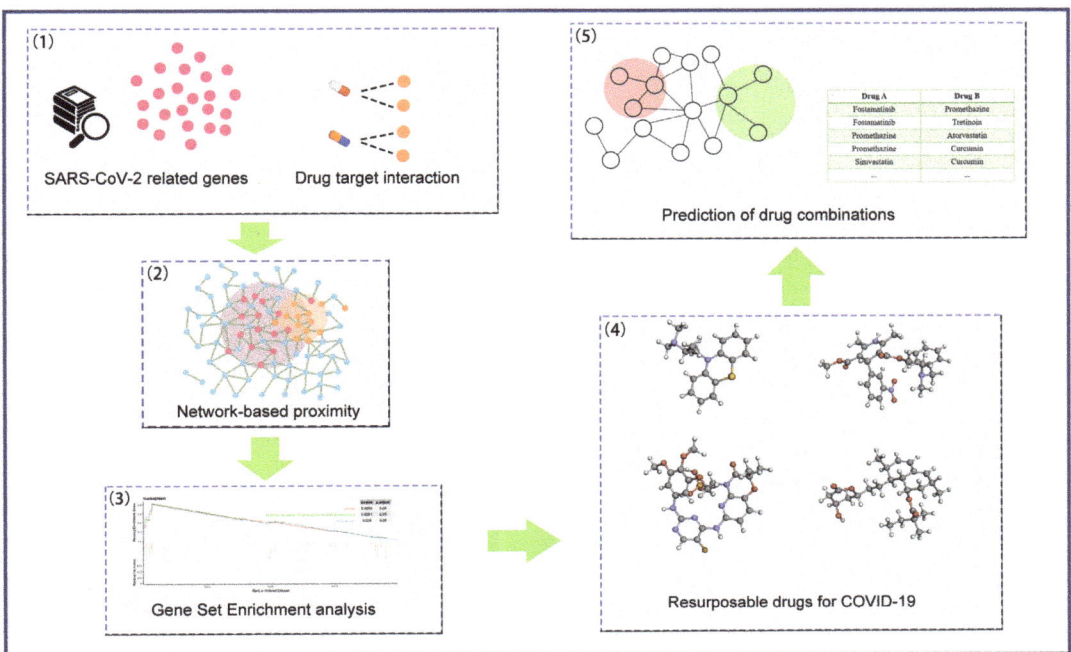

Figure 1. Schematic illustration of the computational framework. (1) Collection of the coronavirus disease 2019 (COVID-19) related genes from published SARS-CoV-2 human host data and differential expression genes (DEGs) from a single-cell study of the peripheral immune response in patients with severe COVID-19 (GSE150728). (2) Drug–target information retrieved from DrugBank and SuperTarget. (3) Quantify the therapeutic effect by computing the proximity between drug targets and COVID-19 related genes. (4) Gene set enrichment analysis (GSEA) to determine whether COVID-19 related genes show significance in drug-induced gene expression profiles. (5) Drug candidates were further prioritized for drug combinations using the "Complementary Exposure" model.

2.1. Genes Related to COVID-19

Genes related to COVID-19 were retrieved from the latest SARS-CoV-2 human host data and a single-cell transcriptomic study of the peripheral immune response to severe COVID-19 (GSE150728). SARS-CoV-2 protein sequences, viral genomes, literature, clinical resources submitted to the National Center for Biotechnology Information (NCBI) on the SARS-CoV-2 special subject have been rapidly evolving [22]. In total, 65 SARS-CoV-2 human host proteins were selected from the coronavirus genomes of NCBI datasets and 1070 potential COVID-19 related genes were obtained from the transcriptomic study by selecting the differential expression genes (DEGs) between individual COVID-19 samples ($n = 7$) and healthy controls ($n = 6$) in 7 cell types, that was 409 genes from CD14+ Monocytes, 257 genes from CD16+ Monocytes, 261 genes from Dendritic Cells, 173 genes from NK (nature killer) cells, 180 genes from CD8+ T cells, 172 genes from CD4+ T cells and 481 genes from B cells (Tables S1 and S2) [23]. All the identified proteins were mapped to the official gene symbols of humans reported by the HUGO Gene Nomenclature Committee (HGNC). Finally, 63 SARS-CoV-2 related genes derived from human host proteins and 971 DEGs were retained as the COVID-19 potential related genes after removing duplicates.

Gene Ontology (GO) enrichment analysis was performed on the potential COVID-19 related genes to identify significant pathways. By using the R package ClusterProfiler [24], all potential COVID-19 related genes were functionally categorized according to their biological processes, cellular components, and molecular functions. Functional term enrichment analysis was performed to provide insights into the biological mechanisms underlying the COVID-19 related genes. Using this approach, only genes involved in the significantly enriched GO terms (p-value < 0.05) were retained for further analysis as COVID-19 related genes in the context of networks.

2.2. Drug–Target Relationship Modules

The drug information was obtained from DrugBank and SuperTarget [25,26]. Briefly, 7485 drugs with 21,335 drug–protein links were selected from DrugBank (version 5.1.6), and 3138 drugs with 16,579 drug–protein links were retrieved from SuperTarget. After removing drugs without targets as well as duplications, and converting all target genes into human gene symbols, 31,139 interactions containing 3121 targets of 7811 drugs were finally identified (Supplemental Table S3). A drug–target relationship module was defined by the drug–target interaction information, where multiple targets share one drug.

2.3. Network-Based Proximity between Drugs and COVID-19

A network-based approach was used to analyze the correlation between drug and disease, in which proximity scores were quantified by calculating the closest distance between the drug–target module and COVID-19 related genes in the context of the human protein-protein interaction (PPI) network. The PPI data were obtained from Pathway Commons (version 12), which contains over 5772 pathways and 2.4 million interactions [27]. Genes (nodes) with interaction (links) constructed a network graph of PPI, while the interaction between two nodes was undirected and unweighted. Here, a proximity score was defined by the average shortest path length between the drug target genes and their nearest disease proteins in the context of PPI to quantify the therapeutic effect of drugs [28,29]. Given the set of COVID-19 related genes sourced from SARS-CoV-2 proteins (S), the group of drug target genes (T), the shortest distance between two genes in the PPI network $d(s,t)$ where $s \in S$ and $t \in T$ (Equation (1)),

$$d(S,T) = \frac{1}{|T|} \sum_{t \in T} min_{s \in S}(d(s,t) + w) \qquad (1)$$

where w is the drug influencing weight, defined as $w = -\ln(D+1)$ if the drug target is one of the COVID-19 related genes sourced from DEGs (D is the connectivity degree of targets) and $w = 0$ otherwise.

A simulated reference distance score distribution corresponding to the drug was generated to assess the significance of the results by linking the drug's random target modules and disease-related genes. Referenced drug modules were constructed by selecting random genes (denoted as R) with the same degree of drug target sets in the network, where the distance $d(S,R)$ indicates the relationship between a simulated drug and COVID-19. The reference distribution was established based on 30,000 replications. A drug with a score lower than 98% of the reference distribution scores was considered significant [28]. The network proximity was converted to Z-score based on permutation tests (Equation (2)):

$$Z(S,T) = \frac{d(S,T) - \mu_{d(S,R)}}{\sigma_{d(S,R)}} \qquad (2)$$

where $\mu_{d(S,R)}$ and $\sigma_{d(S,R)}$ are the mean and standard deviation of the permutation tests.

2.4. Biological Enrichment Analysis of COVID-19 Related Genes on the Drug-Induced Expression Profiles

We performed GSEA as a further prioritization strategy to screen drug candidates by examining the distribution of disease-related genes in drug-induced gene expression profiles. GSEA was utilized to determine whether a priori defined sets of genes showed statistically significant enrichment in a collected gene list [30], which could identify whether drug candidates affected the expression of disease pathways. We first collected perturbation-driven gene expression profiles from LINCS (Library of Integrated Network-based Cellular Signatures), which provided transcriptional responses of human cells to chemical and genetic perturbation [31]. Human myeloid leukemia mononuclear (THP-1) cell line from blood was selected due to the important association of peripheral blood and myelomonocytic cells with COVID-19 [32–34]. The goal of GSEA was to determine whether the COVID-19 related genes sourced from the SARS-CoV-2 related gene set was randomly distributed throughout the drug-induced expression data set sorted by correlation with the phenotype of interest or enriched at either the top or bottom. Drugs with FDR (False Discovery Rate) less than 0.25 and ES (Enrichment Scores) higher than 0 were identified as potential drug candidates for COVID-19.

2.5. GSEA Analysis of Repurposing Drugs in Specific Cell-Types

According to the Seurat data provided by Aaron J. Wilk [23], we chose "Cell type (coarse)" as the standard to select scRNA seq data of seven cell types, including B Cells, CD14+ Monocytes, CD16+ Monocytes, CD4+ T Cells, CD8+ T Cells, Dendritic Cells, NK (natural killer) Cells, and calculated differentially expressed genes between total COVID-19 samples ($n = 7$) and all healthy controls ($n = 6$). Each cell type was divided into two groups, diseased and healthy controls, according to whether the donor had COVID-19. Subsequently, differential gene expression profiles between the diseased and healthy controls in specific cell-types were calculated by using the "FindMarkers" function in Seurat (Supplemental Tables S7–S13) [35]. GSEA analysis of repurposing drug-induced THP-1 differential expression genes (logFC > 1) and specific cell-type transcriptomes were used to assess the enrichment of sets of genes (repurposing drugs DE genes) in each cell type (scRNA seq gene list). For each repurposing drug, a specific cell with FDR < 0.05 and ES < 0 was identified as potential drug-sensitive cell types for COVID-19.

2.6. Network-Based Prediction of Drug Combinations

Drug combination therapies are more beneficial rather than individual drug since the synergistic drug pairs can target more genes and play role in multiple complicated pathways [36]. The Complementary Exposure model has previously been demonstrated as an effective approach to predict useful combinations [37]. The model is based on the following conditions: drug targets and disease genes overlap topologically ($Z_{DA} < 0, Z_{DB} < 0, Z_{DA} < 0, Z_{DB} < 0$), and two sets of drug targets are separated topologically ($S_{AB} > 0$). The Complementary Exposure model network proximity between a drug (A or B) and a disease (D) is defined by the z-score (Equation (3)):

$$Z_{DA} = \frac{d_{DA} - \mu_d}{\sigma_d} \quad (3)$$

The z-score is calculated by randomly sampling both degrees of nodes (drug targets and disease genes) with 1000 replications. The mean distance μ_d and standard deviation σ_d of the reference distribution are used to convert d_{DA} to a normalized distance (Equation (4)), where d_{DA} relies on the average shortest path lengths $d(d, a)$ between disease genes ($d, d \in D$) and drug targets ($a, a \in A$).

$$d_{DA} = \frac{1}{\|D\|} \sum_{d \in D} min_{a \in A} d(d, a) \quad (4)$$

The network-based separation S_{AB} is quantified with two drug targets module A and B by calculating the mean shortest distances d_{AA} and d_{BB} (Equation (5)):

$$d_{AA} = \frac{1}{\|A\|} \sum_{a \in A} min_{a' \in A} d(a, a') \quad (5)$$

where a' ($a' \in A$) is the closet node to a ($a \in A$) within the interactome network. The mean shortest distance d_{AB} between their proteins is defined by the "closest" measure, where $d(a,b)$ is the shortest path length between a ($a \in A$) and b ($b \in B$) in the interactome network (Equation (6)).

$$d_{AB} = \frac{1}{\|A\| + \|B\|} \left(\sum_{a \in A} min_{b \in B} d(a,b) + \sum_{b \in B} min_{a \in A} d(a,b) \right) \quad (6)$$

A networked-based separation of a drug pair, A and B, can be calculated as follows (Equation (7)):

$$S_{AB} = \langle d_{AB} \rangle - \frac{\langle d_{AA} \rangle + \langle d_{BB} \rangle}{2} \quad (7)$$

where $d_{AB} = 0$ if genes are included in both the drug A and B target modules [38].

3. Results

3.1. GO Enrichment Analysis of COVID-19 Related Genes

To obtain meaningful molecular mechanisms underlying COVID-19, GO enrichment analysis classified potential COVID-19 related genes into enriched terms (Supplemental Table S4). All 63 SARS-CoV-2 related genes were categorized functionally into 1035 Gene Ontology terms including biological processes, cellular components, and molecular functions. Among the 971 COVID-19 DEGs, 860 genes were enriched in 1399 Gene Ontology terms. The COVID-19 related genes we identified were significantly enriched in blood pressure regulation (p-value = 5.29×10^{-23}), inflammatory response (p-value = 3.62×10^{-09}), neutrophil activation (p-value = 6.16×10^{-60}), and response to virus (p-value = 8.68×10^{-32}) (Figure 2). The results are consistent with previous studies, indicating that the renin-angiotensin system (RAS) plays an important role in the biological mechanisms of COVID-19 [39,40].

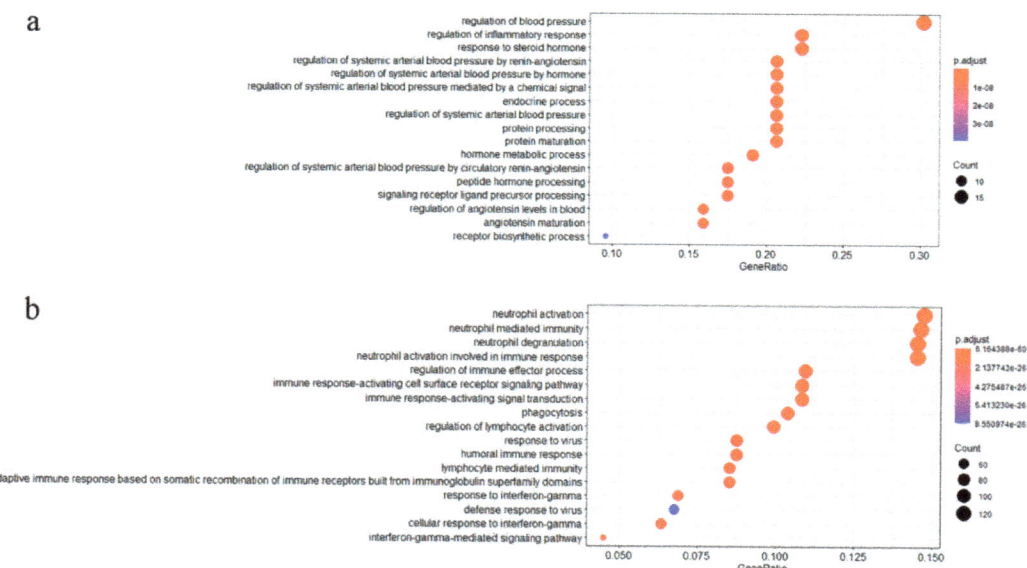

Figure 2. GO enrichment analysis of COVID-19 related genes. The dot plot is used to visualize enriched terms, (**a**) shows the COVID-19 related genes (n = 63) enrichment visualization and category interpretation. (**b**) pathway enrichment analysis visualization of single-cell DEGs (n = 860).

3.2. Network-Based Proximity Scores between Drug–Target Modules and COVID-19 Related Genes

We obtained the drug–disease proximity scores to evaluate the drug effect on COVID-19 through a network-based calculation. Drugs with low proximity scores are more likely to be effective against SARS-CoV-2 infection since the proximity scores reflect the distance between drug target sets and COVID-19 related genes in the interactome networks. Using this approach, we explored the distance of 7811 drug–target modules and COVID-19 related genes. The distance distribution of the drug targets to COVID-19 related genes was in the range of −2.66 to 2.79, and both real drugs and simulated drugs were widely distributed near the point of 1.70 (Figure 3). A ranked list of the potential drugs was clearly distributed in the range of −2.66 to 0.99, suggesting that the targets of existing drugs were closer to the COVID-19 genes than the reference sets (simulated drugs). We selected a distance smaller than 0.99 as the threshold to screen the potential drug candidates for COVID-19, where the corresponding Z-score was approximately −2.33 after converting into the proximity value. Finally, 468 drugs with proximity less than −2.33 were included in further analyses (Supplemental Table S5).

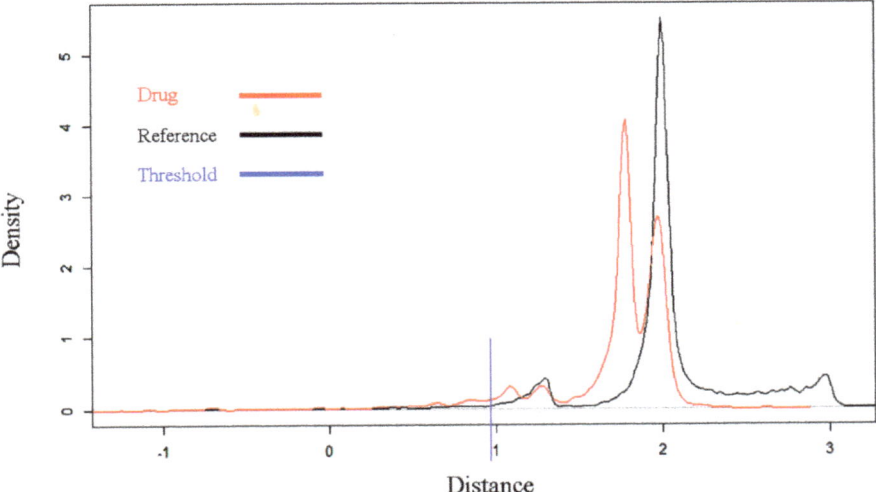

Figure 3. Distance distribution of all 7811 drugs and simulated reference. Peaks suggest that the distance corresponding to most members was around this value. The red line shows the distribution of the distance of the 7811 drugs to COVID-19 related genes. The black line illustrates the distance distribution of the simulated reference based on 30,000 replications. The blue line shows the threshold (distance < 0.99, Z-score < −2.33) to screen the drug candidates for COVID-19.

3.3. GSEA Analysis of COVID-19 Related Genes in Drug-Induced Signatures

To further estimate the drug candidate's efficacy on the disease and explore the underlying signaling pathways, we performed GSEA to examine their impact on the transcriptome of THP-1 cells. Since drugs were not fully matched between DrugBank and LINCS, some drugs were removed during the matching progress. In the total of 7811 drugs included in DrugBank and 377 from LINCS (THP-1 cell line), 112 drugs were matched by common name and 101 were matched by InChI Key (International Chemical Identifier Key). After removing overlaps, 131 drugs were included in both DrugBank and LINCS, 27 of which had low proximity scores (Z < −2.33) and were obtained for further GSEA.

We identified 18 drugs (FDR < 0.25 and ES > 0, Table 1) as potential therapeutic candidates since they significantly affected the expression of COVID-19 related genes in the mononuclear cells (Supplemental Table S6). These candidates included anti-viral agents (curcumin, dexamethasone, chloroquine), anti-diabetic agents (glibenclamide), analgesics (resveratrol), anti-convulsant (valproic acid), anti-cholesteremic agents (simvastatin), anti-carcinogenic agents (phenethyl isothiocyanate), anti-neoplastic agents (tretinoin), immunosuppressive agents (fostamatinib, atorvastatin, cyclosporine), anti-estrogen (tamoxifen), anti-hypertensive (nicardipine, nifedipine), anti-allergic agents (promethazine), and anti-cancer agents (orantinib, tipifarnib).

Table 1. Eighteen repurposable candidates for COVID-19.

DrugBank ID	Z-Score	Drug Name	Structure	Pharmacodynamics	Reported Studies of COVID-19 (PMID)
DB12010	−8.75	Fostamatinib		immunosuppressive agents	32637960
DB12695	−6.64	Phenethyl-isothiocyanate		anti-carcinogenic agents	33131530
DB01069	−5.65	Promethazine		anti-allergic agents	NA [1]
DB00641	−5.49	Simvastatin		anti-cholesteremic agents	32626922
DB00675	−4.75	Tamoxifen		anti-estrogen	32663742
DB01076	−4.74	Atorvastatin		immunosuppressive agents	32664990 32817953
DB11672	−3.65	Curcumin		antiviral agents	32430996 32442323
DB00755	−3.37	Tretinoin		anti-neoplastic agents	32707573
DB01234	−3.21	Dexamethasone		antiviral agents	327065533 2620554
DB00608	−3.14	Chloroquine		antiviral agents	32145363 32147496
DB00313	−2.90	Valproic acid		anti-convulsant	32498007
DB01016	−2.82	Glibenclamide		antiviral agents	32787684
DB00622	−2.75	Nicardipine		anti-hypertensive	NA
DB01115	−2.68	Nifedipine		anti-hypertensive	32226695 32411566
DB00091	−2.65	Cyclosporine		immunosuppressive agents	32376422 32487139
DB02709	−5.63	Resveratrol		analgesics	32412158 32764275
DB12072	−2.54	Orantinib		anti-cancer agents	NA
DB04960	−2.40	Tipifarnib		anti-cancer agents	NA

[1] NA: Not previously been reported as potential treatments for COVID-19.

3.4. Repurposing Drugs Sensitivity in Specific Cell Type

Differential expression analyses in 7 cell types between COVID-19 patients ($n = 7$) and controls ($n = 6$) were performed based on the scRNA-seq data (Tables S7–S13). According to the GSEA analysis, the DE genes of most repurposing drugs were enriched significantly in B cells (Table 2, Table S14). CD14+ Monocytes Cells and Dendritic Cells also showed sensitivity to the repurposing drug treatment. None repurposing drug DE genes were significantly enriched for the Single-cell gene expression spectrum of NK Cells, CD8+ T Cells, CD4+ T Cells.

Table 2. GSEA analysis of drug-induced different expression (DE) genes in scRNA profiles.

Drug Name	B Cells	CD14+ Monocytes Cells	CD16+ Monocytes Cells	Dendritic Cells	NK Cells	CD4+ T Cells	CD8+ T Cells
Chloroquine	NA [1]	NA	NA	NA	NA	NA	NA
Nicardipine	Significant [2]	Significant	NA	NA	NA	NA	NA
Simvastatin	NA	NA	NA	NA	NA	NA	NA
Tamoxifen	Significant	Significant	NA	Significant	NA	NA	NA
Promethazine	NA	NA	NA	NA	NA	NA	NA
Nifedipine	Significant	NA	NA	NA	NA	NA	NA
Resveratrol	Significant	NA	NA	Significant	NA	NA	NA
Tipifarnib	Significant	Significant	NA	Significant	NA	NA	NA
Orantinib	NA	NA	NA	NA	NA	NA	NA
Tretinoin	Significant	Significant	Significant	Significant	NA	NA	NA
Atorvastatin	Significant	NA	NA	NA	NA	NA	NA
Dexamethasone	Significant	Significant	Significant	Significant	NA	NA	NA
Curcumin	NA	NA	NA	NA	NA	NA	NA
Fostamatinib	Significant	Significant	NA	Significant	NA	NA	NA
Valproic-acid	Significant	NA	NA	NA	NA	NA	NA
Glibenclamide	Significant	Significant	NA	NA	NA	NA	NA
Phenethyl Isothiocyanate	Significant	NA	NA	NA	NA	NA	NA
Cyclosporin	Significant	NA	NA	NA	NA	NA	NA

[1] Significant: Drug-induced DE genes statistically significant enrichment in scRNA profile; [2] NA: Drug-induced DE genes statistically no significant enrichment in scRNA profile.

3.5. Identification of Synergistic Drug Combinations

Based on the Complementary Exposure model, we identified 153 drug combinations based on the 18 potential therapeutic candidates for COVID-19. Among these combinations, 123 drug pairs were excluded due to close drug–target modules ($S_{AB} < 0$), while 30 drug combination conformed to the Complementary Exposure Model and may therefore be effective in the treatment of COVID-19 (Table 3).

Table 3. All predicted possible combinations for COVID-19.

Drug A	Drug B	Drug A Common. Name	Drug B Common. Name	S_{AB}	Z_{DA}	Z_{DB}
DB01069	DB12072	Promethazine	Orantinib	0.76	−2.58	−2.53
DB12072	DB00313	Orantinib	Valproic acid	0.67	−2.53	−2.99
DB12072	DB00755	Orantinib	Tretinoin	0.66	−2.53	−2.44
DB00755	DB12010	Tretinoin	Fostamatinib	0.66	−2.44	−3.68
DB00622	DB12072	Nicardipine	Orantinib	0.60	−2.81	−2.53
DB01115	DB12072	Nifedipine	Orantinib	0.57	−2.71	−2.53
DB12072	DB01234	Orantinib	Dexamethasone	0.54	−2.53	−3.40
DB01069	DB04960	Promethazine	Tipifarnib	0.49	−2.58	−2.35

Table 3. Cont.

Drug A	Drug B	Drug A Common. Name	Drug B Common. Name	S_{AB}	Z_{DA}	Z_{DB}
DB12695	DB00091	Phenethyl Isothiocyanate	Cyclosporine	0.43	−3.22	−2.67
DB04960	DB12695	Tipifarnib	Phenethyl Isothiocyanate	0.43	−2.35	−3.22
DB00675	DB12072	Tamoxifen	Orantinib	0.42	−3.40	−2.53
DB01069	DB12010	Promethazine	Fostamatinib	0.42	−2.58	−3.68
DB12072	DB01016	Orantinib	Glyburide	0.40	−2.53	−2.90
DB00641	DB12072	Simvastatin	Orantinib	0.39	−4.37	−2.53
DB12072	DB00091	Orantinib	Cyclosporine	0.37	−2.53	−2.67
DB02709	DB12072	Resveratrol	Orantinib	0.37	−3.91	−2.53
DB12072	DB01076	Orantinib	Atorvastatin	0.37	−2.53	−4.23
DB01069	DB01076	Promethazine	Atorvastatin	0.37	−2.58	−4.23
DB01069	DB12695	Promethazine	Phenethyl Isothiocyanate	0.34	−2.58	−3.22
DB00608	DB12072	Chloroquine	Orantinib	0.34	−3.31	−2.53
DB01069	DB02709	Promethazine	Resveratrol	0.33	−2.58	−3.91
DB12072	DB12695	Orantinib	Phenethyl Isothiocyanate	0.30	−2.53	−3.22
DB01069	DB11672	Promethazine	Curcumin	0.26	−2.58	−2.81
DB01016	DB12695	Glyburide	Phenethyl Isothiocyanate	0.18	−2.90	−3.22
DB12010	DB12695	Fostamatinib	Phenethyl Isothiocyanate	0.17	−3.68	−3.22
DB00622	DB12695	Nicardipine	Phenethyl Isothiocyanate	0.16	−2.81	−3.22
DB04960	DB00755	Tipifarnib	Tretinoin	0.14	−2.35	−2.44
DB01076	DB12695	Atorvastatin	Phenethyl Isothiocyanate	0.11	−4.23	−3.22
DB11672	DB12695	Curcumin	Phenethyl Isothiocyanate	0.06	−2.81	−3.22
DB00608	DB11672	Chloroquine	Curcumin	0.04	−3.31	−2.81

One notable potential drug combination was fostamatinib (F) plus tretinoin (T). Fostamatinib ($Z_{DF} = -3.68$) and tretinoin ($Z_{DT} = -2.44$) targets were both overlapped with the COVID-19 disease module, indicating that the drug combination might have a therapeutic effect on the disease. At the same time, the targets of fostamatinib and tretinoin were independent with network-based separation ($S_{FT} > 0$), and therefore fit the Complementary Exposure pattern (Figure 4a). We also used the Sankey diagram to represent the interactions among drug–target-disease (Figure 4b). Apart from the drug directly targeting COVID-19 related genes, un-targetable drug–disease effects were present due to the drug–target interaction with COVID-19 related genes in the PPI as reflected by the proximity scores. Additionally, take promethazine (P) and nicardipine (N) as a counterexample. Promethazine ($Z_{DP} = -2.58$) and nicardipine ($Z_{DN} = -2.81$) targets fell into the Overlapping Exposure with the COVID-19 disease module. Although promethazine and nicardipine showed effective treatment on the disease, overlapping drug pair ($S_{PN} < 0$) was not a synergistic drug pair due to adverse effects such as overlapping drug toxicity (Figure 4c). Additionally, sharing targets of promethazine and nicardipine meant the drug pair had limits in treatment from different therapeutic pathways (Figure 4d).

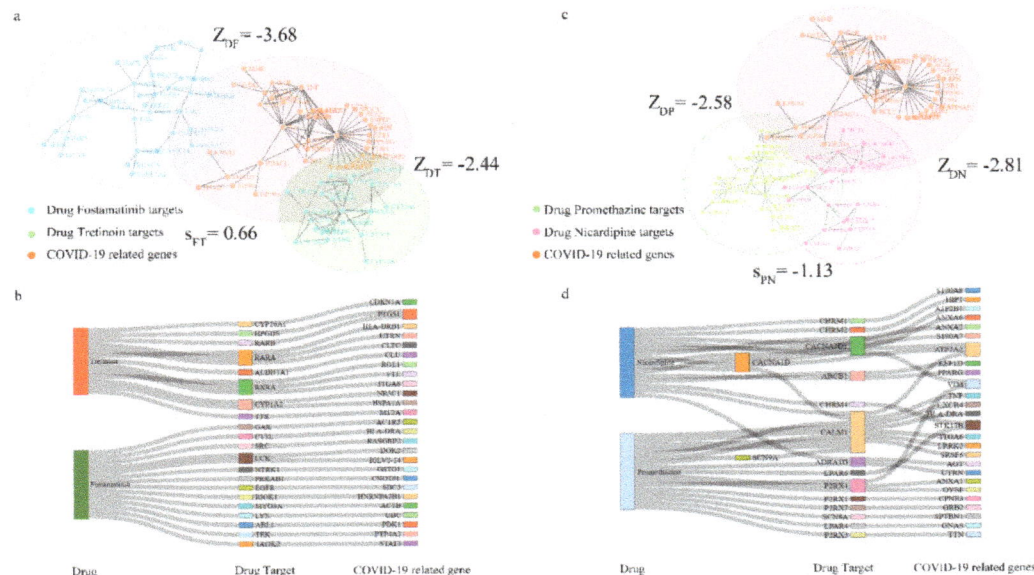

Figure 4. Network-based stratification of hypertensive drug combinations. (**a**) A network-based separation of a drug pair, fostamatinib (F), and tretinoin (T). For $Z_{DF} < 0$ and $Z_{DT} < 0$, the drug–target module of fostamatinib (F) and tretinoin (T) was overlapped with the disease module (D). For $S_{FT} > 0$, the two sets of drug targets are separated topologically. Fostamatinib and tretinoin targets both separately hit the COVID-19 module, which was captured by the Complementary Exposure pattern. The disease module in orange (D) included disease-related genes (nodes) and their undirected and unweighted interactions (links), while the drug module (F or T) in blue (green) included drug–targets (nodes) and their undirected and unweighted interactions (links). (**b**) Sankey diagram visualizes drug pairs' mechanism hypothesis: drugs are on the left, and COVID-19 related genes are right. Links show drugs that were mapped onto COVID-19 related genes through drug–target associations and human protein-protein interaction. (**c**) Nicardipine (N) and Promethazine (P) drug–target modules overlapped the network. For $S_{PN} < 0$, the two sets of drug targets were Overlapping Exposure, which meant more adverse effects and less efficacy compared to the Complementary Exposure pattern. (**d**) Sankey diagram showed how drug–targets of Nicardipine and Promethazine overlapped and interacted with related genes.

4. Discussion

This study used a network-based drug repurposing combined with a transcriptomics strategy to identify potential drug candidates and drug pairs for COVID-19 treatment. The joint analysis of the proximity of drug–target relationship modules, SARS-CoV-2 genomics, transcriptomics, and synergistic drug effects could overcome the limitations of analyzing data from only network distance or transcriptome and improve drug candidate prediction. We proposed 18 drugs and 30 drug combinations including broad-spectrum antiviral agents, receptor antagonists, channel blockers, and renin-angiotensin system agents.

Some medications such as dexamethasone, chloroquine, curcumin [41], glyburide [42], tretinoin [43,44], cyclosporine [45,46], valproic acid [47], fostamatinib [48,49], atorvastatin [50–52], and phenethyl-isothiocyanate [53] have recently received major attention for the treatment of COVID-19 and have been validated by previous studies, supporting the reliability of our findings. Nicardipine, promethazine, orantinib, and tipifarnib have not previously been reported as potential treatments for COVID-19. Therefore, we will discuss these novel drug candidates in the following.

- Nicardipine

With a similar structure to nifedipine (Z = −2.68), nicardipine (Z = −2.75) was initially developed to regulate high blood pressure as a dihydropyridine calcium channel blocker [54]. Nifedipine is indicated to potentially be effective in the treatment regimens of elderly patients with hypertension hospitalized with COVID-19 [55,56]. Therefore, nicardipine might play a similar role with nifedipine in the adjuvant treatment of COVID-19 patients.

- Promethazine

Promethazine (Z = −5.65) antagonizes various receptors including dopaminergic, histamine, and cholinergic receptors, and is commonly used for indications such as allergic conditions, motion sickness, sedation, nausea, and vomiting [57]. The proximity score of promethazine was significantly low partly by targeting genes including CALM1, KCNS1, LPAR4, LPAR6, P2RY12, P2PY8, and P2RX5, which were DEGs between T cell subsets of COVID-19 samples and healthy controls. Characteristics of the bronchoalveolar immune genes have been explored as potential mechanisms underlying pathogenesis in COVID-19 [58]. These findings implied that promethazine might be effective for COVID-19 by regulating the immune cell microenvironment.

- Orantinib and Tipifarnib

Orantinib (Z = −2.54) showed preliminary efficacy and safety in advanced hepatocellular carcinoma [59]. Tipifarnib (Z = −2.40) was studied in the treatment of acute myeloid leukemia (AML) and other types of cancer [60]. Although orantinib and tipifarnib are both not yet approved by the FDA, anticancer drugs identified by our study such as phenethyl isothiocyanate have been reported to be an effective treatment strategy to treat COVID-19 [53]. Drug repurposing against COVID-19 focused on anticancer agents was previously predicted to be effective and it was speculated that drugs interfering with specific cancer cell pathways may be effective in reducing viral replication [61]. Therefore, the anticancer drugs orantinib and tipifarnib might also be potential candidates for the treatment of COVID-19.

In contrast with our results, tamoxifen (Z = −4.75) was reported to increase the COVID-19 risk due to its anti-estrogen and P-glycoprotein inhibitory effects [62]. Data from previous experiments suggested that estrogen could regulate the expression of angiotensin-converting enzyme 2 (ACE2) [63], which was reported to be the critical natural cellular receptor for SARS-CoV-2 and was an important factor for infection. However, a recent study discussed the uncertain effects of RAS blockers on ACE2 levels and activity in humans and proposed an alternative hypothesis that ACE2 might more likely be beneficial than harmful in patients with lung injury [64]. The controversies of ACE2 system inhibition attempt to explain the relationship between the virus and the RAS [65], but existing research is too limited to support or refute these hypotheses. Our research suggested that tamoxifen may influence cytokine storm syndrome by regulating cytokine-mediated signaling pathways (ES = 0.67, P = 0.14), which is a severe clinical symptom of COVID-19 [66,67]. Several studies have indicated that tamoxifen could reduce cytokines to normal levels and it has been demonstrated to be beneficial for inflammation in rats [68,69]. Overall, we recommend that tamoxifen may protect against cytokine storms and alleviate ARDS in COVID-19 patients as well as reduce the incidence of critical illness and mortality.

There are some limitations to our strategy. First, the proximity calculation regards proteins interaction as nodes and links, which may not completely capture important information about the interaction types. Second, the LINCS and DrugBank databases are only partly matched, and therefore many important drug candidates may be ignored. Additionally, some of the potentially interesting drugs, such as alemtuzumab (Z = −3.27), were not able to be included in the final screening. Third, although THP-1 cells might be a useful tool in the research of monocyte and macrophage-related mechanisms [70], heterogeneity still exists in the gene expression profile of the mononuclear cells of COVID-19 patients and THP-1 cells. Additionally, considering that the impaired function of heart, brain, lung, and liver were complications of COVID-19 [71], more types of infection-related cell lines could be taken into account to fully investigate drugs and treatment outcome on COVID-19.

In conclusion, our effective drug repurposing strategy combined network-based pharmacology and transcriptomes methods to identify 18 potential COVID-19 drugs, and recommend 30 drug combinations. Although several candidate repurposing drugs were previously reported to have the anti-COVID-19 effect, four drugs such as nicardipine, promethazine, orantinib, and tipifarnib were recommended for the first time in COVID-19 treatment. Additionally, based on our repurposing drug sensitivity analysis, DE genes of most repurposing drugs were enriched significantly in B cells. Our analysis contributed to guide and accelerate research in COVID-19 drug development, and this method would be kindly applicable for drug repurposing research in future complex diseases. However, the identified drug candidates still require future experimental validation and large-scale clinical trials before their use in COVID-19 management.

Supplementary Materials: The following are available online at https://www.mdpi.com/article/10.3390/pharmaceutics13040545/s1, Table S1: DE genes list compared individual COVID-19 samples with all healthy controls in each cell type; Table S2: Number of DE genes between individual COVID-19 samples and the healthy controls in 7 cell types; Table S3: Drug target interactions from the well-known database; Table S4: GO enrichment of COVID-19 related genes; Table S5: Network-based proximity scores of drug–disease relationships; Table S6: GSEA results on the SARS-CoV-2 related gene set in the THP-1 cells; Table S7: COVID-19 DE genes in CD14+ Monocytes; Table S8: COVID-19 DE genes in Dendritic Cells; Table S9: COVID-19 DE genes in CD8+ T cells; Table S10: COVID-19 DE genes in CD16+ Monocytes; Table S11: COVID-19 DE genes in B cells; Table S12: COVID-19 DE genes in NK cells; Table S13: COVID-19 DE genes in CD4+ T cells; Table S14: GSEA results on the repurposing drugs-related gene set in the specific cells.

Author Contributions: Conceptualization, H.-W.D., L.-J.T. and H.-M.X.; methodology, D.-Y.L., J.-C.L., X.-H.M. and S.L.; software, D.-Y.L.; data analysis, D.-Y.L.; writing—original draft preparation, D.-Y.L.; writing—review and editing, J.-C.L., S.L., L.-J.T., X.-H.M., J.G. and H.-W.D.; visualization, D.-Y.L.; supervision, L.-J.T. and H.-W.D.; funding acquisition, L.-J.T. and H.-W.D. All authors have read and agreed to the published version of the manuscript.

Funding: This study was supported in part by the Natural Science Foundation of China (NSFC; 81570807). HWD was partially was supported by grants from the National Institutes of Health [U19AG05537301, R01AR069055, P20GM109036, R01MH104680, R01AG061917, U54MD007595].

Institutional Review Board Statement: Not applicate.

Informed Consent Statement: Not applicate.

Data Availability Statement: Not applicate.

Acknowledgments: The authors are grateful to Ying Liu and Yun Gong for technical assistance with the data analysis. The authors acknowledge the NCBI and World Health Organization for their work on collecting, processing, and sharing datasets about COVID-19.

Conflicts of Interest: The authors declare no conflict of interest.

References

1. Jin, Y.; Yang, H.; Ji, W.; Wu, W.; Chen, S.; Zhang, W.; Duan, G. Virology, Epidemiology, Pathogenesis, and Control of COVID-19. *Viruses* **2020**, *12*, 372. [CrossRef] [PubMed]
2. Coronavirus Disease (COVID-19)—World Health Organization. Available online: https://www.who.int/emergencies/diseases/novel-coronavirus-2019 (accessed on 14 January 2021).
3. Li, G.; De Clercq, E. Therapeutic Options for the 2019 Novel Coronavirus (2019-NCoV). *Nat. Rev. Drug Discov.* **2020**, *19*, 149–150. [CrossRef]
4. Chen, N.; Zhou, M.; Dong, X.; Qu, J.; Gong, F.; Han, Y.; Qiu, Y.; Wang, J.; Liu, Y.; Wei, Y.; et al. Epidemiological and Clinical Characteristics of 99 Cases of 2019 Novel Coronavirus Pneumonia in Wuhan, China: A Descriptive Study. *Lancet* **2020**, *395*, 507–513. [CrossRef]

5. Wu, J.; Li, W.; Shi, X.; Chen, Z.; Jiang, B.; Liu, J.; Wang, D.; Liu, C.; Meng, Y.; Cui, L.; et al. Early Antiviral Treatment Contributes to Alleviate the Severity and Improve the Prognosis of Patients with Novel Coronavirus Disease (COVID-19). *J. Intern. Med.* **2020**, *288*, 128–138. [CrossRef] [PubMed]
6. Wang, Y.; Zhang, D.; Du, G.; Du, R.; Zhao, J.; Jin, Y.; Fu, S.; Gao, L.; Cheng, Z.; Lu, Q.; et al. Remdesivir in Adults with Severe COVID-19: A Randomised, Double-Blind, Placebo-Controlled, Multicentre Trial. *Lancet* **2020**, *395*, 1569–1578. [CrossRef]
7. Home—ClinicalTrials.Gov. Available online: https://clinicaltrials.gov/ (accessed on 11 March 2021).
8. Warren, T.K.; Jordan, R.; Lo, M.K.; Ray, A.S.; Mackman, R.L.; Soloveva, V.; Siegel, D.; Perron, M.; Bannister, R.; Hui, H.C.; et al. Therapeutic Efficacy of the Small Molecule GS-5734 against Ebola Virus in Rhesus Monkeys. *Nature* **2016**, *531*, 381–385. [CrossRef]
9. Spinner, C.D.; Gottlieb, R.L.; Criner, G.J.; Arribas Lopez, J.R.; Cattelan, A.M.; Soriano Viladomiu, A.; Ogbuagu, O.; Malhotra, P.; Mullane, K.M.; Castagna, A.; et al. Effect of Remdesivir vs. Standard Care on Clinical Status at 11 Days in Patients with Moderate COVID-19: A Randomized Clinical Trial. *JAMA* **2020**, *324*, 1048–1057. [CrossRef] [PubMed]
10. Pan, H.; Peto, R.; Abdool Karim, Q.; Alejandria, M.; Henao Restrepo, A.M.; Hernandez Garcia, C.; Kieny, M.P.; Malekzadeh, R.; Murthy, S.; Preziosi, M.-P.; et al. Repurposed Antiviral Drugs for COVID-19; Interim WHO SOLIDARITY Trial Results. *medRxiv* **2020**. [CrossRef]
11. Luo, Y.; Zhao, X.; Zhou, J.; Yang, J.; Zhang, Y.; Kuang, W.; Peng, J.; Chen, L.; Zeng, J. A Network Integration Approach for Drug-Target Interaction Prediction and Computational Drug Repositioning from Heterogeneous Information. *Nat. Commun.* **2017**, *8*, 573. [CrossRef]
12. Cheng, F.; Desai, R.J.; Handy, D.E.; Wang, R.; Schneeweiss, S.; Barabási, A.-L.; Loscalzo, J. Network-Based Approach to Prediction and Population-Based Validation of in Silico Drug Repurposing. *Nat. Commun.* **2018**, *9*, 2691. [CrossRef] [PubMed]
13. Tu, Y.-F.; Chien, C.-S.; Yarmishyn, A.A.; Lin, Y.-Y.; Luo, Y.-H.; Lin, Y.-T.; Lai, W.-Y.; Yang, D.-M.; Chou, S.-J.; Yang, Y.-P.; et al. A Review of SARS-CoV-2 and the Ongoing Clinical Trials. *Int. J. Mol. Sci.* **2020**, *21*, 2657. [CrossRef]
14. Gordon, D.E.; Jang, G.M.; Bouhaddou, M.; Xu, J.; Obernier, K.; White, K.M.; O'Meara, M.J.; Rezelj, V.V.; Guo, J.Z.; Swaney, D.L.; et al. A SARS-CoV-2 Protein Interaction Map Reveals Targets for Drug-Repurposing. *Nature* **2020**, *583*, 459–468. [CrossRef]
15. Han, H.; Lee, S.; Lee, I. NGSEA: Network-Based Gene Set Enrichment Analysis for Interpreting Gene Expression Phenotypes with Functional Gene Sets. *Mol. Cells* **2019**, *42*, 579–588. [CrossRef]
16. Yu, A.Z.; Ramsey, S.A. A Computational Systems Biology Approach for Identifying Candidate Drugs for Repositioning for Cardiovascular Disease. *Interdiscip. Sci. Comput. Life Sci.* **2018**, *10*, 449–454. [CrossRef]
17. Guney, E.; Menche, J.; Vidal, M.; Barabasi, A.-L. Network-Based in Silico Drug Efficacy Screening. *Nat. Commun.* **2016**, *7*, 10331. [CrossRef] [PubMed]
18. Iorio, F.; Bosotti, R.; Scacheri, E.; Belcastro, V.; Mithbaokar, P.; Ferriero, R.; Murino, L.; Tagliaferri, R.; Brunetti-Pierri, N.; Isacchi, A.; et al. Discovery of Drug Mode of Action and Drug Repositioning from Transcriptional Responses. *Proc. Natl. Acad. Sci. USA* **2010**, *107*, 14621–14626. [CrossRef]
19. Vásquez-Bochm, L.X.; Velázquez-Paniagua, M.; Castro-Vázquez, S.S.; Guerrero-Rodríguez, S.L.; Mondragon-Peralta, A.; De La Fuente-Granada, M.; Pérez-Tapia, S.M.; González-Arenas, A.; Velasco-Velázquez, M.A. Transcriptome-Based Identification of Lovastatin as a Breast Cancer Stem Cell-Targeting Drug. *Pharmacol. Rep.* **2019**, *71*, 535–544. [CrossRef] [PubMed]
20. Zhang, M.; Luo, H.; Xi, Z.; Rogaeva, E. Drug Repositioning for Diabetes Based on "Omics" Data Mining. *PLoS ONE* **2015**, *10*, e0126082. [CrossRef] [PubMed]
21. Kinnings, S.L.; Liu, N.; Buchmeier, N.; Tonge, P.J.; Xie, L.; Bourne, P.E. Drug Discovery Using Chemical Systems Biology: Repositioning the Safe Medicine Comtan to Treat Multi-Drug and Extensively Drug Resistant Tuberculosis. *PLoS Comput. Biol.* **2009**, *5*, e1000423. [CrossRef]
22. Coronaviridae—NCBI Datasets. Available online: https://www.ncbi.nlm.nih.gov/datasets/coronavirus/genomes/ (accessed on 14 January 2021).
23. Wilk, A.J.; Rustagi, A.; Zhao, N.Q.; Roque, J.; Martinez-Colon, G.J.; McKechnie, J.L.; Ivison, G.T.; Ranganath, T.; Vergara, R.; Hollis, T.; et al. A Single-Cell Atlas of the Peripheral Immune Response in Patients with Severe COVID-19. *Nat. Med.* **2020**, *26*, 1070–1076. [CrossRef]
24. Yu, G.; Wang, L.G.; Han, Y.; He, Q.Y. ClusterProfiler: An R Package for Comparing Biological Themes among Gene Clusters. *Omics J. Integr. Biol.* **2012**, *16*, 284–287. [CrossRef]
25. Wishart, D.S.; Feunang, Y.D.; Guo, A.C.; Lo, E.J.; Marcu, A.; Grant, J.R.; Sajed, T.; Johnson, D.; Li, C.; Sayeeda, Z.; et al. DrugBank 5.0: A Major Update to the DrugBank Database for 2018. *Nucleic Acids Res.* **2018**, *46*, D1074–D1082. [CrossRef] [PubMed]
26. SuperTarget. Available online: http://insilico.charite.de/supertarget/index.php?site=drugs (accessed on 14 January 2021).
27. Rodchenkov, I.; Babur, O.; Luna, A.; Aksoy, B.A.; Wong, J.V.; Fong, D.; Franz, M.; Siper, M.C.; Cheung, M.; Wrana, M.; et al. Pathway Commons 2019 Update: Integration, Analysis and Exploration of Pathway Data. *Nucleic Acids Res.* **2020**, *48*, D489–D497. [CrossRef]
28. Misselbeck, K.; Parolo, S.; Lorenzini, F.; Savoca, V.; Leonardelli, L.; Bora, P.; Morine, M.J.; Mione, M.C.; Domenici, E.; Priami, C. A Network-Based Approach to Identify Deregulated Pathways and Drug Effects in Metabolic Syndrome. *Nat. Commun.* **2019**, *10*, 5215. [CrossRef] [PubMed]
29. Peng, Y.; Yuan, M.; Xin, J.; Liu, X.; Wang, J. Screening Novel Drug Candidates for Alzheimer's Disease by an Integrated Network and Transcriptome Analysis. *Bioinformatics* **2020**. [CrossRef]

30. Subramanian, A.; Tamayo, P.; Mootha, V.K.; Mukherjee, S.; Ebert, B.L.; Gillette, M.A.; Paulovich, A.; Pomeroy, S.L.; Golub, T.R.; Lander, E.S.; et al. Gene Set Enrichment Analysis: A Knowledge-Based Approach for Interpreting Genome-Wide Expression Profiles. *Proc. Natl. Acad. Sci. USA* **2005**, *102*, 15545–15550. [CrossRef]
31. Subramanian, A.; Narayan, R.; Corsello, S.M.; Peck, D.D.; Natoli, T.E.; Lu, X.; Gould, J.; Davis, J.F.; Tubelli, A.A.; Asiedu, J.K.; et al. A Next Generation Connectivity Map: L1000 Platform and the First 1,000,000 Profiles. *Cell* **2017**, *171*, 1437–1452.e17. [CrossRef] [PubMed]
32. Sun, D.W.; Zhang, D.; Tian, R.H.; Li, Y.; Wang, Y.S.; Cao, J.; Tang, Y.; Zhang, N.; Zan, T.; Gao, L.; et al. The Underlying Changes and Predicting Role of Peripheral Blood Inflammatory Cells in Severe COVID-19 Patients: A Sentinel? *Clin. Chim. Acta* **2020**, *508*, 122–129. [CrossRef]
33. Han, H.; Yang, L.; Liu, R.; Liu, F.; Wu, K.; Li, J.; Liu, X.; Zhu, C. Prominent Changes in Blood Coagulation of Patients with SARS-CoV-2 Infection. *Clin. Chem. Lab. Med.* **2020**, *58*, 1116–1120. [CrossRef]
34. Laing, A.G.; Lorenc, A.; del Barrio, I.D.M.; Das, A.; Fish, M.; Monin, L.; Munoz-Ruiz, M.; McKenzie, D.R.; Hayday, T.S.; Francos-Quijorna, I.; et al. A Dynamic COVID-19 Immune Signature Includes Associations with Poor Prognosis. *Nat. Med.* **2020**, *26*, 1623–1635. [CrossRef] [PubMed]
35. Stuart, T.; Butler, A.; Hoffman, P.; Hafemeister, C.; Papalexi, E.; Mauck, W.M.; Hao, Y.; Stoeckius, M.; Smibert, P.; Satija, R. Comprehensive Integration of Single-Cell Data. *Cell* **2019**, *177*, 1888–1902.e21. [CrossRef]
36. Sun, X.; Vilar, S.; Tatonetti, N.P. High-Throughput Methods for Combinatorial Drug Discovery. *Sci. Transl. Med.* **2013**, *5*, 205rv1. [CrossRef] [PubMed]
37. Cheng, F.; Kovacs, I.A.; Barabasi, A.L. Network-Based Prediction of Drug Combinations. *Nat. Commun.* **2019**, *10*, 1197. [CrossRef] [PubMed]
38. Menche, J.; Sharma, A.; Kitsak, M.; Ghiassian, S.D.; Vidal, M.; Loscalzo, J.; Barabasi, A.L. Disease Networks. Uncovering Disease-Disease Relationships through the Incomplete Interactome. *Science* **2015**, *347*, 1257601. [CrossRef] [PubMed]
39. Meng, J.; Xiao, G.; Zhang, J.; He, X.; Ou, M.; Bi, J.; Yang, R.; Di, W.; Wang, Z.; Li, Z.; et al. Renin-Angiotensin System Inhibitors Improve the Clinical Outcomes of COVID-19 Patients with Hypertension. *Emerg. Microbes Infect.* **2020**, *9*, 757–760. [CrossRef]
40. Woelfel, R.; Corman, V.M.; Guggemos, W.; Seilmaier, M.; Zange, S.; Mueller, M.A.; Niemeyer, D.; Jones, T.C.; Vollmar, P.; Rothe, C.; et al. Virological Assessment of Hospitalized Patients with COVID-2019. *Nature* **2020**, *581*, 465–469. [CrossRef]
41. Stancioiu, F.; Papadakis, G.Z.; Kteniadakis, S.; Izotov, B.N.; Coleman, M.D.; Spandidos, D.A.; Tsatsakis, A. A Dissection of SARSCoV2 with Clinical Implications (Review). *Int. J. Mol. Med.* **2020**, *46*, 489–508. [CrossRef] [PubMed]
42. Ferraz, W.R.; Gomes, R.A.; S Novaes, A.L.; Goulart Trossini, G.H. Ligand and Structure-Based Virtual Screening Applied to the SARS-CoV-2 Main Protease: An in Silico Repurposing Study. *Future Med. Chem.* **2020**. [CrossRef]
43. Warrell, R.P.; Frankel, S.R.; Miller, W.H.; Scheinberg, D.A.; Itri, L.M.; Hittelman, W.N.; Vyas, R.; Andreeff, M.; Tafuri, A.; Jakubowski, A.; et al. Differentiation Therapy of Acute Promyelocytic Leukemia with Tretinoin (All-Trans-Retinoic Acid). *N. Engl. J. Med.* **1991**, *324*, 1385–1393. [CrossRef] [PubMed]
44. Riva, L.; Yuan, S.; Yin, X.; Martin-Sancho, L.; Matsunaga, N.; Pache, L.; Burgstaller-Muehlbacher, S.; De Jesus, P.D.; Teriete, P.; Hull, M.V.; et al. Discovery of SARS-CoV-2 Antiviral Drugs through Large-Scale Compound Repurposing. *Nature* **2020**. [CrossRef] [PubMed]
45. de Wilde, A.H.; Pham, U.; Posthuma, C.C.; Snijder, E.J. Cyclophilins and Cyclophilin Inhibitors in Nidovirus Replication. *Virology* **2018**, *522*, 46–55. [CrossRef] [PubMed]
46. Glowacka, P.; Rudnicka, L.; Warszawik-Hendzel, O.; Sikora, M.; Goldust, M.; Gajda, P.; Stochmal, A.; Blicharz, L.; Rakowska, A.; Olszewska, M. The Antiviral Properties of Cyclosporine. Focus on Coronavirus, Hepatitis C Virus, Influenza Virus, and Human Immunodeficiency Virus Infections. *Biology* **2020**, *9*, 192. [CrossRef] [PubMed]
47. Unal, G.; Turan, B.; Balcioglu, Y.H. Immunopharmacological Management of COVID-19: Potential Therapeutic Role of Valproic Acid. *Med. Hypotheses* **2020**, *143*, 109891. [CrossRef] [PubMed]
48. Markham, A. Fostamatinib: First Global Approval. *Drugs* **2018**, *78*, 959–963. [CrossRef] [PubMed]
49. Alimova, M.; Sidhom, E.H.; Satyam, A.; Dvela-Levitt, M.; Melanson, M.; Chamberlain, B.T.; Alper, S.L.; Santos, J.; Gutierrez, J.; Subramanian, A.; et al. A High Content Screen for Mucin-1-Reducing Compounds Identifies Fostamatinib as a Candidate for Rapid Repurposing for Acute Lung Injury during the COVID-19 Pandemic. *bioRxiv* **2020**. [CrossRef]
50. Risner, K.H.; Tieu, K.V.; Wang, Y.; Bakovic, A.; Alem, F.; Bhalla, N.; Nathan, S.; Conway, D.E.; Macklin, P.; Narayanan, A. Maraviroc Inhibits SARS-CoV-2 Multiplication and s-Protein Mediated Cell Fusion in Cell Culture. *bioRxiv* **2020**. [CrossRef]
51. Zhang, X.J.; Qin, J.J.; Cheng, X.; Shen, L.; Zhao, Y.C.; Yuan, Y.; Lei, F.; Chen, M.M.; Yang, H.; Bai, L.; et al. In-Hospital Use of Statins Is Associated with a Reduced Risk of Mortality among Individuals with COVID-19. *Cell Metab.* **2020**, *32*, 176–187.e4. [CrossRef] [PubMed]
52. Rodriguez-Nava, G.; Trelles-Garcia, D.P.; Yanez-Bello, M.A.; Chung, C.W.; Trelles-Garcia, V.P.; Friedman, H.J. Atorvastatin Associated with Decreased Hazard for Death in COVID-19 Patients Admitted to an ICU: A Retrospective Cohort Study. *Crit. Care* **2020**, *24*, 429. [CrossRef] [PubMed]
53. Barh, D.; Tiwari, S.; Weener, M.E.; Azevedo, V.; Góes-Neto, A.; Gromiha, M.M.; Ghosh, P. Multi-Omics-Based Identification of SARS-CoV-2 Infection Biology and Candidate Drugs against COVID-19. *Comput. Biol. Med.* **2020**, *126*, 104051. [CrossRef]

54. Sorkin, E.M.; Clissold, S.P. Nicardipine. A Review of Its Pharmacodynamic and Pharmacokinetic Properties, and Therapeutic Efficacy, in the Treatment of Angina Pectoris, Hypertension and Related Cardiovascular Disorders. *Drugs* **1987**, *33*, 296–345. [CrossRef] [PubMed]
55. Solaimanzadeh, I. Acetazolamide, Nifedipine and Phosphodiesterase Inhibitors: Rationale for Their Utilization as Adjunctive Countermeasures in the Treatment of Coronavirus Disease 2019 (COVID-19). *Cureus* **2020**, *12*, e7343. [CrossRef]
56. Solaimanzadeh, I. Nifedipine and Amlodipine Are Associated with Improved Mortality and Decreased Risk for Intubation and Mechanical Ventilation in Elderly Patients Hospitalized for COVID-19. *Cureus* **2020**, *12*, e8069. [CrossRef]
57. Southard, B.T.; Al Khalili, Y. *Promethazine*; StatPearls: Treasure Island, FL, USA, 2020.
58. Liao, M.; Liu, Y.; Yuan, J.; Wen, Y.; Xu, G.; Zhao, J.; Cheng, L.; Li, J.; Wang, X.; Wang, F.; et al. Single-Cell Landscape of Bronchoalveolar Immune Cells in Patients with COVID-19. *Nat. Med.* **2020**, *26*, 842–844. [CrossRef] [PubMed]
59. Ikeda, M.; Shiina, S.; Nakachi, K.; Mitsunaga, S.; Shimizu, S.; Kojima, Y.; Ueno, H.; Morizane, C.; Kondo, S.; Sakamoto, Y.; et al. Phase I Study on the Safety, Pharmacokinetic Profile, and Efficacy of the Combination of TSU-68, an Oral Antiangiogenic Agent, and S-1 in Patients with Advanced Hepatocellular Carcinoma. *Investig. New Drugs* **2014**, *32*, 928–936. [CrossRef]
60. Gilardi, M.; Wang, Z.; Proietto, M.; Chillà, A.; Calleja-Valera, J.L.; Goto, Y.; Vanoni, M.; Janes, M.R.; Mikulski, Z.; Gualberto, A.; et al. Tipifarnib as a Precision Therapy for HRAS-Mutant Head and Neck Squamous Cell Carcinomas. *Mol. Cancer Ther.* **2020**, *19*, 1784–1796. [CrossRef] [PubMed]
61. Ciliberto, G.; Mancini, R.; Paggi, M.G. Drug Repurposing against COVID-19: Focus on Anticancer Agents. *J. Exp. Clin. Cancer Res.* **2020**, *39*. [CrossRef] [PubMed]
62. Vatansev, H.; Kadiyoran, C.; Cumhur Cure, M.; Cure, E. COVID-19 Infection Can Cause Chemotherapy Resistance Development in Patients with Breast Cancer and Tamoxifen May Cause Susceptibility to COVID-19 Infection. *Med. Hypotheses* **2020**, *143*, 110091. [CrossRef] [PubMed]
63. Stelzig, K.E.; Canepa-Escaro, F.; Schiliro, M.; Berdnikovs, S.; Prakash, Y.S.; Chiarella, S.E. Estrogen Regulates the Expression of SARS-CoV-2 Receptor ACE2 in Differentiated Airway Epithelial Cells. *Am. J. Physiol. Lung Cell. Mol. Physiol.* **2020**, *318*, L1280–L1281. [CrossRef]
64. Vaduganathan, M.; Vardeny, O.; Michel, T.; McMurray, J.J.V.; Pfeffer, M.A.; Solomon, S.D. Renin-Angiotensin-Aldosterone System Inhibitors in Patients with Covid-19. *N. Engl. J. Med.* **2020**, *382*, 1653–1659. [CrossRef]
65. South, A.M.; Tomlinson, L.; Edmonston, D.; Hiremath, S.; Sparks, M.A. Controversies of Renin-Angiotensin System Inhibition during the COVID-19 Pandemic. *Nat. Rev. Nephrol.* **2020**, *16*, 305–307. [CrossRef]
66. Mehta, P.; McAuley, D.F.; Brown, M.; Sanchez, E.; Tattersall, R.S.; Manson, J.J. COVID-19: Consider Cytokine Storm Syndromes and Immunosuppression. *Lancet* **2020**, *395*, 1033–1034. [CrossRef]
67. Lin, S.; Zhao, Y.; Zhou, D.; Zhou, F.; Xu, F. Coronavirus Disease 2019 (COVID-19): Cytokine Storms, Hyper-Inflammatory Phenotypes, and Acute Respiratory Distress Syndrome. *Genes Dis.* **2020**, *7*, 520–527. [CrossRef]
68. Yazgan, B.; Yazgan, Y.; Ovey, I.S.; Naziroglu, M. Raloxifene and Tamoxifen Reduce PARP Activity, Cytokine and Oxidative Stress Levels in the Brain and Blood of Ovariectomized Rats. *J. Mol. Neurosci.* **2016**, *60*, 214–222. [CrossRef]
69. Dayan, M.; Zinger, H.; Kalush, F.; Mor, G.; Amir-Zaltzman, Y.; Kohen, F.; Sthoeger, Z.; Mozes, E. The Beneficial Effects of Treatment with Tamoxifen and Anti-Oestradiol Antibody on Experimental Systemic Lupus Erythematosus Are Associated with Cytokine Modulations. *Immunology* **1997**, *90*, 101–108. [CrossRef] [PubMed]
70. Tsuchiya, S.; Yamabe, M.; Yamaguchi, Y.; Kobayashi, Y.; Konno, T.; Tada, K. Establishment and Characterization of a Human Acute Monocytic Leukemia Cell Line (THP-1). *Int. J. Cancer* **1980**, *26*, 171–176. [CrossRef] [PubMed]
71. Wiersinga, W.J.; Rhodes, A.; Cheng, A.C.; Peacock, S.J.; Prescott, H.C. Pathophysiology, Transmission, Diagnosis, and Treatment of Coronavirus Disease 2019 (COVID-19): A Review. *JAMA* **2020**, *324*, 782. [CrossRef] [PubMed]

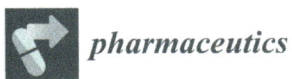

Article

Combination Therapy with Fluoxetine and the Nucleoside Analog GS-441524 Exerts Synergistic Antiviral Effects against Different SARS-CoV-2 Variants In Vitro

Linda Brunotte [1], Shuyu Zheng [2], Angeles Mecate-Zambrano [1], Jing Tang [2], Stephan Ludwig [1], Ursula Rescher [3] and Sebastian Schloer [3,*]

[1] Institute of Virology, Center for Molecular Biology of Inflammation, and "Cells in Motion" Interfaculty Centre, University of Muenster, Von-Esmarch-Str. 56, D-48149 Muenster, Germany; brunotte@uni-muenster.de (L.B.); a_meca01@uni-muenster.de (A.M.-Z.); ludwigs@uni-muenster.de (S.L.)
[2] Research Program in Systems Oncology, Faculty of Medicine, University of Helsinki, Haartmaninkatu 8, 00029 Helsinki, Finland; shuyu.zheng@helsinki.fi (S.Z.); jing.tang@helsinki.fi (J.T.)
[3] Institut-Associated Research Group Regulatory Mechanisms of Inflammation, Institute of Medical Biochemistry, Center for Molecular Biology of Inflammation, and "Cells in Motion" Interfaculty Centre, University of Muenster, Von-Esmarch-Str. 56, D-48149 Muenster, Germany; rescher@uni-muenster.de
* Correspondence: sebastianmaximilian.schloer@ukmuenster.de; Tel.: +49-2518352113; Fax: +49-2518356748

Abstract: The ongoing SARS-CoV-2 pandemic requires efficient and safe antiviral treatment strategies. Drug repurposing represents a fast and low-cost approach to the development of new medical treatment options. The direct antiviral agent remdesivir has been reported to exert antiviral activity against SARS-CoV-2. Whereas remdesivir only has a very short half-life time and a bioactivation, which relies on pro-drug activating enzymes, its plasma metabolite GS-441524 can be activated through various kinases including the adenosine kinase (ADK) that is moderately expressed in all tissues. The pharmacokinetics of GS-441524 argue for a suitable antiviral drug that can be given to patients with COVID-19. Here, we analyzed the antiviral property of a combined treatment with the remdesivir metabolite GS-441524 and the antidepressant fluoxetine in a polarized Calu-3 cell culture model against SARS-CoV-2. The combined treatment with GS-441524 and fluoxetine were well-tolerated and displayed synergistic antiviral effects against three circulating SARS-CoV-2 variants in vitro in the commonly used reference models for drug interaction. Thus, combinatory treatment with the virus-targeting GS-441524 and the host-directed drug fluoxetine might offer a suitable therapeutic treatment option for SARS-CoV-2 infections.

Keywords: combination therapy; SARS-CoV-2; nucleoside GS-441524; fluoxetine; synergy

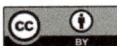

1. Introduction

The Coronavirus Disease 2019 (COVID-19) caused by the Severe Acute Respiratory Syndrome Related Coronavirus 2 (SARS-CoV-2) has resulted in over 2 million deaths within one year and demonstrates the risk of newly emerged pathogens [1,2].

In contrast to other human circulating coronaviruses, SARS-CoV-2 leads to a severe disease with multiple organ failures, especially in elderly patients and those with chronic medical conditions [3–5]. Although vaccines are available, their production, distribution and vaccine hesitancy are critical limiting factors in healthcare. Thus, additional therapeutic strategies to combat the SARS-CoV-2 infection are needed. However, the development and production of new antiviral drugs is a time-consuming process that can be accelerated by the repurposing of already clinically licensed drugs [6,7].

One of the repurposed FDA-approved drugs that has received considerable attention as an antiviral agent against SARS-CoV-2 is remdesivir, a nucleotide monophosphate analogue of adenosine monophosphate (AMP) that interferes with the viral RNA-dependent RNA polymerase [8,9]. Remdesivir was originally developed by Gilead for the treatment of Ebola [10], and is shown to have strong therapeutic efficacy in in vivo models of coronaviruses (MERS-CoV, SARS-CoV, SARS-CoV-2) in mice and primates [11–13]. However, it has a very limited half-life time in the plasma of patients [14–16]. Remdesivir is converted into its predominant serum metabolite GS-441524, which maintains the antiviral properties [12,15–18]. A study conducted in rhesus macaques infected with SARS-CoV-2 treated with remdesivir revealed 1000-fold higher GS-441524 serum levels than those of remdesivir [16]. The benefit of GS-441524 over remdesivir is the lower molecular weight and hydrophilicity, which makes it easier to produce an aerosolized formulation for inhalable therapeutic treatment. An inhalable formulation would allow a high concentration of the drug in lung cells and minimized systemic toxicity [17]. Hence, GS-441524 has a higher potential to be used for antiviral treatments of respiratory pathogens like SARS-CoV-2.

While the majority of antiviral drugs such as remdesivir or GS-441524 are directly targeting viral proteins and are quite efficient to eliminate the pathogen, they pose the risk of emerging viral resistance [19–21]. Thus, combination therapies that include virus- and host-directed drugs are considered to cause less resistance. We recently reported the importance of the endosomal lipid balance for the entry process of enveloped viruses like SARS-CoV-2. The clinically licensed antidepressant fluoxetine, a drug belonging to the class of functional inhibitors of acid sphingomyelinase (FIASMA), blocks the sphingomyelin converting acid sphingomyelinase (ASMase) within the late endosomal/lysosomal (LEL) compartments [22]. The inhibitory effects of fluoxetine relies on its ability to interfere with the endosomal lipid balance, preventing the entry of SARS-CoV-2 [23].

Here, we evaluated the antiviral potential of GS-441524 in a polarized Calu-3 cell culture model when administered alone or in combination with the host-directed drug fluoxetine. The drug combination of fluoxetine and GS-441524 showed stronger antiviral activities against three different SARS-CoV-2 variants compared to the monotherapies. Notably, both drugs act synergistic, as calculated with the commonly used reference models for drug interaction studies.

2. Materials and Methods

2.1. Cells and Compounds

The human bronchial epithelial cell line Calu-3 and the Vero E6 cells derived from the kidney of an African green monkey were cultivated in Dulbecco's modified Eagle's medium (DMEM, Sigma-Aldrich, Darmstadt, Germany) with a 10% standardized fetal bovine serum (FBS Advance; Capricorn, Ebsdorfergrund, Germany), 2 mM L-glutamine, 100 U/mL penicillin, 0.1 mg/mL streptomycin, and 1% non-essential amino acids (Merck, Darmstadt, Germany) in a humidified incubator at 5% CO_2 and 37 °C. Calu-3 monolayers were polarized and cultured as described [24]. Fluoxetine (5 mM, Sigma-Aldrich, Darmstadt, Germany) and GS-441524 (100 mM, Biomol, Hamburg, Germany) were solubilized in DMSO.

2.2. Cytotoxicity Assay

Calu-3 cells were cultured at the indicated concentrations with either the solvent DMSO, GS-441524, fluoxetine or with the combinations of fluoxetine/GS-441524 for 48 h. To estimate cytotoxic effects, a staurosporine solution (1 µM) was used as a positive control. The cell viability was evaluated by adding MTT 3-(4,5-dimethylthiazol-2-yl)-2,5-diphenyltetrazolium bromide (Sigma-Aldrich, Darmstadt, Germany) to the cells for 4 h and OD_{562} measurements according to the manufacturer's protocols (Sigma-Aldrich, Darmstadt, Germany).

2.3. Virus Infection and Drug Treatment

The Muenster SARS-CoV-2 isolate hCoV-19/Germany/FI1103201/2020 (EPI-ISL_463008, mutation D614G in spike protein), and the two newly emerged variants B1.1.7 UK VOC (alpha) and B1.351 SA VOV (beta) were amplified on Vero E6 cells (passage 1) and used for the infection assays. Polarized Calu-3 cells were washed once with PBS and inoculated with the virus diluted in infection-PBS (containing 0.2% BSA, 1% CaCl$_2$, 1% MgCl$_2$, 100 U/mL penicillin and 0.1 mg/mL streptomycin) at a multiplicity of infection (MOI) of 0.1 at 37 °C for 1 h. Following infection, cells were washed with PBS and cultured in infection-DMEM (serum-free DMEM containing 0.2% BSA, 1 mM MgCl$_2$, 0.9 mM CaCl$_2$, 100 U/mL penicillin, and 0.1 mg/mL streptomycin) at 5% CO$_2$ and 37 °C. Calu-3 cells were then treated with the solvent DMSO or the indicated GS-441524 or fluoxetine concentration at 2 h post-infection (hpi) for the entire 48 h infection period. Afterwards, the apical culture supernatants were collected and immediately frozen at -80 °C to determine the number of infectious particles.

2.4. Plaque Assay

The number of infectious particles in the supernatant of treated cells were governed via a standard plaque assay. Briefly, monolayers of Vero E6 cells cultured in six-well dishes were washed with PBS and infected with serial dilutions of the respective supernatants in infection-PBS for 1 h at 37 °C. Subsequently, the inoculum was replaced with 2x MEM (MEM containing 0.2% BSA, 2 mM L-glutamine 1 M HEPES, pH 7.2, 7.5% NaHCO$_3$, 100 U/mL penicillin, 0.1 mg/mL streptomycin, and 0.4% Oxoid agar) and incubated at 37 °C for 72 h. A neutral red staining was performed to visualize virus plaques, and virus titers were calculated and expressed as plaque-forming units (PFU) per mL.

2.5. Data and Statistical Analysis

The required sample sizes (to detect a > 90% reduction in virus titers at a power > 0.8) were determined by using the a priori power analysis G*Power 3.1 (Faul et al., 2007). Data were analyzed using the software GraphPad Prism version 8.00 (GraphPad).

To define dose–response curves, virus titers were normalized to the percentages of titers detected in cells treated with the solvent DMSO (control), and drug concentrations were log-transformed. EC values were calculated from the sigmoidal curve fits using a four-parameter logistic (4PL) model. The combinatory effects of the drug pair fluoxetine/GS-441524 were analyzed by using SynergyFinder, an open-source, free, standalone web application for the analysis of drug combination data [25]. The synergy was evaluated based on the Zero Interaction Potency (ZIP), Bliss independence, and highest single agent (HSA) reference models. Additionally, we analyzed the overall drug combination sensitivity score (CSS) by using the CSS method [26]. For statistical analysis of cytotoxicity assays, values were normalized to the percentages of toxicity detected in the control cells (cells treated with the solvent DMSO); significant differences were evaluated using a one-way ANOVA followed by Dunnett's multiple comparison test. ** $p < 0.01$, *** $p < 0.001$, **** $p \leq 0.0001$.

3. Results

We have recently reported that the clinically used antidepressant fluoxetine in combination with the viral RNA-dependent RNA polymerase inhibitor remdesivir exhibits synergistic antiviral effects against the SARS-CoV-2 infection in vitro [27]. A major drawback for the in vivo use of the prodrug remdesivir is the very short plasma half-life time of approximately 20 min [17]. Remdesivir is converted into its main plasma metabolite GS-441524 when administered to patients [14,17]. Thus, we wanted to assess the antiviral potential of GS-441524 in a polarized Calu-3 cell culture model. We infected Calu-3 cells with the isolate hCoV-19/Germany/FI1103201/2020 at MOI 0.1 for 48 h and quantified the production of infectious SARS-CoV-2 particles by a plaque assay. Control Calu-3 cells that were treated with the solvent DMSO yielded viral titers up to 2×10^6 PFU, whereas treatment with the nucleoside GS-441524 2hpi significantly inhibited the production of the circulating SARS-CoV-2 variant in a dose-depended manner (Figure 1). Fitting of the experimental dose–response values to a nonlinear four-parameter logistic model resulted in a half-maximal inhibitory (EC$_{50}$) and 90% inhibitory concentrations (EC$_{90}$) of 0.28 µM and 1.33 µM, respectively, for the Muenster Isolate (Figure 1). Validation of Calu-3 cell viability after administration of GS-441524 via an MTT assay revealed that only a very high concentration of GS-441524 resulted in detectable cytotoxicity, whereas all concentrations further used in the pharmacological interaction studies had no influence on the cell viability (Figure S1a, Supplementary Material). The calculated 50% cytotoxic concentration (CC_{50}) of the remdesivir metabolite is 47.66 µM with a selectivity index (SI) of 170.21, which emphasizes a safe antiviral treatment window.

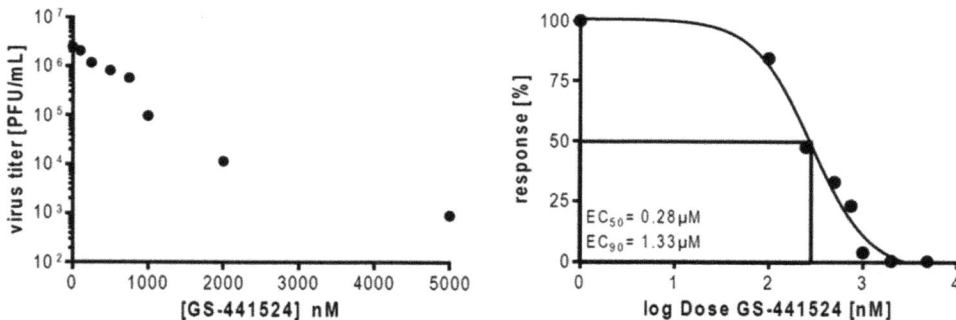

Figure 1. Analysis of GS-441524-mediated reduction of infectious SARS-CoV-2 particle production. Polarized Calu-3 cells were infected with 0.1 MOI of SARS-CoV-2 (hCoV-19/Germany/FI1103201/2020) for 48 h. At 2 hpi, cells were treated with GS-441524 at the indicated concentrations. Data were expressed as mean infectious viral titers ± SEM or as mean percent inhibition ± SEM of SARS-CoV-2 replication (control cells that were treated with the solvent DMSO were set to 100%), $n = 5$. $LogEC_{50}$ and $LogEC_{90}$ values were determined by fitting a four-parameter non-linear regression model.

We next addressed whether a combinatory treatment with the drug pair fluoxetine-GS-441524 had a synergistic interaction to limit the SARS-CoV-2 infection. For studying the antiviral properties of the drug combinations, we used, for both drugs, concentrations that were previously reported to have an individual antiviral activity below 90%, whereas their combination was able to achieve a more than 90% reduction in viral titers [27]. The highest single dose of GS-441524 (1000 nM) was able to achieve 95% inhibition on viral titers, whereas treatment with the highest single dose of fluoxetine reduced viral titers up to 75% (Figure 2).

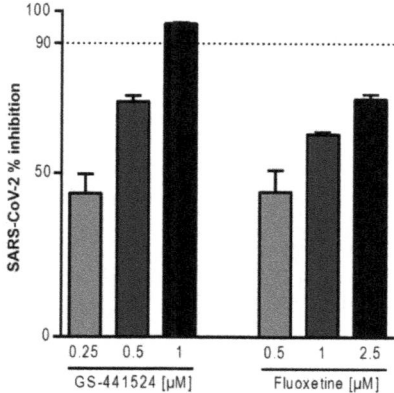

Figure 2. Antiviral activities of a single treatment against SARS-CoV-2. Polarized Calu-3 cells were infected with SARS-CoV-2 and treated with the indicated GS-441524 or fluoxetine concentrations for 48 h. Bars represent mean percent inhibition ± SEM of infectious virus production, with mean virus titer produced in control cells (treated with the solvent DMSO) set to 100%; $n = 5$. Dotted line, 90% reduction in viral titer.

Next, we determined the number of infectious virus particles in Calu-3 cells that were treated with a combination of both drugs. On the basis of our recent publications [27] on the antiviral potential of fluoxetine alone or in combination with remdesivir, we now analyzed the antiviral effects of a combined fluoxetine/GS-441524 treatment (Figure 3A,B). We observed a noticeable increase in the pharmacological inhibition of infectious virus production (>90%) when cells were treated with a concentration of 500 nM GS-441524 and 1000 nM fluoxetine or higher doses of the drug pair (Figure 3A,B), thus showing the great potential of a combination treatment of the remdesivir metabolite GS-441524 with fluoxetine. Additionally, we assessed the cytotoxic effects of the combinatory treatments via an MTT assay to exclude the potential synergistic toxicity of the drug pair. The MTT assay is based on the reduction in 3-(4,5-dimethylthiazol-2-yl)-2,5-diphenyltetrazolium bromide to formazan crystals by NAD(P)H-dependent oxidoreductase enzymes in metabolically active cells, this colorimetric assay measures the metabolic activity as an integrated indicator of changes in the cell viability, cytotoxicity, and proliferation. As the analysis of the combination treatments with fluoxetine and GS-441524 did not reveal any toxicities (Figure S1b), we continued to analyze the drug synergy without the subtraction of cytotoxicity.

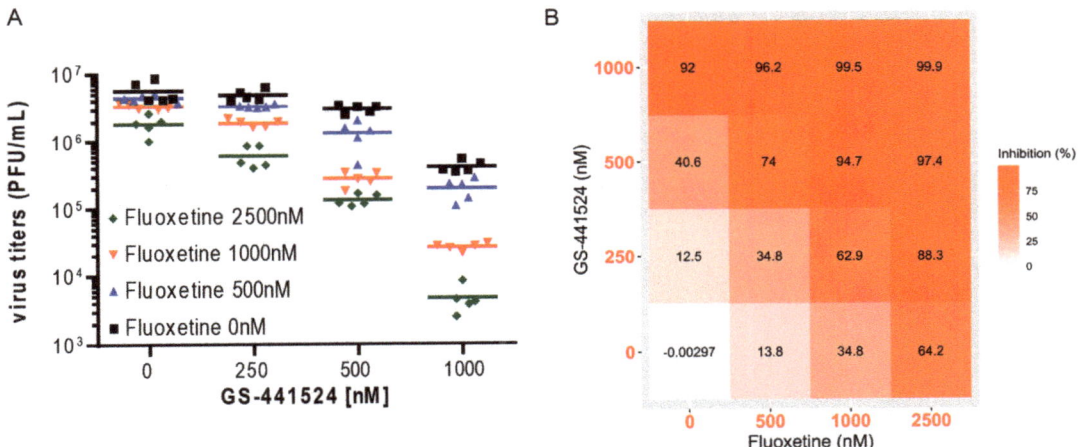

Figure 3. Antiviral activities of combination treatment with fluoxetine and GS-441524. Polarized Calu-3 cells were infected with SARS-CoV-2 and treated with the indicated drug combinations for 48 h. (**A**) Data were expressed as plaque-forming units (PFU) per mL detected in a single experimental sample, lines indicate means; $n = 5$/treatment or as (**B**) percent pharmacological inhibition of infectious virus production for the drug pair fluoxetine and GS-441524 (with mean virus titer produced in control cells (treated with the solvent DMSO) set to 100%).

Although drug synergy is not necessarily required for clinical benefits, synergy scoring remains an important parameter for the evaluation of drug combination therapies. Thus, we next evaluated the drug interaction profile of fluoxetine and GS-441524 by using three commonly used reference synergy models: ZIP, Bliss independence and highest single agent (HSA). Even though these different reference synergy models analyzed the drug interactions based on different basic interaction assumptions, they emphasized a synergistic action of GS-441524 and fluoxetine (Figure 4). The drug interaction relationships and landscape visualizations revealed in all models, a high synergy score when cells were treated with a combination of 500–1000 nM GS-441524 and ~1000 nM fluoxetine. The strong synergy of the combinatory treatment with both drugs led to an overall drug combination sensitivity score (CSS) of 92.42.

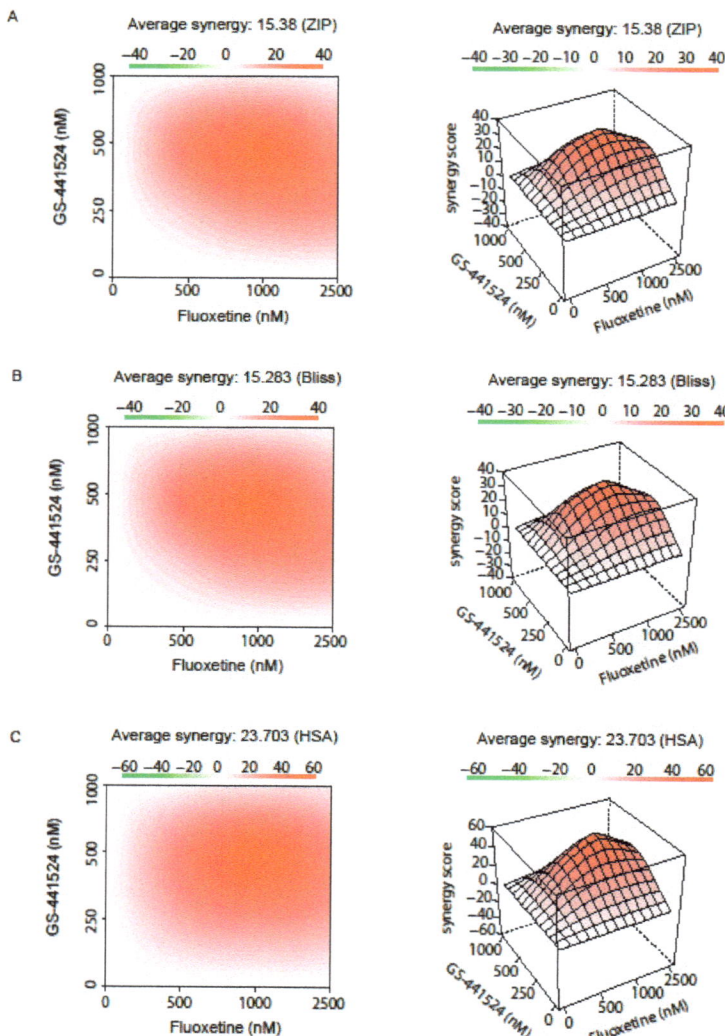

Figure 4. Pharmacological interaction profile of the drug pair GS-441524 and fluoxetine. Drug interactions were analyzed based on the three commonly used reference models: (**A**) Zero Interaction Potency (ZIP), (**B**) Bliss independence, and (**C**) highest single agent (HSA). While the HSA model assumes a synergistic drug combination that produce additional benefits on top of what the drugs can achieve alone, the Bliss independence model uses probabilistic theory to model the effects of individual drugs in a combination as independent yet competing events. Synergy calculations via the ZIP model includes the comparison of potency changes of the dose–response curves between individual drugs and their combinations. A color-coded interaction surface was used to illustrate the synergy scores of the responses, where high synergistic scores are colored in red. Synergy score calculations via the ZIP and Bliss independence model revealed a synergy of ~ 15, while the HSA model showed a higher synergy score of ~23.

We further assessed the antiviral capacity of the combination therapy with GS-441524 and fluoxetine against the SARS-CoV-2 alpha and beta variants of concern (VOC). Both strains have mutations in the spike protein's receptor binding domain (for example, 501Y, a change from asparagine (N) to tyrosine (Y) in amino-acid position 501), which impair angiotensin-converting enzyme 2 (ACE2) binding specificity and lead to an increased transmissibility [28–31]. At least for the beta variant, changes in the spike protein's receptor-binding domain enables a partial immune escape from neutralization induced by vaccination or previous virus infection and is therefore considered to be of concern [28]. Importantly, the combination of GS-441524 and fluoxetine potently reduced viral titers of both VOCs synergistically when compared to monotherapy (Figure 5). While the monotherapy reduced viral titers between 60 to 70% for fluoxetine or up to 90% when treated with GS-441524, the combination of both drugs resulted in a viral inhibition above 99% (Figure 5). Thus, the combination of the host-directed fluoxetine and the virus-targeting GS-441524 showed great antiviral potential against SARS-CoV-2 variants that have significant changes in the spike protein's receptor-binding domain.

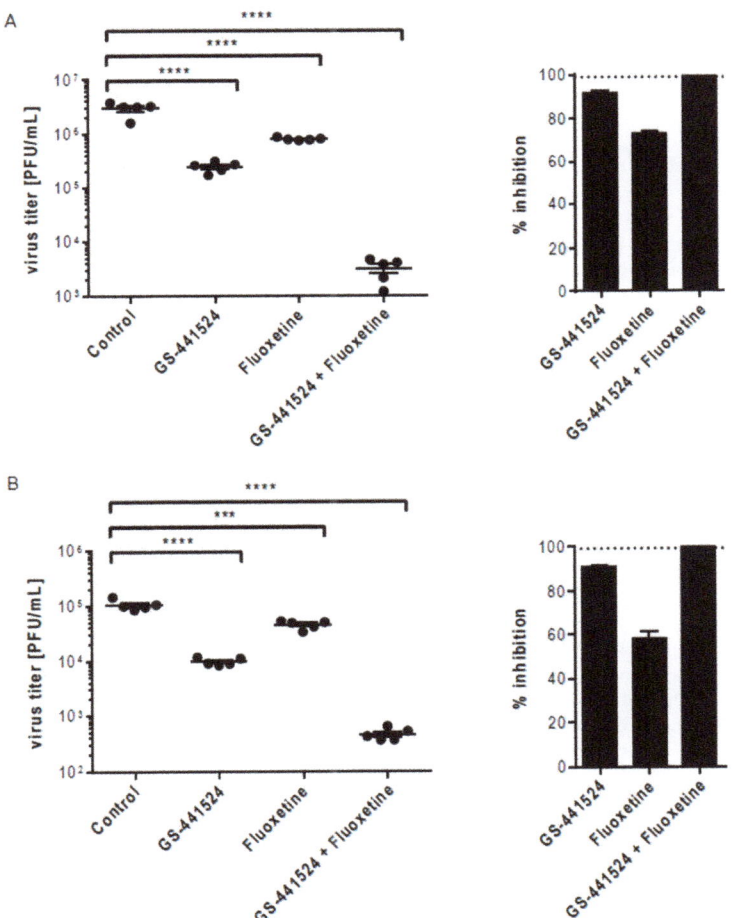

Figure 5. Antiviral effect of the combination therapy with GS-441524 and fluoxetine against two newly emerged SARS-CoV-2 variants. Polarized Calu-3 cells were infected with the (**A**) alpha or (**B**) beta variant of SARS-CoV-2 and treated with 2.5 µM fluoxetine, 1 µM GS-441524 or the combination of both drugs for 48 h. (**A**) Data were expressed as plaque-forming units (PFU) per mL detected in a single experimental sample, lines indicate means; $n = 5$/treatment or as (**B**) percent pharmacological inhibition of infectious virus production for the drug pair fluoxetine and GS-441524 (with mean virus titer produced in control cells (treated with the solvent DMSO) set to 100%, $n = 5$. Dotted line, 99% reduction in viral titer. One-way ANOVA followed by Dunnett's multiple comparison test. *** $p \leq 0.001$, **** $p \leq 0.0001$.

4. Discussion

Emerging zoonotic diseases such as the current SARS-CoV-2 pandemic are global threats to humans and the health care systems. SARS-CoV-2, which causes COVID-19, has already led to more than 2 million deaths within one year. Thus, vaccines and antivirals are urgently needed to decelerate the global spreading and community transmission of SARS-CoV-2. Antiviral therapy often includes a combination of several drugs, each targeting different steps in the virus life-cycle to circumvent the emergence of drug resistance. The benefit of antiviral combinations has been reported in a large number of studies [32–35]. The most significant and latest successes of antiviral combination therapy was achieved in the fight against HIV-1 or HCV, where drugs that interfere with the virus entry and replication were used [36–38]. While host-directed drugs mostly impair the viral replication without a complete eradication of the pathogen, antivirals that directly target viral proteins are much more efficient in eradicating viruses. However, a major concern of direct antiviral therapy is the risk to induce new resistant virus strains [39], an adaptive step that was already observed in the antiviral therapy against influenza or HIV [40,41]. The combination of antivirals with host-directed drugs makes it much more unlikely that a virus can overcome the antiviral barrier and emerge resistances. Thus, the combination of both is routinely explored for enhanced treatment success [42–44].

One critical step in the life cycle of enveloped viruses such as SARS-CoV-2 is the entry into the host cell. SARS-CoV-2, similar to other enveloped viruses, needs to overcome the host cell membrane for transferring the viral genome into the cytosol, a step that is limited by the fusion of viral and cellular membranes [23,45]. SARS-CoV-2 binds via its spike protein, a viral envelope protein, to the host cell receptor ACE2 [46–48]. Attachment of virus particles facilitate a priming of the spike protein via proteolytic cleavage, which is mediated by several host proteases and a prerequisite for membrane fusion. Cleavage by the cellular transmembrane protease serine 2 (TMPRSS2) triggers the fusion with the plasma membrane, whereas other endosome-residing proteases are required for the fusion of endocytosed SARS-CoV-2 particles with endosomes [23,45]. Thus, the endosomal compartment is a critical host/pathogen interface for SARS-CoV-2 [23]. The antiviral mode of action of fluoxetine is most likely based on its inhibitory effect on the endolysosome-residing enzyme sphingomyelin phosphodiesterase ("acid sphingomyelinase", ASM). The blocking of ASM activity results in sphingomyelin accumulation, which negatively affects cholesterol release from the endolysosomal compartment, causing the favored antiviral barrier [22,23].

In our recent study [27], we showed that the combination of the host-directed drug fluoxetine and the viral RNA-dependent RNA-polymerase inhibitor remdesivir results in a synergistic antiviral effect on the production of infectious virus particles. Remdesivir was originally developed for the treatment of Ebola [18], but exerts antiviral activity against a number of other viruses, including Ebolavirus, Marburg virus, MERS-CoV and also SARS-CoV-2 [9,11,15,18,49]. Remdesivir was the first drug that received an FDA emergency use authorization for severe COVID-19 treatment. Since remdesivir has a very short half-life time in the plasma of patients (approximately 20 min) and, moreover, requires activation through pro-drug enzymes (such as carboxylesterases (CES1), cathepsin A (CTSA) and histidinetriad nucleotide binding proteins (HINT)) which are preferentially expressed in the liver [17,50–53], it is unsuitable for a lung-specific delivery and its clinical use remains controversial [17]. Structural similarity studies between the main remdesivir metabolite GS-441524 and human enzymes suggest that the bioactivation of GS-441524 relies on adenosine kinase (ADK) [17]. ADK is moderately expressed across all tissues and, thus, the administration of GS-441524 would be more eligible for systemic and lung-specific delivery. GS-441524 has been reported to potently inhibit SARS-CoV-2 replication in vitro and in a mouse model of SARS-CoV-2 infection and pathogenesis [11,12], implying this metabolite as a promising drug candidate for further evaluation. The favorable safety profile of GS-441524 (shown by the better SI values [10,54] and by animal models [55,56]) suggests an increased therapy window, which allows for a higher dosing of GS-441524 compared to remdesivir without causing adverse side effects.

Our data are consistent with recent studies demonstrating that the monotherapy of the remdesivir metabolite GS-441524 elucidated similar EC_{50} and EC_{90} values similar to remdesivir in polarized Calu-3 cells (GS-441524; EC_{50} = 0.28 µM and EC_{90} = 1.33 µM; remdesivir: EC_{50} = 0.28 µM, EC_{90} = 2.48 µM, ref. [11]).

We further evaluated the overall antiviral effect of the combination GS441524 and fluoxetine, which was larger than the expected sum of the independent drug effects, showing a synergistic effect against three circulating SARS-CoV-2 variants (Figures 4 and 5). Treatment of GS-441524 in combination with fluoxetine indicates a comparable synergistic activity to the recent published combination of fluoxetine and remdesivir [27]. Both combination treatments lead to an average synergy score of ~15 (in the ZIP or Bliss independence reference model) or of ~23 in the HSA reference model with a high synergy score when cells were treated with a combination of 500–1000 nM GS-441524 or remdesivir and 1000–2500 nM fluoxetine [27]. Of note, no cytotoxic effects were observed when the cells were treated with the combination of both drugs. For successful monotherapy of the individual drugs, high drug doses are required, and a prolonged treatment is often associated with poor patient compliance. The synergistic action of fluoxetine and GS-441524 offers the administration of lower concentrations of the individual drugs, which can reduce potential side effects.

The transfer of in vitro data to the in vivo situation is critical in antiviral research. Thus, we compared the concentrations shown to be effective in our in vitro study with reachable plasma concentrations in patients when drugs were administered. The nucleoside analog GS-441524 can reach plasma concentrations up to 1000-fold higher than remdesivir (maximum plasma levels 3 mg/L directly after intravenous infusion and 80–170 µg/L after 1 h when given intravenously) [14], whereas orally administered fluoxetine (20 mg/day) has a high bioavailability with plasma levels of 350 µg/L after two weeks and up to 1055 µg/L for longer treatment periods in patients [57,58]. For both drugs, plasma concentrations are well within the ranges that equal effective drug concentrations in vitro.

Our results demonstrate a strain-independent potential therapeutic capacity of combined treatment with the direct antiviral acting nucleoside analog GS-441524 and the host-directed drug fluoxetine to combat the SARS-CoV-2 infection and limit deleterious COVID-19 outcomes. At least mutations occurring in the spike protein's receptor binding domain had no influence on the antiviral efficacy of the combination or monotherapies with GS-441524 and/or fluoxetine (Figure 5) [28–31]. The eligibility of combining host-directed drugs with antivirals in SARS-CoV-2 therapy was recently confirmed in a double-blind, randomized, placebo-controlled trial where combination therapy with remdesivir and the host-directed Janus kinase inhibitor baricitinib was beneficial in the treatment of hospitalized COVID-19 patients [59,60].

However, combined medications pose the risk of drug–drug interactions which may lead to a reduced therapeutic benefit or even severe adverse effects. Thus, it is indispensable to survey the drug interactions and to carefully evaluate the appropriate treatment strategy against SARS-CoV-2. While clinical data from healthy donors showed that remdesivir and its metabolite GS-4412524 are metabolized through Cytochromes P450 (CYPs) enzymes (CYP2C8, CYP2D6, and CYP3A4), clinical studies that examined drug–drug interactions were not yet complete, although the mathematical prediction of DDI liability suggested that remdesivir and GS-441524 might elevate the levels of co-prescribed drugs that depend on these CYP enzymes [61–63]. However, the influence of remdesivir on CYP-enzyme dependent metabolism is suggested to be weak [61,63]. Thus, simultaneous administration with fluoxetine, another known inhibitor of CYPs (CYP2D6 and CYP2C9/10) should be carefully monitored [64–66]. As fluoxetine is also a serotonin-reuptake inhibitor (SRI), simultaneous administration with other SRIs should also be avoided (including amphetamines and other sympathomimetic appetite suppressants) [67,68]. For further information about possible drug–drug interaction, visit Drugs.com (accessed on 18 February 2021) [69]. Since fluoxetine can exert, in some patients, serious side effects, we do not recommended self-medication. The careful administration of drugs should exclusively rely on medical advice.

Supplementary Materials: The following are available online at https://www.mdpi.com/article/10.3390/pharmaceutics13091400/s1, Figure S1: Analysis of the cytotoxicity of GS-441524 monotherapy and of the combinatory treatment with fluoxetine.

Author Contributions: Conceptualization and methodology, S.S.; validation, formal analysis, investigation, and data curation, L.B., A.M.-Z., S.S. and S.Z.; resources, L.B., S.S., J.T., S.L. and U.R.; writing—original draft preparation, S.S.; writing—review and editing, S.S., L.B., S.L., J.T. and U.R.; visualization, L.B., S.Z. and S.S.; supervision, U.R., S.L., J.T. and S.S., project administration, S.S.; funding acquisition, S.S., L.B., U.R., J.T. and S.L. All authors have read and agreed to the published version of the manuscript.

Funding: This research was funded by grants from the German Research Foundation (DFG), CRC1009 "Breaking Barriers", Project A06 (to U.R.) and B02 (to S.L.), CRC 1348 "Dynamic Cellular Interfaces", Project A11 (to U.R.), DFG Lu477/23-1 (to S.L.), KFO342 TP6, Br5189/3-1 (to L.B.), Lu477/30-1 (to S.L.), the European Research Council No. 716063 (to S.Z. and J.T.), the Academy of Finland No. 317680 (to S.Z. and J.T.), the Interdisciplinary Center for Clinical Research (IZKF) of the Münster Medical School, grant number Re2/022/20 (to U.R.), Bru2/015/19 (to L.B.), the Innovative Medizinische Forschung (IMF) of the Münster Medical School, grant number SC121912 (to S.S.) and from BR111502(to L.B.). Further funding was provided by the German Federal Ministry for Education and Research (BMBF), grant number 01KI20218 (CoIMMUNE) and NUM-COVID-19, Organo-Strat 01KX2021 (to L.B. and S.L.). S.S., S.L. and U.R. are members of the German FluResearchNet, a nationwide research network on zoonotic influenza. S.S. and U.R. are also members of the British Pharmacological Society.

Institutional Review Board Statement: Not applicable.

Informed Consent Statement: Not applicable.

Data Availability Statement: The data presented in this study are available on request from the corresponding author. The data are not publicly available due to privacy or ethical restrictions.

Acknowledgments: We thank Jonathan Hentrey for help with the cell culture. We acknowledge support from the Open Access Publication fund at the University of Muenster.

Conflicts of Interest: The authors declare no conflict of interest. The funders had no role in the design of the study; in the collection, analyses, or interpretation of data; in the writing of the manuscript, or in the decision to publish the results.

References

1. Baud, D.; Qi, X.; Nielsen-Saines, K.; Musso, D.; Pomar, L.; Favre, G. Real estimates of mortality following COVID-19 infection. *Lancet Infect. Dis.* **2020**, *20*, 773. [CrossRef]
2. Rajgor, D.D.; Lee, M.H.; Archuleta, S.; Bagdasarian, N.; Quek, S.C. The many estimates of the COVID-19 case fatality rate. *Lancet Infect. Dis.* **2020**, *20*, 776–777. [CrossRef]
3. Corman, V.M.; Lienau, J.; Witzenrath, M. Coronaviruses as the cause of respiratory infections. *Internist* **2019**, *60*, 1136–1145. [CrossRef]
4. Wang, D.; Hu, B.; Hu, C.; Zhu, F.; Liu, X.; Zhang, J.; Wang, B.; Xiang, H.; Cheng, Z.; Xiong, Y.; et al. Clinical Characteristics of 138 Hospitalized Patients with 2019 Novel Coronavirus-Infected Pneumonia in Wuhan, China. *J. Am. Med. Assoc.* **2020**, *323*, 1061–1069. [CrossRef] [PubMed]
5. Tang, N.; Li, D.; Wang, X.; Sun, Z. Abnormal coagulation parameters are associated with poor prognosis in patients with novel coronavirus pneumonia. *J. Thromb. Haemost.* **2020**, *18*, 844–847. [CrossRef] [PubMed]
6. Pushpakom, S.; Iorio, F.; Eyers, P.A.; Escott, K.J.; Hopper, S.; Wells, A.; Doig, A.; Guilliams, T.; Latimer, J.; McNamee, C.; et al. Drug repurposing: Progress, challenges and recommendations. *Nat. Rev. Drug Discov.* **2018**, *18*, 41–58. [CrossRef]
7. Ianevski, A.; Yao, R.; Fenstad, M.H.; Biza, S.; Zusinaite, E.; Reisberg, T.; Lysvand, H.; Løseth, K.; Landsem, V.M.; Malmring, J.F.; et al. Potential antiviral options against SARS-CoV-2 infection. *Viruses* **2020**, *12*, 642. [CrossRef] [PubMed]
8. Gordon, C.J.; Tchesnokov, E.P.; Woolner, E.; Perry, J.K.; Feng, J.Y.; Porter, D.P.; Götte, M. Remdesivir is a direct-acting antiviral that inhibits RNA-dependent RNA polymerase from severe acute respiratory syndrome coronavirus 2 with high potency. *J. Biol. Chem.* **2020**, *295*, 6785–6797. [CrossRef] [PubMed]
9. Agostini, M.L.; Andres, E.L.; Sims, A.C.; Graham, R.L.; Sheahan, T.P.; Lu, X.; Smith, E.C.; Case, J.B.; Feng, J.Y.; Jordan, R.; et al. Coronavirus susceptibility to the antiviral remdesivir (GS-5734) is mediated by the viral polymerase and the proofreading exoribonuclease. *MBio* **2018**, *9*, e00221-18. [CrossRef]

10. Siegel, D.; Hui, H.C.; Doerffler, E.; Clarke, M.O.; Chun, K.; Zhang, L.; Neville, S.; Carra, E.; Lew, W.; Ross, B.; et al. Discovery and Synthesis of a Phosphoramidate Prodrug of a Pyrrolo[2,1-f][triazin-4-amino] Adenine C-Nucleoside (GS-5734) for the Treatment of Ebola and Emerging Viruses. *J. Med. Chem.* **2017**, *60*, 1648–1661. [CrossRef]
11. Pruijssers, A.J.; George, A.S.; Schäfer, A.; Leist, S.R.; Gralinksi, L.E.; Dinnon, K.H.; Yount, B.L.; Agostini, M.L.; Stevens, L.J.; Chappell, J.D.; et al. Remdesivir Inhibits SARS-CoV-2 in Human Lung Cells and Chimeric SARS-CoV Expressing the SARS-CoV-2 RNA Polymerase in Mice. *Cell Rep.* **2020**, *32*, 107940. [CrossRef]
12. Li, Y.; Cao, L.; Li, G.; Cong, F.; Li, Y.; Sun, J.; Luo, Y.; Chen, G.; Li, G.; Wang, P.; et al. Remdesivir Metabolite GS-441524 Effectively Inhibits SARS-CoV-2 Infection in Mice Models. *bioRxiv* **2020**. [CrossRef]
13. Goldman, J.D.; Lye, D.C.B.; Hui, D.S.; Marks, K.M.; Bruno, R.; Montejano, R.; Spinner, C.D.; Galli, M.; Ahn, M.-Y.; Nahass, R.G.; et al. Remdesivir for 5 or 10 Days in Patients with Severe COVID-19. *N. Engl. J. Med.* **2020**, *383*, 1827–1837. [CrossRef]
14. Tempestilli, M.; Caputi, P.; Avataneo, V.; Notari, S.; Forini, O.; Scorzolini, L.; Marchioni, L.; Bartoli, T.A.; Castilletti, C.; Lalle, E.; et al. Pharmacokinetics of remdesivir and GS-441524 in two critically ill patients who recovered from COVID-19. *J. Antimicrob. Chemother.* **2020**, *75*, 2977–2980. [CrossRef] [PubMed]
15. Sheahan, T.P.; Sims, A.C.; Graham, R.L.; Menachery, V.D.; Gralinski, L.E.; Case, J.B.; Leist, S.R.; Pyrc, K.; Feng, J.Y.; Trantcheva, I.; et al. Broad-spectrum antiviral GS-5734 inhibits both epidemic and zoonotic coronaviruses. *Sci. Transl. Med.* **2017**, *9*, eaal3653. [CrossRef] [PubMed]
16. Williamson, B.N.; Feldmann, F.; Schwarz, B.; Meade-White, K.; Porter, D.P.; Schulz, J.; van Doremalen, N.; Leighton, I.; Yinda, C.K.; Pérez-Pérez, L.; et al. Clinical benefit of remdesivir in rhesus macaques infected with SARS-CoV-2. *Nature* **2020**, *585*, 273–276. [CrossRef] [PubMed]
17. Yan, V.C.; Muller, F.L. Advantages of the Parent Nucleoside GS-441524 over Remdesivir for COVID-19 Treatment. *ACS Med. Chem. Lett.* **2020**, *11*, 1361–1366. [CrossRef]
18. Warren, T.K.; Jordan, R.; Lo, M.K.; Ray, A.S.; Mackman, R.L.; Soloveva, V.; Siegel, D.; Perron, M.; Bannister, R.; Hui, H.C.; et al. Therapeutic efficacy of the small molecule GS-5734 against Ebola virus in rhesus monkeys. *Nature* **2016**, *531*, 381–385. [CrossRef]
19. Schwegmann, A.; Brombacher, F. Host-directed drug targeting of factors hijacked by pathogens. *Sci. Signal.* **2008**, *1*, re8. [CrossRef]
20. Zumla, A.; Rao, M.; Wallis, R.S.; Kaufmann, S.H.E.; Rustomjee, R.; Mwaba, P.; Vilaplana, C.; Yeboah-Manu, D.; Chakaya, J.; Ippolito, G.; et al. Host-directed therapies for infectious diseases: Current status, recent progress, and future prospects. *Lancet Infect. Dis.* **2016**, *16*, e47–e63. [CrossRef]
21. Zumla, A.; Hui, D.S.; Azhar, E.I.; Memish, Z.A.; Maeurer, M. Reducing mortality from 2019-nCoV: Host-directed therapies should be an option. *Lancet* **2020**, *395*, e35–e36. [CrossRef]
22. Kornhuber, J.; Tripal, P.; Reichel, M.; Mühle, C.; Rhein, C.; Muehlbacher, M.; Groemer, T.W.; Gulbins, E. Functional Inhibitors of Acid Sphingomyelinase (FIASMAs): A Novel Pharmacological Group of Drugs with Broad Clinical Applications. *Cell. Physiol. Biochem.* **2010**, *25*, 9–20. [CrossRef] [PubMed]
23. Schloer, S.; Brunotte, L.; Goretzko, J.; Mecate-Zambrano, A.; Korthals, N.; Gerke, V.; Ludwig, S.; Rescher, U. Targeting the endolysosomal host-SARS-CoV-2 interface by clinically licensed functional inhibitors of acid sphingomyelinase (FIASMA) including the antidepressant fluoxetine. *Emerg. Microbes Infect.* **2020**, 1–26. [CrossRef]
24. Schloer, S.; Goretzko, J.; Pleschka, S.; Ludwig, S.; Rescher, U. Combinatory Treatment with Oseltamivir and Itraconazole Targeting Both Virus and Host Factors in Influenza A Virus Infection. *Viruses* **2020**, *12*, 703. [CrossRef] [PubMed]
25. Ianevski, A.; He, L.; Aittokallio, T.; Tang, J. SynergyFinder: A web application for analyzing drug combination dose-response matrix data. *Bioinformatics* **2017**, *33*, 2413–2415. [CrossRef]
26. Malyutina, A.; Majumder, M.M.; Wang, W.; Pessia, A.; Heckman, C.A.; Tang, J. Drug combination sensitivity scoring facilitates the discovery of synergistic and efficacious drug combinations in cancer. *PLoS Comput. Biol.* **2019**, *15*, e1006752. [CrossRef]
27. Schloer, S.; Brunotte, L.; Mecate-Zambrano, A.; Zheng, S.; Tang, J.; Ludwig, S.; Rescher, U. Drug synergy of combinatory treatment with remdesivir and the repurposed drugs fluoxetine and itraconazole effectively impairs SARS-CoV-2 infection in vitro. *Br. J. Pharmacol.* **2021**, *178*, 2339–2350. [CrossRef] [PubMed]
28. Yi, C.; Sun, X.; Ye, J.; Ding, L.; Liu, M.; Yang, Z.; Lu, X.; Zhang, Y.; Ma, L.; Gu, W.; et al. Key residues of the receptor binding motif in the spike protein of SARS-CoV-2 that interact with ACE2 and neutralizing antibodies. *Cell. Mol. Immunol.* **2020**, *17*, 621–630. [CrossRef] [PubMed]
29. Davies, N.G.; Jarvis, C.I.; van Zandvoort, K.; Clifford, S.; Sun, F.Y.; Funk, S.; Medley, G.; Jafari, Y.; Meakin, S.R.; Lowe, R.; et al. Increased mortality in community-tested cases of SARS-CoV-2 lineage B.1.1.7. *Nature* **2021**, *593*, 270–274. [CrossRef]
30. Tegally, H.; Wilkinson, E.; Giovanetti, M.; Iranzadeh, A.; Fonseca, V.; Giandhari, J.; Doolabh, D.; Pillay, S.; San, E.J.; Msomi, N.; et al. Emergence and rapid spread of a new severe acute respiratory syndrome-related coronavirus 2 (SARS-CoV-2) lineage with multiple spike mutations in South Africa. *medRxiv* **2020**. [CrossRef]
31. Kirby, T. New variant of SARS-CoV-2 in UK causes surge of COVID-19. *Lancet. Respir. Med.* **2021**, *9*, e20–e21. [CrossRef]
32. Palella, F.J.; Delaney, K.M.; Moorman, A.C.; Loveless, M.O.; Fuhrer, J.; Satten, G.A.; Aschman, D.J.; Holmberg, S.D. Declining Morbidity and Mortality among Patients with Advanced Human Immunodeficiency Virus Infection. *N. Engl. J. Med.* **1998**, *338*, 853–860. [CrossRef]
33. Naggie, S.; Muir, A.J. Oral Combination Therapies for Hepatitis C Virus Infection: Successes, Challenges, and Unmet Needs. *Annu. Rev. Med.* **2017**, *68*, 345–358. [CrossRef] [PubMed]
34. Hayden, F.G. Combination antiviral therapy for respiratory virus infections. *Antiviral Res.* **1996**, *29*, 45–48. [CrossRef]

35. Korba, B.E.; Cote, P.; Hornbuckle, W.; Schinazi, R.; Gerin, J.L.; Tennant, B.C. Enhanced antiviral benefit of combination therapy with lamivudine and famciclovir against WHV replication in chronic WHV carrier woodchucks. *Antiviral Res.* **2000**, *45*, 19–32. [CrossRef]
36. Qian, X.J.; Zhu, Y.Z.; Zhao, P.; Qi, Z.T. Entry inhibitors: New advances in HCV treatment. *Emerg. Microbes Infect.* **2016**, *5*, e3. [CrossRef] [PubMed]
37. Crouchet, E.; Wrensch, F.; Schuster, C.; Zeisel, M.B.; Baumert, T.F. Host-targeting therapies for hepatitis C virus infection: Current developments and future applications. *Therap. Adv. Gastroenterol.* **2018**, *11*, 1–15. [CrossRef] [PubMed]
38. Pirrone, V.; Thakkar, N.; Jacobson, J.M.; Wigdahl, B.; Krebs, F.C. Combinatorial approaches to the prevention and treatment of HIV-1 infection. *Antimicrob. Agents Chemother.* **2011**, *55*, 1831–1842. [CrossRef]
39. Strasfeld, L.; Chou, S. Antiviral drug resistance: Mechanisms and clinical implications. *Infect. Dis. Clin. N. Am.* **2010**, *24*, 809–833. [CrossRef]
40. Kim, S.G.; Hwang, Y.H.; Shin, Y.H.; Kim, S.W.; Jung, W.S.; Kim, S.M.; Oh, J.M.; Lee, N.Y.; Kim, M.J.; Cho, K.S.; et al. Occurrence and characterization of oseltamivir-resistant influenza virus in children between 2007–2008 and 2008–2009 seasons. *Korean J. Pediatr.* **2013**, *56*, 165–175. [CrossRef]
41. Kuritzkes, D.R. Drug resistance in HIV-1. *Curr. Opin. Virol.* **2011**, *1*, 582–589. [CrossRef]
42. Kiso, M.; Yamayoshi, S.; Kawaoka, Y. Triple combination therapy of favipiravir plus two monoclonal antibodies eradicates influenza virus from nude mice. *Commun. Biol.* **2020**, *3*, 1–7. [CrossRef] [PubMed]
43. Zumla, A.; Memish, Z.A.; Maeurer, M.; Bates, M.; Mwaba, P.; Al-Tawfiq, J.A.; Denning, D.W.; Hayden, F.G.; Hui, D.S. Emerging novel and antimicrobial-resistant respiratory tract infections: New drug development and therapeutic options. *Lancet Infect. Dis.* **2014**, *14*, 1136–1149. [CrossRef]
44. Mhamdi, Z.; Fausther-Bovendo, H.; Uyar, O.; Carbonneau, J.; Venable, M.-C.; Abed, Y.; Kobinger, G.; Boivin, G.; Baz, M. Effects of Different Drug Combinations in Immunodeficient Mice Infected with an Influenza A/H3N2 Virus. *Microorganisms* **2020**, *8*, 1968. [CrossRef]
45. Hoffmann, M.; Kleine-Weber, H.; Schroeder, S.; Krüger, N.; Herrler, T.; Erichsen, S.; Schiergens, T.S.; Herrler, G.; Wu, N.H.; Nitsche, A.; et al. SARS-CoV-2 Cell Entry Depends on ACE2 and TMPRSS2 and Is Blocked by a Clinically Proven Protease Inhibitor. *Cell* **2020**, *181*, 271–280.e8. [CrossRef] [PubMed]
46. Li, W.; Moore, M.J.; Vasllieva, N.; Sui, J.; Wong, S.K.; Berne, M.A.; Somasundaran, M.; Sullivan, J.L.; Luzuriaga, K.; Greeneugh, T.C.; et al. Angiotensin-converting enzyme 2 is a functional receptor for the SARS coronavirus. *Nature* **2003**, *426*, 450–454. [CrossRef] [PubMed]
47. Lan, J.; Ge, J.; Yu, J.; Shan, S.; Zhou, H.; Fan, S.; Zhang, Q.; Shi, X.; Wang, Q.; Zhang, L.; et al. Structure of the SARS-CoV-2 spike receptor-binding domain bound to the ACE2 receptor. *Nature* **2020**, *581*, 215–220. [CrossRef]
48. Ou, X.; Liu, Y.; Lei, X.; Li, P.; Mi, D.; Ren, L.; Guo, L.; Guo, R.; Chen, T.; Hu, J.; et al. Characterization of spike glycoprotein of SARS-CoV-2 on virus entry and its immune cross-reactivity with SARS-CoV. *Nat. Commun.* **2020**, *11*, 1–12. [CrossRef]
49. Brown, A.J.; Won, J.J.; Graham, R.L.; Dinnon, K.H.; Sims, A.C.; Feng, J.Y.; Cihlar, T.; Denison, M.R.; Baric, R.S.; Sheahan, T.P. Broad spectrum antiviral remdesivir inhibits human endemic and zoonotic deltacoronaviruses with a highly divergent RNA dependent RNA polymerase. *Antiviral Res.* **2019**, *169*, 104541. [CrossRef]
50. Murakami, E.; Wang, T.; Babusis, D.; Lepist, E.I.; Sauer, D.; Park, Y.; Vela, J.E.; Shih, R.; Birkus, G.; Stefanidis, D.; et al. Metabolism and pharmacokinetics of the anti-hepatitis C virus nucleotide prodrug GS-6620. *Antimicrob. Agents Chemother.* **2014**, *58*, 1943–1951. [CrossRef]
51. Wichmann, D.; Sperhake, J.P.; Lütgehetmann, M.; Steurer, S.; Edler, C.; Heinemann, A.; Heinrich, F.; Mushumba, H.; Kniep, I.; Schröder, A.S.; et al. Autopsy Findings and Venous Thromboembolism in Patients With COVID-19: A Prospective Cohort Study. *Ann. Intern. Med.* **2020**, *173*, 268–277. [CrossRef]
52. Bieganowski, P.; Garrison, P.N.; Hodawadekar, S.C.; Faye, G.; Barnes, L.D.; Brenner, C. Adenosine monophosphoramidase activity of Hint and Hnt1 supports function of Kin28, Ccl1, and Tfb3. *J. Biol. Chem.* **2002**, *277*, 10852–10860. [CrossRef] [PubMed]
53. Chou, T.F.; Baraniak, J.; Kaczmarek, R.; Zhou, X.; Cheng, J.; Ghosh, B.; Wagner, C.R. Phosphoramidate pronucleotides: A comparison of the phosphoramidase substrate specificity of human and Escherichia coli histidine triad nucleotide binding proteins. *Mol. Pharm.* **2007**, *4*, 208–217. [CrossRef]
54. Lo, M.K.; Jordan, R.; Arvey, A.; Sudhamsu, J.; Shrivastava-Ranjan, P.; Hotard, A.L.; Flint, M.; McMullan, L.K.; Siegel, D.; Clarke, M.O.; et al. GS-5734 and its parent nucleoside analog inhibit Filo-, Pneumo-, and Paramyxoviruses. *Sci. Rep.* **2017**, *7*, 1–7. [CrossRef] [PubMed]
55. Yan, V.C.; Khadka, S.; Arthur, K.; Pham, C.-D.; Yan, A.J.; Ackroyd, J.J.; Georgiou, D.K. Pharmacokinetics of Orally Administered GS-441524 in Dogs. *bioRxiv* **2021**. [CrossRef]
56. Pedersen, N.C.; Perron, M.; Bannasch, M.; Montgomery, E.; Murakami, E.; Liepnieks, M.; Liu, H. Efficacy and safety of the nucleoside analog GS-441524 for treatment of cats with naturally occurring feline infectious peritonitis. *J. Feline Med. Surg.* **2019**, *21*, 271–281. [CrossRef]
57. Preskorn, S.H.; Silkey, B.; Beber, J.; Dorey, C. Antidepressant response and plasma concentrations of fluoxetine. *Ann. Clin. Psychiatry* **1991**, *3*, 147–151. [CrossRef]
58. Pope, S.; Zaraa, S.G. Serum fluoxetine and norfluoxetine levels support the safety of fluoxetine in overdose. *Ann. Gen. Psychiatry* **2016**, *15*, 30. [CrossRef] [PubMed]

59. Beigel, J.H.; Tomashek, K.M.; Dodd, L.E.; Mehta, A.K.; Zingman, B.S.; Kalil, A.C.; Hohmann, E.; Chu, H.Y.; Luetkemeyer, A.; Kline, S.; et al. Remdesivir for the Treatment of COVID-19—Final Report. *N. Engl. J. Med.* **2020**, *383*, 1813–1826. [CrossRef] [PubMed]
60. Kalil, A.C.; Patterson, T.F.; Mehta, A.K.; Tomashek, K.M.; Wolfe, C.R.; Ghazaryan, V.; Marconi, V.C.; Ruiz-Palacios, G.M.; Hsieh, L.; Kline, S.; et al. Baricitinib plus Remdesivir for Hospitalized Adults with COVID-19. *N. Engl. J. Med.* **2020**, *384*, 795–807. [CrossRef]
61. Kumar, D.; Trivedi, N. Disease-drug and drug-drug interaction in COVID-19: Risk and assessment. *Biomed. Pharmacother.* **2021**, *139*, 111642. [CrossRef] [PubMed]
62. Yang, K. What Do We Know About Remdesivir Drug Interactions? *Clin. Transl. Sci.* **2020**, *13*, 842–844. [CrossRef] [PubMed]
63. Humeniuk, R.; Mathias, A.; Kirby, B.J.; Lutz, J.D.; Cao, H.; Osinusi, A.; Babusis, D.; Porter, D.; Wei, X.; Ling, J.; et al. Pharmacokinetic, Pharmacodynamic, and Drug-Interaction Profile of Remdesivir, a SARS-CoV-2 Replication Inhibitor. *Clin. Pharmacokinet.* **2021**, *60*, 569–583. [CrossRef]
64. Sager, J.E.; Lutz, J.D.; Foti, R.S.; Davis, C.; Kunze, K.L.; Isoherranen, N. Fluoxetine- and norfluoxetine-mediated complex drug-drug interactions: In vitro to in vivo correlation of effects on CYP2D6, CYP2C19, and CYP3A4. *Clin. Pharmacol. Ther.* **2014**, *95*, 653–662. [CrossRef]
65. Deodhar, M.; Al Rihani, S.B.; Darakjian, L.; Turgeon, J.; Michaud, V. Assessing the Mechanism of Fluoxetine-Mediated CYP2D6 Inhibition. *Pharmaceutics* **2021**, *13*, 148. [CrossRef] [PubMed]
66. Plasencia-García, B.O.; Rico-Rangel, M.I.; Rodríguez-Menéndez, G.; Rubio-García, A.; Torelló-Iserte, J.; Crespo-Facorro, B. Drug-drug Interactions between COVID-19 Treatments and Antidepressants, Mood Stabilizers/Anticonvulsants, and Benzodiazepines: Integrated Evidence from 3 Databases. *Pharmacopsychiatry* **2021**. [CrossRef] [PubMed]
67. Brambilla, P.; Cipriani, A.; Hotopf, M.; Barbui, C. Side-effect profile of fluoxetine in comparison with other SSRIs, tricyclic and newer antidepressants: A meta-analysis of clinical trial data. *Pharmacopsychiatry* **2005**, *38*, 69–77. [CrossRef]
68. Cooper, G.L. The safety of fluoxetine—An update. *Br. J. Psychiatry* **1988**, *153*, 77–86. [CrossRef]
69. Drugs.com. Drug Interaction Checker from Drugs.com; c1996–2018 [Last Updated: 2 Nov 2020]. Available online: https://www.drugs.com/drug_interactions.html (accessed on 21 January 2021).

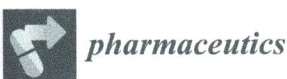

Article

3D-ALMOND-QSAR Models to Predict the Antidepressant Effect of Some Natural Compounds

Speranta Avram [1,†], Miruna Silvia Stan [1,2], Ana Maria Udrea [2,3,†], Cătălin Buiu [4,*], Anca Andreea Boboc [5,6] and Maria Mernea [1]

1. Department of Anatomy, Animal Physiology and Biophysics, Faculty of Biology, University of Bucharest, SplaiulIndependentei, No 91-95, 050095 Bucharest, Romania; speranta.avram@gmail.com (S.A.); miruna.stan@bio.unibuc.ro (M.S.S.); maria.mernea@bio.unibuc.ro (M.M.)
2. Research Institute of the University of Bucharest–ICUB, University of Bucharest, 91–95, SplaiulIndependentei, 050095 Bucharest, Romania; ana.udrea@inflpr.ro
3. Laser Department, National Institute for Laser, Plasma and Radiation Physics, 077125 Magurele, Romania
4. Department of Automatic Control and Systems Engineering, Politehnica University of Bucharest, 313 SplaiulIndependenței, 060042 Bucharest, Romania
5. "Maria Sklodowska Curie" Emergency Children's Hospital, 20, Constantin Brancoveanu Bd., 077120 Bucharest, Romania; anca.orzan@gmail.com
6. Department of Pediatrics 8, "Carol Davila" University of Medicine and Pharmacy, EroiiSanitari Bd., 020021 Bucharest, Romania
* Correspondence: catalin.buiu@upb.ro; Tel.: +40-021-402-9167
† These authors contributed equally to this work.

Abstract: The current treatment of depression involves antidepressant synthetic drugs that have a variety of side effects. In searching for alternatives, natural compounds could represent a solution, as many studies reported that such compounds modulate the nervous system and exhibit antidepressant effects. We used bioinformatics methods to predict the antidepressant effect of ten natural compounds with neuroleptic activity, reported in the literature. For all compounds we computed their drug-likeness, absorption, distribution, metabolism, excretion (ADME), and toxicity profiles. Their antidepressant and neuroleptic activities were predicted by 3D-ALMOND-QSAR models built by considering three important targets, namely serotonin transporter (SERT), 5-hydroxytryptamine receptor 1A (5-HT1A), and dopamine D2 receptor. For our QSAR models we have used the following molecular descriptors: hydrophobicity, electrostatic, and hydrogen bond donor/acceptor. Our results showed that all compounds present drug-likeness features as well as promising ADME features and no toxicity. Most compounds appear to modulate SERT, and fewer appear as ligands for 5-HT1A and D2 receptors. From our prediction, linalyl acetate appears as the only ligand for all three targets, neryl acetate appears as a ligand for SERT and D2 receptors, while 1,8-cineole appears as a ligand for 5-HT1A and D2 receptors.

Keywords: antidepressant; natural compounds; QSAR; molecular docking

1. Introduction

Depression is a common mental disorder, 264 million persons being affected worldwide, according to the WHO. A severe consequence of depression is suicide, and near 800,000 people commit suicide every year [1]. Depression can be treated by psychotherapy and medication involving antidepressant and antipsychotic drugs. Although these drugs have beneficial effects in the management of depression, their usage could lead to severe side effects like hepatotoxicity, weight gain, sexual dysfunction, cardiovascular disorders, central nervous system disturbances, etc. [2].

Natural compounds may represent a viable alternative in depression treatment with possibly fewer side effects, supporting their administration even in patients with comorbidities [3,4]. Here we used an in silico approach to predict the antidepressant activity of

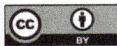

the following natural compounds: resveratrol, quercetin, limonene, sabinene, 1,8-cineole, chamazulene, linalyl acetate, germacrene D, nerol, and neryl acetate.

Resveratrol is a polyphenol with benefits in inflammation, brain diseases, and depression [4]. A study on irritable bowel syndrome rat model shows that resveratrol had inhibitory activity on the 5-hydroxytryptamine receptor 1A (5-HT1A), thus improving the brain–gut axis [5]. A review of twenty-two studies concludes that resveratrol has positive effects on animal models with depression, comparable with those of antidepressant drugs. Regarding safety, the same review concludes that resveratrol has an exceptional safety profile and only a few side effects [6].

Quercetin is a flavonoid whose antidepressant activity was studied on diabetic mice and compared with antidepressants fluoxetine and imipramine. Results show that quercetin had similar results with those drugs in diabetic mice but not in naive mice [7]. Another study on mice concludes that pre-administrated quercetin decreases stress-induced behaviour, regulates cholinergic and serotoninergic functions, has an anxiolytic and antidepressant effect, and boosts memory function [8]. Quercetin also inhibits the behavioral effects induced by corticotropin-releasing factor (anxiety and depression) in mice model study [9].

Limonene is a monocyclic monoterpene known for its antiviral, antibacterial, anticancer, and anti-inflammatory activities [10]. This compound also shows neuroprotective effects in a *Drosophila* model [11] and antidepressant-like activity (mediated by its anti-neuroinflammatory action and by lowering hippocampal nitrite levels) in a mice model [12]. Studies on mice models showed that limonene regulates dopamine levels and 5-HT function [13] and increases dopamine and norepinephrine levels [14].

Sabinene is a monoterpene with antimicrobial and antifungal activity, with possible effects on the central nervous system [15,16]. Sabinene is a component of *Origanum vulgare* (oregano) essential oil (4.95%), and it may show antidepressant-like activity in a rat model [17].

Eucalyptol, 1,8-cineole, is a monoterpenoid with benefits as an anti-mucolytic or antispasmolytic [18]. Additionally, 1,8-cineole inhalation shows an anxiolytic effect in both mice and humans [19,20]. Eucalyptol is found in various plants, including *Rosmarinus officinalis* (rosemary) aerial plants oil (8.58%). This oil shows inhibitory activity on 5-HT1A [21]. Even if this compound had antidepressant effects, the mechanism of action is not clear yet [14].

Chamazulene is an aromatic compound found in *Matricaria chamomilla* (chamomile) and is known as a compound with antioxidant, anti-inflammatory, and hepatoprotective effects [22]. Chamomile is known for its benefits in generalized anxiety and insomnia [23].

The monoterpene linalyl acetate is the main constituent of *Lavandula angustifolia* (lavander) essential oil. Lavender essential oil is known for its antidepressant and anxiolytic properties [24,25]. Linalyl acetate's mechanism of action as an antidepressant is well studied: this compound has binding affinity for N-methyl-D-aspartate (NMDA) receptor [26], and reduces the activity of 5-HT1A receptor [24], but not of serotonin transporter (SERT) [26]. Nerol monoterpene can also be found in *Lavandula angustifolia* essential oil [27] or in *Rosa damascene* (damask rose) oil. It can decrease the lipid peroxidation levels, a process occurring under chronic mild stress [28].

Germacrene D is a sesquiterpenoid found in *Anthriscus nemorosa* (chervil) essential oil in a proportion of 5.6%. Studies on rats revealed that scopolamine-induced memory impairment, anxiety, and depression can be improved using chervil essential oil [14]. Neryl acetate is one of the main constituents of *Cananga odorata* (ilang-ilang) essential oil. This oil decreases dopamine levels and increases serotonin levels in mice [29].

The compounds that we have chosen to analyze are indexed in FooDB, a resource on food constituents, comprising detailed descriptions of compound, including their physiological and presumed health effects [30]. Except for sabiene, linalyl acetate, nerol, and neryl acetate, the compounds are also indexed in DrugBank, a database comprising extensive information on drugs and drugs targets, including natural compounds and herbs used in therapeutic products [31]. The applications of selected compounds as indexed in the two databases are summarized in Table 1. It is essential to highlight that DrugBank—or any other database, for that matter—does not index the considered compounds as antidepressants. Taking into account their promising benefits in depression, as revealed mostly by studies conducted in animal models, we considered here the possibility to reposition some of these compounds as antidepressants and even as neuroleptics to be used in the treatment of humans.

Table 1. Applications of the natural compounds indexed in the critical data bases DrugBank 5.1.8 [31] and Foodb [30].

Compound	DrugBank Accession Number	Medical Applications	Foodb Accession Number	Medical Applications
resveratrol	DB02709	anti-inflammatory, antioxidant, anticancer effects	FDB031212	suppresses NF-kappa B activation in HSV infected cells
quercetin	DB04216	specific quinone reductase 2 (QR2) inhibitor, may contribute to killing the malaria causing parasites	FDB011904	non-specific protein kinase enzyme inhibitor, agonist of the G protein-coupled estrogen receptor in human breast cancer cell lines
limonene	DB08921	common in cosmetic products, a flavoring to mask the bitter taste of alkaloids, a fragrance in perfumery	FDB013567	antimicrobial, expectorant
sabinene	not available	not available	FDB001456	not available
1,8-cineole	DB03852	controls airway mucus hypersecretion and asthma via anti-inflammatory cytokine inhibition, eucalyptol reduces inflammation and pain	FDB014616	antibronchitis, antiallergic
chamazulene	DB15931	not available	FDB015363	analgesic, antioxidant
linalyl acetate	not available	not available	FDB019133	antimicrobial, antioxidant, flavor
germacrene D	DB11276	as component of pine needle oil is used as disinfectant, lubricant, sanitizer, antimicrobial, insecticide	FDB003856	pesticide
nerol	not available	not available	FDB014945	antimicrobial, flavor, perfumery
neryl acetate	not available	not available	FDB013794	antimicrobial, flavor, perfumery

Previously, we used structure-activity relationship (SAR) models to investigate the potential of natural compounds from *Mentha spicata* essential oil to modulate acetylcholinesterase and NMDA receptor, two important targets considered in Alzheimer's disease therapy [32]. A similar approach can be applied in the case of other nervous system diseases, like depression. In depression, important therapy targets are SERT, dopamine receptor 2 (D2), and 5-HT1A [33,34]. In our previous work, we built quantitative structure-activity relationship (QSAR) models to predict the effect of candidate compounds against these targets [33,34].

Particularly useful in drug design, discovery, and development is 3D-QSAR methodology, which helps to understand the relationship between spatial parameters of molecules and their biological properties [35]. Recent studies have used 3D-QSAR as a screening step in drug repositioning strategies, some examples being [36–39]. In these cases, QSAR models were used to screen compounds from: (i) DrugBank database [31] in order to identify promising candidates that modulate histone deacetylases [37] or inhibit SARS-CoV main protease [38]; (ii) FDA approved drugs from ZINC database [40] that inhibit Sirt2 [39]; or (iii) FDA approved drugs from e-Drug3D database [41] to identify druggable compounds for iatrogenic botulism treatment [36]. 3D-QSAR is valuable in drug repositioning, being complementary to other methods like molecular docking, because it predicts the activity of compounds (high/low activity) and yields the molecular features important for their effect [39].

In the present study we built three QSAR models to screen our collection of natural compounds identified from the literature against SERT, D2, and 5-HT1A receptor in order to identify the most promising compound with antidepressant and neuroleptic activity. Additionally, we analyzed the interactions between receptors and lead ligands using molecular docking.

2. Materials and Methods

2.1. Preparation of Natural Compounds Structures

The present study looked at ten natural compounds, including resveratrol, quercetin, limonene, sabinene, 1,8-cineole, chamazulene, linalyl acetate, germacrene D, nerol, and neryl acetate, based on their potential antidepressant effects identified in the literature, as described in the Section 1. The antidepressant efficacy of these drugs is determined using SERT and 5-HT1A receptors, as well as the neuroleptic effect on the D2 receptor.

MOE software was used to model and optimize the 3D structures of molecules. We minimized the energy using the MMFF94x force field at a 0.005 gradient and Gasteiger-type charges [42].

2.2. Prediction of Compounds Drug- and Lead-Likeness Features

The Lipinski [43], Veber [44], Ghose [45], and Egan [46] filters, which were predicted in the SwissADME online tool [47], were used to evaluate the drug-likeness of the natural compounds. The analyzed compounds should not violate more than three of these rules. According to the Lipinski criteria, compounds must have a molecular weight lower than 500 Daltons, no more than 10 hydrogen bond acceptors, no more than 5 hydrogen bond donors, and a log octanol/water (Log P(o/w)) lower than 5.

The molecular weight must be between 160 and 480, the Log P(o/w) must be between 0.4 and 5.6, the molar refractivity must be between 40 and 130, and the number of atoms must be between 20 and 70, according to the Ghose filter.

If the total polar surface area is less than 140 and the number of rotatable bonds is less than 10, the Veber rule applies. The Log P(o/w) must be less than 5.88, and the total polar surface area must be less than 131, according to the Egan filter.

2.3. Computational Pharmacokinetics and Pharmacogenomics Profiles of Natural Compounds

The SMILES files of natural compounds were used to predict their absorption, distribution, metabolism, excretion, and toxicity (ADMET) profiles using the pkCSM database [48].

We started by calculating all of the ADMET entries that the bioinformatics portal sent us. The following were chosen as related to our research: (i) intestinal absorption (percentage)—a molecule with an absorption rate of less than 30% is deemed poorly absorbed; (ii) permeability of the blood-brain barrier (BBB) represented as log BBB (logarithm of the brain to plasma drug concentration ratio)—higher than 0.3 indicates high BBB permeability, while lower than 1 indicates low BBB permeability; (iii) central nervous system (CNS) permeability—a compound with a permeability-surface area product (logPS) higher than -2 can penetrate the CNS; (iv) fraction unbound (human) is represented by the ratio of the unbounded compound on plasmatic proteins; (v) substrate of renal organic cation transporter 2 (OCT2), the main renal uptake transporter that is expressed on the basolateral side of the proximal tubule.

We investigated the potential of the compounds to serve as inhibitors or substrates for cytochromes involved in the metabolization of neuropsychiatric medications, such as CYP2D6, CYP3A4, CYP1A2, CYP2C19, and CYP2C9, to predict their pharmacogenomic profile. The prediction of toxicity was a significant aspect of our research.

We assessed AMES toxicity, hepatotoxicity, LD50 (median lethal dose), and maximum tolerated dose (human).

2.4. Building 3D-ALMOND-QSAR to Predict Natural Compounds Effects

We used Pentacle software to create three 3D-QSAR-ALMOND models to predict the action of natural compounds on SERT, D2, and 5-HT1A receptors [33,49]. The three models are further called QSAR-SERT, QSAR-D2, and QSAR-5-HT1A in correlation with the target they address.

For each molecule, we computed several molecular descriptors. Each descriptor's contribution to biological activity was assessed singly or in groups of different combinations. The hydrophobicity, electrostatic, and hydrogen bond donor/acceptor features were found to be the most important statistical combination of molecular descriptors for all QSAR models.

The chemometric analysis was made using the regression analysis, partial least squares (PLS) within PENTACLE. The number of PLS components (latent variables, LVs = 5) was chosen to achieve optimum values of statistical parameters. These are $r^2 > 0.8$ (fitted correlation coefficient) and $q^2 > 0.6$ (cross-validated correlation coefficient). Additionally, SDEP (standard deviation of error prediction) and SDEC (standard deviation of error calculation) were evaluated.

The generation of consistent statistical models depends on the quality of training, validation, and testing sets in terms of structural diversity and property values distribution.

QSAR-SERT model has amitriptyline, citalopram, clomipramine, desipramine, doxepin, escitalopram, fluoxetine, imipramine, lofepramine, paroxetine, sertraline, trazodone, venlafaxine, aripiprazole, chlorpromazine, clozapine, fluphenazine, haloperidol, risperidone, sertindole, and zotepine in the training set and, in the validation set, bupropion, olanzapine, quetiapine, thioridazine, ziprasidone, and fluvoxamine.

QSAR-5-HT1A model has amitriptyline, desipramine, doxepin, escitalopram, fluoxetine, trazodone, aripiprazole, chlorpromazine, fluphenazine, haloperidol, iloperidone, loxapine, olanzapine, prochlorperazine, quetiapine, risperidone, spiperone, trifluoperazine, and ziprasidone in the training set and, in the validation set, clozapine, sertindole, thioridazine, and zotepine.

QSAR-D2 model has amitriptyline, despyramine, flufenazine, haloperidol, iloperidone, loxapine, prochlorperazine, risperidone, spiperone, trifluoperazine, clomipramine, clozapine, mesoridazine, olanzapine, promazine, remoxipride, sertindole, thioridazine, and zotepine in the training set and, in the validation set, doxepine, aripriprazole, quetiapine, chlorpromazine, and ziprasidone.

The test set used in all QSAR models is represented by the ten natural compounds that we investigated.

The biological activities of compounds in training and validation sets expressed as Ki values (inhibition constants) were retrieved from PDSP Ki Database—Psychoactive Drug Screening Program [50]. The three models that we built predict the biological activities of compounds as pKi values (log 1/Ki) for a better statistical analysis.

2.5. Molecular Docking Protocol

The interactions of the lead compounds identified using our QSAR models with SERT, D2, and 5-HT1A receptors were predicted using molecular docking.

The 3D protein structures were imported from Protein Data Bank in the case of SERT (PDB ID: 6VRH [51]) and D2 (PDB ID:6CM4 [52]) receptors; the structure of the 5-HT1A receptor was imported from AlphaFold [53].

The molecular docking was performed using the CDOCKER algorithm [54] implemented in Biovia Discovery Studio v16.1.0.15350 (BIOVIA Dassault Systemes, San Diego, CA, USA).

The ligands were docked in the drug binding cavities according to the PDB files used [51,52]. In the case of 5-HT1A, the binding site was identified by similarity with the site of the D2 receptor [52]. The Docking protocol was applied as described in the study of Rao et al. [55].

3. Results

3.1. Drug-Likeness, Pharmacokinetics, and Pharmacogenomics Profiles of Compounds

The structures of compounds were retrieved from PubChem database [56] as SMILES (Simplified Molecular Input Line Entry) files, as presented in Table 2.

Table 2. The name of natural compounds and PubChem ID, 2D structure, SMILES [56], natural source, compound FooDB ID [30], and the druglikness features [47].

Compound	Smiles	Natural Source/ FooDB Id	Lipinski	Veber	Ghose	Egan
1,8-cineole [PubChem ID = 2758]	CC1(C2CCC(O1)(CC2)C)C	eucalyptus, sage [FDB014616]	YES	YES	No; 1 violation: MW < 160	YES
limonene [PubChem ID = 22311]	CC1=CCC(CC1)C(=C)C	peppermint, spearmint [FDB013567]	YES	YES	No; 1 violation: MW < 160	YES
sabinene [PubChem ID = 18818]	CC(C)C12CCC(=C)C1C2	lemon, mint [FDB001454]	YES	YES	No; 1 violation: MW < 160	YES

Table 2. Cont.

Compound	Smiles	Natural Source/ FooDB Id	Lipinski	Veber	Ghose	Egan
resveratrol [PubChem ID = 445154]	C1=CC(=CC= C1C=CC2=CC (=CC(=C2)O)O)O	skin of grapes [FDB031212]	YES	YES	YES	YES
chamazulene [PubChem ID = 10719]	CCC1=CC2=C (C=CC2=C (C=C1)C)C	german chamomile, roman chamomile [FDB015363]	YES	YES	YES	YES
germacrene D [PubChem ID = 5317570]	CC1=CCCC (=C)C=CC (CC1)C(C)C	Peppermint [FDB003856]	YES	YES	YES	YES
linalyl acetate [PubChem ID = 8294]	CC(=CCCC (C)(C=C)OC (=O)C)C	sage [FDB019133]	YES	YES	YES	YES
nerol [PubChem ID = 643820]	CC(=CCCC (=CCO)C)C	common grapes [FDB014945]	YES	YES	YES	YES

Table 2. Cont.

Compound	Smiles	Natural Source/ FooDB Id	Lipinski	Veber	Ghose	Egan
neryl acetate PubChem [ID = 1549025]	CC(=CCC/C (=C\COC (=O)C)/C)C	lemon balm, peppermint [FDB014946]	YES	YES	YES	YES
quercetin [PubChem ID = 5280343]	C1=CC(=C (C=C1C2=C(C (=O)C3=C(C=C (C=C3O2)O) O)O)O)O	Grape [FDB011904]	YES	YES	YES	YES

To determine the drug-likeness of compounds, we applied different filters, as presented in Table 2. As can be seen, all compounds comply with Lipinski, Veber, and Egan rules. In the case of the Ghose rule, only 1,8-cineole, limonene, and sabiene present one violation of the rule. These results show that the compounds present drug-likeness features and could present a good bioavailability.

ADME and toxicity profiles of compounds were computed, with an emphasis on human intestinal absorption (HIA), BBB and CNS permeabilities, human fraction unbound (HFU), renal OCT2 substrate, mutagenesis features-AMES, hepatotoxicity, maximum of tolerated dose (human), and LD50 (Table 3).

Table 3. Computed human intestinal absorption (HIA), blood-brain barrier permeability (log BBB), CNS permeability, human fraction unbound (HFU), maximum tolerated dose (human), and LD50 for selected compounds.

Compound	HIA	Log BBB	CNS Permeability	HFU	Max. Tolerated Dose (Human)	LD50
1,8-cineole	96.50	0.36	−2.97	0.55	0.55	2.01
limonene	95.89	0.72	−2.37	0.48	0.77	1.88
sabinene	95.35	0.83	−1.46	0.29	0.36	1.54
resveratrol	89.05	−0.04	−2.09	0.18	0.48	1.79
chamazulene	94.50	0.79	−1.82	0.24	0.05	1.45
germacrene D	95.59	0.72	−2.13	0.26	0.49	1.63
linalyl acetate	95.27	0.51	−2.37	0.42	0.54	1.72
nerol	93.46	0.62	−2.17	0.44	0.85	1.71
neryl acetate	96.06	0.56	−2.19	0.37	0.74	1.95
quercetin	77.20	−1.09	−3.06	0.20	0.49	2.47

Here, we also computed the biological activities of considered natural compounds at some very important human cytochromes involved in neuropsychiatric disorders, namely CYP2D6, CYP3A4, CYP1A2, CYP2C19, and CYP2C9 [57].

The biological activities of natural compounds were expressed as inhibitors or substrates of human cytochromes, as presented in Table 4.

Table 4. The inhibitor/substrate features of natural compounds at CYP2D6, CYP3A4, CYP1A2, CYP2C19 and CYP2C9.

Compound	CYP2D6 Substrate/Inhibitor	CYP3A4 Substrate/Inhibitor	CYP1A2 Inhibitor	CYP2C19 Inhibitor	CYP2C9 Inhibitor
1,8-cineole	no/no	no/no	no	no	no
limonene	no/no	no/no	no	no	no
sabinene	no/no	no/no	no	no	no
resveratrol	no/yes	no/yes	yes	yes	yes
chamazulene	no/no	no/no	no	no	no
germacrene d	no/no	no/no	no	no	no
linalyl acetate	no/no	no/no	no	no	no
nerol	no/no	no/no	no	no	no
neryl acetate	no/no	no/no	no	no	no
quercetin	no/no	no/no	yes	no	no

We intended to generate a pharmacogenomic pathway of natural compounds through these predictions, establishing if these are metabolized by the same cytochromes as classical antidepressants or neuroleptics, which is relevant when a combinatorial therapy involving classical antidepressants, classical neuroleptics, and natural compounds is indicated.

3.2. Natural Compounds' Antidepressant Activities Predicted by 3D-ALMOND-QSAR

Three QSAR models (QSAR-SERT, QSAR-D2, and QSAR-5-HT1A) were built to predict the biological effect of natural compounds against SERT, 5-HT1A, and D2 receptors. In building the models we initially considered individual descriptors like hydrophobicity, hydrogen bond donor/acceptor, electrostatic, or steric. These models could not predict biological activities in correlation with experimental activities.

Further, we considered the contribution of several descriptors at the same time, which led to a significant improvement of the prediction accuracy of our models ($r^2 > 0.9$, $q^2 > 0.8$, SDEP < 0.5), the statistical parameters being given in Table 5.

Table 5. Summary of the ALMOND statistical parameters in QSAR-SERT, QSAR-5-HT1A, and QSAR-D2.

Statistical Parameters	QSAR-SERT	QSAR-5HT-1A	QSAR-D2
No. of molecules in a training set	21	19	19
q^2	0.80	0.90	0.83
r^2	0.96	0.95	0.95
SDEP	0.50	0.29	0.40

The predicted activity of classical neuropsychiatric drugs in the training and validation sets was calculated according to the QSAR equations previously generated and was compared with experimental activity on SERT, 5-HT1A, and D2 receptors (Table 6).

Our QSAR models are described by very good statistical parameters, which allow us to predict the biological activities of 1,8-cineole, limonene, sabinene, resveratrol, chamazulene, germacrene D, linalyl acetate, nerol, neryl acetate, and quercetin at SERT, 5-HT1A, and D2 by following the QSAR equation generated in ALMOND-Pentacle (Table 6).

Table 6. Predicted and experimental biological activities of compounds at SERT, 5-HT1A, and D2 receptors. The biological activities of molecules in the validation set are in italics. In brackets are the predicted biological activities of natural compounds versus the most active compounds of each QSAR model (paroxetine in QSAR-SERT; ziprasidone in QSAR-5HT-1A; spiperone in QSAR-D2).

Compounds	pKiSERT$_{exp}$/ pKiSERT$_{predicted}$	pKi 5-HT1A$_{exp}$/ pKi 5-HT1A$_{predicted}$	pKi D2$_{exp}$/ pKi D2$_{predicted}$
amitriptyline	8.55/8.68	6.34/6.62	6.70/7.17
citalopram	9.00/8.74	-	-
clomipramine	9.85/9.66	-	7.11/7.29
desipramine	7.75/8.07	5.19/5.29	5.80/5.42
doxepin	7.16/7.58	6.55/6.45	6.44/7.35
escitalopram	8.95/8.85	5.00/5.06	-
fluoxetine	9.09/9.23	5.00/4.96	-
imipramine	9.82/9.31	-	-
lofepramine	7.15/7.19	-	-
paroxetine	10.09/9.83	-	-
sertraline	9.58/9.57	-	-
trazodone	6.79/6.72	7.00/6.91	-
venlafaxine	8.12/8.02	-	-
aripiprazole	5.74/5.87	8.25/8.40	*9.18/8.53*
chlorpromazine	8.88/9.23	6.93/6.78	9.18/8.22
clozapine	6.00/5.49	6.97/5.32	7.55/8.23
fluphenazine	5.22/5.22	6.83/6.68	9.69/9.95
haloperidol	6.00/5.51	5.92/5.97	9.45/9.38
risperidone	6.00/6.04	6.72/6.87	9.52/9.65
sertindole	6.00/6.42	*6.55/7.19*	9.02/9.11
zotepine	6.82/7.35	*6.89/6.26*	8.09/8.06
bupropion	*5.04/5.62*	-	-
olanzapine	*6.00/5.69*	5.68/5.61	8.52/8.13
quetiapine,	*6.00/5.20*	6.63/6.47	7.79/8.66
thioridazine	*5.89/7.29*	6.96/6.50	9.39/8.69
ziprasidone	*7.27/6.57*	8.72/8.80	*8.92/8.67*
fluvoxamine	*8.79/8.64*	-	-
iloperidone	-	7.48/7.52	9.45/9.38
loxapine	-	5.60/5.73	8.28/8.22
prochlorperazine	-	5.22/5.30	9.69/9.07
spiperone	-	7.76/7.50	10.15/10.06
trifluoperidine	-	6.02/5.93	-
mesoridazine	-	-	8.36/8.52
promazine	-	-	6.79/7.07
remoxipride	-	-	7.79/7.72
trifluoperazine	-	-	8.92/9.16
Natural compounds			
1,8-cineole	8.57 (−1.52)	7.09 (−1.63)	8.11 (−2.04)
limonene	9.45 (−0.64)	6.73 (−1.99)	7.99 (−2.16)
sabinene	9.37 (−0.72)	6.68 (−2.04)	7.98 (−2.17)
resveratrol	8.68 (−1.41)	5.23 (−3.49)	6.72 (−3.43)
chamazulene	9.50 (−0.59)	6.51 (−2.21)	7.96 (−2.19)
germacrene D	9.52 (−0.57)	6.49 (−2.23)	7.90 (−2.25)
linalyl acetate	9.40 (−0.69)	6.89 (−1.83)	8.11 (−2.04)
nerol	9.74 (−0.35)	6.17 (−2.55)	8.05 (−2.10)
neryl acetate	10.61 (0.52)	6.06 (−2.66)	8.14 (−2.01)
quercetin	6.42 (−3.67)	5.87 (−2.85)	8.39 (−1.76)

The correlation between the training and validation sets of our QSAR models is also represented in Figure 1.

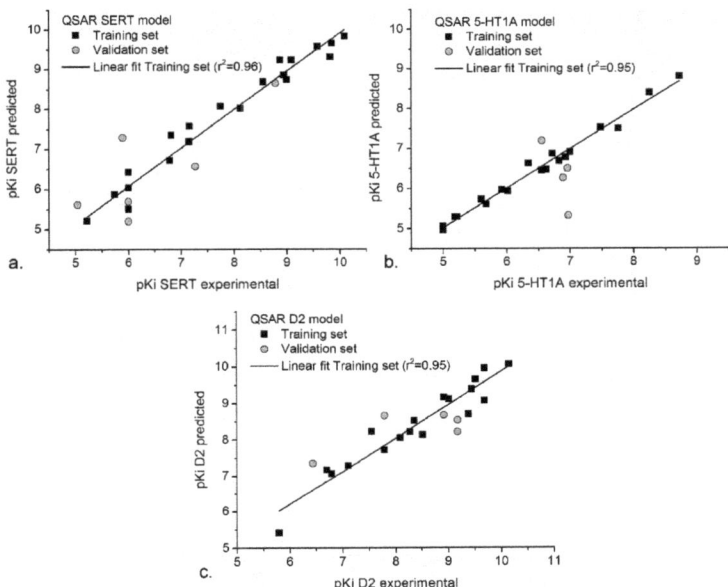

Figure 1. The correlation between experimental and predicted values of QSAR SERT (**a**), QSAR 5-HT1A (**b**), and QSAR D2 (**c**) models. Data were plotted and fitted using Origin Pro, version 9.2 (2015), OriginLab Corporation, Northampton, MA, USA.

3.3. Molecular Docking

The interaction of the most promising compounds acting on the three protein targets were investigated by molecular docking. Therefore, we docked linalyl acetate at SERT, D2, and 5-HT1A; neryl acetate was docked at SERT and 5-HT1A; and 1,8-cineole was docked at D2 and 5-HT1A (see Section 4.3). The binding of ligands was evaluated based on CDOCKER energy and CDOCKER interaction energy; values are presented in Table 7.

Table 7. Molecular docking predictions of interactions between molecular targets in depression, natural compounds linalyl acetate, neryl acetate, and 1,8-cineole and CDOCKER scores calculated for analyzed ligands.

Compound	Target	-CDOCKER_ENERGY	-CDOCKER_INTERACTION_ENERGY
linalyl acetate	SERT	4.65	31.46
linalyl acetate	D2	−3.94	30.82
linalyl acetate	5-HT1A	−1.96	27.17
neryl acetate	SERT	−11.64	31.29
neryl acetate	5-HT1A	−9.79	33.85
1,8-cineole	D2	−14.66	17.25
1,8-cineole	5-HT1A	−8.22	19.07

We further analyzed the structural basis of the interaction between ligands and targets. The 2D interaction maps are presented in Figure 2.

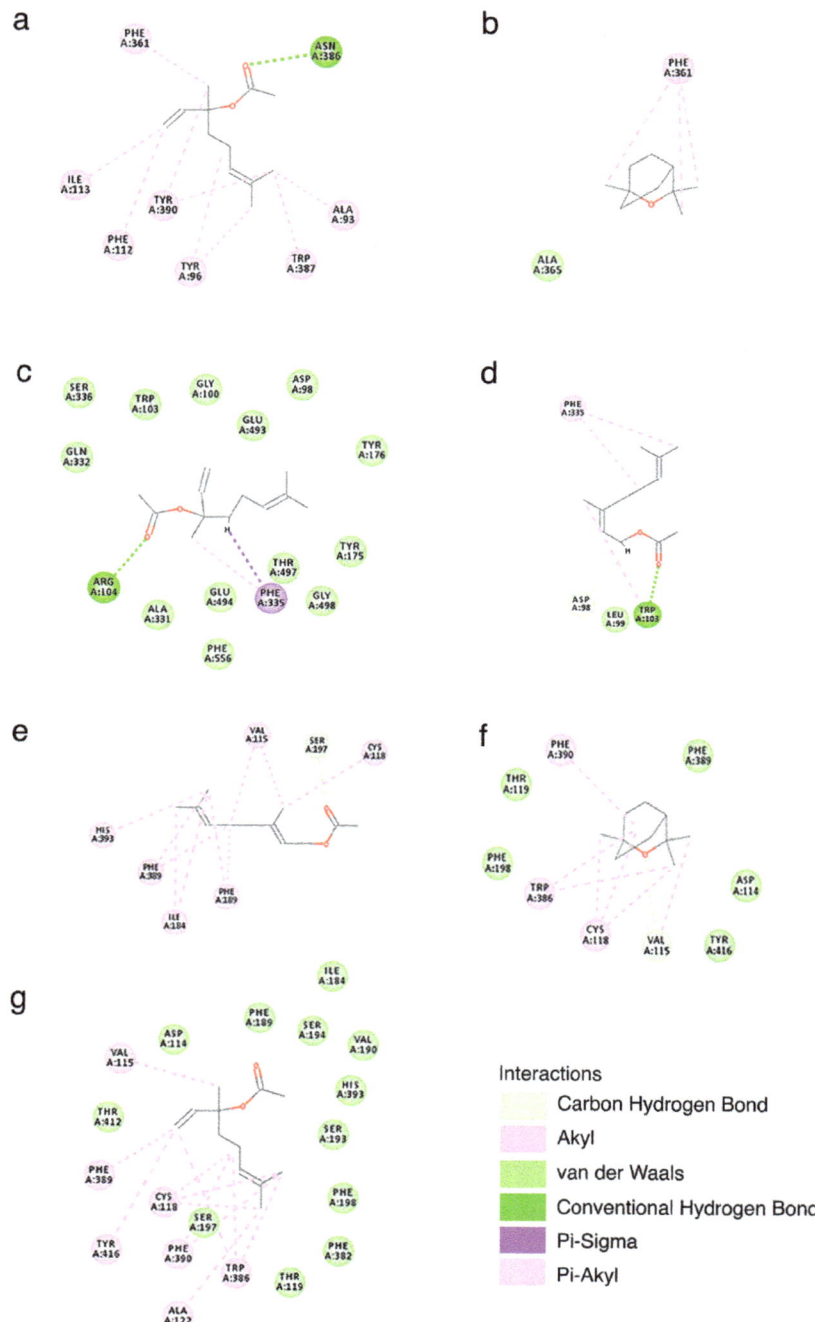

Figure 2. Interaction maps (2D) calculated based on the complexes formed by linalyl acetate with 5-HT1A (**a**), SERT (**c**), or D2 (**g**); 1,8-cineole with 5-HT1A (**b**) or D2 (**f**) and neryl acetate with SERT (**d**) or D2 (**e**). The maps were generated using Discovery Studio Visualizer v21.1.0.20298 (BIOVIA Dassault Systemes, San Diego, CA, USA).

4. Discussion

Drug repositioning involves the identification of novel treatments for diseases based on "old" drugs or compounds [58]. Several strategies were developed to achieve the identification of druggable compounds against novel targets, like QSAR studies, in conjunction with molecular docking [36], with molecular docking and molecular dynamics [37,38], and even with quantum mechanics/molecular mechanics methods [39]. High performance QSAR models can be obtained by using machine learning approaches to classify the molecular descriptors of compounds from large datasets [59]. Repositioning drug candidates can be identified using drug-drug interaction networks [60]; the method even allows the ranking of compounds into simple and complex multi-pathology therapies [61]. Unsupervised machine learning approaches can be used to establish dug–drug similarity networks based on drug–target interactions, which also lead to the identification of repositioning candidates [62]. Other approaches in drug repositioning, as well as limitations and recommendations, are presented in [58].

In the present study we performed a computational investigation on the possibility of repositioning some natural compounds as antidepressants and neuroleptics. Our tentative hypotheses were supported by previous experimental studies that report their antidepressant effects mainly in animals, as presented in the Section 1. Our strategy involved an initial filtering of compounds based on their drug-like properties, their predicted pharmacokinetic, and pharmacogenomic profiles (Sections 4.1 and 4.2). In the following step, QSAR models were built to predict the most active inhibitors of three druggable targets in depression, namely SERT, 5-HT1A, and D2 receptors. We selected the potent compounds that modulate three or at least two targets at once (Section 4.3). The interactions between lead compounds and the targets were addressed by molecular docking (Section 4.4).

4.1. Assessment of Compounds Drug-Likeness Features

Generally, all the natural compounds studied here are in agreement with the medicinal chemistry rules (Table 2). One rule of the Ghose filter (MW < 160) was violated only by 1,8-cineole, limonene, and sabinene. The molecular descriptors of resveratrol, chamazulene, germacrene D, linalyl acetate, nerol, neryl acetate, and quercetin presented values within the ranges defined by Lipinski, Veber, Ghose, and Egan rules. Our results suggest that the natural compounds considered here present drug-likeness features and should be further characterized by computing their pharmacokinetic and pharmacodynamic profiles.

4.2. Computational Pharmacokinetics and Pharmacogenomics Profiles of Natural Compounds

The ADME profiles predicted for the compounds showed that the human intestinal absorption parameter lies in the 77.20% (quercitin) to 96.50% (1,8-cineole) range, as shown in Table 3. Very good human intestinal absorption values were recorded for 1,8-cineole, neryl acetate, and limonene.

Regarding the distribution of the natural compounds in the human body, the human fraction unbound parameter presented a large variation, from 0.18 (resveratrol) to 0.55 (1,8-cineole). Unfortunately, the selected natural compounds presented low human fraction unbound percents. Other critical parameters for describing the natural compounds' distribution in the body are BBB and CNS permeabilities. As shown in Table 3, the considered natural compounds recorded very good BBB permeability values, log BBB ranging from 0.83 (sabinene) to -1.09 (quercitin). An easy BBB penetration was recorded for sabinene, limonene, chamazulene, germacrene D, and nerol, our results being in good agreement with the experimental studies [14,63]. The predicted CNS permeability values range from -1.46 (sabinene) to -3.06 (quercitin). These suggest that the considered natural compounds should have a good CNS permeability, the most permeable compounds being sabinene, chamazulene, resveratrol, germacrene D, and nerol (Table 3). These results are supported by experimental studies showing a possible activity of these compounds at CNS level [15].

The metabolism of compounds was addressed by predicting their affinities for human cytochrome P450 proteins (CYPs): CYP2D6, CYP3A4, CYP1A2, CYP2C19, and

CYP2C9 (Table 4). Our results revealed that resveratrol inhibits CYP2D6, CYP3A4, CYP1A2, CYP2C19, and CYP2C9, quercitin and chamazulene inhibit CYP1A2. Our results are in agreement with an experimental study mentioning that resveratrol modified the metabolism of aripiprazole by CYP2D6 and CYP3A4 [64]. The predicted inhibitory activity of quercetin on CYP1A2 is supported by a previous study [65] showing that quercetin is able to change the metabolism of melatonin by CYP1A2. Quercetin was also reported to be a strong inhibitor of CYP2D6 and a moderate inhibitor of CYP3A4 [66]. Chamazulene was experimentally proved to be a potent inhibitor of CYP1A2, CYP4A4, and CYP2D6 [67].

Important results were recorded for the elimination rate: none of the ten natural compounds are renal OCT2 substrates. In our study, high importance was given to predicting the toxicity of compounds. Our results predict that none of the compounds should present hepatotoxicity, cardiotoxicity, or AMES features. Additionally, we evaluated the maximum tolerated dose (human) and LD50 of natural compounds. Predicted LD50 values vary in a short range, from 1.54 (sabinene) to 2.47 (quercetin). A significant fluctuation was recorded for the maximum tolerated dose, from 0.05 mol/Kg (chamazulene) to 0.85 mol/Kg (nerol). Taken together, our results suggest that none of the natural compounds that we considered are toxic.

4.3. Predicted Pharmacodynamic Profiles of Natural Compounds on SERT, 5H-T1A, and D2 Active Sites by 3D-ALMOND-QSAR

The application of the QSAR-SERT model to molecules from the training and testing sets resulted in a suitable correlation between experimental and calculated biological activities. The differences between experimental and predicted biological activities for the molecules in the training set vary from 0.00 (fluphenazine) and −0.53 (zotepine), while the differences between experimental and predicted biological activities for the molecules in the validation set vary from 0.15 (fluvoxamine) and −1.40 (thioridazine). The statistical parameters (Table 5) and the good correlation between experimental and predicted biological activities of classical neuropsychiatric drugs support the strong power of prediction of QSAR-SERT model. Therefore, the model was used to predict the biological activities of natural compounds against SERT. These are presented in Table 6.

In order to evaluate the potency of natural compounds against SERT, their predicted biological effects were subtracted from the value obtained for paroxetine, the most active compound from the training set (pKi experimental = 10.09). The results show that natural compounds such as limonene ($pKi_{paroxetine}$-$pKi_{limonene}$ = −0.64), sabinene ($pKi_{paroxetine}$-$pKi_{sabinene}$ = −0.72), chamazulene ($pKi_{paroxetine}$-$pKi_{chamazulene}$ = −0.59), germacrene D ($pKi_{paroxetine}$-$pKi_{germacrene\ D}$ = −0.57), linalyl acetate ($pKi_{paroxetine}$-$pKi_{linalyl\ acetate}$ = −0.69), nerol ($pKi_{paroxetine}$-pKi_{nerol} = −0.35), and neryl acetate ($pKi_{paroxetine}$-$pKi_{neryl\ acetate}$ = 0.52) have a strong antidepressant character.

Our results are in accord with other studies [14,68] which mention that limonene and sabinene reduce the depression-related behaviors in a similar manner with fluoxetine [69], linalyl acetate increases 5-HT levels in the amygdala, hypothalamus, and hippocampus of mice [70] and nerol effectively reduces the symptoms of depression and sensitivity.

In QSAR-5-HT1A model, a good correlation between predicted and experimental biological activities was noticed for molecules from the training set, where residual value varies from 0.04 (fluoxetine, iloperidone) to −0.28 (amitriptyline) and also for the validation set, where the residual value varies from 0.46 (thioridazine) to 1.65 (clozapine). The biological activities of natural compounds at 5-HT1A were evaluated relative to the activity of ziprasidone, the most active compound of the training set (pKi experimental = 8.72). We noticed that the natural compounds presented a middle antidepressant activity. A good affinity was predicted in the case of 1,8-cineole ($pKi_{ziprasidone}$-$pKi_{1,8-cineole}$ = 1.83) and linalyl acetate ($pKi_{ziprasidone}$-$pKi_{linalyl\ acetate}$ = 1.83) (Table 6).

The neuroleptic activity of natural compounds was evaluated by their affinity at D2 receptor. The power of prediction of QSAR-D2 model was sustained by the good statistical parameters (Table 5). Similar to previous QSAR models, a good correlation between predicted and experimental biological activities were obtained in both training and validation sets (Table 6). The neuroleptic activity of natural compounds was evaluated versus spiperone (pKi experimental = 10.15) and we noticed that a good neuroleptic activity is recorded by quercetin ($pKi_{spiperone}-pKi_{quercetin} = -1.76$), neryl acetate ($pKi_{spiperone}-pKi_{neryl\ acetate} = -2.01$), linalyl acetate ($pKi_{spiperone}-pKi_{linalyl\ acetate} = -2.04$), and 1,8-cineole ($pKi_{spiperone}-pKi_{1,8-cineole} = -2.04$). The affinity of quercitin at D2 is close to the affinity of mesoridazine, loxapine, and olanzapine, our results being supported by experimental studies [71].

4.4. Molecular Basis of the Interaction between Lead Compounds and Targets

The docking scores that we calculated were CDOKER energy (calculated based on ligand strain energy and receptor-ligand interaction energy) and CDOCKER interaction energy (calculated based on ligand-receptor nonbonded interaction energy). In the case of linalyl acetate acting on the three targets, neryl acetate acting on SERT, and 5-HT1A and 1,8-cineole acting on D2 and 5-HT1A we obtained negative CDOCKER interaction energies, confirming that the ligands present favorable interaction energies with the targets (Table 7). The most favorable interaction energies were obtained for linalyl acetate and neryl acetate, while less favorable energies were calculated for 1,8-cinole.

By analyzing the 2D interaction maps presented in Figure 2 we observe that compounds form hydrogen bonds with the targets in the case of linalyl acetate with SERT and 5-HT1A or in the case of neryl acetate and SERT. Other types of interactions established by the compounds and the targets fall in the category of: (i) van der Waals interactions—important for the binding of linalyl acetate to SERT, linalyl acetate to D2, or 1,8-cineole to D2; (ii) alkyl or π-alkyl interactions—important for the binding of linalyl acetate to 5-HT1A or D2, neryl acetate to D2, or 1,8-cineole to D2; and (iii) μ-σ interactions—which appear only in the case of linalyl acetate binding to SERT. The types of interactions that we identified are consistent with the molecular properties relevant for target binding that we identified using our QSAR models.

5. Conclusions

Medication repositioning is a quick way to employ an existing drug to treat new diseases [72–74]. The present study has investigated the opportunity to reposition ten natural compounds identified from the literature, namely resveratrol, quercetin, limonene, sabinene, 1,8-cineole, chamazulene, linalyl acetate, germacrene D, nerol, and neryl acetate, as antidepressants and even as neuroleptics. These compounds are found in common fruits, spices, and tea herbs. All compounds are indexed in databases (DrugBank, FooDB) with different effects like anti-inflammatory, antioxidant, antimicrobial, antiallergic, or anti cancer, but none of them are indexed as antidepressants. Several experimental studies conducted mostly in animal models point toward their antidepressive effects. Therefore, we used computational methods to address the ability of compounds to modulate three major targets in depression, namely SERT, 5-HT1A, and D2 receptors and compared their predicted effect with the effect of potent drugs used in clinics.

All ten compounds present drug-likeness features and no toxicity, meaning that they could be used in therapy. Their ADME features showed a very good intestinal absorption, as well as a good BBB and CNS permeability, suggesting that the compounds can reach the brain, where they should exert their biological effects.

Their biological activities relevant to depression were determined against SERT, 5-HT1A, and D2 receptors. For each target, we built powerful QSAR models that were trained and validated based on synthesis drugs that modulate their function. When predicting the effect of natural compounds, we determined that most compounds, namely limonene, sabiene, chamazulene, germacrene D, linalyl acetate, nerol, and neryl acetate, should inhibit SERT to an extent similar to paroxetine. Only two compounds appear as candidates to modulate 5-HT1A, namely 1,8-cineole and linalyl acetate, in a manner comparable with fluoxetine. Concerning the neuroleptic effect of compounds, quercetin, neryl acetate, linalyl acetate, and 1,8-cineole could be active against D2 receptors, in a similar manner with ziprasidone. Overall, we identified linalyl acetate as a strong affinity ligand for all three targets (SERT, 5-HT1A, and D2 receptor), and we consider it to be a promising antidepressant compound. Neryl acetate appeared as a promising ligand for both SERT and D2, while 1,8-cineole appears as a common ligand for 5-HT1A and D2 receptors. Molecular docking results confirm the favorable interaction between lead compounds and the targets.

The results obtained here show that linalyl acetate, neryl acetate, and 1,8-cineole target the proteins relevant in depression and present drug-likeness features, suitable ADME profiles, and no toxicity, suggesting they represent viable candidates for repurposing as antidepressants. Our simulation study offers evidence on the molecular mechanism of these compounds and the results should be confirmed experimentally. Results obtained here can be the starting point for studies on the repositioning of natural compounds and plants for an alternative treatment of depression, with significant efficiency, but reduced side effects, that can be administered even to patients with comorbidities or during pregnancy.

Author Contributions: Conceptualization, S.A.; methodology, S.A.; software, S.A. and C.B.; investigation, S.A. and A.M.U.; formal analysis, C.B. and A.A.B.; writing—original draft preparation, A.M.U. and S.A.; writing—review and editing, M.M. and M.S.S. All authors have read and agreed to the published version of the manuscript.

Funding: The study was supported by UEFISCDI through the projects PN-III-P2-2.1-PED-2019-1471, PN-III-P1-1.2-PCCDI-2017-0728, PN-III-P2-2.1-PED-2019-4771, PN-III-P2-2.1-PED-2019-1264, and PN-III-P4-ID-PCE-2020-0620.

Institutional Review Board Statement: Not applicable.

Informed Consent Statement: Not applicable.

Conflicts of Interest: The authors declare no conflict of interest. The funders had no role in the design of the study; in the collection, analyses, or interpretation of data; in the writing of the manuscript, or in the decision to publish the results.

References

1. World Health Organization (WHO) Depression. Available online: https://www.who.int/news-room/fact-sheets/detail/depression (accessed on 24 April 2021).
2. Carvalho, A.F.; Sharma, M.S.; Brunoni, A.R.; Vieta, E.; Fava, G.A. The Safety, Tolerability and Risks Associated with the Use of Newer Generation Antidepressant Drugs: A Critical Review of the Literature. *Psychother. Psychosom.* **2016**, *85*, 270–288. [CrossRef]
3. Yeung, K.S.; Hernandez, M.; Mao, J.J.; Haviland, I.; Gubili, J. Herbal medicine for depression and anxiety: A systematic review with assessment of potential psycho-oncologic relevance. *Phytother. Res.* **2018**, *32*, 865–891. [CrossRef]
4. Udrea, A.-M.; Puia, A.; Shaposhnikov, S.; Avram, S. Computational approaches of new perspectives in the treatment of depression during pregnancy. *Target* **2018**, *3*, 680–687. [CrossRef]
5. Yu, Y.-C.; Li, J.; Zhang, M.; Pan, J.-C.; Yu, Y.; Zhang, J.-B.; Zheng, L.; Si, J.-M.; Xu, Y. Resveratrol improves brain-gut axis by regulation of 5-HT-dependent signaling in the rat model of irritable bowel syndrome. *Front. Cell. Neurosci.* **2019**, *13*, 30. [CrossRef] [PubMed]
6. Moore, A.; Beidler, J.; Hong, M.Y. Resveratrol and depression in animal models: A systematic review of the biological mechanisms. *Molecules* **2018**, *23*, 2197. [CrossRef]
7. Anjaneyulu, M.; Chopra, K.; Kaur, I. Antidepressant Activity of Quercetin, a Bioflavonoid, in Streptozotocin-Induced Diabetic Mice. *J. Med. Food* **2003**, *6*, 391–395. [CrossRef]
8. Samad, N.; Saleem, A.; Yasmin, F.; Shehzad, M. Quercetin protects against stress-induced anxiety-and depression-like behavior and improves memory in male mice. *Physiol. Res.* **2018**, *67*, 795–808. [CrossRef] [PubMed]
9. Bhutada, P.; Mundhada, Y.; Bansod, K.; Ubgade, A.; Quazi, M.; Umathe, S.; Mundhada, D. Reversal by quercetin of corticotrophin releasing factor induced anxiety- and depression-like effect in mice. *Prog. Neuro-Psychopharmacol. Biol. Psychiatry* **2010**, *34*, 955–960. [CrossRef] [PubMed]
10. Mukhtar, Y.M.; Adu-Frimpong, M.; Xu, X.; Yu, J. Biochemical significance of limonene and its metabolites: Future prospects for designing and developing highly potent anticancer drugs. *Biosci. Rep.* **2018**, *38*, BSR20181253. [CrossRef]
11. Shin, M.; Liu, Q.F.; Choi, B.; Shin, C.; Lee, B.; Yuan, C.; Song, Y.J.; Yun, H.S.; Lee, I.-S.; Koo, B.-S. Neuroprotective effects of limonene (+) against Aβ42-induced neurotoxicity in a Drosophila model of Alzheimer's disease. *Biol. Pharm. Bull.* **2020**, *43*, 409–417. [CrossRef]
12. Lorigooini, Z.; Boroujeni, S.N.; Sayyadi-Shahraki, M.; Rahimi-Madiseh, M.; Bijad, E.; Amini-Khoei, H. Limonene through Attenuation of Neuroinflammation and Nitrite Level Exerts Antidepressant-Like Effect on Mouse Model of Maternal Separation Stress. *Behav. Neurol.* **2021**, *2021*, 8817309. [CrossRef] [PubMed]

13. Yun, J. Limonene inhibits methamphetamine-induced locomotor activity via regulation of 5-HT neuronal function and dopamine release. *Phytomedicine* **2014**, *21*, 883–887. [CrossRef] [PubMed]
14. Zhang, Y.; Long, Y.; Yu, S.; Li, D.; Yang, M.; Guan, Y.; Zhang, D.; Wan, J.; Liu, S.; Shi, A. Natural volatile oils derived from herbal medicines: A promising therapy way for treating depressive disorder. *Pharmacol. Res.* **2020**, *164*, 105376. [CrossRef]
15. Caputo, L.; Nazzaro, F.; Souza, L.F.; Aliberti, L.; De Martino, L.; Fratianni, F.; Coppola, R.; De Feo, V. Laurus nobilis: Composition of essential oil and its biological activities. *Molecules* **2017**, *22*, 930. [CrossRef] [PubMed]
16. Fidan, H.; Stefanova, G.; Kostova, I.; Stankov, S.; Damyanova, S.; Stoyanova, A.; Zheljazkov, V.D. Chemical composition and antimicrobial activity of Laurus nobilis L. essential oils from Bulgaria. *Molecules* **2019**, *24*, 804. [CrossRef] [PubMed]
17. Amiresmaeili, A.; Roohollahi, S.; Mostafavi, A.; Askari, N. Effects of oregano essential oil on brain TLR4 and TLR2 gene expression and depressive-like behavior in a rat model. *Res. Pharm. Sci.* **2018**, *13*, 130. [PubMed]
18. Juergens, U. Anti-inflammatory properties of the monoterpene 1.8-cineole: Current evidence for co-medication in inflammatory airway diseases. *Drug Res.* **2014**, *64*, 638–646. [CrossRef]
19. Kim, K.Y.; Seo, H.J.; Min, S.S.; Park, M.; Seol, G.H. The effect of 1, 8-cineole inhalation on preoperative anxiety: A randomized clinical trial. *Evid.-Based Complementary Altern. Med.* **2014**, *2014*, 820126. [CrossRef]
20. Dougnon, G.; Ito, M. Inhalation administration of the bicyclic ethers 1, 8-and 1, 4-cineole prevent anxiety and depressive-like behaviours in mice. *Molecules* **2020**, *25*, 1884. [CrossRef] [PubMed]
21. Martínez, A.L.; González-Trujano, M.E.; Pellicer, F.; López-Muñoz, F.J.; Navarrete, A. Antinociceptive effect and GC/MS analysis of Rosmarinus officinalis L. essential oil from its aerial parts. *Planta Med.* **2009**, *75*, 508–511. [CrossRef]
22. Wang, X.; Dong, K.; Ma, Y.; Jin, Q.; Yin, S.; Wang, S. Hepatoprotective effects of chamazulene against alcohol-induced liver damage by alleviation of oxidative stress in rat models. *Open Life Sci.* **2020**, *15*, 251–258. [CrossRef] [PubMed]
23. Mao, J.J.; Xie, S.X.; Keefe, J.R.; Soeller, I.; Li, Q.S.; Amsterdam, J.D. Long-term chamomile (Matricaria chamomilla L.) treatment for generalized anxiety disorder: A randomized clinical trial. *Phytomedicine* **2016**, *23*, 1735–1742. [CrossRef] [PubMed]
24. Malcolm, B.J.; Tallian, K. Essential oil of lavender in anxiety disorders: Ready for prime time? *Ment. Health Clin.* **2017**, *7*, 147–155. [CrossRef]
25. Donelli, D.; Antonelli, M.; Bellinazzi, C.; Gensini, G.F.; Firenzuoli, F. Effects of lavender on anxiety: A systematic review and meta-analysis. *Phytomedicine* **2019**, *65*, 153099. [CrossRef]
26. López, V.; Nielsen, B.; Solas, M.; Ramírez, M.J.; Jäger, A.K. Exploring pharmacological mechanisms of lavender (Lavandula angustifolia) essential oil on central nervous system targets. *Front. Pharmacol.* **2017**, *8*, 280. [CrossRef]
27. Saki, K.; Bahmani, M.; Rafieian-Kopaei, M. The effect of most important medicinal plants on two importnt psychiatric disorders (anxiety and depression)-a review. *Asian Pac. J. Trop. Med.* **2014**, *7*, S34–S42. [CrossRef]
28. Nazıroğlu, M.; Kozlu, S.; Yorgancıgil, E.; Uğuz, A.C.; Karakuş, K. Rose oil (from Rosa × damascena Mill.) vapor attenuates depression-induced oxidative toxicity in rat brain. *J. Nat. Med.* **2013**, *67*, 152–158. [CrossRef]
29. Zhang, N.; Zhang, L.; Feng, L.; Yao, L. The anxiolytic effect of essential oil of Cananga odorata exposure on mice and determination of its major active constituents. *Phytomedicine* **2016**, *23*, 1727–1734. [CrossRef]
30. FooDB, Version 1.0. Available online: www.foodb.ca (accessed on 24 June 2021).
31. Wishart, D.S.; Knox, C.; Guo, A.C.; Shrivastava, S.; Hassanali, M.; Stothard, P.; Chang, Z.; Woolsey, J. DrugBank: A comprehensive resource for in silico drug discovery and exploration. *Nucleic Acids Res.* **2006**, *34*, D668–D672. [CrossRef]
32. Avram, S.; Mernea, M.; Bagci, E.; Hritcu, L.; Borcan, L.C.; Mihailescu, D.F. Advanced Structure-activity Relationships Applied to Mentha spicata L. Subsp. spicata Essential Oil Compounds as AChE and NMDA Ligands, in Comparison with Donepezil, Galantamine and Memantine—New Approach in Brain Disorders Pharmacology. *CNS Neurol. Disord.-Drug Targets* **2017**, *16*, 800–811. [CrossRef] [PubMed]
33. Avram, S.; Duda-Seiman, D.; Borcan, F.; Wolschann, P. QSAR-CoMSIA applied to antipsychotic drugs with their dopamine D2 and serotonine 5HT2A membrane receptors. *J. Serb. Chem. Soc.* **2011**, *76*, 263–281. [CrossRef]
34. Avram, S.; Buiu, C.; Duda-Seiman, D.M.; Duda-Seiman, C.; Mihailescu, D. 3D-QSAR design of new escitalopram derivatives for the treatment of major depressive disorders. *Sci. Pharm.* **2010**, *78*, 233–248. [CrossRef]
35. Silverman, R.B. Chapter 2-Drug Discovery, Design, and Development. In *The Organic Chemistry of Drug Design and Drug Action*, 2nd ed.; Silverman, R.B., Ed.; Academic Press: San Diego, CA, USA, 2004; pp. 7–120.
36. Floresta, G.; Patamia, V.; Gentile, D.; Molteni, F.; Santamato, A.; Rescifina, A.; Vecchio, M. Repurposing of FDA-Approved Drugs for Treating Iatrogenic Botulism: A Paired 3D-QSAR/Docking Approach. *Chem. Med. Chem.* **2020**, *15*, 256–262. [CrossRef]
37. Liu, J.; Zhu, Y.; He, Y.; Zhu, H.; Gao, Y.; Li, Z.; Zhu, J.; Sun, X.; Fang, F.; Wen, H.; et al. Combined pharmacophore modeling, 3D-QSAR and docking studies to identify novel HDAC inhibitors using drug repurposing. *J. Biomol. Struct. Dyn.* **2020**, *38*, 533–547. [CrossRef]
38. Tejera, E.; Munteanu, C.R.; López-Cortés, A.; Cabrera-Andrade, A.; Pérez-Castillo, Y. Drugs repurposing using QSAR, docking and molecular dynamics for possible inhibitors of the SARS-CoV-2 Mpro protease. *Molecules* **2020**, *25*, 5172. [CrossRef] [PubMed]
39. Bharadwaj, S.; Dubey, A.; Kamboj, N.K.; Sahoo, A.K.; Kang, S.G.; Yadava, U. Drug repurposing for ligand-induced rearrangement of Sirt2 active site-based inhibitors via molecular modeling and quantum mechanics calculations. *Sci. Rep.* **2021**, *11*, 10169. [CrossRef] [PubMed]
40. Irwin, J.J.; Shoichet, B.K. ZINC—A free database of commercially available compounds for virtual screening. *J. Chem. Inf. Model.* **2005**, *45*, 177–182. [CrossRef]

41. Douguet, D. Data Sets Representative of the Structures and Experimental Properties of FDA-Approved Drugs. *ACS Med. Chem. Lett.* **2018**, *9*, 204–209. [CrossRef]
42. Molecular Operating Environment (MOE), 2019.01; Chemical Computing Group ULC: Montreal, QC, Canada, 2021.
43. Lipinski, C.A.; Lombardo, F.; Dominy, B.W.; Feeney, P.J. Experimental and computational approaches to estimate solubility and permeability in drug discovery and development settings. *Adv. Drug Deliv. Rev.* **1997**, *23*, 3–25. [CrossRef]
44. Veber, D.F.; Johnson, S.R.; Cheng, H.Y.; Smith, B.R.; Ward, K.W.; Kopple, K.D. Molecular properties that influence the oral bioavailability of drug candidates. *J. Med. Chem.* **2002**, *45*, 2615–2623. [CrossRef]
45. Ghose, A.K.; Viswanadhan, V.N.; Wendoloski, J.J. A Knowledge-Based Approach in Designing Combinatorial or Medicinal Chemistry Libraries for Drug Discovery. 1. A Qualitative and Quantitative Characterization of Known Drug Databases. *J. Comb. Chem.* **1999**, *1*, 55–68. [CrossRef] [PubMed]
46. Egan, W.J.; Merz, K.M.; Baldwin, J.J. Prediction of Drug Absorption Using Multivariate Statistics. *J. Med. Chem.* **2000**, *43*, 3867–3877. [CrossRef] [PubMed]
47. Daina, A.; Michielin, O.; Zoete, V. SwissADME: A free web tool to evaluate pharmacokinetics, drug-likeness and medicinal chemistry friendliness of small molecules. *Sci. Rep.* **2017**, *7*, 42717. [CrossRef] [PubMed]
48. Pires, D.E.; Blundell, T.L.; Ascher, D.B. pkCSM: Predicting Small-Molecule Pharmacokinetic and Toxicity Properties Using Graph-Based Signatures. *J. Med. Chem.* **2015**, *58*, 4066–4072. [CrossRef]
49. Durán, Á.; Zamora, I.; Pastor, M. Suitability of GRIND-Based Principal Properties for the Description of Molecular Similarity and Ligand-Based Virtual Screening. *J. Chem. Inf. Modeling* **2009**, *49*, 2129–2138. [CrossRef]
50. PDSP (Psychoactive Drug Screening Program) Ki Database. Available online: https://pdsp.unc.edu/databases/kidb.php (accessed on 24 June 2021).
51. Coleman, J.A.; Navratna, V.; Antermite, D.; Yang, D.; Bull, J.A.; Gouaux, E. Chemical and structural investigation of the paroxetine-human serotonin transporter complex. *Elife* **2020**, *9*, e56427. [CrossRef]
52. Wang, S.; Che, T.; Levit, A.; Shoichet, B.K.; Wacker, D.; Roth, B.L. Structure of the D2 dopamine receptor bound to the atypical antipsychotic drug risperidone. *Nature* **2018**, *555*, 269–273. [CrossRef]
53. Jumper, J.; Evans, R.; Pritzel, A.; Green, T.; Figurnov, M.; Ronneberger, O.; Tunyasuvunakool, K.; Bates, R.; Žídek, A.; Potapenko, A.; et al. Highly accurate protein structure prediction with AlphaFold. *Nature* **2021**, *596*, 583–589. [CrossRef]
54. Gagnon, J.K.; Law, S.M.; Brooks, C.L., 3rd. Flexible CDOCKER: Development and application of a pseudo-explicit structure-based docking method within CHARMM. *J. Comput. Chem.* **2016**, *37*, 753–762. [CrossRef]
55. Rao, P.P.; Pham, A.T.; Shakeri, A.; El Shatshat, A.; Zhao, Y.; Karuturi, R.C.; Hefny, A.A. Drug repurposing: Dipeptidyl peptidase IV (DPP4) inhibitors as potential agents to treat SARS-CoV-2 (2019-nCov) infection. *Pharmaceuticals* **2021**, *14*, 44. [CrossRef] [PubMed]
56. Kim, S.; Chen, J.; Cheng, T.; Gindulyte, A.; He, J.; He, S.; Li, Q.; Shoemaker, B.A.; Thiessen, P.A.; Yu, B.; et al. PubChem in 2021: New data content and improved web interfaces. *Nucleic Acids Res.* **2020**, *49*, D1388–D1395. [CrossRef]
57. Höfer, P.; Schosser, A.; Calati, R.; Serretti, A.; Massat, I.; Kocabas, N.A.; Konstantinidis, A.; Linotte, S.; Mendlewicz, J.; Souery, D.; et al. The impact of Cytochrome P450 CYP1A2, CYP2C9, CYP2C19 and CYP2D6 genes on suicide attempt and suicide risk-a European multicentre study on treatment-resistant major depressive disorder. *Eur. Arch. Psychiatry Clin. Neurosci.* **2013**, *263*, 385–391. [CrossRef] [PubMed]
58. Pushpakom, S.; Iorio, F.; Eyers, P.A.; Escott, K.J.; Hopper, S.; Wells, A.; Doig, A.; Guilliams, T.; Latimer, J.; McNamee, C.; et al. Drug repurposing: Progress, challenges and recommendations. *Nat. Rev. Drug Discov.* **2019**, *18*, 41–58. [CrossRef] [PubMed]
59. Cañizares-Carmenate, Y.; Mena-Ulecia, K.; MacLeod Carey, D.; Perera-Sardiña, Y.; Hernández-Rodríguez, E.W.; Marrero-Ponce, Y.; Torrens, F.; Castillo-Garit, J.A. Machine learning approach to discovery of small molecules with potential inhibitory action against vasoactive metalloproteases. *Mol. Divers.* **2021**, 1–15. [CrossRef]
60. Udrescu, M.; Udrescu, L. A Drug Repurposing Method Based on Drug-Drug Interaction Networks and Using Energy Model Layouts. *Methods Mol. Biol.* **2019**, *1903*, 185–201.
61. Udrescu, L.; Sbârcea, L.; Topîrceanu, A.; Iovanovici, A.; Kurunczi, L.; Bogdan, P.; Udrescu, M. Clustering drug-drug interaction networks with energy model layouts: Community analysis and drug repurposing. *Sci. Rep.* **2016**, *6*, 32745. [CrossRef]
62. Udrescu, L.; Bogdan, P.; Chiş, A.; Sîrbu, I.O.; Topîrceanu, A.; Văruţ, >R.-M.; Udrescu, M. Uncovering New Drug Properties in Target-Based Drug–Drug Similarity Networks. *Pharmaceutics* **2020**, *12*, 879. [CrossRef]
63. Sánchez-Martínez, J.D.; Bueno, M.; Alvarez-Rivera, G.; Tudela, J.; Ibañez, E.; Cifuentes, A. In Vitro neuroprotective potential of terpenes from industrial orange juice by-products. *Food Funct.* **2021**, *12*, 302–314. [CrossRef]
64. Zhan, Y.Y.; Liang, B.Q.; Li, X.Y.; Gu, E.M.; Dai, D.P.; Cai, J.P.; Hu, G.X. The effect of resveratrol on pharmacokinetics of aripiprazole in vivo and in vitro. *Xenobiotica* **2016**, *46*, 439–444. [CrossRef]
65. Yim, S.K.; Kim, K.; Chun, S.; Oh, T.; Jung, W.; Jung, K.; Yun, C.H. Screening of Human CYP1A2 and CYP3A4 Inhibitors from Seaweed In Silico and In Vitro. *Mar. Drugs* **2020**, *18*, 603. [CrossRef]
66. Elbarbry, F.; Ung, A.; Abdelkawy, K. Studying the Inhibitory Effect of Quercetin and Thymoquinone on Human Cytochrome P450 Enzyme Activities. *Pharmacogn. Mag.* **2018**, *13*, S895–S899.
67. Ganzera, M.; Schneider, P.; Stuppner, H. Inhibitory effects of the essential oil of chamomile (Matricaria recutita L.) and its major constituents on human cytochrome P450 enzymes. *Life Sci.* **2006**, *78*, 856–861. [CrossRef]

68. Koyama, S.; Heinbockel, T. The Effects of Essential Oils and Terpenes in Relation to Their Routes of Intake and Application. *Int. J. Mol. Sci.* **2020**, *21*, 1558. [CrossRef]
69. Saiyudthong, S.; Mekseepralard, C. Effect of Inhaling Bergamot Oil on Depression-Related Behaviors in Chronic Stressed Rats. *J. Med Assoc. Thail.* **2015**, *98* (Suppl. 9), S152–S159.
70. Garzoli, S.; Turchetti, G.; Giacomello, P.; Tiezzi, A.; Laghezza Masci, V.; Ovidi, E. Liquid and Vapour Phase of Lavandin (Lavandula × intermedia) Essential Oil: Chemical Composition and Antimicrobial Activity. *Molecules* **2019**, *24*, 2701. [CrossRef] [PubMed]
71. Jamal, M.; Ameno, K.; Ameno, S.; Morishita, J.; Wang, W.; Kumihashi, M.; Ikuo, U.; Miki, T.; Ijiri, I. Changes in cholinergic function in the frontal cortex and hippocampus of rat exposed to ethanol and acetaldehyde. *Neuroscience* **2007**, *144*, 232–238. [CrossRef] [PubMed]
72. Tozar, T.; Santos Costa, S.; Udrea, A.-M.; Nastasa, V.; Couto, I.; Viveiros, M.; Pascu, M.L.; Romanitan, M.O. Anti-staphylococcal activity and mode of action of thioridazine photoproducts. *Sci. Rep.* **2020**, *10*, 18043. [CrossRef] [PubMed]
73. Udrea, A.-M.; Avram, S.; Nistorescu, S.; Pascu, M.-L.; Romanitan, M.O. Laser irradiated phenothiazines: New potential treatment for COVID-19 explored by molecular docking. *J. Photochem. Photobiol. B Biol.* **2020**, *211*, 111997. [CrossRef]
74. Avram, S.; Puia, A.; Udrea, A.M.; Mihailescu, D.; Mernea, M.; Dinischiotu, A.; Oancea, F.; Stiens, J. Natural Compounds Therapeutic Features in Brain Disorders by Experimental, Bioinformatics and Cheminformatics Methods. *Curr. Med. Chem.* **2020**, *27*, 78–98. [CrossRef]

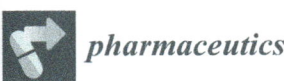 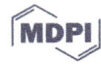

Article

Exploring Drugs and Vaccines Associated with Altered Risks and Severity of COVID-19: A UK Biobank Cohort Study of All ATC Level-4 Drug Categories Reveals Repositioning Opportunities

Yong Xiang [1], Kenneth Chi-Yin Wong [1] and Hon-Cheong So [1,2,3,4,5,6,7,*]

1. Lo Kwee-Seong Integrated Biomedical Sciences Building, School of Biomedical Sciences, Faculty of Medicine, The Chinese University of Hong Kong, Shatin, Hong Kong, China; xyong11@link.cuhk.edu.hk (Y.X.); mail@cywong.hk (K.C.-Y.W.)
2. KIZ-CUHK Joint Laboratory of Bioresources and Molecular Research of Common Diseases, Kunming Institute of Zoology, Kunming 650223, China
3. CUHK Shenzhen Research Institute, Shenzhen 518172, China
4. Department of Psychiatry, Faculty of Medicine, The Chinese University of Hong Kong, Shatin, Hong Kong, China
5. Margaret K.L. Cheung Research Centre for Management of Parkinsonism, The Chinese University of Hong Kong, Shatin, Hong Kong, China
6. Brain and Mind Institute, The Chinese University of Hong Kong, Shatin, Hong Kong, China
7. Hong Kong Branch of the Chinese Academy of Sciences Center for Excellence in Animal Evolution and Genetics, The Chinese University of Hong Kong, Shatin, Hong Kong, China
* Correspondence: hcso@cuhk.edu.hk; Tel.: +852-3943-9255

Citation: Xiang, Y.; Wong, K.C.-Y.; So, H.-C. Exploring Drugs and Vaccines Associated with Altered Risks and Severity of COVID-19: A UK Biobank Cohort Study of All ATC Level-4 Drug Categories Reveals Repositioning Opportunities. *Pharmaceutics* **2021**, *13*, 1514. https://doi.org/10.3390/pharmaceutics13091514

Academic Editors: Lucreţia Udrescu, Ludovic Kurunczi, Paul Bogdan and Mihai Udrescu

Received: 13 August 2021
Accepted: 10 September 2021
Published: 18 September 2021

Publisher's Note: MDPI stays neutral with regard to jurisdictional claims in published maps and institutional affiliations.

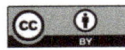

Copyright: © 2021 by the authors. Licensee MDPI, Basel, Switzerland. This article is an open access article distributed under the terms and conditions of the Creative Commons Attribution (CC BY) license (https://creativecommons.org/licenses/by/4.0/).

Abstract: Effective therapies for COVID-19 are still lacking, and drug repositioning is a promising approach to address this problem. Here, we adopted a medical informatics approach to repositioning. We leveraged a large prospective cohort, the UK-Biobank (UKBB, $N \sim 397{,}000$), and studied associations of prior use of all level-4 ATC drug categories ($N = 819$, including vaccines) with COVID-19 diagnosis and severity. Effects of drugs on the risk of infection, disease severity, and mortality were investigated separately. Logistic regression was conducted, controlling for main confounders. We observed strong and highly consistent protective associations with statins. Many top-listed protective drugs were also cardiovascular medications, such as angiotensin-converting enzyme inhibitors (ACEI), angiotensin receptor blockers (ARB), calcium channel blocker (CCB), and beta-blockers. Some other drugs showing protective associations included biguanides (metformin), estrogens, thyroid hormones, proton pump inhibitors, and testosterone-5-alpha reductase inhibitors, among others. We also observed protective associations by influenza, pneumococcal, and several other vaccines. Subgroup and interaction analyses were also conducted, which revealed differences in protective effects in various subgroups. For example, protective effects of flu/pneumococcal vaccines were weaker in obese individuals, while protection by statins was stronger in cardiovascular patients. To conclude, our analysis revealed many drug repositioning candidates, for example several cardiovascular medications. Further studies are required for validation.

Keywords: COVID-19; drug repositioning; UK Biobank; vaccine

1. Introduction

Coronavirus disease 2019 (COVID-19) has resulted in a pandemic affecting more than a hundred countries worldwide [1–3]. More than 220 million confirmed infections and 4.56 million fatalities have been reported worldwide as of 6 September 2021 (https://coronavirus.jhu.edu/map.html, accessed on 6 September 2021). Besides the burden due to the disease itself, COVID-19 has created heavy burdens on the medical systems in many countries and has led to delays in the diagnosis and treatment of other types of diseases [4,5]. Therefore, it is of urgent public interest to gain deeper understanding into the disease, including identifying risk factors (RFs) for infection and severe disease, and uncovering new treatment strategies.

Although vaccines have been developed for COVID-19, its distribution is highly uneven and only a small proportion of the world's population has been fully vaccinated so far. In addition, vaccine hesitancy remains a major issue that has led to suboptimal vaccination coverage [6,7]. Inadequate knowledge and awareness of COVID-19, especially among the younger population, may also contribute to the continuous rise in the number of cases [8]. Coupled with viral variants that may be associated with increased transmission and reduced vaccine effectiveness [9], the search for drugs that may reduce susceptibility to disease and/or disease severity remains highly important.

A number of clinical risk factors (e.g., age, obesity, cardiometabolic disorders, renal diseases, presence of multiple comorbidities) [10–15] have been found to increase the risk of infection or complications. However, it is less well-known how different drugs may affect the risks of COVID-19 or its severity. Importantly, drugs with protective effects may be potentially repurposed for the prevention or treatment of the disease, as development of a new drug is often extremely lengthy and costly.

Drug repositioning by computational or statistical approaches for COVID-19 is an area of intense interest. Please refer to other reviews (e.g., [16–18]) for an overview of recent studies. For instance, one widely used methodology is the network-based approach, which can integrate different data sources, including omics data and drug–protein–disease interaction networks [16,19–21]. Another methodology is the structure-based approach, which enables a large number of compounds to be screened for their ability to bind to known or predicted molecular targets for COVID-19 treatment [16,22–25]. These methodologies are promising but may have their limitations. For example, they generally do not provide direct evidence for the candidates' effectiveness in real-world or clinical settings. In addition, these approaches may be limited by inadequate knowledge of the pathophysiology and molecular basis of COVID-19. Another limitation is that most drug repositioning studies did not consider patient characteristics; for example, a drug may be more effective within a certain age group or in those with a certain comorbidity. In addition, the effect size (e.g., relative risk reduction) of individual drugs and the level of statistical significance usually cannot be easily estimated by network/structure-based approaches.

Here, we employed a different methodology *not* previously applied to drug repositioning studies for COVID-19. We adopted a medical informatics approach which involves screening a large number of drugs for their associations with the disease, leveraging a large-scale population cohort. In brief, we performed a comprehensive study on all Anatomical Therapeutic Chemical Classification System (ATC) level-4 drug categories ($N = 819$) and assessed their associations with susceptibility to, and severity of, COVID-19 in the UK Biobank (UKBB), controlling for possible confounders. Vaccines were also included for analysis. To our knowledge, this is the most comprehensive analysis to date to screen for drug associations and repositioning candidates for COVID-19, leveraging real-world population data.

While pharmacoepidemiology studies are typically focused on one or a few drugs, COVID-19 is a new disease, and we still have limited understanding of its pathophysiology and treatment. As a result, a hypothesis-driven approach may have important limitations of missing potential drug associations and new repositioning candidates. In the field of genetic epidemiology, it has been observed that hypothesis-driven candidate gene studies are not as reliable as genome-wide association studies (GWAS) [26] which are relatively unbiased, indicating merits of the latter approach. In the same vein, here we adopted a "drug-wide" association study approach, which provides a systematic and unbiased assessment of drug associations and repositioning candidates. This approach has also been advocated before [27].

In the present study, we performed rigorous analyses on the impact of medications/vaccinations on the risk of infection, disease severity, and mortality. Analyses were also conducted within infected patients, tested subjects, and the whole population respectively, and for five different time windows of prescriptions. We also performed further subgroup and interaction analyses to reveal differential effects of the drugs in people with different clinical background. This may enable more "personalized" drug repositioning, i.e., prioritizing drug candidates for specific patient subgroups.

2. Methods

2.1. UK Biobank Data

The UK Biobank is a large-scale prospective cohort comprising over 500,000 subjects aged 40–69 years who were recruited in 2006–2010 [28]. In this study, subjects with recorded mortality before 31 January 2020 (N = 28,930) were excluded, as it was the date for the first recorded case in UK. This study was conducted under project 28732.

2.2. COVID-19 Phenotypes

COVID-19 outcome data were downloaded from UKBB data portal. Information regarding COVID-19 data in the UKBB can be viewed at http://biobank.ndph.ox.ac.uk/showcase/exinfo.cgi?src=COVID19 (accessed on 3 November 2020). Briefly, the latest COVID test results were downloaded on 6 November 2020 (last update 3 November 2020). We consider inpatient (hospitalization) status at testing as a proxy for severity. Data on date and cause of mortality were also extracted (latest update on 21 October 2020). Cases indicated by U07.1 were considered to be (laboratory-confirmed) COVID-19-related fatalities.

A case was considered as having "severe COVID-19" if the subject was hospitalized and/or if the cause of mortality was U07.1. We required both test result and origin to be 1 (positive test and inpatient origin) to be considered as a hospitalized case. For a small number of subjects with initial outpatient origin and positive test result, but changed to inpatient origin and negative result within 2 weeks, we still considered these subjects inpatient cases (i.e., assume the hospitalization was related to the infection).

For a minority of subjects (N = 19) whose mortality cause was U07.1 but test results were negative within one week, to be conservative, they were excluded from subsequent analyses.

2.3. Medication Data

Medication data was obtained from the primary care data for COVID-19 research in UKBB (details available at https://biobank.ndph.ox.ac.uk/showcase/showcase/docs/gp4covid19.pdf, accessed on 9 November 2020). We made use of the latest release of General Practice (GP) records released by UKBB, which contains prescription data from two electronic health record (EHR) systems (TPP or EMIS) for ~397,000 UKBB participants. The drug code and issue date of each drug are available. Please also refer to Figure 1 for an overview of our analysis workflow.

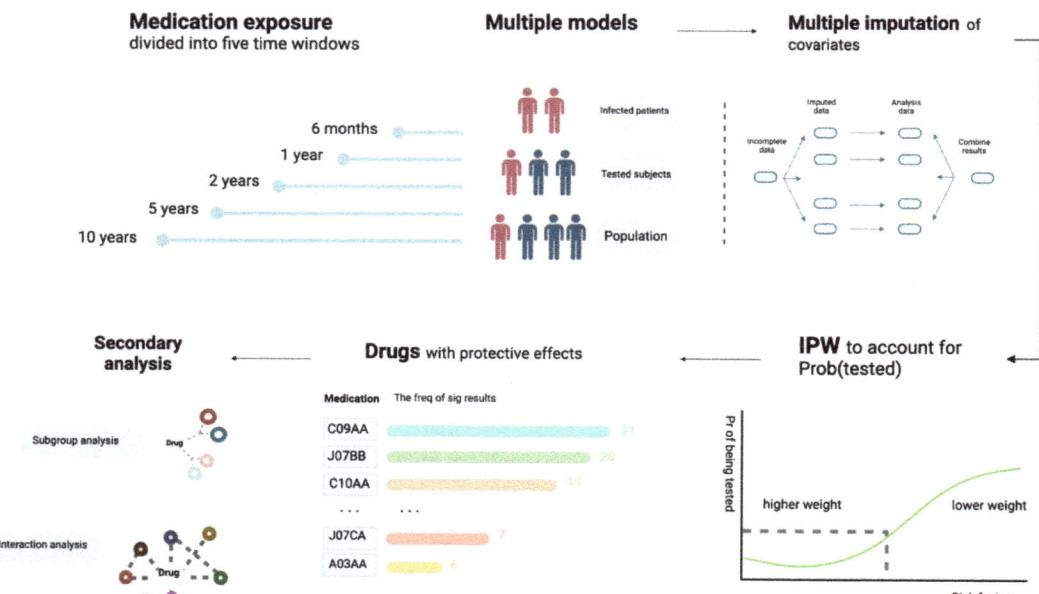

Figure 1. An overview of the analytic workflow. We considered five exposure time windows and multiple statistical models. We conducted analyses within infected patients, tested subjects, and the whole population, respectively. Effects of prescribed medications/vaccinations on the risk of infection, severity of disease (hospitalization as proxy) and mortality were investigated separately. Missing data were accounted for by multiple imputation. Inverse probability weighting (IPW) of the probability of being tested (Prob(tested)) was employed to reduce testing bias. Multivariable logistic regression was conducted, controlling for main confounders. We primarily focused on drugs with protective effects, as residual confounding tends to bias towards harmful effects. In addition, we performed further subgroup and interaction analysis to identify factors that may modify the drug effects.

2.3.1. Time Window of Prescriptions

Since the GP records cover many years of prescriptions, we set time windows to restrict prescriptions with a certain time period as the "exposure". The "index date" was defined as (1) the date of the first positive COVID-19 test for infected subjects (for U07.1 cases, the mortality date was regarded as the index date if no test record was found); or (2) the date of last test for those who were tested negative; or (3) 3 November 2020 (the date of the latest update of COVID-19 test results) for those who were untested.

The issue date of each prescription was available, but the duration was not. Time windows were determined by whether the drug was issued within a specified period before the index date. The following windows were considered for medications: 6 months, 1 year, 2 years, and 5 years. Narrower time windows (<6 months) may not be desirable and may lead to many prescriptions being missed, as the latest issue date was 25 July 2020, but the latest index date was 3 November 2020.

As for vaccines, unlike many medications, vaccines are not prescribed regularly, and most vaccines only need to be given once or less than a few times; hence, a narrow time window is not optimal due to sparsity of data. For seasonal vaccines, namely flu vaccines, they are usually given in autumn (September to November) or early winter in the UK. A time window of 6 months will lead to missing most of the flu vaccines given. On the other hand, it is also reasonable to consider a longer time window (e.g., 10 years) as vaccine effects can be more long-lasting [29]. In view of the above, we considered time windows of 1, 2, 5, and 10 years for vaccinations. For flu vaccines, we defined "past 1 year" as prescriptions from 1 September 2019 onwards (and similarly for past k years) to account for the seasonal nature of vaccination.

2.3.2. Mapping to ATC

All the medications were mapped to the ATC Classification (https://www.genome.jp/kegg-bin/get_htext?br08303, accessed on 9 November 2020). Drug categories were defined by the fourth level of ATC classification.

2.4. Covariate Data

We performed multivariable regression analysis with adjustment for potential confounders including basic demographic variables (age, sex, ethnic group), comorbidities (coronary artery disease (CAD), diabetes (DM), hypertension, asthma, chronic obstructive pulmonary disease (COPD), depression, dementia, history of cancer, blood urea and creatinine reflecting renal function), indicators of general health (number of medications taken, number of non-cancer illnesses), anthropometric measures (body mass index (BMI)), socioeconomic status (Townsend deprivation index) and lifestyle risk factor (smoking status). For disease traits, we included information from ICD-10 diagnoses (code 41270) and self-reported illnesses (code 20002), and incorporated data from all waves of follow-ups. Subjects with no records of the relevant disease from either self-report or ICD-10 were regarded as having no history of the disease.

2.5. Sets of Analysis

We performed a total of eight sets of analysis (Table 1). The impact of prescribed medication/vaccination on the risk of infection (Models E and F), severity of infection (Models A, C, and G) and risk of mortality (Models B, D, and H) from COVID-19 were investigated separately. Both hospitalized and fatal cases were grouped under the "severe" category.

Table 1. The eight sets of analyses based on infected patients (model A, B), tested subjects (models F, G, H) and the population (models C, D, E).

Model	Cohort 1	Cohort 2
A	Hospitalized or fatal infection (U07.1) (Severe)	Non-hospitalized COVID-19 (Mild)
B	U07.1 cases	All other COVID-19 cases
C	Hospitalized or fatal infection (U07.1) (Severe)	UKBB subjects without COVID-19 Dx or tested-ve
D	U07.1 cases	UKBB subjects without COVID-19 Dx or tested-ve
E	Infected	UKBB subjects without COVID-19 Dx or tested-ve
F	Infected	Tested-ve
G	Hospitalized or fatal infection (U07.1) (Severe)	Tested-ve
H	U07.1 cases	Tested-ve

U07.1 is the code for fatal (laboratory-confirmed) COVID-19 infection based on the latest ICD coding. Dx, diagnosis; -ve, negative.

We also considered different study designs and conducted our analyses with different comparison samples. Models A and B are restricted to the infected subjects, while models C, D, and E involve comparison of severe, fatal and general infected cases to the general population (with no known diagnosis of COVID-19). On the other hand, models F, G, and H compared infected, severe, and fatal cases, respectively, against subjects who were tested negative for SARS-CoV-2.

There were 397,000 subjects in the UKBB with available GP prescription records. Among them, 30,835 subjects have received at least one COVID-19 test, and 3858 had been tested positive. There were 1318 cases classified as "severe" (hospitalized or mortality from COVID-19) and 170 fatal cases. In total 393,142 UKBB participants did not have a known diagnosis of COVID-19. The detailed count of participants for each model is listed in Table 2.

Table 2. Number of available subjects for analysis for the 8 models.

Model	Cohort 1	Cohort 2	Total
A	1318	2540	3858
B	170	3688	3858
C	1318	393,142	394,460
D	170	393,142	393,312
E	3858	393,142	397,000
F	3858	26,977	30,835
G	1318	26,977	28,295
H	170	26,977	27,147

Only subjects with available GP prescription records are shown.

2.6. Statistical Analysis Methods

Logistic regression (using the R package speedglm) was used to examine the impact of medication on different outcomes in the eight sets of analysis. For more stable estimates, analysis was not performed if the number of subjects taking the drug in the affected or unaffected group was less than five. All statistical analyses were conducted using R. The false discovery rate (FDR) approach by Benjamini and Hochberg [30] was performed to control for multiple testing. This approach controls the expected proportion of false positives among the rejected null hypotheses.

2.7. Imputation of Missing Data

Missing values of remaining features were imputed with the R package "missRanger". The program is based on missForest, which is an iterative imputation approach based on random forest (RF). It has been widely used and shown to produce low imputation errors and good performance in predictive models [31]. The program missRanger is largely based on the algorithm of missForest, but uses the R package "ranger" [32] to build RF for improvement in speed (we found that other packages, such as MICE and missForest, are computationally too slow to produce results for the large-scale analyses here). Predictive mean matching (pmm) was employed to avoid imputation of values not present in the original data, and to increase variance to more realistic levels for multiple imputation (MI). We followed the default settings with pmm.k = 5 and num.trees = 100. We performed the analyses on multiply imputed datasets (imputed for 10 times) and combined the results by Rubin's rules [33] using the function "mi.meld" under the R package "amelia". Another advantage of missRanger is that out-of-bag errors (in terms of classification errors or normalized root-mean-squared error) could be computed, which provides an estimate of imputation accuracy.

2.8. Inverse Probability Weighting of the Probability of Being Tested

Bias due to non-random testing has been discussed previously in other works [34,35]. As a person has to be tested to be diagnosed with COVID-19, factors leading to increased probability of being tested will also lead to an apparent increase in the risk of infection [35]. In addition, it has been raised that collider bias can occur when conditioned on the tested group. This could result in spurious associations, for example, between a risk factor and COVID-19 severity if both increases the probability of being tested (Pr(tested)). One way to reduce this kind of bias is to employ inverse probability weighting (IPW) of Pr(tested). Essentially, we wish to create a pseudo-population, or mimic a scenario under which testing is random instead of selected for certain subgroups. The IPW approach up-weighs those who are less likely to be tested and down-weighs those who have a high chance of being tested. This may create more unbiased estimates of the effects of drugs.

We took reference to the approach described in [34] to analyze the data with IPW. Following our recent work [36] which aims to predict COVID-19 severity with machine learning (ML), here we also employed an ML model (XGboost) to predict Pr(tested) based on a range of factors. An advantage of using ML models is that nonlinear and complex interactions can be considered, which may improve predictive performance over logistic models. We employed the same set of predictors as in our previous work [36], and followed the same analysis strategy of hyper-parameter tuning and cross-validation to obtain predicted probabilities (please refer to [36] for details). Beta-calibration [37] was performed, and the resulting average AUC was 0.622. The predicted probabilities (i.e., Pr(tested)) were used to construct weights for IPW. Stabilized weights [38] were used.

2.9. Subgroup Analysis

For selected drugs showing tentative protective effects, we also performed further subgroup and interaction analyses. These drugs included cardiovascular medications listed in Table 3, four vaccines with protective associations (influenza, pneumococcal, typhoid, and combined bacterial/viral vaccines), and other top drugs with consistent protective associations across multiple models/time windows as listed in Table 4.

Table 3. Cardiometabolic medications showing significant protective associations (limited to FDR < 0.05) within time windows of 6, 12, and 24 months.

Window	Model	ATC Code	OR	conf.low	conf.high	p	FDR.BH	Full Name
1 year	C	A10BA	0.67	0.51	0.88	4.01×10^{-3}	1.11×10^{-2}	Biguanides
2 years	C	A10BA	0.68	0.52	0.90	5.79×10^{-3}	1.68×10^{-2}	Biguanides
0.5 year	F	C07AB	0.78	0.68	0.89	3.56×10^{-4}	7.40×10^{-3}	Beta blocking agents, selective
1 year	F	C07AB	0.80	0.70	0.91	7.59×10^{-4}	1.29×10^{-2}	Beta blocking agents, selective
2 years	F	C07AB	0.78	0.69	0.88	9.10×10^{-5}	2.15×10^{-3}	Beta blocking agents, selective
1 year	C	C08CA	0.76	0.64	0.90	1.31×10^{-3}	4.23×10^{-3}	Dihydropyridine derivatives
2 years	C	C08CA	0.78	0.66	0.92	3.27×10^{-3}	1.11×10^{-2}	Dihydropyridine derivatives
0.5 year	A	C09AA	0.68	0.53	0.87	2.11×10^{-3}	1.43×10^{-2}	ACE inhibitors, plain
0.5 year	C	C09AA	0.75	0.62	0.91	3.15×10^{-3}	6.48×10^{-3}	ACE inhibitors, plain
0.5 year	G	C09AA	0.68	0.56	0.83	1.13×10^{-4}	1.54×10^{-3}	ACE inhibitors, plain
1 year	A	C09AA	0.68	0.54	0.86	1.15×10^{-3}	1.03×10^{-2}	ACE inhibitors, plain
1 year	C	C09AA	0.61	0.51	0.74	1.59×10^{-7}	1.25×10^{-6}	ACE inhibitors, plain
1 year	D	C09AA	0.57	0.36	0.92	2.22×10^{-2}	4.31×10^{-2}	ACE inhibitors, plain
1 year	E	C09AA	0.79	0.72	0.88	1.40×10^{-5}	8.63×10^{-5}	ACE inhibitors, plain
1 year	G	C09AA	0.71	0.59	0.85	2.80×10^{-4}	4.00×10^{-3}	ACE inhibitors, plain
2 years	A	C09AA	0.67	0.54	0.84	5.87×10^{-4}	1.10×10^{-2}	ACE inhibitors, plain
2 years	C	C09AA	0.63	0.53	0.75	2.84×10^{-7}	2.60×10^{-6}	ACE inhibitors, plain
2 years	E	C09AA	0.81	0.73	0.90	5.38×10^{-5}	3.41×10^{-4}	ACE inhibitors, plain
2 years	G	C09AA	0.71	0.59	0.85	1.40×10^{-4}	2.81×10^{-3}	ACE inhibitors, plain
1 year	C	C09CA	0.68	0.54	0.85	7.58×10^{-4}	2.61×10^{-3}	Angiotensin II receptor blockers, plain
1 year	G	C09CA	0.69	0.55	0.87	1.95×10^{-3}	1.85×10^{-2}	Angiotensin II receptor blockers, plain
2 years	C	C09CA	0.73	0.58	0.90	3.97×10^{-3}	1.25×10^{-2}	Angiotensin II receptor blockers, plain
2 years	G	C09CA	0.72	0.58	0.90	3.93×10^{-3}	4.80×10^{-2}	Angiotensin II receptor blockers, plain
0.5 year	A	C10AA	0.57	0.47	0.68	3.37×10^{-9}	8.37×10^{-8}	HMG CoA reductase inhibitors
0.5 year	C	C10AA	0.79	0.68	0.91	1.20×10^{-3}	2.63×10^{-3}	HMG CoA reductase inhibitors
0.5 year	E	C10AA	1.14	1.05	1.24	1.64×10^{-3}	4.26×10^{-3}	HMG CoA reductase inhibitors
0.5 year	G	C10AA	0.66	0.57	0.76	2.55×10^{-8}	9.03×10^{-7}	HMG CoA reductase inhibitors
1 year	A	C10AA	0.50	0.42	0.60	2.87×10^{-13}	5.17×10^{-11}	HMG CoA reductase inhibitors
1 year	C	C10AA	0.49	0.42	0.57	2.97×10^{-21}	7.42×10^{-20}	HMG CoA reductase inhibitors
1 year	D	C10AA	0.50	0.34	0.74	5.28×10^{-4}	1.57×10^{-3}	HMG CoA reductase inhibitors
1 year	E	C10AA	0.83	0.77	0.91	1.69×10^{-5}	1.00×10^{-4}	HMG CoA reductase inhibitors
1 year	G	C10AA	0.63	0.54	0.73	4.15×10^{-10}	2.77×10^{-8}	HMG CoA reductase inhibitors
2 years	A	C10AA	0.49	0.40	0.58	1.55×10^{-14}	3.19×10^{-12}	HMG CoA reductase inhibitors
2 years	C	C10AA	0.49	0.43	0.57	7.09×10^{-21}	2.60×10^{-19}	HMG CoA reductase inhibitors
2 years	D	C10AA	0.50	0.34	0.74	4.38×10^{-4}	1.63×10^{-3}	HMG CoA reductase inhibitors
2 years	E	C10AA	0.86	0.79	0.93	3.09×10^{-4}	1.52×10^{-3}	HMG CoA reductase inhibitors
2 years	G	C10AA	0.63	0.54	0.72	2.65×10^{-10}	2.92×10^{-8}	HMG CoA reductase inhibitors

For space limits, only results with FDR < 0.05 are shown. Please refer to Tables S3 and S6 for full results. OR, odds ratio; conf.low, lower 95% CI for OR; conf.high, upper 95% CI for OR; FDR.BH, false discovery rate by the Benjamini–Hochberg method.

Table 4. Drugs showing consistent protective associations across 4 time-windows and 8 models (ranked by the frequency of being nominally significant, i.e., $p < 0.05$).

	ATC Code	Drug Name	Freq
1	C09AA	ACE inhibitors, plain	21
2	J07BB	Influenza vaccines	20
3	C10AA	HMG CoA reductase inhibitors	19
4	H03AA	Thyroid hormones	17
5	C09CA	Angiotensin II receptor blockers, plain	15
6	G04CB	Testosterone-5-alpha reductase inhibitors	12
7	A02BC	Proton pump inhibitors	11
8	C08CA	Dihydropyridine derivatives	11
9	R03BA	Glucocorticoids	9
10	C07AB	Beta blocking agents, selective	8
11	A10BA	Biguanides	7
12	B01AC	Platelet aggregation inhibitors excl. heparin	7
13	G03CA	Natural and semisynthetic estrogens, plain	7
14	J07CA	Bacterial and viral vaccines, combined	7
15	A03AA	Synthetic anticholinergics, esters with tertiary amino group	6

Frequency (freq) calculated based on results from time windows of 6 months to 5 years. Ophthalmological and dermatological agents are not listed in the above table.

Subgroup analysis was performed with respect to main demographic features (age, sex, and ethnicity) and main comorbidities (same as the diseases listed under "covariate data"). We also compared log(OR) estimates across the subgroups with or without the risk factor of interest. The test statistic was obtained by $z = (\beta_1 - \beta_2)/\sqrt{var(\beta_1) + var(\beta_2)}$, where β_1 and β_2 refer to the coefficients under the two independent subgroups.

2.10. Interaction Analysis

As a complementary approach, we also performed analysis with a logistic model including an interaction term (drug*risk_factor). The same set of drugs and risk factors were studied. The two approaches are similar in principle; however, stratified analysis yields more unbiased estimates if confounders have subgroup-dependent associations, while the interaction term approach produces more precise (lower-SE) estimates (hence higher power to detect interactions) [39].

2.11. Controlling for Other Drugs

We also performed additional regression analyses controlling for other top-ranked drugs. Two sets of analyses were conducted. In the first set of analysis, we controlled for the top 10 or 20 protective and harmful drugs in each time window and model. As for the second analysis, for drugs with protective associations, we controlled all other protective drugs with FDR < 0.05 or 0.1 (this analysis was performed for protective drugs only, as there were too many drugs associated with harmful effects to be included as covariates).

3. Results

Due to the large number of models and drugs being studied, we highlight the main results and findings from different sensitivity analysis.

Confounding by indication and other comorbidities is unavoidable, and, in particular, drugs showing harmful effects may possibly be explained by such confounding. On the other hand, as it is expected that most diseases tend to *increase* the risk/severity of infection, drugs showing *protective* effects are much less likely to be affected by confounding, and such associations may be relatively more reliable. We therefore place a greater emphasis on protective drugs in the sections below; this is also in line with our primary objective to prioritize repositioning candidates. Drugs with harmful effects are briefly discussed for comprehensiveness.

A summary of the demographic and covariate data of the original UKBB dataset is shown in Table S1. The missing rates and out-of-bag (OOB) errors for different variables from multiple imputations are shown in Table S2.

3.1. Primary Analysis with Multiple Imputation of Covariates

Full results of all drug categories across all time windows (including 6, 12, 24, 60, and 120 months; the last time window only for vaccines) are shown in Tables S6–S10. All protective associations (with at least nominal significance, i.e., $p < 0.05$) are shown in Table S3, while all association results with vaccines are presented in Table S4. For drugs associated with increased odds of infection/severity, we also summarize the top 10 drugs (ranked by p-value) from each model and time window, and organize them together in Table S5.

3.1.1. Overview

Across all categories, statins showed the strongest and most consistent protective associations. Highly significant protective effects were seen across infected subjects, tested subjects, or the whole population, especially in reducing the severity or mortality of infection. Albeit with smaller effect sizes, we also observed that statins might be linked to lower susceptibility to infection (model E). Interestingly, a number of top-listed drugs are also cardiovascular medications, such as angiotensin-converting enzyme inhibitors (ACEI), angiotensin receptor blockers (ARB), calcium channel blocker (CCB), and beta-blockers.

For simplicity, odds ratios (OR) are presented for a time horizon of 1 year if not further specified.

3.1.2. Drugs for Cardiometabolic Disorders

Significant protective associations with FDR < 0.05 are shown in Table 3. Statins showed protective effects across models A, C, D, E, and G. Significant protective effects against severe infection were seen among infected subjects (OR for prescriptions within a 12-month window, same below: 0.50, 95% CI: 0.42–0.60), tested subjects (OR = 0.63, 0.54–0.73), or when comparing severe cases to the general population (OR = 0.49, 0.42–0.57). In addition, protective association against fatal infection was observed (OR = 0.51, CI 0.34–0.74). Statins was also associated with lower susceptibility to infection, with ORs of 0.83 (CI: 0.77–0.91) and 0.86 (CI: 0.79–0.93) for prescriptions within 1 year and 2 years, respectively.

Another group of drugs with highly consistent protective associations were *ACEI and ARB*. ACEI showed protective associations against severe disease among infected subjects (model A: OR for 1-year time window, same below: 0.68, CI: 0.54–0.86), and when compared to the general population (model C: OR 1 year = 0.61, CI: 0.51–0.74) or test-negative subjects (model G: OR 1 year = 0.71, CI: 0.59–0.85). We also observed association with lower odds of infection at a population level (model E: OR 1 year = 0.81, CI: 0.73–0.90); the effect size seemed to decrease over longer time windows. ARBs also showed protective associations against severe disease in the population (model C: OR 1 year = 0.68, CI: 0.54–0.85) or among tested individuals (model G: OR 1 year = 0.68, CI: 0.55–0.87).

Biguanides (mainly metformin) were associated with lower odds of severe illness among the infected (model A: OR for 2-year time window = 0.60, CI: 0.42–0.86) and in the population (model C; OR 1 year = 0.67, CI: 0.51–0.88). Other drugs of interest include beta-blockers, which were associated with lower risk of infection among tested subjects (model F, OR 1 year = 0.80, CI: 0.70–0.91), and CCBs (C08CA) which were associated with lower odds of severe disease in the population (model C, OR 1 year: 0.76, CI: 0.64–0.90).

3.1.3. Vaccines

Significant associations for vaccines with FDR < 0.05 are shown in Table 5. One of the most consistent associations was observed for influenza vaccines. Protective associations were observed across almost all models (B to H), and across all time windows. Flu vaccination was associated with lower odds of infection when compared to population controls (model E; OR 1 year = 0.73, CI: 0.65–0.83) or compared to test-negative individuals (model F; OR 1 year = 0.60, CI: 0.53–0.68). Similar protective effects were also observed when restricting the cases to severe cases (model C: OR 1 year = 0.74; CI: 0.60–0.91; model G: OR 1 year = 0.61, CI: 0.50–0.76). Association with lower odds of mortality was also observed, although the confidence interval is wide as the number of fatal cases was small (model D: OR 1 year = 0.28, CI: 0.13–0.63; model H: OR 1 year = 0.23, CI: 0.11–0.52). The effect sizes in general became weaker with longer time windows.

Table 5. Vaccines with significant protective associations (limited to FDR < 0.05) within time windows of 1, 2, 5, and 10 years.

Window	Model	ATC Code	OR	conf.low	conf.high	p	FDR.BH	Full Name
1 year	F	J07AL	0.50	0.31	0.82	5.29×10^{-3}	4.65×10^{-2}	Pneumococcal vaccines
2 years	F	J07AL	0.59	0.42	0.82	1.59×10^{-3}	2.17×10^{-2}	Pneumococcal vaccines
5 years	E	J07AL	0.70	0.55	0.89	3.81×10^{-3}	1.62×10^{-2}	Pneumococcal vaccines
5 years	F	J07AL	0.61	0.47	0.79	1.47×10^{-4}	3.27×10^{-3}	Pneumococcal vaccines
10 years	E	J07AL	0.78	0.67	0.91	1.89×10^{-3}	8.52×10^{-3}	Pneumococcal vaccines
10 years	F	J07AL	0.67	0.57	0.78	9.39×10^{-7}	4.23×10^{-6}	Pneumococcal vaccines
10 years	G	J07AL	0.67	0.51	0.87	3.32×10^{-3}	9.20×10^{-3}	Pneumococcal vaccines
5 years	F	J07AM	0.45	0.29	0.68	1.93×10^{-4}	3.73×10^{-3}	Tetanus vaccines
10 years	E	J07AM	0.65	0.45	0.92	1.60×10^{-2}	4.23×10^{-2}	Tetanus vaccines
10 years	F	J07AM	0.49	0.34	0.71	1.69×10^{-4}	3.80×10^{-4}	Tetanus vaccines
5 years	F	J07AP	0.70	0.58	0.84	1.60×10^{-4}	3.30×10^{-3}	Typhoid vaccines
10 years	E	J07AP	0.86	0.76	0.97	1.88×10^{-2}	4.23×10^{-2}	Typhoid vaccines
10 years	F	J07AP	0.76	0.67	0.88	1.18×10^{-4}	3.55×10^{-4}	Typhoid vaccines
10 years	G	J07AP	0.74	0.58	0.95	1.61×10^{-2}	2.82×10^{-2}	Typhoid vaccines
1 year	C	J07BB	0.74	0.60	0.91	3.80×10^{-3}	1.08×10^{-2}	Influenza vaccines
1 year	D	J07BB	0.28	0.13	0.63	1.92×10^{-3}	4.68×10^{-3}	Influenza vaccines
1 year	E	J07BB	0.73	0.65	0.83	5.93×10^{-7}	4.50×10^{-6}	Influenza vaccines
1 year	F	J07BB	0.60	0.53	0.68	2.94×10^{-15}	6.97×10^{-13}	Influenza vaccines
1 year	G	J07BB	0.61	0.50	0.76	4.35×10^{-6}	1.09×10^{-4}	Influenza vaccines
1 year	H	J07BB	0.23	0.11	0.52	4.04×10^{-4}	3.32×10^{-3}	Influenza vaccines
2 years	C	J07BB	0.75	0.62	0.90	2.01×10^{-3}	7.27×10^{-3}	Influenza vaccines
2 years	D	J07BB	0.30	0.15	0.60	7.22×10^{-4}	2.30×10^{-3}	Influenza vaccines
2 years	E	J07BB	0.75	0.68	0.84	4.83×10^{-7}	4.83×10^{-6}	Influenza vaccines
2 years	F	J07BB	0.62	0.55	0.70	4.38×10^{-16}	1.14×10^{-13}	Influenza vaccines
2 years	G	J07BB	0.62	0.52	0.75	8.86×10^{-7}	2.78×10^{-5}	Influenza vaccines
2 years	H	J07BB	0.25	0.12	0.50	9.64×10^{-5}	9.11×10^{-4}	Influenza vaccines
5 years	D	J07BB	0.53	0.32	0.86	9.80×10^{-3}	3.83×10^{-2}	Influenza vaccines
5 years	E	J07BB	0.80	0.73	0.88	7.01×10^{-6}	5.79×10^{-5}	Influenza vaccines
5 years	F	J07BB	0.66	0.60	0.73	7.67×10^{-16}	1.11×10^{-13}	Influenza vaccines
5 years	G	J07BB	0.69	0.59	0.81	8.14×10^{-6}	2.93×10^{-4}	Influenza vaccines
5 years	H	J07BB	0.44	0.27	0.72	1.12×10^{-3}	1.07×10^{-2}	Influenza vaccines
10 years	D	J07BB	0.59	0.39	0.90	1.51×10^{-2}	4.54×10^{-2}	Influenza vaccines
10 years	E	J07BB	0.82	0.75	0.89	6.70×10^{-6}	6.03×10^{-5}	Influenza vaccines
10 years	F	J07BB	0.67	0.61	0.74	5.16×10^{-17}	4.64×10^{-16}	Influenza vaccines
10 years	G	J07BB	0.69	0.59	0.80	9.82×10^{-7}	6.87×10^{-6}	Influenza vaccines
10 years	H	J07BB	0.50	0.32	0.76	1.44×10^{-3}	4.31×10^{-3}	Influenza vaccines
1 year	F	J07CA	0.56	0.38	0.84	4.30×10^{-3}	3.97×10^{-2}	Bacterial and viral vaccines, combined
2 years	F	J07CA	0.71	0.57	0.89	3.05×10^{-3}	3.59×10^{-2}	Bacterial and viral vaccines, combined
10 years	F	J07CA	0.85	0.78	0.94	7.85×10^{-4}	1.41×10^{-3}	Bacterial and viral vaccines, combined
10 years	G	J07CA	0.78	0.66	0.92	3.94×10^{-3}	9.20×10^{-3}	Bacterial and viral vaccines, combined

For space limits, only results with FDR < 0.05 are shown. Please refer to Table S4 for full results.

In view of the significant findings, we repeated the analyses on flu vaccines with other ways to define the exposure (Table S14). First, we defined the exposure based on the actual season of vaccination instead of any vaccines received in the past k years. For people who had received flu vaccination in 2019–2020 (regardless of vaccination in other years), the OR for infection was 0.60 (CI: 0.53–0.68), compared to those who had not (test-negative subjects as controls, model F; same below). The OR was attenuated to 0.76 (CI: 0.67–0.87) if the exposure was defined as flu vaccination in 2015–2016 (regardless of vaccination in other years). We then narrowed down the exposure as receiving flu vaccine in the last season (2019–2020) but *not* in 2018–2019; the resulting OR was 0.67 (CI: 0.53–0.83). On the other hand, if we considered exposure as vaccination in 2018–19 but not 2019–20, the OR became weaker and nonsignificant (OR = 0.80, CI: 0.63–1.01). Those who received the vaccine consecutively for the last two seasons had similar but slightly stronger protection from infection (OR = 0.59, CI: 0.51–0.69); however, the CI overlaps with other estimates. A similar pattern of association was observed for model E (population controls). In general, more recent vaccination was associated with stronger protective effects.

Pneumococcal vaccines were also associated with protection against infection, especially within tested subjects (model F: OR 1 year = 0.50, CI: 0.31–0.82), which shows a trend of attenuation with longer time windows (OR for 10-year window = 0.67, CI: 0.51–0.87). Another group of vaccines showing protective effects is J07CA (bacterial and viral vaccines), which was significant under model F (OR for 1-year window: 0.56, CI: 0.38–0.84); it also showed weakening of effect over time. Other significant associations included tetanus and typhoid vaccines, which were observed to be protective against infections.

3.1.4. Other Drugs Showing Protective Associations

Significant results for other drugs having protective effects and FDR < 0.05 are shown in Table 6. As for other drugs, proton pump inhibitors (PPI) were associated with lower odds of infection when we compared test-positive against test-negative patients (model F: OR 1 year = 0.77, CI: 0.71–0.83); the ORs showed a gradient with largest effect within 6 month of use (OR = 0.72) and became weaker at the 5-year time window (OR = 0.87). PPI was also significantly associated with lower severity of disease.

Natural and semisynthetic estrogens (ATC G03CA) were linked to lower risk of infection and severity in the tested population (model F: OR 1 year = 0.67, CI: 0.58–0.78), which showed attenuation of effect over time. The largest effect size was noted within 6 months of use (OR = 0.63), which was attenuated for a 5-year time window (OR = 0.73). Similar protective associations were observed under model G, with severity as the outcome.

Prior use of thyroid hormones was consistently associated with lower risk of infection and severity, no matter whether the general population or test-negative individuals were considered as controls. The ORs were similar across all time windows. For model E (infected vs. population), the OR for 1-year time window was 0.80 (CI 0.71 to 0.92), which was close to the effect size under model F (infected vs. test-negative). For model C (hospitalized/fatal cases vs. population), the OR for 1-year time window was 0.62 (CI 0.48 to 0.79), and it was similar when constrained to tested subjects.

Table 6. Other drugs with significant protective associations (limited to FDR < 0.05) within time windows of 6, 12, and 24 months.

Window	Model	ATC Code	OR	conf.low	conf.high	p	FDR.BH	Full Name
0.5 year	F	A02BC	0.72	0.67	0.79	1.05×10^{-13}	2.18×10^{-11}	Proton pump inhibitors
0.5 year	G	A02BC	0.70	0.61	0.81	1.06×10^{-6}	2.08×10^{-5}	Proton pump inhibitors
1 year	A	A02BC	0.77	0.65	0.91	2.37×10^{-3}	1.78×10^{-2}	Proton pump inhibitors
1 year	F	A02BC	0.77	0.71	0.83	2.01×10^{-11}	2.38×10^{-9}	Proton pump inhibitors
1 year	G	A02BC	0.66	0.58	0.76	1.56×10^{-9}	7.80×10^{-8}	Proton pump inhibitors
2 years	A	A02BC	0.77	0.66	0.90	1.05×10^{-3}	1.80×10^{-2}	Proton pump inhibitors
2 years	F	A02BC	0.80	0.74	0.86	2.94×10^{-9}	2.55×10^{-7}	Proton pump inhibitors
2 years	G	A02BC	0.68	0.59	0.77	1.81×10^{-9}	9.96×10^{-8}	Proton pump inhibitors
2 years	F	A03FA	0.51	0.37	0.70	3.67×10^{-5}	1.19×10^{-3}	Propulsives
1 year	F	A09AA	0.24	0.09	0.64	4.19×10^{-3}	3.97×10^{-2}	Enzyme preparations
2 years	F	A09AA	0.23	0.09	0.60	2.81×10^{-3}	3.48×10^{-2}	Enzyme preparations
0.5 year	F	A12AX	0.80	0.69	0.93	2.74×10^{-3}	3.49×10^{-2}	Calcium, combinations with vitamin D and/or other drugs
1 year	F	A12AX	0.83	0.72	0.94	4.36×10^{-3}	3.97×10^{-2}	Calcium, combinations with vitamin D and/or other drugs
1 year	F	B03AA	0.74	0.60	0.91	4.00×10^{-3}	3.97×10^{-2}	Iron bivalent, oral preparations
2 years	F	C05AE	0.33	0.16	0.69	3.18×10^{-3}	3.59×10^{-2}	Muscle relaxants
0.5 year	F	G03CA	0.63	0.52	0.76	3.03×10^{-6}	1.58×10^{-4}	Natural and semisynthetic estrogens, plain
1 year	F	G03CA	0.67	0.58	0.78	4.08×10^{-7}	2.42×10^{-5}	Natural and semisynthetic estrogens, plain
2 years	F	G03CA	0.70	0.61	0.80	1.89×10^{-7}	9.83×10^{-6}	Natural and semisynthetic estrogens, plain
2 years	G	G03CA	0.66	0.51	0.86	2.43×10^{-3}	3.35×10^{-2}	Natural and semisynthetic estrogens, plain
0.5 year	F	G04CB	0.63	0.46	0.85	3.02×10^{-3}	3.49×10^{-2}	Testosterone-5-alpha reductase inhibitors
0.5 year	F	H03AA	0.80	0.69	0.92	2.24×10^{-3}	3.11×10^{-2}	Thyroid hormones
0.5 year	G	H03AA	0.66	0.51	0.86	2.10×10^{-3}	1.96×10^{-2}	Thyroid hormones
1 year	C	H03AA	0.62	0.48	0.79	1.77×10^{-4}	6.57×10^{-4}	Thyroid hormones
1 year	E	H03AA	0.80	0.71	0.92	9.47×10^{-4}	4.23×10^{-3}	Thyroid hormones
1 year	F	H03AA	0.81	0.71	0.93	2.51×10^{-3}	2.98×10^{-2}	Thyroid hormones
1 year	G	H03AA	0.64	0.49	0.82	5.53×10^{-4}	6.50×10^{-3}	Thyroid hormones
2 years	C	H03AA	0.62	0.48	0.79	1.50×10^{-4}	7.36×10^{-4}	Thyroid hormones
2 years	E	H03AA	0.80	0.70	0.91	5.94×10^{-4}	2.81×10^{-3}	Thyroid hormones
2 years	F	H03AA	0.81	0.71	0.93	2.57×10^{-3}	3.35×10^{-2}	Thyroid hormones
2 years	G	H03AA	0.64	0.50	0.83	6.06×10^{-4}	9.52×10^{-3}	Thyroid hormones
1 year	F	J01MA	0.49	0.34	0.72	2.40×10^{-4}	5.93×10^{-3}	Fluoroquinolones
2 years	F	J01MA	0.59	0.46	0.76	5.39×10^{-5}	1.56×10^{-3}	Fluoroquinolones
0.5 year	F	L02AE	0.29	0.14	0.60	9.84×10^{-4}	1.86×10^{-2}	Gonadotropin releasing hormone analogues
1 year	F	L02AE	0.41	0.23	0.72	2.02×10^{-3}	2.62×10^{-2}	Gonadotropin releasing hormone analogues
2 years	F	L02AE	0.42	0.25	0.70	9.73×10^{-4}	1.49×10^{-2}	Gonadotropin releasing hormone analogues
0.5 year	F	M01AE	0.68	0.56	0.82	4.61×10^{-5}	1.37×10^{-3}	Propionic acid derivatives
1 year	F	M01AE	0.79	0.70	0.91	6.65×10^{-4}	1.29×10^{-2}	Propionic acid derivatives
0.5 year	F	N02AX	0.56	0.41	0.76	1.88×10^{-4}	4.33×10^{-3}	Other opioids
1 year	F	N02AX	0.63	0.49	0.80	1.63×10^{-4}	4.84×10^{-3}	Other opioids
2 years	F	N02AX	0.68	0.56	0.83	1.14×10^{-4}	2.29×10^{-3}	Other opioids
0.5 year	F	N03AX	0.68	0.58	0.81	1.72×10^{-5}	5.96×10^{-4}	Other antiepileptics
1 year	F	N03AX	0.70	0.60	0.82	1.00×10^{-5}	3.95×10^{-4}	Other antiepileptics
2 years	F	N03AX	0.73	0.64	0.84	7.15×10^{-6}	3.10×10^{-4}	Other antiepileptics
0.5 year	F	N06AA	0.77	0.65	0.92	3.99×10^{-3}	4.15×10^{-2}	Nonselective monoamine reuptake inhibitors
1 year	F	N06AA	0.79	0.68	0.92	1.98×10^{-3}	2.62×10^{-2}	Nonselective monoamine reuptake inhibitors
2 years	F	N06AA	0.79	0.70	0.90	2.67×10^{-4}	4.96×10^{-3}	Nonselective monoamine reuptake inhibitors
1 year	A	R03BA	0.48	0.31	0.73	7.44×10^{-4}	7.44×10^{-3}	Glucocorticoids
2 years	A	R03BA	0.55	0.38	0.81	2.44×10^{-3}	3.36×10^{-2}	Glucocorticoids
0.5 year	F	R05DA	0.69	0.55	0.87	1.46×10^{-3}	2.33×10^{-2}	Opium alkaloids and derivatives
1 year	F	R05DA	0.74	0.62	0.88	5.47×10^{-4}	1.18×10^{-2}	Opium alkaloids and derivatives
2 years	F	R05DA	0.80	0.70	0.91	7.02×10^{-4}	1.22×10^{-2}	Opium alkaloids and derivatives

For space limits, only results with FDR < 0.05 are shown. Please refer to Tables S3 and S6 for full results. Ophthalmological and other topical agents are not listed in the above table.

3.1.5. Drugs Ranked by Consistency of Protective Associations

We also ranked the drugs in term of their *consistency* of protective associations. Briefly, drugs were ranked by their frequency of being at least nominally significant ($p < 0.05$) across the four time windows and eight models (Table 4). This serves as an alternative approach to prioritize drugs. For some drugs, the results may not be significant after FDR correction. Nevertheless, if a drug showed consistent associations (at least nominally) across multiple models or time-frames, it may also be worthy of further investigation.

3.1.6. Drug Associated with Increased Odds of Risk/Severity of Infection

Among the drugs with harmful associations, the more frequently top-listed ones include laxatives, opioids (N02AA), benzodiazepines, tetracycline, penicillins, other antipsychotics (N05AX), and antidementia drugs (N06DA/DX). The full results are presented in Tables S6–S10, and a summary is also provided in Table S5.

3.2. Analysis Restricted to Subjects with Complete Covariate Data, and Models with/without IPW

As a sensitivity analysis, for the above analysis with imputed covariates, we also repeated models A to H *without* IPW of Pr(tested). In addition, we also repeated the analyses, limiting to subjects with complete covariate data, with or without the IPW approach. In general, we observed similar drugs with significant results, and the top-ranked protective or harmful drugs were similar to the above. Comparing results with and without IPW, the list of significant drugs remained similar although the OR estimates and SE were adjusted. The full results are presented in Tables S7 and S8 (complete covariate data with and without IPW) and Table S9 (imputed covariates without IPW).

3.3. Subgroup Analysis

The proportion of subjects falling into each subgroup is presented in Table S10, while full results are presented in Table S11. We performed a statistical test to compare the log(OR) across the two subgroups with and without the risk factor; drugs with protective effect in one subgroup but significantly different OR in the other subgroup are listed in Table 7. For example, the protective effects of pneumococcal and flu vaccines were significantly weaker in obese (BMI > 30) subjects under model F. With regards to age, several drugs, such as PPI and ACEI, showed larger protective effects in those with age > 70 under models F and E, respectively. Statins, ACEIs, and PPI showed stronger protective associations in hypertensive patients under models C, E, and F, respectively. Regarding ethnicity as a subgroup, a number of drugs, including several vaccines, appeared to have stronger protective effects in the white compared to non-white subjects. However, only <10% of the UKBB subjects included here were non-white, and the non-white subgroup was heterogeneous and composed of several different ethnicities. We did not observe clear evidence of sex-specific effects in this analysis.

Table 7. Summary of subgroup analysis, showing drugs having significant protective association in one subgroup but significantly different OR in the other subgroup (FDR < 0.2).

Subgp	Windows	Model	OR_Y	OR_N	sig_Y	sig_N	z_OR_cmp	p_OR_cmp	p.adjust_OR_cmp	Name
AGE > 70	5 years	F	0.81	0.99	1	0	−2.65	8.15×10^{-3}	1.47×10^{-1}	A02BC Proton pump inhibitors
AGE > 70	1 year	E	1.19	0.49	0	1	2.11	3.47×10^{-2}	1.56×10^{-1}	A10AE Insulins and analogues for injection, long-acting
AGE > 70	1 year	E	0.81	1.04	1	0	−2.38	1.72×10^{-2}	1.55×10^{-1}	C09AA ACE inhibitors, plain
Asthma	5 years	E	0.60	0.86	1	1	−2.66	7.76×10^{-3}	1.40×10^{-1}	J07BB Influenza vaccines
Asthma	10 years	E	0.61	0.87	1	1	−2.95	3.22×10^{-3}	1.29×10^{-2}	J07BB Influenza vaccines
BMI > 30	1 year	F	1.04	0.31	0	1	2.42	1.56×10^{-2}	1.40×10^{-1}	J07AL Pneumococcal vaccines
BMI > 30	1 year	F	0.76	0.54	1	1	2.52	1.17×10^{-2}	1.40×10^{-1}	J07BB Influenza vaccines
BMI > 30	2 years	F	0.79	0.56	1	1	2.75	6.01×10^{-3}	1.08×10^{-1}	J07BB Influenza vaccines
BMI > 30	6 months	F	0.92	0.16	0	1	2.68	7.40×10^{-3}	1.26×10^{-1}	R03BA Glucocorticoids
CAD	5 years	H	0.36	1.32	1	0	−2.39	1.71×10^{-2}	1.53×10^{-1}	C08CA Dihydropyridine derivatives
CAD	5 years	H	1.72	0.18	0	1	2.42	1.53×10^{-2}	1.53×10^{-1}	G04CB Testosterone-5-alpha reductase inhibitors
CAD	5 years	C	1.92	0.56	0	1	2.38	1.72×10^{-2}	1.55×10^{-1}	J07AL Pneumococcal vaccines
CAD	5 years	F	1.55	0.56	0	1	2.55	1.07×10^{-2}	1.92×10^{-1}	J07AL Pneumococcal vaccines

Table 7. Cont.

Subgp	Windows	Model	OR_Y	OR_N	sig_Y	sig_N	z_OR_cmp	p_OR_cmp	p.adjust_OR_cmp	Name
Depression	1 yearr	B	0.07	0.73	1	0	-2.60	9.36×10^{-3}	1.50×10^{-1}	C10AA HMG CoA reductase inhibitors
HT	2 years	F	0.75	0.93	1	0	-2.69	7.20×10^{-3}	1.30×10^{-1}	A02BC Proton pump inhibitors
HT	5 years	F	0.76	1.00	1	0	-3.36	7.92×10^{-4}	1.43×10^{-2}	A02BC Proton pump inhibitors
HT	1 year	E	0.86	1.07	1	0	-2.11	3.49×10^{-2}	1.26×10^{-1}	C09AA ACE inhibitors, plain
HT	1 year	C	0.71	1.02	1	0	-2.58	9.90×10^{-3}	8.91×10^{-2}	C10AA HMG CoA reductase inhibitors

OR_Y, odds ratio within the subgroup defined in the 1st column; OR_N, OR in the other subgroup. Sig_Y, sig_N, significance in the two subgroups, 1 denotes significant protective effect, 0 denotes nonsignificant effect, -1 denotes significant harmful effect. p_OR_cmp, p-value based on comparison of ORs; p.adjust_OR_cmp, corresponding FDR. Ethnicity as a subgroup is not shown here; please refer to Table S11 for details. CAD, coronary artery disease, HT, hypertension.

3.4. Interaction Analysis

A summary of results (results with FDR < 0.2) is presented in Table 8, while a fuller version is given in Table S12. Full results are given in Table S13. More significant results (at FDR < 0.2) are observed compared to stratified analysis, presumably due to the higher power of this approach. For example, we found that most vaccines showing protective effects, including influenza and pneumococcal vaccines, interacted with BMI and obesity significantly. Higher BMI was associated with *reduced* protective effects, in line with evidence from subgroup analysis.

On the other hand, statins, biguanides (metformin), and antiplatelet drugs showed positive interactions with BMI. For CAD, significant interaction was observed with several cardiometabolic drugs, including beta-blockers (nonselective), antiplatelet drugs, and statins, suggesting larger protective effects for such drugs in CAD patients. In a similar vein, most cardiometabolic medications showed interaction with HT, indicating more prominent protective associations in HT patients.

Considering age as an interacting variable, interaction was observed with a large number of drugs, most suggesting weaker protection as age increases. Considering specific medications, statins interact with multiple risk factors and demonstrate larger protective effects with CAD, obesity, DM, CAD, HT, dementia, and in males. However, its effect tends to be weaker with increasing age. Interaction analysis with flu vaccines showed that its effect may be weaker in the obese and with increasing age, but was stronger in the white population and asthmatic subgroup. ACEI and ARB showed stronger protective effects in the white and HT patients, but weaker effects with advanced age.

3.5. Controlling for Other Medications

We primarily focused on protective drugs, as the number of drugs with significant negative effects is large and is hard to control for all. Overall, most drugs with protective effects remain significant (at least for a subset of models), despite controlling for other medications (Table S15). However, biguanides (A10BA), CCB (C08CA), and platelet aggregation inhibitors, excluding heparin (B01AC), showed a relatively consistent trend of nonsignificant association with outcome when other protective drugs were controlled for. The findings are similar when controlling for top-10/20 drugs or all protective drugs having FDR < 0.05/0.1.

Table 8. Summary of interaction analysis, showing pairs of variables with significant interactions (FDR < 0.2).

ATC Code	Interacting Factor	Drug Name	Interaction Term	ATC Code	Interacting Factor	Drug Name	Interaction Term
A02BC	AGE	Proton pump inhibitors	1/−1	A02BC	CAD	Proton pump inhibitors	1
A03AA	AGE	Synthetic anticholinergics, esters with tertiary amino group	−1	A03AA	CAD	Synthetic anticholinergics, esters with tertiary amino group	1
A10AE	AGE	Insulins and analogues for injection, long-acting	−1	B01AC	CAD	Platelet aggregation inhibitors excl. heparin	1
B01AC	AGE	Platelet aggregation inhibitors excl. heparin	−1	C07AB	CAD	Beta blocking agents, selective	1
C07AB	AGE	Beta blocking agents, selective	−1	C10AA	CAD	HMG CoA reductase inhibitors	1
C08CA	AGE	Dihydropyridine derivatives	−1	J07AL	CAD	Pneumococcal vaccines	−1
C09AA	AGE	ACE inhibitors, plain	−1	C10AA	Dementia	HMG CoA reductase inhibitors	1
C09CA	AGE	Angiotensin II receptor blockers, plain	−1	J07CA	Dementia	Bacterial and viral vaccines, combined	−1
C10AA	AGE	HMG CoA reductase inhibitors	−1	C08CA	COPD	Dihydropyridine derivatives	−1
G04CB	AGE	Testosterone-5-alpha reductase inhibitors	−1	J07AP	COPD	Typhoid vaccines	−1
J07AL	AGE	Pneumococcal vaccines	−1	A03AA	Depression	Synthetic anticholinergics, esters with tertiary amino group	−1
R03BA	AGE	Glucocorticoids	1	C10AA	DM	HMG CoA reductase inhibitors	1
A02BC	AGE > 70	Proton pump inhibitors	−1	A02BC	Dx_cancer	Proton pump inhibitors	−1
A10AE	AGE > 70	Insulins and analogues for injection, long-acting	−1	J07AL	Dx_cancer	Pneumococcal vaccines	−1
A10BA	AGE > 70	Biguanides	−1	A10BA	Ethnic (White)	Biguanides	1
B01AC	AGE > 70	Platelet aggregation inhibitors excl. heparin	−1	C08CA	Ethnic (White)	Dihydropyridine derivatives	1
C07AB	AGE > 70	Beta blocking agents, selective	−1	C09AA	Ethnic (White)	ACE inhibitors, plain	1
C08CA	AGE > 70	Dihydropyridine derivatives	−1	C09CA	Ethnic (White)	Angiotensin II receptor blockers, plain	1
C09AA	AGE > 70	ACE inhibitors, plain	−1	H03AA	Ethnic (White)	Thyroid hormones	1
C10AA	AGE > 70	HMG CoA reductase inhibitors	−1	J07AL	Ethnic (White)	Pneumococcal vaccines	1
G04CB	AGE > 70	Testosterone-5-alpha reductase inhibitors	−1	J07AP	Ethnic (White)	Typhoid vaccines	1
J07AL	AGE > 70	Pneumococcal vaccines	−1	J07BB	Ethnic (White)	Influenza vaccines	1
J07BB	AGE > 70	Influenza vaccines	−1	A02BC	Hypertension	Proton pump inhibitors	−1
R03BA	AGE > 70	Glucocorticoids	−1	A03AA	Hypertension	Synthetic anticholinergics, esters with tertiary amino group	1
A10AE	Asthma	Insulins and analogues for injection, long-acting	−1	B01AC	Hypertension	Platelet aggregation inhibitors excl. heparin	1
A10BA	Asthma	Biguanides	−1	C07AB	Hypertension	Beta blocking agents, selective	1
C08CA	Asthma	Dihydropyridine derivatives	−1	C08CA	Hypertension	Dihydropyridine derivatives	1
C09CA	Asthma	Angiotensin II receptor blockers, plain	−1	C09AA	Hypertension	ACE inhibitors, plain	1
J07AL	Asthma	Pneumococcal vaccines	−1	C09CA	Hypertension	Angiotensin II receptor blockers, plain	1
J07BB	Asthma	Influenza vaccines	1	C10AA	Hypertension	HMG CoA reductase inhibitors	1
A02BC	BMI	Proton pump inhibitors	1	J07AL	Hypertension	Pneumococcal vaccines	−1
A03AA	BMI	Synthetic anticholinergics, esters with tertiary amino group	−1	B01AC	Obesity	Platelet aggregation inhibitors excl. heparin	1

Table 8. *Cont.*

ATC Code	Interacting Factor	Drug Name	Interaction Term	ATC Code	Interacting Factor	Drug Name	Interaction Term
A10BA	BMI	Biguanides	1	C10AA	Obesity	HMG CoA reductase inhibitors	1
B01AC	BMI	Platelet aggregation inhibitors excl. heparin	1	J07AL	Obesity	Pneumococcal vaccines	−1
C10AA	BMI	HMG CoA reductase inhibitors	1	J07BB	Obesity	Influenza vaccines	−1
J07AL	BMI	Pneumococcal vaccines	−1	A02BC	Sex (male)	Proton pump inhibitors	1
J07AP	BMI	Typhoid vaccines	−1	C10AA	Sex (male)	HMG CoA reductase inhibitors	1
J07BB	BMI	Influenza vaccines	−1	J07AL	Sex (male)	Pneumococcal vaccines	−1
J07CA	BMI	Bacterial and viral vaccines, combined	−1	J07AP	Sex (male)	Typhoid vaccines	1

We added an interaction term drug*interacting factor in the regression model. For "interaction term", 1 denotes significant interaction effects towards protection (i.e., presence of the interacting factor tends to increase the protective effect of the drug); −1 denotes significant interaction effects towards harmful side (presence of the interacting factor tends to reduce the protective effect of the drug). We consider significant results in any model or time window. For age and BMI, they were modeled as continuous variables unless otherwise specified. For full results, please refer to Tables S12 and S13.

4. Discussion

In this work, we performed a thorough and rigorous analysis on the effect of drugs and vaccines on COVID-19 susceptibility and severity. We uncovered a number of drugs with potentially protective effects, which may be further explored as candidates for drug repositioning.

As an approach based on observational data, different kinds of bias, such as confounding and selection bias, may affect the results. We performed analysis on infected subjects (models A and B), the whole population (models C, D, E) and the tested population (models F, G, H) to obtain a more comprehensive picture of drug effects under different settings, and to avoid limitations (e.g., selection bias, collider bias, unscreened controls) of some designs.

4.1. Highlights of Relevant Drugs

Below, we highlight drugs that are tentatively associated with altered risk or severity of infection. We preferentially consider drugs that showed significant associations across multiple models and time windows, those with stronger statistical significance, and those with protective effects, as confounding by indication is much less likely.

4.1.1. Drugs for Cardiometabolic Disorders with Protective Effects

Interestingly, many drugs with potential protective effects are indicated for cardiometabolic (CM) disorders. Cardiometabolic risk factors, such as obesity, hypertension, DM, and CAD, have consistently been shown to be associated with risk and severity of infection [15,40]; as such, it is biologically plausible that drugs for treating CM disorders may be beneficial.

Among all drugs, the strongest and most consistent protective association was observed for statins. The beneficial effects of statins are supported by several previous studies. For example, a recent meta-analysis of four retrospective studies of COVID-19 patients [41] showed a significantly decreased hazard of severity or mortality of infection (pooled HR = 0.70) when comparing statin users against nonusers. Another retrospective study by Tan et al. [42] also reported lower risk of intensive care unit (ICU) admission among statin users in infected patients. Yet another work showed that statins may be effective in reducing in-hospital mortality among diabetic patients [43]. Potential mechanisms for the protective actions of statins have been discussed elsewhere [44–46]. It has been postulated that, besides reducing CVD risks, statins may reduce risk/severity of infection by inhibiting inflammation and excessive immune response, producing direct antiviral effects, improving endothelial function, and exerting an antithrombotic effect, among other actions [44–46].

Another group of drugs worth highlighting is ACEI and ARB. There have been intense discussions on whether ACEI/ARB may affect risk or severity of infection from early on, as ACE2 is a receptor for SARS-CoV-2. Nevertheless, a recent study showed that ACE2 is localized in respiratory cilia, and the use of ARB/ACEI does not change its expression [47]. Recent systemic reviews and meta-analysis (for example, see [48] with continuous updates) of observational studies do not support an association between ACEI/ARB prior use and severity of infection. However, several studies [47,49–55] reported protective effects of ACEI/ARB on severity or mortality of disease. Here, we observed consistent association of prior use of ACEI/ARB with reduced risks of severe/fatal infection (models A, C, G) and overall infection risk in the population (model E).

For several other kinds of cardiometabolic drugs, the associations were not as strong, but may still be worthy of further studies. Biguanides (mainly metformin) are observed to be protective for severe COVID-19 infection, both among the infected and at a population level. For example, in a meta-analysis on four observational studies of hospitalized patients mostly with type 2 DM, the use of metformin was associated with a lower risk of mortality (OR = 0.75, 95% CI = 0.67–0.85) [56]. A number of mechanisms have been proposed [56,57]. For example, besides improving glycemic control and weight reduction, metformin may lead to AMPK activation which potentially reduces viral entry by phosphorylation of ACE2 receptor. It may also lead to mTOR pathway inhibition and prevents hyperactivation of the immune system [56].

Other drugs of interest may include beta-blockers and calcium channel blockers (C08CA, dihydropyridine derivatives). It was suggested that beta-blockers may be useful in preventing hyperinflammation and hence beneficial for COVID-19 [58]. For calcium channel blockers (CCBs), a study using cell culture suggested that CCBs, especially amlodipine and nifedipine, were useful in blocking viral entry and infection in epithelial lung cells [59]. In another retrospective study [60], both beta-blockers and CCBs were associated with lower mortality. Another relevant study in the UK [61] utilized data from the UK Clinical Practice Research Datalink (CPRD) and found that ACEI/ARB, CCBs, and thiazide diuretics were all associated with lower odds of diagnosis, while beta-blockers do not show any association after adjusting for consultation frequency. None of the above drugs were associated with mortality in that study [61].

4.1.2. Vaccines

There has been intense interest in whether vaccines indicated for other diseases may protect against COVID-19. Here, we observed that a number of vaccines showed protection against infection or severe infection. For example, pneumococcal vaccines were protective against infection in the population and tested subjects, and risk of severe infection (model G). Significant protective associations were also observed for tetanus and typhoid vaccines at a time horizon of 10 years (the power to detect associations is likely stronger over longer periods due to larger number of people having received the vaccine; it does not exclude the possibility that the vaccines may have effects over shorter time windows). We also observed associations with the J07CA category, which contains various bacterial and viral vaccines (see https://www.whocc.no/atc_ddd_index/?code=J07CA, accessed on 9 November 2020).

For influenza vaccines, we observed highly consistent protective associations. It has been proposed that "trained innate immunity", which may involve epigenetic reprogramming of innate immune cells, may enable a vaccine to protect against other diseases [62,63]. Interestingly, two studies in Italy reported that higher coverage rate of flu vaccine was associated with lower rate of infection, hospitalization, and mortality from COVID-19. Another larger-scale study, based on electronic records of 137,037 subjects who have received viral PCR tests, showed that a number of vaccines (given in the past 1, 2, or 5 years) were associated with lower risks of infection [64]. These included flu and pneumococcal vaccines also implicated in the present study. Another recent study in the Netherlands [65] also showed a reduced risk (Relative risk = 0.61, 95% CI: 0.46–0.82) of infection among recipients of flu vaccine, and this effect size was similar to that observed here. In vitro studies by the same authors showed that the vaccine was able to induce a trained immunity response, including an increase of cytokine responses after stimulation of immune cells with SARS-CoV-2.

We note that this is an observational study, and residual confounding may be present. For example, it is possible that people receiving flu vaccines are more health-conscious and observe preventive measures better. However, we observed waning protective effects over time, which makes sense biologically but could not be entirely explained by the above confounder alone. In addition, the vaccine appears to have stronger effect sizes if fatal infection is considered as the outcome (although the confidence interval is large), which cannot be easily explained by health-consciousness. On the other hand, as flu vaccines are more likely to be received by the elderly and those with chronic illnesses, residual confounding of these factors tend to push the effects towards the harmful side.

Taken together, we believe that the protective effects of vaccines may not be easily and fully explained away by other confounders. Further experimental and clinical studies are warranted to investigate the nonspecific effects of flu and other vaccines, especially since COVID-19 vaccines may not be easily available to many people (especially those in low-income countries) in a short timeframe.

4.1.3. Other Potential Protective Drugs

We briefly highlight a few other drugs with potential protective effects. Estrogens (G03CA) were among the drugs showing protective associations. As many studies reported higher risks of severe disease in men than in women, it has been hypothesized that estrogen may play a part in the sex-discordant outcomes, for example via its effects on immune response to infections [66–68].

Thyroid hormones (TH) were also among the top-ranked drugs. It was postulated that TH may ameliorate tissue injury due to hypoxia by suppression of p38 MAPK [69]. Clinical trials on TH are ongoing [69,70], and our findings support a protective role of TH in COVID-19.

Another drug category of note is proton pump inhibitors (PPI). Several studies have suggested harmful effects of PPI on disease severity, which may be related to reduced gastric acid production with subsequent bacterial overgrowth [71–73]. However, an in vitro screening study revealed that PPIs may serve as a potent inhibitor of SARS-CoV-2 replication [74]. The difference in findings between the current study and previous works may be due to heterogeneity in study samples and designs, differences in the outcome studied (e.g., hospitalization vs. ICU admission used in some other studies; infection risk vs. severity of disease, etc.), and variations in the covariates being adjusted for. Residual confounding, such as by other comorbidities and drugs given, may also affect the results. Interestingly, we observed that effects of PPI may be stronger in certain subgroups (e.g., older age, HT), which may also account for the discrepancy in results across different studies.

Several other top-ranked drug categories in Table 4 may also be worth discussing. Testosterone-5-alpha reductase inhibitors (5ARis) were recently shown in a small randomized controlled trial (RCT) to reduce the time to remission [75]. Two earlier observational studies also reported lower risk of ICU admission and frequency of symptoms [76,77]; 5ARis block the conversion of testosterone to its more potent form, dihydrotestosterone. Of note, one of the key receptors for the SAR-CoV-2 virus is TMPRSS2 [78], and the only known promoter of the gene is an androgen response element in the promoter region [79].

Another drug category of interest is platelet aggregation inhibitors (B01AC). It has been reported that COVID-19 is associated with higher risk of thrombotic events, including deep vein thrombosis and pulmonary embolism [80]. Antithrombotic therapies have been hypothesized to reduce thrombo-inflammatory processes as a result of endothelial dysfunction related to viral infection [81]. An observational study reported that aspirin is associated with reduced risk of mechanical ventilation and mortality in hospitalized patients [82]; however, RCTs are lacking.

For some of the protective drugs highlighted above, we note that their significance weakened (or became nonsignificant) when controlling for other medications. However, we expect multicollinearity among the drug variables, as cardiometabolic disorders are highly comorbid and one patient often takes multiple medications. Multicollinearity may render interpretation of individual predictors difficult due to unstable coefficient estimates [83].

In our secondary analyses, we also considered *subgroup and interaction effects*. While this is a more exploratory analysis and further replications are required, it shed light on how the effects of drugs/vaccines may differ in people with different clinical background and may contribute to more "personalized" drug repositioning in the future. For instance, we observed a consistent trend that the protective associations of flu and pneumococcal vaccines were weaker in obese individuals. As an example, comparing those who received flu vaccine in the past season (2019–2020) against those who did not, the estimated OR for infection was 0.76 in the obese group and 0.54 in the non-obese group (model F). It has been observed before that obese individuals respond less well to flu and other vaccines due to impaired immunological responses [84,85]. As another example, statins were observed to have more prominent protective effects in those with cardiometabolic abnormalities, such as DM, HT, CAD, and obesity. This is also supported by a recent study [43] which showed mortality reduction in statin users in diabetic patients only.

4.1.4. Drugs with Potentially Harmful Effects

We noted a number of drugs with potentially harmful effects, but we caution that residual confounding, such as confounding by indication, other comorbidities, and general poor health, may lead to bias towards an increased odds of infection or severe disease.

For example, people who have poorer health in general may visit their GPs more often and be prescribed drugs (e.g., laxatives, antibiotics, painkillers), which may lead to confounding. Nevertheless, it is possible that some of the top-ranked drugs may indeed increase the risk/severity of infection. For instance, it is slightly unexpected that laxatives were highly significant across multiple models and time windows. It has recently been postulated that dysregulation of gut microbiome may be associated with susceptibility or resilience to infection [86,87], and laxatives represent a main category of drugs that affect the gut microbiome [88]. Interestingly, several associations involve psychiatric medications such as benzodiazepines, antipsychotics, and antidementia drugs. The association may be due to underlying neuropsychiatric conditions (e.g., anxiety, psychosis, dementia, etc.), or the effect of the drugs, or a combination of both. Some of the above drugs overlap with those revealed in a recent study using primary care data in Scotland. In a univariate analysis restricted to nonresidents in care homes and those without major conditions, laxatives, anxiolytics, penicillins, and opioid analgesics were significantly associated with ICU admission or mortality from COVID-19 when compared to population controls [89]. These drugs were also top-listed as drugs with harmful effects in this study.

Patients taking immunosuppressants are more susceptible to viral infections in general, and it is possible that these drugs are also associated with increased vulnerability to COVID-19 infection [90]. On the other hand, such drugs may dampen excessive immune responses ("cytokine storm") that may occur in severe infections [91]. However, here we did not find consistent evidence of associations between immunosuppressive agents and COVID-19. Across immunosuppressive drugs (ATC category L04), we only found two significant associations (FDR < 0.05). Interleukin inhibitors were associated with higher susceptibility to infection (model E) and selective immunosuppressants (L04AA) were associated with higher risk of severe infection (model C), respectively, when compared to population controls (Table S6). No other significant associations were observed. Of note, a few preclinical studies reported that thiopurines, a type of immunosuppressant, may lead to reduced viral replication [92,93] via other mechanisms, although clinical studies suggested possible harmful effects [94,95]. However, the number of patients taking such drugs was too small for meaningful analysis in this study.

4.1.5. Different Results under Different Models

We note that sometimes the different models may yield different results. One main observation is that analysis on the tested population appears to result in more findings of drugs with protective effects. We also observed that some drugs in model F (infected vs. tested negative) may show different effects under model E (infected vs. general population). Several reasons may explain this finding. First, confounding by indication is inevitable and may play a more important role when analyzing general population samples. It is possible that apparent harmful effects of drugs are due to the diseases/conditions that the prescription is related to, or poorer health in general. Based on a machine learning model for predicting testing probability (see Figure S1), we observed that people who are older, having more comorbidities and taking more medications, suffering from cardiovascular conditions, etc. were more likely to be tested. Compared to the general population, the tested group may represent a more "homogeneous" population, enriched for people with poorer health and more comorbidities in general. Therefore, a proportion of confounders which overlap with factors associated with higher Pr(tested) are essentially controlled for by stratification, if we only study the tested subjects. On the other hand, in the general population, as there is a higher proportion of healthy subjects, the effect of confounding by indication may be stronger. Another possibility is collider bias due to conditioning on a subgroup of subjects. For example, a drug may be associated with certain conditions which, in turn, are associated with higher chance of being tested; on the other hand, those who have more severe symptoms or complications are more likely to be tested. Conditioning on testing may result in spurious associations between the drug and severity of infection. However, we have tried to minimize this type of bias by the IPW approach, and we did not observe substantial difference in results with or without IPW correction for most drugs. However, we note that, even with adjustment by IPW, there is still chance for residual selection or collider bias. For example, some factors associated with Pr(tested) may not be captured in the prediction model. A third possibility to consider is that a drug may truly produce different effects in different subgroups, due to effect modification by other factors or diseases. For instance, a recent study reported that the protective effect of statins is more marked in patients with diabetes [43]. The fact that risk factor associations may differ between a whole-population- or tested-population-based study has also been noted previously, for example in [35].

4.2. Strengths and Limitation

This study has a number of strengths. First and foremost, the study was performed on a large cohort with a sample size close to half a million. The sample was not limited to one or a few medical centers, and covered the entire UK population, although this is not an entirely random sample and participation bias still exists [34]. The large and well-characterized sample also enables analysis of infected and tested, as well as the whole population. We have studied *all* level-4 ATC drug categories, allowing an unbiased and systematic analysis on the association of different drugs with COVID-19 risks or outcomes. This avoids the risk of publication bias, especially negative results to be unreported. Drugs showing null associations can still be of important public health interest, as this may suggest that patients on such medications may not need to change their regimen in view of the pandemic. In addition, medication history was retrieved from GP records, which minimize recall bias and errors from self-reporting. Another strength is that we performed a variety of statistical analysis to reduce bias, including control for potential confounders, multiple imputation, IPW to reduce effects of testing bias, and study of different time windows and multiple models. Some of our findings were also corroborated by previous studies. Many previous clinical studies were limited to hospitalized or infected individuals, which cannot study the effect of drugs on susceptibility to infection. Selection on hospitalized/infected subjects may also be prone to selection/collider bias, as discussed elsewhere [34]; therefore, we included multiple models with infected and tested, as well the whole population as samples, which aims to reduce limitations due to specific designs.

There are also various limitations, some of which have been mentioned above. First and foremost, this is an observational study based on a retrospective cohort of UKBB. As this is not a randomized controlled trial, confounding is inevitable, especially confounding by indication. Although we have controlled for main confounders in the regression model, residual confounding is still likely. Since confounding by indication will likely bias towards *increased* odds of infection or severe disease, null or protective associations may be more reliable. Confounding by the use of other types of drugs is also possible. In addition, the UKBB cohort is not random, and participants are on average healthier than the general population [96]. The majority of participants are of European descent, so the findings may not be generalizable to other ethnicities. In addition, the subjects are mostly >50 years old, and drug effects in younger individuals may be different.

Regarding drug history, it is worth noting that vaccination records are not complete, as individuals may receive vaccination outside GP practices. Over-the-counter prescriptions were not counted, and it cannot be guaranteed that all drugs issued are dispensed by the pharmacy (see https://biobank.ctsu.ox.ac.uk/crystal/crystal/docs/tppgp4covid19.pdf, accessed on 9 November 2020). However, if this misclassification is nondifferential (unrelated to outcome), the bias will be towards the null. There is a relatively high missing rate of GP prescription records for deceased COVID-19 patients, which leads to reduced power to detect associations. While the UKBB cohort sample is large, we still have low power to detect associations for drugs that are uncommonly prescribed. Another limitation with the GP records is that only the issue date, but no duration or dosage, is available.

As for the outcome, hospitalization is a rough proxy for severity only. For models comparing to the general population, it is likely that a proportion of the population may be infected but were not tested. This tends to lead to bias on the conservative side (akin to the use of unscreened controls in genetic studies [97,98]), especially under model E. Patients with more severe symptoms are less likely to remain untested, so other models may be less affected by this bias. We note that this study focuses on prior (or pre-diagnostic) use of drugs and their association with infection risk/severity, and does not provide direct evidence for whether newly prescribed drugs to recently diagnosed patients will be useful or not. The current study represents one approach to drug repositioning with real-world population data, yet integrating results from other repositioning approaches (e.g., network/structure-based) may further improve the reliability of candidates.

4.3. Clinical Implications

We highlight a few clinical implications here, although we stress that further studies are required to confirm our findings. We discovered a number of drugs with potential protective effects that, if replicated and tested in further trials, may represent promising repurposing candidates (for prevention or treatment of disease). As CM disorders are a major risk factor for severe infection, this study also provides further support for the safety of CM medications and reinforces the need to continue these drugs for those indicated. In a similar vein, negative findings (nonsignificant associations with COVID-19) in this study may also be of value, given that some patients or physicians may have concerns over the risk of COVID-19 induced by existing drugs.

Another important finding is that flu (and possibly others, e.g., pneumococcal) vaccines may be associated with lower odds of infection and severity of disease. If further confirmed, the finding is clinically important as COVID-19 vaccines are not fully available yet to a large part of the world's population (especially those in developing countries), some may be hesitant to take the new vaccine, and the efficacy of existing vaccines varies and is less than perfect. At least, the present work supports that flu and other vaccinations should be continued and encouraged amid the pandemic. For any vaccines/drugs that may be repurposed for COVID-19, we believe that even a modest reduction in the risk/severity of infection may still be highly useful, given the huge number of people at risk for COVID-19 and its complications.

5. Conclusions

Here, we observed that a number of drugs, including many for cardiometabolic disorders, may be associated with lower odds of infection/severity of COVID-19. Several existing vaccines, especially flu vaccines, may be beneficial against COVID-19 as well. Due to the observational nature of the study, confounding cannot be excluded, and other limitations may be present. We understand that causal relationship between drugs and disease cannot be reliably concluded from this study alone, and shall regard the findings as more exploratory than confirmatory. Nevertheless, to our knowledge, this is the most comprehensive study to date on drug/vaccine associations with COVID-19. We believe that the current work provides a valuable resource to prioritize repositioning candidates for future meta-analyses, clinical trials, and/or experimental studies.

Supplementary Materials: The following are available online at https://www.mdpi.com/article/10.3390/pharmaceutics13091514/s1, All supplementary Tables and notes are available at the journal's website and at https://drive.google.com/drive/folders/1_noITkBAsef_7Kb6bUd_RI_3VQK5jafH?usp=sharing (accessed on 28 January 2021) or https://doi.org/10.6084/m9.figshare.14828112 (accessed on 23 June 2021). Table S1: Demographic and other characteristics of the original UKBB data, Table S2: Out-of-bag (OOB) errors for different variables from multiple imputations, Table S3: (a) All protective associations with at least nominal significance ($p < 0.05$) (6 month to 5 years), Table S4: All association results with vaccines (time windows of 1, 2, 5 and 10 years), Table S5: (a) Top 10 drugs with harmful effects (ranked by p-value) from each model and time window (time window of 6 month to 5 years) (b) Summary table by frequency of being listed among the top 10, Table S6: All association results based on subjects with available GP prescription records, with multiple imputation of covariates and inverse probability weighting (IPW) of probability of being tested, Table S7: Analysis restricted to subjects with complete covariate data, with IPW, Table S8: Analysis restricted to subjects with complete covariate data, without IPW, Table S9: Analysis with imputed covariates without IPW, Table S10: Proportion of subjects in each subgroup, Table S11: Full results of subgroup analysis, Table S12: Summary table of interaction analyses (results with FDR < 0.2), Table S13: Full results of interaction analyses, Table S14: Further analysis on associations of flu vaccine and risks/severity of infection, according to the season of vaccination, Table S15: Results of analyses after controlling for other top medications. Figure S1: Shapley dependence plot of top 15 variables contributing to Pr(tested) from the XGboost prediction model. Variables are ranked by absolute mean Shapley value. Please refer to Lundberg et al. (https://doi.org/10.1038/s42256-019-0138-9) for details on Shapley values.

Author Contributions: Conceptualization, H.-C.S.; Data curation, Y.X. and K.C.-Y.W.; Formal analysis, Y.X. (lead) and K.C.-Y.W.; Funding acquisition, H.-C.S.; Methodology, H.-C.S. (lead) and Y.X.; Project administration, Y.X.; Supervision, H.-C.S.; Writing—original draft, H.-C.S. and Y.X.; Writing—review & editing, Y.X., K.C.-Y.W. and H.-C.S. All authors have read and agreed to the published version of the manuscript.

Funding: This research was funded by National Natural Science Foundation of China, grant number 81971706; KIZ-CUHK Joint Laboratory of Bioresources and Molecular Research of Common Diseases, Kunming Institute of Zoology and The Chinese University of Hong Kong, China; Lo Kwee Seong Biomedical Research Fund, The Chinese University of Hong Kong.

Institutional Review Board Statement: The UK Biobank study has received ethical approval from the NHS National Research Ethics Service North West (16/NW/0274). Details of UK Biobank research ethics approval can be found at https://www.ukbiobank.ac.uk/learn-more-about-uk-biobank/about-us/ethics.

Informed Consent Statement: Informed consent was obtained from all subjects involved in the study.

Data Availability Statement: UK Biobank data are available to eligible researchers after completing an application procedure (https://www.ukbiobank.ac.uk/enable-your-research).

Acknowledgments: We thank Pak SHAM for support on data access. We thank Carlos CHAU for help with data presentation, Liangying YIN for help with data cleaning and Shitao RAO and Jinghong QIU for help in manuscript preparation.

Conflicts of Interest: The authors declare no conflict of interest.

References

1. Li, Q.; Guan, X.; Wu, P.; Wang, X.; Zhou, L.; Tong, Y.; Ren, R.; Leung, K.S.M.; Lau, E.H.Y. Early Transmission Dynamics in Wuhan, China, of Novel Coronavirus-Infected Pneumonia. *N. Engl. J. Med.* **2020**, *382*, 1199–1207. [CrossRef]
2. Novel-Coronavirus-Pneumonia-Emergency-Response-Epidemiology-Team. The epidemiological characteristics of an outbreak of 2019 novel coronavirus diseases (COVID-19) in China. *Zhonghua Liu Xing Bing Xue Za Zhi* **2020**, *41*, 145–151.
3. Guan, W.-J.; Ni, Z.-Y.; Hu, Y.; Liang, W.-H.; Ou, C.-Q.; He, J.-X.; Liu, L.; Shan, H.; Lei, C.-L.; Hui, D.S.; et al. Clinical Characteristics of Coronavirus Disease 2019 in China. *N. Engl. J. Med.* **2020**, *382*, 1708–1720. [CrossRef]
4. di Gennaro, F.; Gualano, G.; Timelli, L.; Vittozzi, P.; di Bari, V.; Libertone, R.; Cerva, C.; Pinnarelli, L.; Nisii, C.; Ianniello, S.; et al. Increase in tuberculosis diagnostic delay during first wave of the COVID-19 pandemic: Data from an Italian in-fectious disease referral hospital. *Antibiotics* **2021**, *10*, 272. [CrossRef] [PubMed]
5. Czeisler, M.; Marynak, K.; Clarke, K.E.N.; Salah, Z.; Shakya, I.; Thierry, J.M.; Ali, N.; McMillan, H.; Wiley, J.F.; Weaver, M.D.; et al. Delay or avoidance of medical care because of COVID-19–related concerns—United States, June 2020. *Morb. Mortal. Wkly. Rep.* **2020**, *69*, 1250. [CrossRef] [PubMed]
6. di Gennaro, F.; Murri, R.; Segala, F.V.; Cerruti, L.; Abdulle, A.; Saracino, A.; Bavaro, D.F.; Fantoni, M. Attitudes towards Anti-SARS-CoV2 Vaccination among Healthcare Workers: Results from a National Survey in Italy. *Viruses* **2021**, *13*, 371. [CrossRef] [PubMed]
7. Sallam, M. COVID-19 Vaccine Hesitancy Worldwide: A Concise Systematic Review of Vaccine Acceptance Rates. *Vaccines* **2021**, *9*, 160. [CrossRef] [PubMed]
8. Marotta, C.; Nacareia, U.; Estevez, A.; Tognon, F.; Genna, G.; De Meneghi, G.; Occa, E.; Ramirez, L.; Lazzari, M.; Di Gennaro, F.; et al. Mozambican Adolescents and Youths during the COVID-19 Pandemic: Knowledge and Awareness Gaps in the Provinces of Sofala and Tete. *Healthcare* **2021**, *9*, 321. [CrossRef]
9. Pouwels, K.B.; Pritchard, E.; Matthews, P.C.; Stoesser, N.; Eyre, D.W.; Vihta, K.; House, T.; Hay, J.; Bell, J.I.; Newton, J.N.; et al. Impact of Delta on viral burden and vaccine effectiveness against new SARS-CoV-2 infections in the UK. *medRxiv* **2021**. [CrossRef]
10. Kwok, S.; Adam, S.; Ho, J.H.; Iqbal, Z.; Turkington, P.; Razvi, S.; Le Roux, C.W.; Soran, H.; Syed, A.A. Obesity: A critical risk factor in the COVID-19 pandemic. *Clin. Obes.* **2020**, *10*, e12403. [CrossRef]
11. Zhou, F.; Yu, T.; Du, R.; Fan, G.; Liu, Y.; Liu, Z.; Xiang, J.; Wang, Y.; Song, B.; Gu, X.; et al. Clinical course and risk factors for mortality of adult inpatients with COVID-19 in Wuhan, China: A retrospective cohort study. *Lancet* **2020**, *395*, 1054–1062. [CrossRef]
12. Maddaloni, E.; D'Onofrio, L.; Alessandri, F.; Mignogna, C.; Leto, G.; Pascarella, G.; Mezzaroma, I.; Lichtner, M.; Pozzilli, P.; Agrò, F.E.; et al. Cardiometabolic multimorbidity is associated with a worse COVID-19 prognosis than individual cardiometabolic risk factors: A multicentre retrospective study (CoViDiab II). *Cardiovasc. Diabetol.* **2020**, *19*, 1–11. [CrossRef]
13. Gansevoort, R.T.; Hilbrands, L.B. CKD is a key risk factor for COVID-19 mortality. *Nat. Rev. Nephrol.* **2020**, *16*, 705–706. [CrossRef] [PubMed]
14. Zhou, Y.; Yang, Q.; Chi, J.; Dong, B.; Lv, W.; Shen, L.; Wang, Y. Comorbidities and the risk of severe or fatal outcomes associated with coronavirus disease 2019: A systematic review and meta-analysis. *Int. J. Infect. Dis.* **2020**, *99*, 47–56. [CrossRef] [PubMed]
15. Di Castelnuovo, A.; Bonaccio, M.; Costanzo, S.; Gialluisi, A.; Antinori, A.; Berselli, N.; Blandi, L.; Bruno, R.; Cauda, R.; Guaraldi, G.; et al. Common cardiovascular risk factors and in-hospital mortality in 3894 patients with COVID-19: Survival analysis and machine learning-based findings from the multicentre Italian CORIST Study. *Nutr. Metab. Cardiovasc. Dis.* **2020**, *30*, 1899–1913. [CrossRef] [PubMed]
16. Dotolo, S.; Marabotti, A.; Facchiano, A.; Tagliaferri, R. A review on drug repurposing applicable to COVID-19. *Brief. Bioinform.* **2020**, *22*, 726–741. [CrossRef] [PubMed]
17. Jarada, T.N.; Rokne, J.G.; Alhajj, R. A review of computational drug repositioning: Strategies, approaches, opportunities, challenges, and directions. *J. Cheminform.* **2020**, *12*, 46. [CrossRef]
18. Zhou, Y.; Hou, Y.; Shen, J.; Huang, Y.; Martinl, W.; Cheng, F. Network-based drug repurposing for novel coronavirus 2019-nCoV/SARS-CoV-2. *Cell Discov.* **2020**, *6*, 14. [CrossRef]
19. Gysi, D.M.; Valle, D.; Zitnik, M.; Ameli, A.; Gan, X.; Varol, O.; Ghiassian, S.D.; Patten, J.J.; Davey, R.A.; Loscalzo, J.; et al. Network medicine framework for identifying drug-repurposing opportunities for COVID-19. *Proc. Natl. Acad. Sci. USA* **2021**, *118*, e2025581118. [CrossRef]
20. Zhou, Y.; Hou, Y.; Shen, J.; Mehra, R.; Kallianpur, A.; Culver, D.A.; Gack, M.U.; Farha, S.; Zein, J.; Comhair, S.; et al. A network medicine approach to investigation and population-based validation of disease manifestations and drug repurposing for COVID-19. *PLoS Biol.* **2020**, *18*, e3000970. [CrossRef] [PubMed]
21. Liu, D.-Y.; Liu, J.-C.; Liang, S.; Meng, X.-H.; Greenbaum, J.; Xiao, H.-M.; Tan, L.-J.; Deng, H.-W. Drug Repurposing for COVID-19 Treatment by Integrating Network Pharmacology and Transcriptomics. *Pharmaceutics* **2021**, *13*, 545. [CrossRef]
22. Panda, P.K.; Arul, M.N.; Patel, P.; Verma, S.K.; Luo, W.; Rubahn, H.; Mishra, Y.K.; Suar, M.; Ahuja, R. Structure-based drug designing and immunoinformatics approach for SARS-CoV-2. *Sci. Adv.* **2020**, *6*, eabb8097. [CrossRef]
23. Daoud, S.; Alabed, S.J.; Dahabiyeh, L.A. Identification of potential COVID-19 main protease inhibitors using structure-based pharmacophore approach, molecular docking and repurposing studies. *Acta Pharm.* **2020**, *71*, 163–174. [CrossRef]

24. Jang, W.D.; Jeon, S.; Kim, S.; Lee, S.Y. Drugs repurposed for COVID-19 by virtual screening of 6218 drugs and cell-based assay. *Proc. Natl. Acad. Sci. USA* **2021**, *118*, e2024302118. [CrossRef]
25. Masoudi-Sobhanzadeh, Y.; Salemi, A.; Pourseif, M.M.; Jafari, B.; Omidi, Y.; Masoudi-Nejad, A. Structure-based drug repurposing against COVID-19 and emerging infectious diseases: Methods, resources and discoveries. *Brief. Bioinform.* **2021**, bbab113. [CrossRef]
26. Marigorta, U.M.; Rodríguez, J.A.; Gibson, G.; Navarro, A. Replicability and Prediction: Lessons and Challenges from GWAS. *Trends Genet.* **2018**, *34*, 504–517. [CrossRef]
27. Gurwitz, D. Repurposing current therapeutics for treating COVID-19: A vital role of prescription records data mining. *Drug Dev. Res.* **2020**, *81*, 777–781. [CrossRef]
28. Sudlow, C.; Gallacher, J.; Allen, N.; Beral, V.; Burton, P.; Danesh, J.; Downey, P.; Elliott, P.; Green, J.; Landray, M.; et al. UK Biobank: An Open Access Resource for Identifying the Causes of a Wide Range of Complex Diseases of Mid-dle and Old Age. *PLoS Med.* **2015**, *12*, e1001779. [CrossRef] [PubMed]
29. Antia, A.; Ahmed, H.; Handel, A.; Carlson, N.E.; Amanna, I.J.; Antia, R.; Slifka, M. Heterogeneity and longevity of antibody memory to viruses and vaccines. *PLoS Biol.* **2018**, *16*, e2006601. [CrossRef] [PubMed]
30. Benjamini, Y.; Hochberg, Y. Controlling the False Discovery Rate: A Practical and Powerful Approach to Multiple Testing. *J. R. Stat. Soc. Ser. B (Stat. Methodol.)* **1995**, *57*, 289–300. [CrossRef]
31. Waljee, A.K.; Mukherjee, A.; Singal, A.G.; Zhang, Y.; Warren, J.; Balis, U.; Marrero, J.; Zhu, J.; Higgins, P.D. Comparison of imputation methods for missing laboratory data in medicine. *BMJ Open* **2013**, *3*, e002847. [CrossRef] [PubMed]
32. Wright, M.N.; Ziegler, A. ranger: A Fast Implementation of Random Forests for High Dimensional Data in C++ and R. *J. Stat. Softw.* **2017**, *77*, 1–17. [CrossRef]
33. Rubin, D.B. *Multiple Imputation for Nonresponse in Surveys*; John Wiley & Sons: New York, NY, USA, 2004.
34. Griffith, G.J.; Morris, T.T.; Tudball, M.J.; Herbert, A.; Mancano, G.; Pike, L.; Sharp, G.C.; Sterne, J.; Palmer, T.M.; Smith, G.D.; et al. Collider bias undermines our understanding of COVID-19 disease risk and severity. *Nat. Commun.* **2020**, *11*, 5749. [CrossRef] [PubMed]
35. Yates, T.; Zaccardi, F.; Razieh, C.; Gillies, C.L.; Rowlands, A.; Kloecker, D.E.; Chudasama, Y.V.; Davies, M.J.; Khunti, K. Framework to aid analysis and interpretation of ongoing COVID-19 research [version 1; peer review: 1 approved with reservations]. *Wellcome Open Res.* **2020**, *5*, 208. [CrossRef]
36. Wong, K.C.Y.; Xiang, Y.; So, H. Uncovering clinical risk factors and prediction of severe COVID-19: A machine learning approach based on UK Biobank data. *medRxiv* **2020**. [CrossRef]
37. Kull, M.; Silva Filho, T.; Flach, P. Beta calibration: A well-founded and easily implemented improvement on logistic calibration for binary classifiers. In Proceedings of the 20th International Conference on Artificial Intelligence and Statistics, Ft. Lauderdale, FL, USA, 20–22 April 2017; pp. 623–631.
38. Xu, S.; Ross, C.; Raebel, M.A.; Shetterly, S.; Blanchette, C.; Smith, D. Use of Stabilized Inverse Propensity Scores as Weights to Directly Estimate Relative Risk and Its Confidence Intervals. *Value Health* **2010**, *13*, 273–277. [CrossRef]
39. Buckley, J.P.; Doherty, B.T.; Keil, A.P.; Engel, S.M. Statistical Approaches for Estimating Sex-Specific Effects in Endocrine Disruptors Research. *Environ. Health Perspect.* **2017**, *125*, 067013. [CrossRef] [PubMed]
40. Nishiga, M.; Wang, D.W.; Han, Y.; Lewis, D.B.; Wu, J.C. COVID-19 and cardiovascular disease: From basic mechanisms to clinical perspectives. *Nat. Rev. Cardiol.* **2020**, *17*, 543–558. [CrossRef] [PubMed]
41. Kow, C.S.; Hasan, S.S. Meta-analysis of Effect of Statins in Patients with COVID-19. *Am. J. Cardiol.* **2020**, *134*, 153–155. [CrossRef]
42. Tan, W.Y.T.; Young, B.E.; Lye, D.C.; Chew, D.E.K.; Dalan, R. Statin use is associated with lower disease severity in COVID-19 infection. *Sci. Rep.* **2020**, *10*, 17458. [CrossRef]
43. Saeed, O.; Castagna, F.; Agalliu, I.; Xue, X.; Patel, S.; Rochlani, Y.; Kataria, R.; Vukelic, S.; Sims, D.B.; Alvarez, C.; et al. Statin Use and In-Hospital Mortality in Diabetics with COVID-19. *J. Am. Heart Assoc.* **2020**, *9*, e018475. [CrossRef]
44. Ganjali, S.; Bianconi, V.; Penson, P.; Pirro, M.; Banach, M.; Watts, G.F.; Sahebkar, A. Commentary: Statins, COVID-19, and coronary artery disease: Killing two birds with one stone. *Metabolism* **2020**, *113*, 154375. [CrossRef] [PubMed]
45. Minz, M.M.; Bansal, M.; Kasliwal, R.R. Statins and SARS-CoV-2 disease: Current concepts and possible benefits. *Diabetol. Metab. Syndr.* **2020**, *14*, 2063–2067. [CrossRef] [PubMed]
46. Lee, K.C.H.; Sewa, D.W.; Phua, G.C. Potential role of statins in COVID-19. *Int. J. Infect. Dis.* **2020**, *96*, 615–617. [CrossRef]
47. Lee, I.T.; Nakayama, T.; Wu, C.-T.; Goltsev, Y.; Jiang, S.; Gall, P.A.; Liao, C.-K.; Shih, L.-C.; Schürch, C.M.; McIlwain, D.R.; et al. ACE2 localizes to the respiratory cilia and is not increased by ACE inhibitors or ARBs. *Nat. Commun.* **2020**, *11*, 5453. [CrossRef]
48. Mackey, K.; Kansagara, D.; Vela, K. Update Alert 4: Risks and Impact of Angiotensin-Converting Enzyme Inhibitors or Angioten-sin-Receptor Blockers on SARS-CoV-2 Infection in Adults. *Ann. Intern. Med.* **2020**, *173*, W147–W148. [CrossRef]
49. Barochiner, J.; Martínez, R. Use of inhibitors of the renin-angiotensin system in hypertensive patients and COVID-19 severity: A systematic review and meta-analysis. *J. Clin. Pharm. Ther.* **2020**, *45*, 1244–1252. [CrossRef]
50. Hippisley-Cox, J.; Young, D.; Coupland, C.; Channon, K.M.; Tan, P.S.; Harrison, D.A.; Rowan, K.; Aveyard, P.; Pavord, I.D.; Watkinson, P.J. Risk of severe COVID-19 disease with ACE inhibitors and angiotensin receptor blockers: Cohort study in-cluding 8.3 million people. *Heart* **2020**, *106*, 1503–1511. [CrossRef]
51. Megaly, M.; Glogoza, M. Renin-angiotensin system antagonists are associated with lower mortality in hypertensive patients with COVID-19. *Scott. Med. J.* **2020**, *65*, 123–126. [CrossRef]

52. Pan, W.; Zhang, J.; Wang, M.; Ye, J.; Xu, Y.; Shen, B.; He, H.; Wang, Z.; Ye, D.; Zhao, M.; et al. Clinical Features of COVID-19 in Patients with Essential Hypertension and the Impacts of Ren-in-angiotensin-aldosterone System Inhibitors on the Prognosis of COVID-19 Patients. *Hypertension* **2020**, *76*, 732–741. [CrossRef] [PubMed]
53. Bean, D.M.; Kraljevic, Z.; Searle, T.; Bendayan, R.; Kevin, O.G.; Pickles, A.; Folarin, A.; Roguski, L.; Noor, K.; Shek, A.; et al. ACE-inhibitors and Angiotensin-2 Receptor Blockers are not associated with severe SARS-COVID19 infection in a multi-site UK acute Hospital Trust. *Eur. J. Heart Fail.* **2020**, *22*, 967–974. [CrossRef]
54. Feng, Y.; Ling, Y.; Bai, T.; Xie, Y.; Huang, J.; Li, J.; Xiong, W.; Yang, D.; Chen, R.; Lu, F.; et al. COVID-19 with Different Severities: A Multicenter Study of Clinical Features. *Am. J. Respir. Crit. Care Med.* **2020**, *201*, 1380–1388. [CrossRef]
55. Zhang, P.; Zhu, L.; Cai, J.; Lei, F.; Qin, J.-J.; Xie, J.; Liu, Y.-M.; Zhao, Y.-C.; Huang, X.; Lin, L.; et al. Association of Inpatient Use of Angiotensin-Converting Enzyme Inhibitors and Angiotensin II Receptor Blockers with Mortality among Patients with Hypertension Hospitalized with COVID-19. *Circ. Res.* **2020**, *126*, 1671–1681. [CrossRef] [PubMed]
56. Scheen, A. Metformin and COVID-19: From cellular mechanisms to reduced mortality. *Diabetes Metab.* **2020**, *46*, 423–426. [CrossRef]
57. Sharma, S.; Ray, A.; Sadasivam, B. Metformin in COVID-19: A possible role beyond diabetes. *Diabetes Res. Clin. Pract.* **2020**, *164*, 108183. [CrossRef]
58. Barbieri, A.; Robinson, N.; Palma, G.; Maurea, N.; Desiderio, V.; Botti, G. Can Beta-2-Adrenergic Pathway Be a New Target to Combat SARS-CoV-2 Hyperinflammatory Syn-drome?—Lessons Learned from Cancer. *Front. Immunol.* **2020**, *11*, 2615. [CrossRef]
59. Straus, M.R.; Bidon, M.; Tang, T.; Whittaker, G.R.; Daniel, S. FDA approved calcium channel blockers inhibit SARS-CoV-2 infec-tivity in epithelial lung cells. *bioRxiv* **2020**, 214577. [CrossRef]
60. Chouchana, L.; Beeker, N.; Garcelon, N.; Rance, B.; Paris, N.; Salamanca, E.; Polard, E.; Burgun, A.; Treluyer, J.; Neuraz, A. Association of antihypertensive agents with the risk of in-hospital death in patients with COVID-19. *Cardiovasc. Drugs Ther.* **2021**, *35*, 1–6.
61. Rezel-Potts, E.; Douiri, A.; Chowienczyk, P.J.; Gulliford, M.C. Antihypertensive Medications and COVID-19 Diagnosis and Mortal-ity: Population-based Case-Control Analysis in the United Kingdom. *Br. J. Clin. Pharm.* **2021**, *87*. [CrossRef]
62. Blok, B.A.; Arts, R.J.W.; Van Crevel, R.; Benn, C.S.; Netea, M.G. Trained innate immunity as underlying mechanism for the long-term, nonspecific effects of vaccines. *J. Leukoc. Biol.* **2015**, *98*, 347–356. [CrossRef] [PubMed]
63. Jensen, K.J.; Benn, C.S.; van Crevel, R. Unravelling the nature of non-specific effects of vaccines-A challenge for innate immu-nologists. *Semin. Immunol.* **2016**, *28*, 377–383. [CrossRef]
64. Pawlowski, C.; Puranik, A.; Bandi, H.; Venkatakrishnan, A.J.; Agarwal, V.; Kennedy, R.; O'Horo, J.C.; Gores, G.J.; Williams, A.W.; Halamka, J.; et al. Exploratory analysis of immunization records highlights decreased SARS-CoV-2 rates in individuals with recent non-COVID-19 vaccinations. *Sci. Rep.* **2021**, *47*, 335–340.
65. Debisarun, P.A.; Struycken, P.; Domínguez-Andrés, J.; Moorlag, S.J.C.F.M.; Taks, E.; Gössling, K.L.; Ostermann, P.N.; Müller, L.; Schaal, H.; Oever, J.T.; et al. The effect of influenza vaccination on trained immunity: Impact on COVID-19. *medRxiv* **2020**. [CrossRef]
66. Strope, J.D.; Chau, C.H.; Figg, W.D. Are sex discordant outcomes in COVID-19 related to sex hormones? *Semin. Oncol.* **2020**, *47*, 335–340. [CrossRef]
67. Mauvais-Jarvis, F.; Klein, S.L.; Levin, E.R. Estradiol, Progesterone, Immunomodulation, and COVID-19 Outcomes. *Endocrinology* **2020**, *161*, bqaa127. [CrossRef] [PubMed]
68. Brandi, M.L.; Giustina, A. Sexual Dimorphism of Coronavirus 19 Morbidity and Lethality. *Trends Endocrinol. Metab.* **2020**, *31*, 918–927. [CrossRef] [PubMed]
69. Pantos, C.; Tseti, I.; Mourouzis, I. Use of triiodothyronine to treat critically ill COVID-19 patients: A new clinical trial. *Crit. Care* **2020**, *24*, 209. [CrossRef]
70. Pantos, C.; Kostopanagiotou, G.; Armaganidis, A.; Trikas, A.; Tseti, I.; Mourouzis, I. Triiodothyronine for the treatment of critically ill patients with COVID-19 infection: A structured summary of a study protocol for a randomised controlled trial. *Trials* **2020**, *21*, 573. [CrossRef]
71. Luxenburger, H.; Sturm, L.; Biever, P.; Rieg, S.; Duerschmied, D.; Schultheiss, M.; Neumann-Haefelin, C.; Thimme, R.; Bettinger, D. Treatment with proton pump inhibitors increases the risk of secondary infections and ARDS in hospitalized patients with COVID-19: Coincidence or underestimated risk factor? *J. Intern. Med.* **2020**, *289*, 121–124. [CrossRef]
72. Kow, C.S.; Hasan, S.S. Use of proton pump inhibitors and risk of adverse clinical outcomes from COVID-19: A meta-analysis. *J. Intern. Med.* **2020**, *289*, 125–128. [CrossRef]
73. Flory, C.M.; Norris, B.J.; Larson, N.A.; Coicou, L.G.; Koniar, B.L.; Mysz, M.A.; Rich, T.P.; Ingbar, D.H.; Schumacher, R.J. A Preclinical Safety Study of Thyroid Hormone Instilled into the Lungs of Healthy Rats—An Investigational Therapy for ARDS. *J. Pharmacol. Exp. Ther.* **2020**, *376*, 74–83. [CrossRef] [PubMed]
74. Touret, F.; Gilles, M.; Barral, K.; Nougairède, A.; van Helden, J.; Decroly, E.; de Lamballerie, X.; Coutard, B. In vitro screening of a FDA approved chemical library reveals potential inhibitors of SARS-CoV-2 replication. *Sci. Rep.* **2020**, *10*, 13093. [CrossRef] [PubMed]
75. Cadegiani, F.A.; McCoy, J.; Wambier, C.G.; Goren, A. 5-Alpha-Reductase Inhibitors Reduce Remission Time of COVID-19: Re-sults From a Randomized Double Blind Placebo Controlled Interventional Trial in 130 SARS-CoV-2 Positive Men. *medRxiv* **2020**. [CrossRef]

76. Tan, M.H.E.; Li, J.; Xu, H.E.; Melcher, K.; Yong, E.-L. Androgen receptor: Structure, role in prostate cancer and drug discovery. *Acta Pharmacol. Sin.* **2014**, *36*, 3–23. [CrossRef]
77. Goren, A.; Wambier, C.G.; Herrera, S.; McCoy, J.; Vaño-Galván, S.; Gioia, F.; Comeche, B.; Ron, R.; Serrano-Villar, S.; Ramos, P.M.; et al. Anti-androgens may protect against severe COVID-19 outcomes: Results from a prospective cohort study of 77 hospitalized men. *J. Eur. Acad. Dermatol. Venereol.* **2020**, *34*. [CrossRef]
78. Hoffmann, M.; Kleine-Weber, H.; Schroeder, S.; Krüger, N.; Herrler, T.; Erichsen, S.; Schiergens, T.S.; Herrler, G.; Wu, N.; Nitsche, A.; et al. SARS-CoV-2 Cell Entry Depends on ACE2 and TMPRSS2 and Is Blocked by a Clinically Proven Protease Inhibitor. *Cell* **2020**, *181*, 271–280. [CrossRef]
79. Lucas, J.M.; Heinlein, C.; Kim, T.; Hernandez, S.A.; Malik, M.S.; True, L.D.; Morrissey, C.; Corey, E.; Montgomery, B.; Mostaghel, E.; et al. The Androgen-Regulated Protease TMPRSS2 Activates a Proteolytic Cascade Involving Components of the Tumor Microenvironment and Promotes Prostate Cancer Metastasis. *Cancer Discov.* **2014**, *4*, 1310–1325. [CrossRef] [PubMed]
80. Al-Ani, F.; Chehade, S.; Lazo-Langner, A. Thrombosis risk associated with COVID-19 infection. A scoping review. *Thromb. Res.* **2020**, *192*, 152–160. [CrossRef]
81. Godino, C.; Scotti, A.; Maugeri, N.; Mancini, N.; Fominskiy, E.; Margonato, A.; Landoni, G. Antithrombotic therapy in patients with COVID-19? -Rationale and Evidence-. *Int. J. Cardiol.* **2020**, *324*, 261–266. [CrossRef]
82. Chow, J.H.; Khanna, A.; Kethireddy, S.; Yamane, D.; Levine, A.; Jackson, A.M.; Mccurdy, M.T.; Tabatabai, A.; Kumar, G.; Park, P.; et al. Aspirin Use is Associated with Decreased Mechanical Ventilation, ICU Admission, and In-Hospital Mortality in Hospitalized Patients with COVID-19. *Anesth. Analg.* **2020**, *132*, 930–941. [CrossRef]
83. Goldstein, R. Conditioning Diagnostics: Collinearity and Weak Data in Regression. *Technometrics* **1993**, *35*, 85–86. [CrossRef]
84. Neidich, S.D.; Green, W.D.; Rebeles, J.; Karlsson, E.; Schultz-Cherry, S.; Noah, T.L.; Chakladar, S.; Hudgens, M.G.; Weir, S.S.; Beck, M.A. Increased risk of influenza among vaccinated adults who are obese. *Int. J. Obes.* **2017**, *41*, 1324–1330. [CrossRef]
85. Frasca, D.; Blomberg, B.B. The Impact of Obesity and Metabolic Syndrome on Vaccination Success. *Interdiscip. Top. Gerontol. Geriatr.* **2020**, *43*, 86–97. [CrossRef]
86. Donati, Z.S.; Agostini, D.; Piccoli, G.; Stocchi, V.; Sestili, P. Gut Microbiota Status in COVID-19: An Unrecognized Player? *Front. Cell. Infect. Microbiol.* **2020**, *10*, 576551. [CrossRef] [PubMed]
87. Zuo, T.; Zhang, F.; Lui, G.C.; Yeoh, Y.K.; Li, A.Y.; Zhan, H.; Wan, Y.; Chung, A.C.; Cheung, C.P.; Chen, N.; et al. Alterations in Gut Microbiota of Patients With COVID-19 during Time of Hospitalization. *Gastroenterology* **2020**, *159*, 944–955. [CrossRef]
88. Vila, A.V.; Collij, V.; Sanna, S.; Sinha, T.; Imhann, F.; Bourgonje, A.; Mujagic, Z.; Jonkers, D.M.A.E.; Masclee, A.A.M.; Fu, J.; et al. Impact of commonly used drugs on the composition and metabolic function of the gut microbiota. *Nat. Commun.* **2020**, *11*, 362. [CrossRef]
89. McKeigue, P.M.; Kennedy, S.; Weir, A.; Bishop, J.; McGurnaghan, S.J.; McAllister, D.; Robertson, C.; Wood, R.; Lone, N.; Murray, J.; et al. Associations of severe COVID-19 with polypharmacy in the REACT-SCOT case-control study. *medRxiv* **2020**. [CrossRef]
90. Barlow-Pay, F.; Htut, T.W.; Khezrian, M.; Myint, P.K. Systematic review of immunosuppressant guidelines in the COVID-19 pan-demic. *Adv. Drug. Saf.* **2021**, *12*. [CrossRef]
91. Schoot, T.S.; Kerckhoffs, A.P.M.; Hilbrands, L.B.; Van Marum, R.J. Immunosuppressive Drugs and COVID-19: A Review. *Front. Pharmacol.* **2020**, *11*. [CrossRef] [PubMed]
92. Slaine, P.D.; Kleer, M.; Duguay, B.A.; Pringle, E.S.; Kadijk, E.; Ying, S.; Balgi, A.; Roberge, M.; McCormick, C.; Khaperskyy, D.A. Thiopurines Activate an Antiviral Unfolded Protein Response That Blocks Influenza A Virus Glycoprotein Accumulation. *J. Virol.* **2021**, *95*, e00453-21. [CrossRef]
93. Swaim, C.D.; Perng, Y.; Zhao, X.; Canadeo, L.A.; Harastani, H.H.; Darling, T.L.; Boon, A.C.M.; Lenschow, D.J.; Huibregtse, J.M. 6-Thioguanine blocks SARS-CoV-2 replication by inhibition of PLpro protease activities. *bioRxiv* **2020**. [CrossRef]
94. Ungaro, R.C.; Brenner, E.J.; Gearry, R.B.; Kaplan, G.G.; Kissous-Hunt, M.; Lewis, J.D.; Ng, S.C.; Rahier, J.-F.; Reinisch, W.; Steinwurz, F.; et al. Effect of IBD medications on COVID-19 outcomes: Results from an international registry. *Gut* **2020**, *70*, 725–732. [CrossRef] [PubMed]
95. Nørgård, B.M.; Nielsen, J.; Knudsen, T.; Nielsen, R.G.; Larsen, M.D.; Jølving, L.R.; Kjeldsen, J. Hospitalization for COVID-19 in patients treated with selected immunosuppressant and immunomodulating agents, compared to the general population: A Danish cohort study. *Br. J. Clin. Pharmacol.* **2021**, *87*, 2111–2120. [CrossRef] [PubMed]
96. Fry, A.; Littlejohns, T.J.; Sudlow, C.; Doherty, N.; Adamska, L.; Sprosen, T.; Collins, R.; Allen, N.E. Comparison of Sociodemographic and Health-Related Characteristics of UK Biobank Participants with Those of the General Population. *Am. J. Epidemiol.* **2017**, *186*, 1026–1034. [CrossRef] [PubMed]
97. Moskvina, V.; Holmans, P.; Schmidt, K.M.; Craddock, N. Design of Case-controls Studies with Unscreened Controls. *Ann. Hum. Genet.* **2005**, *69*, 566–576. [CrossRef]
98. Peyrot, W.J.; Boomsma, D.I.; Penninx, B.W.; Wray, N.R. Disease and Polygenic Architecture: Avoid Trio Design and Appropriately Account for Unscreened Control Subjects for Common Disease. *Am. J. Hum. Genet.* **2016**, *98*, 382–391. [CrossRef]

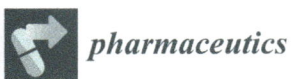

Article

Discovery of a Potent Candidate for RET-Specific Non-Small-Cell Lung Cancer—A Combined In Silico and In Vitro Strategy

Priyanka Ramesh [1], Woong-Hee Shin [2,3,*] and Shanthi Veerappapillai [1,*]

1. Department of Biotechnology, School of Bio Sciences and Technology, Vellore Institute of Technology, Vellore 632014, India; priyanka.r@vit.ac.in
2. Department of Chemical Science Education, College of Education, Sunchon National University, Suncheon 57922, Korea
3. Department of Advanced Components and Materials Engineering, Sunchon National University, Suncheon 57922, Korea
* Correspondence: whshin@scnu.ac.kr (W.-H.S.); shanthi.v@vit.ac.in (S.V.)

Abstract: Rearranged during transfection (RET) is a tyrosine kinase oncogenic receptor, activated in several cancers including non-small-cell lung cancer (NSCLC). Multiple kinase inhibitors vandetanib and cabozantinib are commonly used in the treatment of RET-positive NSCLC. However, specificity, toxicity, and reduced efficacy limit the usage of multiple kinase inhibitors in targeting RET protein. Thus, in the present investigation, we aimed to figure out novel and potent candidates for the inhibition of RET protein using combined in silico and in vitro strategies. In the present study, screening of 11,808 compounds from the DrugBank repository was accomplished by different hypotheses such as pharmacophore, e-pharmacophore, and receptor cavity-based models in the initial stage. The results from the different hypotheses were then integrated to eliminate the false positive prediction. The inhibitory activities of the screened compounds were tested by the glide docking algorithm. Moreover, RF score, Tanimoto coefficient, prime-MM/GBSA, and density functional theory calculations were utilized to re-score the binding free energy of the docked complexes with high precision. This procedure resulted in three lead molecules, namely DB07194, DB03496, and DB11982, against the RET protein. The screened lead molecules together with reference compounds were then subjected to a long molecular dynamics simulation with a 200 ns time duration to validate the inhibitory activity. Further analysis of compounds using MM-PBSA and mutation studies resulted in the identification of potent compound DB07194. In essence, a cell viability assay with RET-specific lung cancer cell line LC-2/ad was also carried out to confirm the in vitro biological activity of the resultant compound, DB07194. Indeed, the results from our study conclude that DB07194 can be effectively translated for this new therapeutic purpose, in contrast to the properties for which it was originally designed and synthesized.

Keywords: LC-2/ad cell line; drug discovery; docking; MM-GBSA calculation; molecular dynamics; cytotoxicity assay

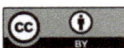

1. Introduction

Targeted therapies using tailored inhibitors against oncogenic driver kinases have transformed the landscape of cancer management, including non-small-cell lung cancer (NSCLC) [1]. Notably, first-generation inhibitors against oncogenic drivers such as gefitinib, erlotinib (EGFR mutations), and crizotinib (ALK rearrangement) have established a novel treatment paradigm for the use of targeted inhibitors in genetically defined NSCLC patients [2,3]. Despite the earlier success of these strategies, the emergence of acquired resistance against the therapy has become a significant challenge in developing selective and more potent next-generation inhibitors.

Rearranged during transfection (RET), a transmembrane tyrosine kinase receptor was found to be overexpressed in 1–2% of never-smoking NSCLC patients [4]. In general, it plays a vital role in the development of neural crest cells in the nervous system and kidney morphogenesis. RET consists of three domains: adhesion, tyrosine kinase, and extracellular domain. Activation of RET involves autophosphorylation of a fusion protein complex with a glial cell line derived from neurotrophic factors (GDNF) and GFR-α, a cell membrane-bound coreceptor [5,6]. The downstream signaling of RET assists in cell migration, proliferation, and differentiation. Nevertheless, genetic alteration of RET oncogenes promotes ligand-independent activation of driver kinases, resulting in tumorigenesis. A study in late 2011 revealed that pericentric inversion, rearrangement, dimerization, and activation of RET proteins with KIF5B and CCD6C in NSCLC were analogous to the mechanism of ALK [7]. Multiple Kinase Inhibitors (MKIs), including cabozantinib and vandetanib, gave the first glimmer of hope for the treatment of RET-positive NSCLC patients. However, these nonselective MKIs demonstrated limited response durability and off-target side effects in NSCLC patients [8]. Thus, selective inhibitors such as selpercatinib and pralsetinib were developed to offset the debility of the multiple kinase inhibitors.

Recently, the emergence of solvent front mutations and gatekeeper mutations in RET-positive NSCLC patients has been reported as the primary cause for the development of acquired resistance against the targeted kinase inhibitors [9]. A similar pattern of the solvent front and gatekeeper mutations was observed in several types of oncogenic driven NSCLCs. A typical example of other proteins associated with resistance in NSCLC includes ALK rearrangement, ROS-1 positive, and EGFR mutations. A significant number of reports are available to tackle resistance caused by the above genes [10]. However, studies on RET mutations in NSCLC are very minimal and are not satisfactory [11]. In addition, it is to be noted that MKIs were the only choice of drug to treat RET-driven NSCLC. Recently, the selective inhibitor pralsetinib was administered in both naïve and platinum-based chemotherapy-treated patients. Among the cohort, 10% of the patients were detected with solvent front mutations (G810C/S), 15% were detected with MET amplification and 5% of the cohort were detected with KRAS amplification [12]. Although the study ended up with satisfactory results and was found to have overcome gatekeeper mutations during the clinical trials, the adverse side effects of the drug limit its efficacy and it failed to overcome solvent front mutations [13]. Moreover, the resistance mechanism of solvent front mutations to selective inhibitors is not yet reported in the literature [14]. Hence, developing next-generation targeted kinase inhibitors particularly against RET solvent front mutations is desperately needed to overcome the acquired resistance.

Virtual screening of active compounds for hit identification and lead optimization has been made possible by advancements in bioinformatics and computer modeling in modern drug research [15]. For instance, Misra et al. identified two potent human great wall kinase inhibitors using the ZINC database that mitigate mitotic division in various types of cancer [16]. Similarly, Tamta et al. identified and validated three natural inhibitors against Mpro of SARS-CoV-2 using different in silico strategies including molecular docking, dynamics and MM-PBSA analysis [17]. In view of the successful evidence mentioned above, we implemented an integrated approach using pralsetinib as the reference inhibitor towards the screening of potent candidates against RET protein. Three different models were generated for performing a virtual screening process using FDA approved, experimental and investigative subsets of the DrugBank database, followed by docking analysis, to identify potent and highly selective RET inhibitors. The combined assessment in this study provides a highly potent drug-like candidate tailored for RET oncogenic drivers that can overcome acquired resistance in NSCLC patients.

2. Materials and Methods

2.1. Dataset Retrieval and Structural Refinement

The 3D conformation of RET tyrosine kinase with PDB ID: 2IVU and resolution of 2.5 Å were retrieved from Protein Data Bank (PDB) (www.rcsb.org/pdb, accessed on 27 August 2021). RET protein was prepared using the protein preparation wizard of the Schrödinger suite [18]. This process involves eliminating water molecules and impurities and incorporating hydrogen bonds and ionization states to the protein. The optimization and minimization of 2IVU were performed using the optimized potential for liquid simulation _2005 (OPLS_2005) force field, to increase the protein's binding efficiency during docking analysis.

Table S1 (see Supplementary Materials) represents the existing RET inhibitors retrieved from various literature. They were utilized for pharmacophore hypothesis generation [19–21]. In addition, the spatial data file (SDF) of molecules in a different subset of the DrugBank repository containing a total of 11,808 compounds was extracted for proceeding with standalone library generation and the virtual screening process. The existing inhibitors and generated library were refined by attaching the hydrogen bonds, generating the stereoisomer, and identifying the significant ionization state using the LigPrep module of Schrödinger. Finally, the OPLS_2005 force field was used to optimize the ligand structures considered in our study [22].

2.2. Hypothesis Generation and Molecular Docking

The screening hypotheses were generated based on three different approaches, such as ligands, protein structure, and energetics of protein–ligand interactions with the aid of the Phase module of Schrödinger (version 5.3). Initially, the reference ligands were divided into actives and inactives based on their IC_{50} values (Table S1, see Supplementary Materials). Compounds with IC50 values higher than 5.0 µM were classified as inactive molecules. Consequently, the ligand-based pharmacophoric hypothesis was generated based on the common features of the active ligands using a tree-based partitioning algorithm [23]. Each common pharmacophore hypothesis (CPH) undergoes a rigorous scoring function based on alignment score, volume score, and vector score of the active ligands. The best CPH with high survival score was chosen for the virtual screening analysis. In the e-pharmacophore strategy, CPH was generated by docking the reference ligand pralsetinib and by mapping the energetic scores onto the atoms [24]. Similarly, receptor cavity-based CPH was developed based on the potential binding site of the RET protein using the SiteMap module of Schrödinger. Altogether, the chosen CPH contained four basic pharmacophoric features, namely a hydrophobic group (H), aromatic ring (R), hydrogen bond acceptor (A), and donor (D) [25]. Finally, the above-generated high precision CPH was used independently to screen the subsets of the DrugBank database. The resultant set in each screening was subjected to three hierarchical docking strategies, namely high-throughput virtual screening (HTVS), standard precision (SP), and extra precision (XP), which were implemented using the Glide module to identify the binders from nonbinders [26]. It is worth nothing that pralsetinib was used as the reference inhibitor throughout the investigation. Finally, the interaction pattern and the essential pharmacokinetic parameters such as stars, central nervous system response (CNS), and human oral absorption (HOA) were analyzed using the Qikprop module of Schrödinger.

2.3. Machine Learning-Based Standalone Rescoring Function

Random Forest score (RF score) based the rescoring function was implemented to determine the binding affinity between the ligand and RET for virtual screening using the open drug discovery toolkit available in https://github.com/oddt/rfscorevs, accessed on 27 August 2021. This scoring function is built using an RF algorithm with descriptors generated based on the distance between the atoms of the protein and the ligand that lie within 12 Å [27]. Compounds that have an RF score greater than the pralsetinib score were considered for further evaluation.

2.4. Chemical Similarity Calculations

Tanimoto coefficient (T_c) was similarly calculated based on the MACCS fingerprint to evaluate the structural similarities of all the compounds. A higher value of T_c depicts the high structural similarity of the compounds with the reference molecule. Hence, the cut-off T_c value of >0.4 was considered in this analysis to quantify the fraction of compounds that exhibit structural similarity to pralsetinib [28]. In the present study, RDKit of the python library was implemented to generate the MACCS fingerprint and to calculate the T_c of the compounds.

2.5. Binding Free Energy and DFT Calculations

The prime module of the Schrödinger suite was used to determine the binding free energy of RET protein–ligand complexes. It is interesting to note that the binding free energies that were calculated using the MM-GBSA method correlated with the experimental study most of the time. The pose viewer file of the protein–ligand complex generated during Glide XP docking was used as a query for binding free-energy calculations. Further, the prime module utilizes the VSGB 2.0 solvation model to optimize hydrogen bonds, hydrophobic interactions, π–π interactions, and self-contact interactions [29]. The energy terms such as electronic interactions, Van der Waal's interaction, entropy terms, polar and nonpolar contributions were considered for the binding free-energy calculations in the Prime package of Schrödinger.

Density functional theory (DFT) was calculated for the hit compounds obtained during the virtual screening process. Jaguar v8.7 was employed to calculate the nature of the interaction between the protein and ligand and molecular electrostatic properties such as highest occupied molecular orbital (HOMO) and lowest unoccupied molecular orbital (LUMO). Frontier orbital gaps of the hit compounds were calculated to analyze the kinetic stability and chemical activity [30].

2.6. Assessing the Stability and Binding Mode of 2IVU–Ligand Complex

A molecular dynamics (MD) simulation of the RET–ligand complex was used in this study to assess the stability and conformational changes of a protein–ligand complex. GROMACS v5.1.2 (Virginia Tech Department of Biochemistry, Blacksburg, VA, United States) with GROMOS96 43a1 force field was used for the simulation. The topology files and the parameters for the ligands were developed using the PRODRG server. Dodecahedron box with dimensions of 1 nm × 1 nm × 1 nm was configured using editconf inbuilt tool of GROMACS. Subsequently, the Simple Point Charge model was explicitly used for solvating the complex system in a dodecahedron box. During the solvation process, the system exhibited a total charge of +8. Hence, eight chlorine counter ions were added to neutralize the protein system. The weak Van der Waals linkages were removed using the Steepest Descent algorithm to minimize the energy of the complex. Electrostatic interactions were enlightened by applying the Particle-Mesh Ewald method. LINCS algorithm was implemented for constraining the hydrogen bonds and for truncating the Van der Waals interactions. The canonical calculations of NVT (Number of particles, Volume, and Temperature) and NPT (Number of particles, Pressure, and Temperature) ensembles were executed for restraining the position. The complex system was heated using a Berendsen thermostat at 300 K with a lapsing time of 0.1 ps and pressure of 1 bar. Precedent to MD simulation, a pre-run was performed with a 1000 kJ mol^{-1} nm^{-2} force constant as a positional restraint for 50 ps. Ultimately, final MD for the apoprotein (without ligand) and protein–ligand complex were carried out for 200 ns [31]. Trajectories for the complex system were saved every 2 fs. Root Mean Square Deviation (RMSD), Root Mean Square Fluctuation (RMSF), H-bond linkages, free-energy landscape, and the salt bridge between the ligand and the protein were also evaluated using GROMACS utilities. In essence, the MM-PBSA strategy was also implemented to calculate the empirical free energies between the RET receptor and the identified potential ligands with high precision [32].

2.7. In Vitro Analysis

The anticancer activities of the potential compounds together with pralsetinib were determined using MTT assay [33]. The LC-2/ad cell was purchased from the European Collection of Authenticated Cell Cultures (Catalogue number: ECACC 94072247, Merck KGaA, Darmstadt, Germany) and grown in high-glucose Dulbecco's Modified Eagle Medium (AL149, Himedia, Mumbai, India) for 24 h. The cell line contains CCDC6-RET driver gene fusion isolated from the lung of a 51-year-old adenocarcinoma Japanese patient. This cell line is widely used to study intracellular signaling pathways, resistance mechanisms, and drug sensitivity against RET fusion in NSCLC samples. The chemical compounds pralsetinib and DB07194 were purchased from MolPort (Catalogue number: HY-112301, Molprot, Riga, Latvia) and Merck (Catalogue number: 574715-2mg, MercK KGaA, Darmstadt, Germany), respectively. Consequently, the grown LC-2/ad cells were exposed to reference and hit compound concentrations ranging from 6.25 µM/mL to 100 µM/mL for four days at 37 °C in a 5% CO_2 atmosphere. The absorbance of the samples was read at 570 nm and 630 nm as the reference wavelength to correct the nonspecific background values. The experiment was performed in triplets, and the mean value of the assays was considered in our analysis. Finally, the IC_{50} of the compound was determined using a linear regression equation and viability graph. In addition, a statistical comparison of cell viability between control and drug candidates was carried out using one-way ANOVA. For all comparisons, a *p*-value of less than 0.05 was regarded as statistically significant.

3. Results and Discussion

3.1. Pharmacophore Modeling and Virtual Screening

A pharmacophore is a collection of chemical features and spatial properties required for the ligand to interact with a macromolecular target and elicit a biological response [34]. In the present investigation, about 193 ligand-based pharmacophore hypotheses were developed with the assistance of actives and inactives (Table S1, see Supplementary Materials) using the Phase module of Schrödinger (v5.3). Depending on the survival score, a five feature CPH containing one hydrogen bond acceptor (A), one hydrogen bond donor (D), one hydrophobic group (H), and two aromatic rings (R) were selected. Likewise, two other hypotheses, DHRRR and ADDHR, were generated from the e-pharmacophore and receptor cavity-based strategies, respectively. A total of 3673, 1198, and 4595 compounds were obtained after phase screening using pharmacophore, e-pharmacophore, and receptor cavity-based hypotheses, respectively. The screened compounds were subjected to three tiers of docking such as HTVS, SP and XP using pralsetinib (−7.79 kcal/mol) as a reference compound. In each stage, 50% of high-scoring leads were passed on to further analysis. This process yielded a total of 887 (Pharmacophore-208; e-Pharmacophore-103; Receptor cavity-576) compounds possessing better binding capability than the reference compound which were carried for further analysis.

3.2. Rescoring Methodologies

Random Forest scoring is a novel machine-learning algorithm implemented extensively in virtual screening to forecast binding affinity on a varied range of targets, using descriptors based on RF Score version v1-3. Despite being less precise on physicochemical properties, the RF scoring function typically outperformed conventional scoring systems in estimating binding affinity [35]. Hence, in the current investigation, rescoring was conducted using a random forest approach for all the hit molecules obtained in the screening process. The results from our algorithm depict that 500 out of 887 compounds had a higher RF score than pralsetinib. Further, T_c was calculated between the reference ligand and the hit molecules to measure the structural similarity [36]. The results indicate that 406 molecules were highly similar to pralsetinib with a T_c threshold value greater than 0.4. RF score and T_c values of compounds obtained from pharmacophore, e-pharmacophore and receptor cavity-based strategy are tabulated in Tables S2–S4, respectively (see Supplementary Materials). On comparing the RF score and T_c results of all the hit molecules, 78,

39, and 59 compounds were found to possess better similarities and RF scores, respectively from pharmacophore, e-pharmacophore, and receptor cavity-based strategies. The results from all three hypotheses were then integrated to eliminate false positive prediction. Notably, only 18 lead molecules were found to be in common among all the three approaches with high similarities and RF scores. The combined result of 18 lead molecules and their scores are tabulated in Table 1.

Table 1. Docking and rescoring evaluation of lead molecules using different strategies.

S. No	DrugBank ID	XP GScore (kcal/mol)	RF Score	Tanimoto Coefficient (T_c)
Reference	Pralsetinib	−7.79	5.962	1.000
1	DB07194	−9.556	5.974	0.418
2	DB08583	−9.012	6.235	0.423
3	DB12672	−9.579	6.986	0.435
4	DB03496	−10.791	7.108	0.48
5	DB07606	−9.291	7.099	0.502
6	DB12848	−8.066	5.978	0.405
7	DB11982	−9.001	6.644	0.436
8	DB04751	−8.395	6.955	0.432
9	DB07981	−8.117	6.054	0.484
10	DB07248	−8.133	6.268	0.413
11	DB08052	−9.398	7.098	0.451
12	DB07474	−8.133	6.219	0.447
13	DB11665	−9.034	5.99	0.48
14	DB07382	−9.381	6.071	0.4
15	DB02933	−9.169	6.084	0.429
16	DB04338	−9.691	7.005	0.401
17	DB06852	−9.327	6.589	0.432
18	DB02282	−9.108	6.048	0.436

3.3. Postdocking MM-GBSA Analysis

The binding free energies of complexes were determined to validate the binding ability of the ligands to the target protein. The summary of the binding free energy of each complex is tabulated in Table 2. It can be observed that the ΔG_{bind} of the complexes varied from between −69.235 kcal/mol and −39.610 kcal/mol. Note that only eight compounds resulted in a binding free-energy value above −55 kcal/mol. The Van der Waals energy for all the compounds was observed to be highly favorable to the overall binding energy. The coulomb energy provided the second-highest contribution to the interaction in all the compounds; however, the high solvation energy compensated coulomb contribution in ΔG_{bind}. The contribution of covalent energy is almost unfavorable or negligible to the binding of the compounds DB08583, DB07606, and DB04751. Additionally, ligand strain energy depicts the deformation of ligands during the interaction, which is considered one of the most important parameters during the MM/GBSA analysis [37,38]. It is clear from the table that almost all the predicted compounds undergo less deformation than pralsetinib during interaction with the target protein except DB08583, DB07606, and DB04751. Although, the compounds DB08583, DB07606, and DB04751 exhibited better binding free energy. Higher ligand strain energy decreases the binding efficacy of the compounds with target receptors. Eventually, DB07194, DB03496, DB11982, DB12672, and DB12848 showed more satisfactory Coulombic potential and ligand strain energy than the other compounds, facilitating tight binding to the RET protein. Of note, these compounds exhibited minimal covalent energy contributions towards ΔG_{bind}, a key factor for forming a thermostable complex with RET protein.

Table 2. The predicted binding free energy of RET-complex structures calculated using MM-GBSA approach.

S. No	DrugBank ID	dG Bind (kcal/mol)	Van der Waal's Energy (kcal/mol)	Ligand Strain Energy (kcal/mol)	Electrostatic Potential (kcal/mol)	Lipophilicity (kcal/mol)	Covalent Interaction (kcal/mol)	Solvation Energy
Reference	Pralsetinib	−63.348	−58.387	6.20432	−12.472	−19.969	−0.4283	37.3355
1	DB07194	−69.235	−46.133	3.22011	−46.443	−17.32	2.77209	40.7179
2	DB08583	−61.769	−48.94	6.4073	−11.888	−18.303	7.34065	36.8761
3	DB12672	−60.017	−51.402	5.56562	−23.095	−20.949	3.90398	33.2395
4	DB03496	−55.502	−46.937	4.2076	−21.81	−20	2.56844	31.9131
5	DB07606	−55.367	−42.62	8.36976	−10.801	−25.237	4.99298	28.2519
6	DB12848	−55.33	−43.57	5.76015	−27.463	−23.935	0.53004	21.6655
7	DB11982	−55.102	−41.865	5.45963	−30.654	−16.496	2.69688	30.5778
8	DB04751	−55.091	−53.348	13.4545	−16.888	−18.303	11.9706	24.1207

3.4. HOMO–LUMO Theory Analysis

All five compounds with high binding free energy and lower ligand strain energy were optimized using B3LYP-D3 theory and LACVP++ basis set (Schrödinger, Bangalore, India). Since the reactivity of a compound is directly related to the energy gap, the parameters HOMO and LUMO had are significant [39]. The molecule with a minimal energy gap between frontier orbitals is usually accompanied by a substantial chemical reactivity and weak kinetic stability which depicts the highly favorable potential reactions [40]. The energy gap between HOMO and LUMO is shown in Figure 1. It is observed that DB07194, DB03496, and DB11982 exhibited a lower or equivalent gap to pralsetinib than DB12672 and DB12848. These results imply that compounds such as DB07194, DB03496, and DB11982 exhibit better biological activities than pralsetinib.

3.5. Interaction Pattern and Pharmacokinetic Analysis

The interaction pattern of hit compounds in the binding pocket of the receptor is represented in Figure S1 (see Supplementary Materials). On analyzing the binding pattern of pralsetinib, two hydrogen bonds were found between the cyclohexane carbomide group and the ALA807 residue of RET, and one additional hydrogen link was observed between the pyridine ring of pralsetinib and the SER811 residue of the protein. The ligand interaction diagram of DB07194 clearly shows the formation of two hydrogen bonds between the amino pyrimidine group of DB07194 and the residues ASN879, ASP892 of the RET protein. Likewise, the N-methylpiperidinyl and flavone group of DB03496 displayed hydrogen bonds with ARG878 and ALA807 residues of the receptor. In addition, a salt bridge was formed between the tertiary amino group of N-methylpiperidinyl and the residue ASP892 in the DB03496-RET complex. In the case of DB11982, a hydrogen bond formation between the pyridine carboxamide and ARG878 of RET protein was observed. It is interesting to note that the anticancer property of these functional groups of the hit compounds involved in the interaction with the RET protein has been reported recently [41–43]. The existence of interactions by the key residues ASN879 and ASP892 of hydrophobic pockets in RET proteins has also been observed in the other approved drugs, crizotinib, and sorafenib, respectively. The interaction pattern of the drugs is given in supplementary Figure S2.

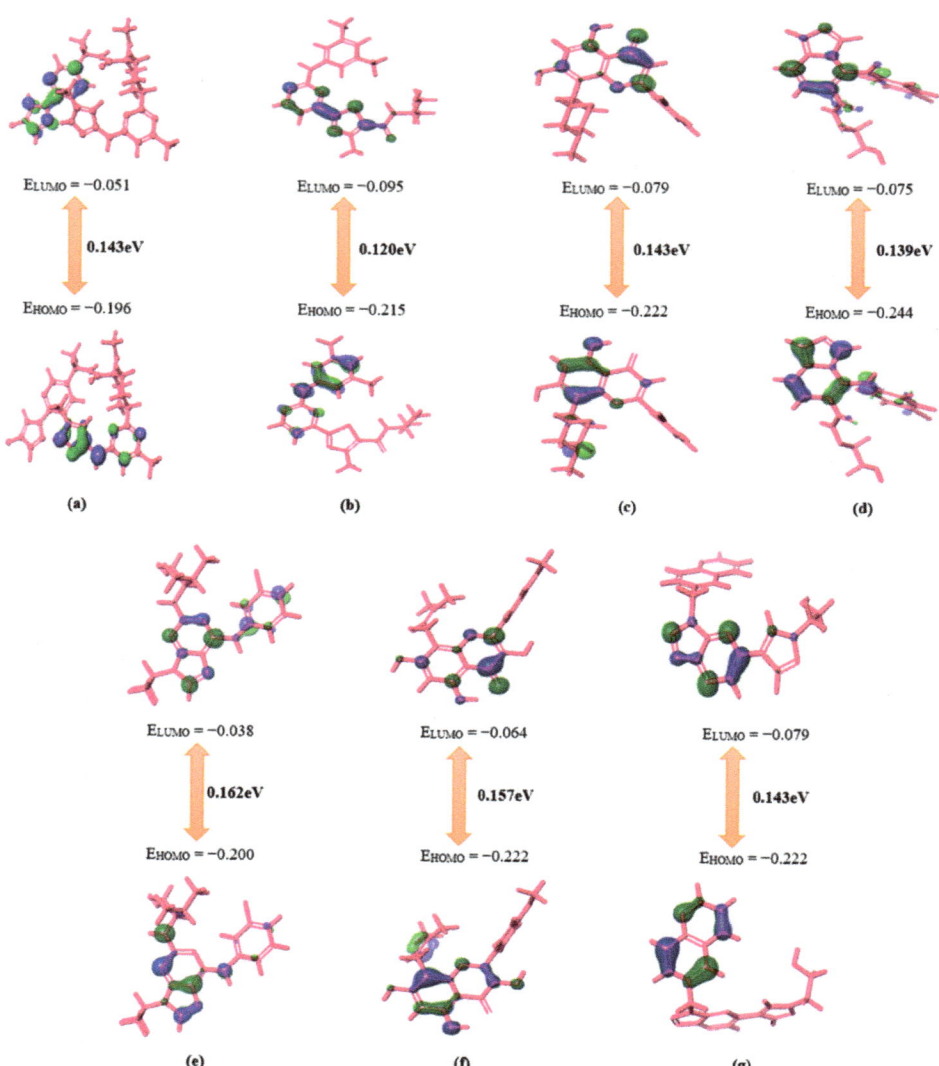

Figure 1. Graphical representation of HOMO–LUMO energy gap calculation for reference (**a**) Pralsetinib and hit compounds (**b**) DB07194, (**c**) DB03496, (**d**) DB11982, (**e**) DB04751, (**f**) DB12672 and (**g**) DB12848.

Furthermore, the essential pharmacokinetic parameters were analyzed to prevent the elimination of the compounds during clinical trials in the future. Table S5 (see Supplementary Materials) characterizes the interaction patterns and pharmacokinetic features of the lead compounds. The hit compounds displayed satisfactory pharmacokinetic and pharmacodynamics properties. Of note, key properties such as solubility, blood–brain barrier, stars, human oral absorption, and CNS activity were found to be in the acceptable range Stars denote the number of pharmacokinetic features that lie outside the required range. Interestingly, none of the hit compounds were found to have outliers based on the star values. Moreover, the capability of stimulating the central nervous system response by the hit molecules was comparatively similar to pralsetinib (CNS = −2). Undeniably, the

HOA of all the predicted molecules was higher than pralsetinib (HOA = 2), which shows the efficacy of a drug that can be attained easily through oral administration in humans.

3.6. Protein–Ligand Complex Stability Analysis

The stability and dynamic characteristics of protein-lead inhibitor complexes were investigated using MD simulations. It provides precise insights on protein–ligand interactions, allowing for the visualization of the influence of ligand binding on protein and its contribution to their stable, bound conformation [32]. The RET protein complexed with three hit compounds alongside the reference complex was analyzed using 200 ns MD simulations. The extent of deviation of atoms in the protein-lead complex during the simulation process is explained using RMSD plots. It is interesting to note that the obtained results correlate well with our initial findings. The results are shown in Figure 2a–d. Figure 2 reveals that all the compounds showed an increased RMSD deviation within the interval of 0–30 ns simulation time. A minimal deviation in the pattern was observed between 30 ns and 75 ns. Consequently, all the compounds maintained a stable equilibrium of ~0.30 nm from 75 ns to the end of the simulation process. Towards the end of the simulation, minimal RMSD values of 0.345 nm, 0.323 nm, and 0.371 nm were observed for DB07194, DB03496, and DB11982, respectively, smaller than pralsetinib (0.385 nm) and apoprotein (0.414 nm). In all the cases, the RMSD data corresponding to apoprotein was significantly higher than the ligand-bound structure investigated in our analysis. This suggests that the hit compound could adapt to a more stable conformation than pralsetinib in the binding pocket of RET protein. Moreover, the overall deviation of hit molecules was less than ~5 nm, depicting the stability of the RET protein in the presence of lead molecules. Thus, we hypothesize that the predicted DB07194 compound could have a higher inhibitory potential against RET protein than pralsetinib.

Guterres and Im showed that active compounds have less RMSD than inactive compounds in 100 ns MD simulations [44] From the DUD-E set, they randomly selected 56 targets. For each target, 10 compounds, five actives and five decoys were selected. They observed that the active compounds have a unimodal RMSD distribution centered at 4 Å, whereas the decoys have a skewed-right distribution, showing that a lot of them leave the binding pocket during the simulation. As mentioned, our molecules including pralsetinib have RMSD ~0.3 nm, which is consistent with the work of Guterres and Im. This implies that the three compounds could act as active compounds.

3.7. Residue Mobility Analysis (RMSF)

RMSF depicts the flexibility of protein residues within the protein–ligand complex. As demonstrated in Figure 3, a similar pattern of fluctuation in the backbone was observed among all four systems. The region between Val871–Asp898 exhibited the least fluctuation, with less than ~0.05 nm, indicating the contribution of these residues to stable binding of predicted inhibitors with the RET receptor. Notably, important residues such as Asn879 and Asp892 showed fluctuations of ~0.04 nm, which were found within the conserved interaction region. It is to be noted that the presence of a highly stable protein–ligand complex was due to the formation of hydrogen bonds between these residues and the inhibitors. The other residues, Met700–Lys722 and Pro957–Arg982, showed high flexibility of about ~0.1 nm, suggesting that these residues contributed less to the RET–ligand interaction. These results are correlated well with the ligand interaction pattern discussed earlier. Moreover, a lower RMSF value depicts the well-organized region whereas a high RMSF value indicates loosely structured terminal ends of the complex [33]. In the present study, the apoprotein exhibited an RMSF value of 0.0696 nm whereas the complexes RET–Pralsetinib, RET–DB07194, RET–DB03496, and RET–DB11982 showed 0.069, 0.0665, 0.0773, and 0.033 nm RMSF values, respectively. The RET–DB07194 and RET–DB11982 complexes showed decreased RMSF values in comparison with the apoprotein and RET–pralsetinib complexes. This clearly depicts that the binding of lead molecules resulted in decreased flexibility of the catalytic residues. Hence, the identified lead compounds were very well positioned in the binding pocket of RET protein compared with other compounds considered in our analysis.

3.8. Hydrogen Bond Analysis

The stability of a protein–ligand complex is usually analyzed based on different types of transient interactions, including electrostatic interaction, Van der Waals, hydrogen bonds, and many others [45]. Among them, the hydrogen bond is regarded as an important transient interaction facilitating the binding of ligands with protein. The existence of hydrogen bonds in the complex structures was calculated from the MD trajectory. The RET–DB7194, RET–DB03496, and RET–DB11982 showed 0–8, 0–4, and 0–6 H-bonds, respectively (Figure 4). These observations demonstrated that the predicted hits showed a higher number of H-bonds than the reference drug during simulation. From the results of the H-bond analysis, it can be concluded that the predicted compounds form a more stable interaction with the RET protein than pralsetinib.

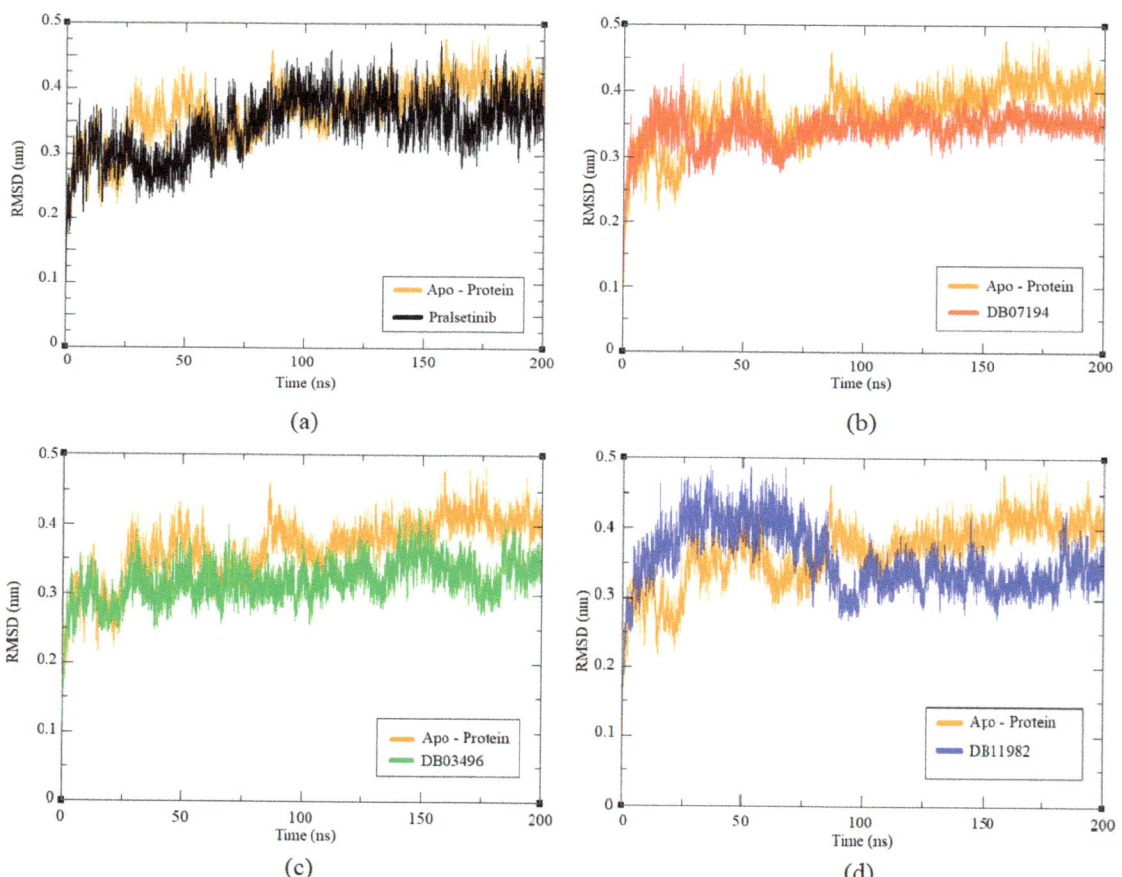

Figure 2. Time evolution of RMSD values for the apoprotein and protein–ligand complexes: (**a**) Pralsetinib, (**b**) DB07194, (**c**) DB03496 and (**d**) DB11982.

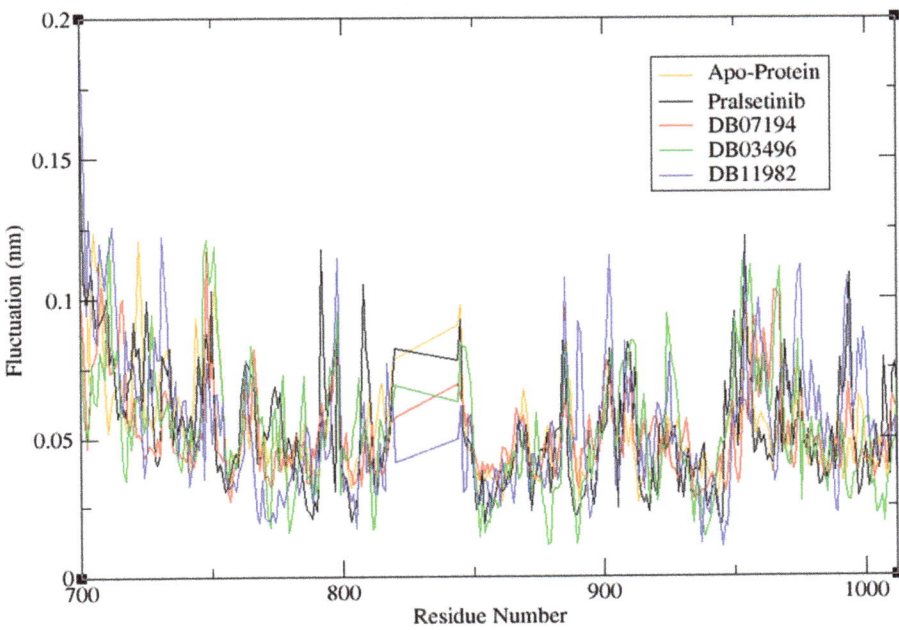

Figure 3. RMSF values for apoprotein and the protein–ligand complexes system during MD simulations.

3.9. Free Energy Landscape (FEL)

An inbuilt GROMACS tool gmx_sham was employed further to investigate the conformational stability of the protein–ligand complex. The exchange of heat in a closed protein–ligand complex system is measured in Gibbs free energy [46]. This analysis provides information on energy minima confirmation and molecular fluctuation. Initially, the covariance matrix containing the eigenvalues was constructed using gmx_covar tool of GROMACS. Subsequently, the eigenvectors were obtained by diagonalizing the constructed matrix. Finally, the first two principal components (PC 1 and PC2) mapping the eigenvector to its corresponding eigenvalues were obtained using gmx_anaeig tool [47]. Figure 5 was plotted using the obtained PC1 and PC2, demonstrating the free energy landscape of the complexes. A dark blue color corresponds to the energetically stable and energy-minima favored complex conformation whereas a yellow color demonstrates the unfavorable conformation. The deep energy basin observed during the MD simulation process indicates the high stability of the complex system, while the shallow basin denotes the lower stability of the complex. The RET–pralsetinib complex contained two connected energy minima and one distinct energy minima. In the case of RET–DB03496 and DB11982, one deep energy basin as well as one shallow energy basin was observed, whereas, in the case of RET–DB07194, three deep energy basins were observed. Moreover, the Gibbs free energy of the two compounds (DB07194 and DB03496) was 14.8 kJ/mol and 14.4 kJ/mol, respectively, which were similar to the Gibbs free energy of pralsetinib (14.8 kJ/mol). Nevertheless, the Gibbs free energy of DB11982 was higher (16.2 kJ/mol) than the other two complexes. From Figure 5, it is evident that the energy basins were broad, clear, and distinct in all three compounds, and exhibited lower Gibbs free energy, which shows the stable confirmation of all three protein–ligand complexes.

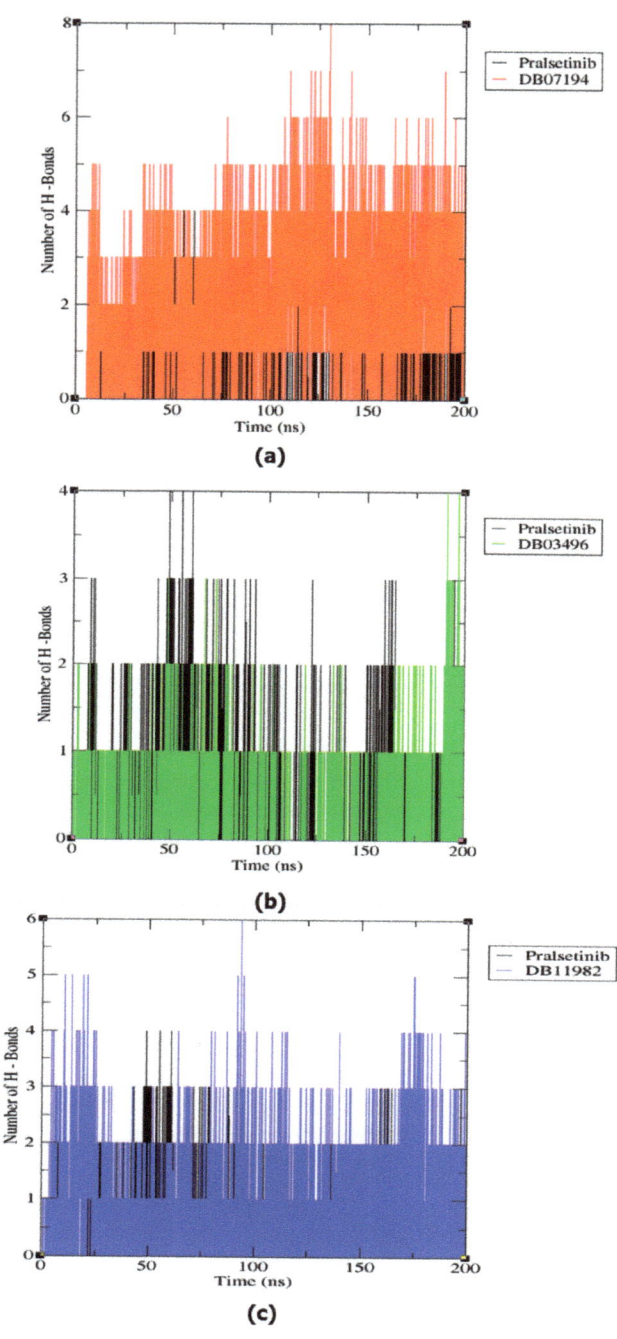

Figure 4. Comparative H-Bond analysis of pairs within 0.35 nm of the complex structures from MD simulation: (**a**) Pralsetinib and DB07194, (**b**) Pralsetinib and DB03496, and (**c**) Pralsetinib and DB11982.

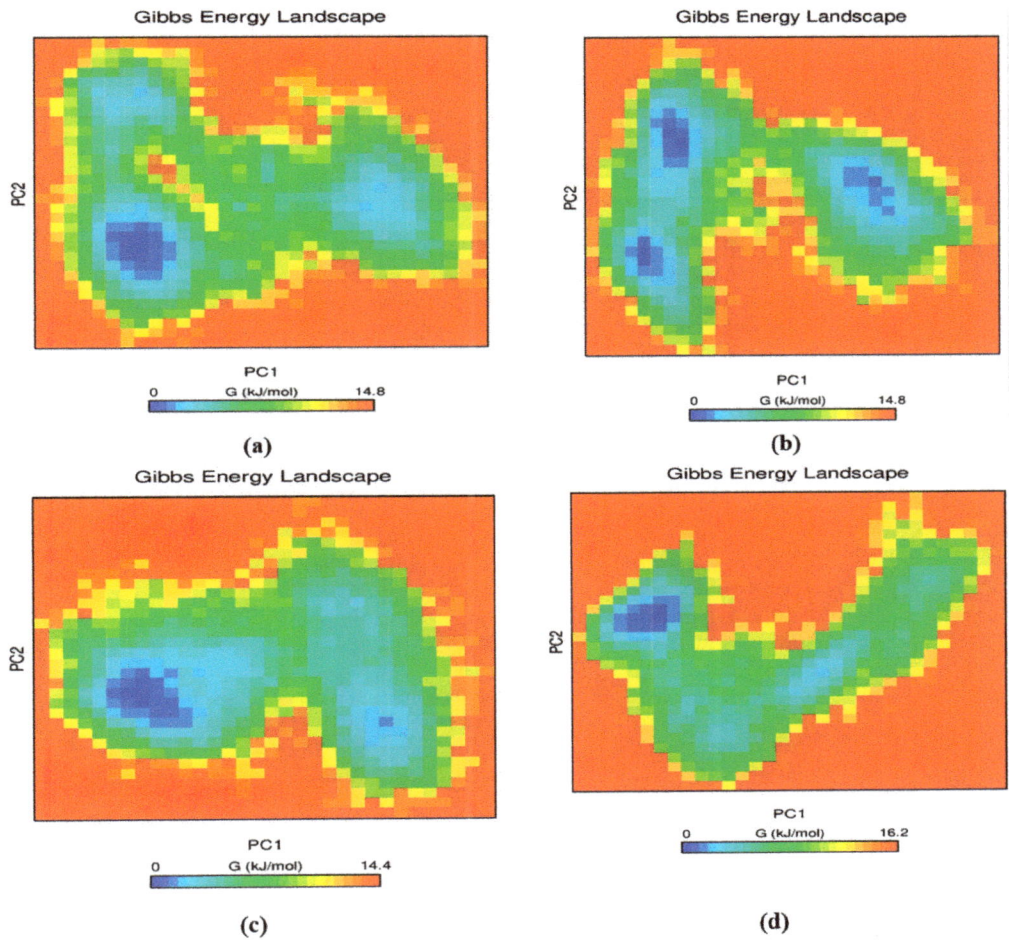

Figure 5. Contour plot demonstrating free energy landscapes of (**a**) RET–Pralsetinib, (**b**) RET–DB07194, (**c**) RET–DB03496 and (**d**) RET–DB11982 during 200 ns MD simulation.

3.10. MM-PBSA

The binding free energy analysis of the three hit compounds and the reference molecule were calculated using the trajectories pulled out from the last 10 ns of the simulation process. The binding energy for RET–pralsetinib (-9.445 ± 65.091 kJ/mol), RET–DB07194 (-111.920 ± 17.179 kJ/mol), RET–DB03496 (-74.514 ± 77.458 kJ/mol) and RET0–DB11982 (-37.949 ± 42.465 kJ/mol) were demonstrated in Table 3. RET–DB07194 exhibited a stable conformation with the least binding energy among all other compounds screened from our study. The total binding energy is composed of Van der Waals energy, electrostatic energy, polar solvation, and solvent accessible surface area energy. Among them, Van der Waals energy has the highest contribution to the overall binding energy, followed by polar solvation energy, SASA, and electrostatic energy, respectively. It is to be noted that the estimated pattern of binding free energies was similar to that of the MM-GBSA strategy. The predicted binding energies were well correlated with RMSD and hydrogen-bond analysis.

Table 3. Total binding energy of the lead molecules against RET protein obtained from MM-PBSA analysis.

S. No	DrugBank ID	Binding Energy (kJ/mol)	Van der Waal Energy (kJ/mol)	Electrostatic Energy (kJ/mol)	Polar Solvation Energy (kJ/mol)	SASA Energy (kJ/mol)
Reference	Pralsetinib	−9.445 ± 65.091	−23.022 ± 53.334	−0.074 ± 3.936	15.905 ± 55.514	−2.254 ± 6.035
1	DB07194	−111.920 ± 17.179	−141.170 ± 11.926	−13.371 ± 9.680	55.122 ± 16.524	−12.500 ± 1.161
2	DB03496	−74.514 ± 77.458	−73.039 ± 94.546	1.261 ± 3.289	2.851 ± 61.775	−5.587 ± 7.630
3	DB11982	−37.949 ± 42.565	−90.713 ± 51.388	−43.922 ± 25.645	106.888 ± 52.148	−10.202 ± 6.052

3.11. In Silico Evaluation of Lead Compounds against Point Mutant RET Receptor

As reported by Solomon et al., point mutations at different locations of RET resulted in the development of acquired resistance against the existing inhibitors. Specifically, the development of resistance due to solvent front mutations prevented the inhibitors from accessing the binding pocket of the protein [9,10]. Hence, we evaluated the binding capability of lead compounds against the mutant RET receptor using docking studies and MM-GBSA analysis. The results of docking and MM-GBSA analysis are tabulated in Table S6 (see Supplementary Materials). About 11 points mutated the RET-protein structure, containing 4 point mutations at the gatekeeper region, 4 mutations at the solvent front region, and 3 mutations at other regions, were generated using the homology modeling suite of Schrödinger. The docking analysis of the three lead compounds against RET mutants revealed that DB07194 had overcome G810C and G810V solvent front mutations with higher binding free energy than pralsetinib and the other two hit molecules. On the other hand, the compound DB03496 exhibited significant inhibitory activity against the G810R solvent front mutation. In addition, both the compounds DB07194 and DB03496 inhibited M918T mutation with high binding free energy, at −74.11 kcal/mol and −87.16 kcal/mol, respectively.

In some cases, including V804M mutational study, all the three lead compounds exhibited a high docking score. In contrast, the binding free energy of the lead compounds was lower than the pralsetinib, preventing them from overcoming resistance. Unfortunately, DB11982 did not overcome the acquired resistance in any RET mutant structures investigated in our study. On analyzing the interaction pattern of DB07194, three hydrogen bonds formed between the amino pyrimidine group and ARG874, ARG878, ASN879 had assisted the compounds in overcoming the acquired resistance caused by the G810C mutation in RET. Interestingly, a similar pattern of interaction was observed against the G810V mutation. In the case of M918T mutation, three hydrogen bonds were formed between DB07194, SER811 and ALA807 of the RET protein. Overall, DB07194 showed higher inhibitory activity against RET mutants, including G810C, G810V, and M918T, than DB03496 and DB11982. It is to be noted that pralsetinib has a comparatively lower potential than DB07194 to overcome the solvent front mutation, which might be due to the absence of an amino pyrimidine group in its structure.

3.12. Cell Viability Analysis of DB07194 against LC-2/ad

Finally, the inhibitory activity of pralsetinib and DB07194 was assessed against LC-2/ad cell lines using a colorimetric MTT assay. The compounds were examined and compared at five different concentrations, 6.25, 12.5, 25, 50, and 100 μM/mL, respectively. The experiment was performed in triplet to overcome the experimental error. Figure 6 and supplementary Table S7 (see Supplementary Materials) represent the comparative cell viability upon treatment with pralsetinib and DB07194. A similar pattern of inhibition was observed between pralsetinib and DB07194 at concentrations 6.25 and 12.5 μM/mL. Interestingly, a sudden rise in the inhibition of LC-2/ad cell using DB07194 was noted at 25 μM/mL, whereas only a smaller variation was observed on using pralsetinib at the same concentration. The inhibitory action does not show much deviation after 50 μM/mL of drugs, which shows the saturation level of inhibition. Overall, LC-2/ad showed higher sensitivity to DB07194 (IC_{50} = 12.48 μM) than pralsetinib (IC_{50} = 23.31 μM). Consistent with its anti-cancer activity, both pralsetinib and DB07194 can decrease the cell viability more significantly than control. Moreover, the anticancer property of DB07194 reveals different pharmacological properties of the compound tested earlier in the experiments as an SYK inhibitor [48,49]. Subsequently, one-way ANOVA analysis was implemented to examine the significance of the difference in cell viability between the control and drug-treated samples. A p-value of less than 0.001 is observed between the control and drug-treated sample. This highlights the statistical significance of the experimental data carried out in our study. In addition, no literature evidence has been reported on the toxicity and side effects of the compound. Hence, the toxicity of the hit molecule was also assessed using the ProTox II server and compared against pralsetinib [50]. For instance, predicted LD50 values of pralsetinib and DB07194 were found to be 800 mg/kg and 681 mg/kg, respectively, and thus fall into the class four (slightly toxic) category of compounds. All these data are evidence that the identified hit molecule, DB07194, belongs to an experimental subset of the DrugBank database, displaying favorable drug-like properties and potential progression into clinical application. Thus, it could be considered for the treatment of RET-positive NSCLC, a contrast to the properties for which it was originally designed and synthesized.

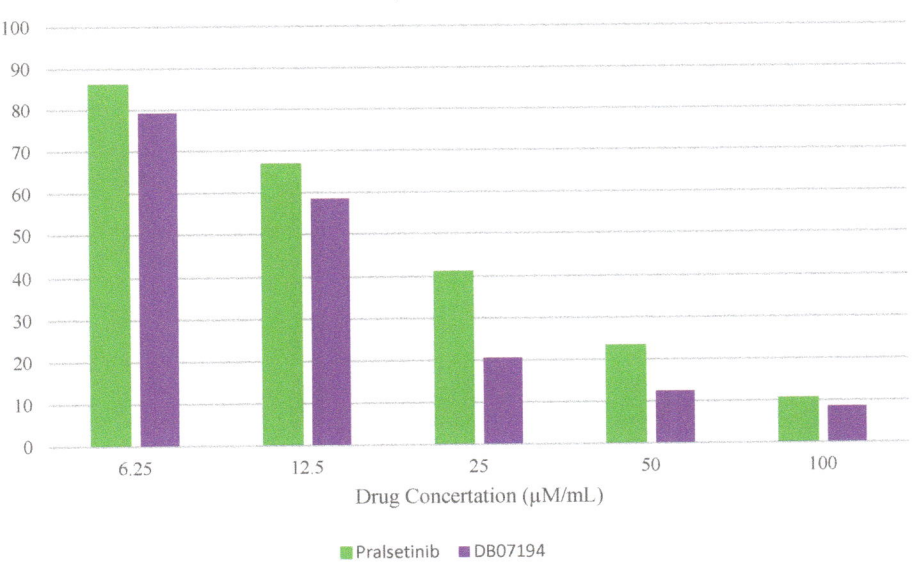

Figure 6. In vitro evaluation of DB07194 inhibitory activity against LC-2/ad cell lines.

4. Limitations and Future Prospective

Acquired drug resistance is the major restraint among RET inhibitors resulting in reduced efficacy of drugs in NSCLC patients. Therefore, we examined the activity of the hit compound against 11 different REF mutations in this study. Although the identified hit can demonstrate potent activity against solvent front mutations (G810C, G810V, and M918T), experimental validation of the compound activity using mutant cell lines is certainly needed to validate this finding. The toxicity studies of this compound either by in vivo micronucleus assays or in vitro genotoxicity assays are also interesting future directions. The in vitro activity of the compound identified by the LC-2/ad cell line in our study opens up a new avenue for biologists to explore the synergistic activity of the compound. Finally, the results of our study will facilitate hit-to-lead optimization to reach novel compounds with economic value in the near future.

5. Conclusions

The current research focuses on the identification of potential candidates against RET and its associated solvent frontline mutations using high-throughput drug discovery strategies. Different pharmacophore models were employed along with docking, Tanimoto coefficient calculations, rescoring with RF score, and MM-GBSA to deduce the structural characteristics and binding poses that govern the activity of inhibitors against the RET receptor. Comparative DFT analysis was carried out, and it was observed that the lead molecules exhibited a lower energy gap than pralsetinib, depicting more inhibitory potential against the protein. Furthermore, the stability and flexibility of the complex system were analyzed using molecular dynamics for 200 ns. The interaction surface of the protein Val871–Asp898 was found to be conserved, and contained a series of important residues and thus formed hydrogen bonds with the lead molecules. Moreover, the aminopyrimidine group in DB07194 facilitated inhibition of both native and mutant forms of RET with higher binding free energy than pralsetinib. Ultimately, the cell line studies proved the efficiency of the predicted RET inhibitor, showing a lower required minimal drug concentration for inhibiting the RET protein than the existing FDA-approved drug pralsetinib. J.L. Kutok's patent, namely WO2017223422A1 also mentions the chemical compound DB07194 as a potential third chemotherapeutic agent used in combinations with phosphoinositide 3-kinase inhibitors for cancer treatment. Taken together, the results from our study provide a new gateway for developing DB07194 as a potent anticancer agent targeting RET protein and overcoming the RET-associated solvent front mutations.

Supplementary Materials: The following contents are available at https://www.mdpi.com/article/10.3390/pharmaceutics13111775/s1. Table S1. List of existing RET inhibitors retrieved from literature. Table S2. Rescoring and structure similarity analysis of screened compounds obtained using pharmacophore based strategy. Table S3. Rescoring and structure similarity analysis of screened compounds obtained using e-pharmacophore based strategy. Table S4. Rescoring and structure similarity analysis of screened compounds obtained using receptor cavity based strategy. Table S5. Interaction and pharmacokinetic evaluation of screened RET inhibitors. Table S6. Mutational analysis of predicted compounds using docking and MM-GBSA studies. Table S7. Examination of cell viability at different drug concentrations (μM/mL) against LC-2/ad cell line. Figure S1. Binding mode analysis of reference compound (a) Pralsetinib, (b) DB07194, (C) DB03496 and (d) DB11982 with the target RET protein. Figure S2. Comparative interaction analysis of (a) crizotinib and (b) Sorafenib with RET protein.

Author Contributions: P.R. performed the data collection, machine learning model generation, and validation. S.V. and W.-H.S. conceived this study and are responsible for the overall design, interpretation, manuscript preparation, and communication. All authors have read and agreed to the published version of the manuscript.

Funding: W.-H.S. acknowledges the supports from the National Research Foundation of Korea (NRF), the grand funded by the Korea government (MSIT) (No. 2020R1F1A1075998, 2020R1A4A1016695).

Institutional Review Board Statement: Not applicable.

Informed Consent Statement: Not applicable.

Data Availability Statement: Not applicable.

Acknowledgments: The authors (P.R. and S.V.) thank the management of Vellore Institute of Technology for providing the necessary facility to carry out this research work.

Conflicts of Interest: We wish to confirm that there is no known conflict of interest associated with this publication and there has been no significant financial support for this work that could have influenced its outcome.

References

1. Subbiah, V.; Gainor, J.F.; Rahal, R.; Brubaker, J.D.; Kim, J.L.; Maynard, M.; Hu, W.; Cao, Q.; Sheets, M.P.; Wilson, D.; et al. Precision targeted therapy with BLU-667 for RET-driven cancers. *Cancer Discov.* **2018**, *8*, 836–849. [CrossRef] [PubMed]
2. Shaw, A.T.; Kim, D.W.; Nakagawa, K.; Seto, T.; Crinó, L.; Ahn, M.J.; De Pas, T.; Besse, B.; Solomon, B.J.; Blackhall, F.; et al. Crizotinib versus chemotherapy in advanced ALK-positive lung cancer. *N. Engl. J. Med.* **2013**, *368*, 2385–2394. [CrossRef] [PubMed]
3. Zhou, C.; Wu, Y.L.; Chen, G.; Feng, J.; Liu, X.Q.; Wang, C.; Zhang, S.; Wang, J.; Zhou, S.; Ren, S.; et al. Erlotinib versus chemotherapy as first-line treatment for patients with advanced EGFR mutation-positive non-small-cell lung cancer (OPTIMAL, CTONG-0802): A multicentre, open-label, randomised, phase 3 study. *Lancet Oncol.* **2011**, *12*, 735–742. [CrossRef]
4. Ju, Y.S.; Lee, W.C.; Shin, J.Y.; Lee, S.; Bleazard, T.; Won, J.K.; Kim, Y.T.; Kim, J.I.; Kang, J.H.; Seo, J.S. A transforming KIF5B and RET gene fusion in lung adenocarcinoma revealed from whole-genome and transcriptome sequencing. *Genome Res.* **2012**, *22*, 436–445. [CrossRef] [PubMed]
5. Gainor, J.F.; Shaw, A.T. Novel targets in non-small cell lung cancer: ROS1 and RET fusions. *Oncologist* **2013**, *18*, 865–875. [CrossRef]
6. Kohno, T.; Ichikawa, H.; Totoki, Y.; Yasuda, K.; Hiramoto, M.; Nammo, T.; Sakamoto, H.; Tsuta, K.; Furuta, K.; Shimada, Y.; et al. KIF5B-RET fusions in lung adenocarcinoma. *Nat. Med.* **2012**, *18*, 375. [CrossRef] [PubMed]
7. Borrello, M.G.; Ardini, E.; Locati, L.D.; Greco, A.; Licitra, L.; Pierotti, M.A. RET inhibition: Implications in cancer therapy. *Expert Opin. Ther. Targets* **2013**, *17*, 403–419. [CrossRef] [PubMed]
8. Lu, C.; Zhou, Q. Diagnostics, therapeutics and RET inhibitor resistance for RET fusion-positive non-small cell lung cancers and future perspectives. *Cancer Treat. Rev.* **2021**, *96*, 102153. [CrossRef]
9. Solomon, B.J.; Tan, L.; Lin, J.J.; Wong, S.Q.; Hollizeck, S.; Ebata, K.; Tuch, B.B.; Yoda, S.; Gainor, J.F.; Sequist, L.V.; et al. RET solvent front mutations mediate acquired resistance to selective RET inhibition in RET-driven malignancies. *J. Thorac. Oncol.* **2020**, *15*, 541–549. [CrossRef]
10. Liu, W.J.; Du, Y.; Wen, R.; Yang, M.; Xu, J. Drug resistance to targeted therapeutic strategies in non-small cell lung cancer. *Pharmacol. Ther.* **2020**, *206*, 107438. [CrossRef]
11. Fancelli, S.; Caliman, E.; Mazzoni, F.; Brugia, M.; Castiglione, F.; Voltolini, L.; Pillozzi, S.; Antonuzzo, L. Chasing the target: New phenomena of resistance to novel selective RET inhibitors in lung cancer. Updated evidence and future perspectives. *Cancers* **2021**, *13*, 1091. [CrossRef] [PubMed]
12. Lin, J.J.; Liu, S.V.; McCoach, C.E.; Zhu, V.W.; Tan, A.C.; Yoda, S.; Peterson, J.; Do, A.; Prutisto-Chang, K.; Dagogo-Jack, I.; et al. Mechanisms of resistance to selective RET tyrosine kinase inhibitors in RET fusion-positive non-small-cell lung cancer. *Ann. Oncol.* **2020**, *31*, 1725–1733. [CrossRef]
13. Subbiah, V.; Shen, T.; Terzyan, S.S.; Liu, X.; Hu, X.; Patel, K.P.; Hu, M.; Cabanillas, M.; Behrang, A.; Meric-Bernstam, F.; et al. Structural basis of acquired resistance to selpercatinib and pralsetinib mediated by non-gatekeeper RET mutations. *Ann. Oncol.* **2021**, *32*, 261–268. [CrossRef]
14. Newton, R.; Waszkowycz, B.; Seewooruthun, C.; Burschowsky, D.; Richards, M.; Hitchin, S.; Begum, H.; Watson, A.; French, E.; Hamilton, N.; et al. Discovery and Optimization of wt-RET/KDR-Selective Inhibitors of RETV804M Kinase. *ACS Med. Chem. Lett.* **2020**, *11*, 497–505. [CrossRef] [PubMed]
15. Selvaraj, C.; Dinesh, D.C.; Panwar, U.; Abhirami, R.; Boura, E.; Singh, S.K. Structure-based virtual screening and molecular dynamics simulation of SARS-CoV-2 Guanine-N7 methyltransferase (nsp14) for identifying antiviral inhibitors against COVID-19. *J. Biomol. Struct. Dyn.* **2021**, *39*, 4582–4593. [CrossRef]
16. Ammarah, U.; Kumar, A.; Pal, R.; Bal, N.C.; Misra, G. Identification of new inhibitors against human Great wall kinase using in silico approaches. *Sci. Rep.* **2018**, *8*, 4894. [CrossRef]
17. Sharma, P.; Joshi, T.; Mathpal, S.; Joshi, T.; Pundir, H.; Chandra, S.; Tamta, S. Identification of natural inhibitors against Mpro of SARS-CoV-2 by molecular docking, molecular dynamics simulation, and MM/PBSA methods. *J. Biomol. Struct. Dyn.* **2020**, 1–2. [CrossRef] [PubMed]
18. Lipinski, C.A.; Lombardo, F.; Dominy, B.W.; Feeney, P.J. Experimental and computational approaches to estimate solubility and permeability in drug discovery and development setting. *Adv. Drug Deliv. Rev.* **1997**, *23*, 3–25. [CrossRef]
19. Kohno, T.; Tsuta, K.; Tsuchihara, K.; Nakaoku, T.; Yoh, K.; Goto, K. RET fusion gene: Translation to personalized lung cancer therapy. *Cancer Sci.* **2013**, *104*, 1396–1400. [CrossRef]
20. Iams, W.T.; Lovly, C.M. Stop fRETting the target: Next-generation RET inhibitors have arrived. *Cancer Discov.* **2018**, *8*, 797–799. [CrossRef] [PubMed]
21. Ferrara, R.; Auger, N.; Auclin, E.; Besse, B. Clinical and Translational Implications of RET Rearrangements in Non–Small Cell Lung Cancer. *J. Thorac. Oncol.* **2018**, *13*, 27–45. [CrossRef] [PubMed]
22. Thangapandian, S.; John, S.; Sakkiah, S.; Lee, K.W. Potential virtual lead identification in the discovery of renin inhibitors: Application of ligand and structure-based pharmacophore modeling approaches. *Eur. J. Med. Chem.* **2011**, *46*, 2469–2476. [CrossRef] [PubMed]
23. Dixon, S.L.; Smondyrev, A.M.; Rao, S.N. PHASE: A novel approach to pharmacophore modeling and 3D database searching. *Chem. Biol. Drug Des.* **2006**, *67*, 370–372. [CrossRef] [PubMed]
24. Maryam, A.; Khalid, R.R.; Siddiqi, A.R.; Ece, A. E-pharmacophore based virtual screening for identification of dual specific PDE5A and PDE3A inhibitors as potential leads against cardiovascular diseases. *J. Biomol. Struct. Dyn.* **2021**, *39*, 2302–2317. [CrossRef]

25. Ali, R.; Badshah, S.L.; Faheem, M.; Abbasi, S.W.; Ullah, R.; Bari, A.; Jamal, S.B.; Mahmood, H.M.; Haider, A.; Haider, S. Identification of potential inhibitors of Zika virus NS5 RNA-dependent RNA polymerase through virtual screening and molecular dynamic simulations. *Saudi Pharm. J.* **2020**, *28*, 1580–1591.
26. Murali, P.; Verma, K.; Rungrotmongkol, T.; Thangavelu, P.; Karuppasamy, R. Targeting the Autophagy Specific Lipid Kinase VPS34 for Cancer Treatment: An Integrative Repurposing Strategy. *Protein J.* **2021**, *40*, 41–53. [CrossRef] [PubMed]
27. Rácz, A.; Bajusz, D.; Héberger, K. Life beyond the Tanimoto coefficient: Similarity measures for interaction fingerprints. *J. Cheminformatics* **2018**, *10*, 48. [CrossRef] [PubMed]
28. Cheng, T.; Li, Q.; Zhou, Z.; Wang, Y.; Bryant, S.H. Structure-based virtual screening for drug discovery: A problem-centric review. *AAPS J.* **2012**, *14*, 133–141. [CrossRef]
29. Shaikh, F.; Siu, S.W. Identification of novel natural compound inhibitors for human complement component 5a receptor by homology modeling and virtual screening. *Med. Chem. Res.* **2016**, *25*, 1564–1573. [CrossRef]
30. Sankar, M.; Jeyachandran, S.; Pandi, B. Screening of inhibitors as potential remedial against Ebolavirus infection: Pharmacophore-based approach. *J. Biomol. Struct. Dyn.* **2021**, *39*, 395–408. [CrossRef]
31. Shukla, R.; Shukla, H.; Sonkar, A.; Pandey, T.; Tripathi, T. Structure-based screening and molecular dynamics simulations offer novel natural compounds as potential inhibitors of Mycobacterium tuberculosis isocitrate lyase. *J. Biomol. Struct. Dyn.* **2018**, *36*, 2045–2057. [CrossRef] [PubMed]
32. Singh, R.; Bhardwaj, V.; Purohit, R. Identification of a novel binding mechanism of Quinoline based molecules with lactate dehydrogenase of Plasmodium falciparum. *J. Biomol. Struct. Dyn.* **2021**, *39*, 348–356. [CrossRef]
33. Van Meerloo, J.; Kaspers, G.J.; Cloos, J. Cell sensitivity assays: The MTT assay. In *Cancer Cell Culture*; Humana Press: Totowa, NJ, USA, 2011; pp. 237–245.
34. Kaserer, T.; Beck, K.R.; Akram, M.; Odermatt, A.; Schuster, D. Pharmacophore models and pharmacophore-based virtual screening: Concepts and applications exemplified on hydroxysteroid dehydrogenases. *Molecules* **2015**, *20*, 22799–22832. [CrossRef] [PubMed]
35. Singh, N.; Chaput, L.; Villoutreix, B.O. Fast re-scoring protocols to improve the performance of structure-based virtual screening performed on protein–protein interfaces. *J. Chem. Inf. Model.* **2020**, *60*, 3910–3934. [CrossRef]
36. Wang, D.; Cui, C.; Ding, X.; Xiong, Z.; Zheng, M.; Luo, X.; Jiang, H.; Chen, K. Improving the virtual screening ability of target-specific scoring functions using deep learning methods. *Front. Pharmacol.* **2019**, *10*, 924. [CrossRef]
37. Aaldering, L.J.; Vasanthanathan Poongavanam, D.; Langkjær, N.; Murugan, N.A.; Jørgensen, P.T.; Wengel, J.; Veedu, R.N. Development of an Efficient G-Quadruplex-Stabilised Thrombin-Binding Aptamer Containing a Three-Carbon Spacer Molecule. *ChemBioChem* **2017**, *18*, 755. [CrossRef]
38. Madhavaram, M.; Nampally, V.; Gangadhari, S.; Palnati, M.K.; Tigulla, P. High-throughput virtual screening, ADME analysis, and estimation of MM/GBSA binding-free energies of azoles as potential inhibitors of Mycobacterium tuberculosis H37Rv. *J. Recept. Signal Transduct.* **2019**, *39*, 312–320. [CrossRef] [PubMed]
39. Khalid, M.; Ullah, M.A.; Adeel, M.; Khan, M.U.; Tahir, M.N.; Braga, A.A. Synthesis, crystal structure analysis, spectral IR, UV–Vis, NMR assessments, electronic and nonlinear optical properties of potent quinoline based derivatives: Interplay of experimental and DFT study. *J. Saudi Chem. Soc.* **2019**, *23*, 546–560. [CrossRef]
40. Hoque, M.J.; Ahsan, A.; Hossain, M.B. Molecular Docking, Pharmacokinetic, and DFT Calculation of Naproxen and its Degradants. *Biomed. J. Sci. Tech. Res.* **2018**, *9*, 7360–7365.
41. Kopustinskiene, D.M.; Jakstas, V.; Savickas, A.; Bernatoniene, J. Flavonoids as anticancer agents. *Nutrients* **2020**, *12*, 457. [CrossRef]
42. Osafo, N.; Boakye, Y.D.; Agyare, C.; Obeng, S.; Foli, J.E.; Minkah, P.A. African plants with antiproliferative properties. In *Natural Products and Cancer Drug Discovery*; IntechOpen: London, UK, 2017; Volume 1.
43. Al-Majid, A.M.; Islam, M.S.; Atef, S.; El-Senduny, F.F.; Badria, F.A.; Elshaier, Y.A.; Ali, M.; Barakat, A.; Motiur Rahman, A.F. Synthesis of pyridine-dicarboxamide-cyclohexanone derivatives: Anticancer and α-glucosidase inhibitory activities and in silico study. *Molecules* **2019**, *24*, 1332. [CrossRef] [PubMed]
44. Guterres, H.; Im, W. Improving protein-ligand docking results with high-throughput molecular dynamics simulations. Journal of chemical information and modeling. *J. Chem. Inf. Model.* **2020**, *60*, 2189–2198. [CrossRef] [PubMed]
45. Swapna, L.S.; Bhaskara, R.M.; Sharma, J.; Srinivasan, N. Roles of residues in the interface of transient protein-protein complexes before complexation. *Sci. Rep.* **2012**, *2*, 1–9. [CrossRef] [PubMed]
46. Londhe, A.M.; Gadhe, C.G.; Lim, S.M.; Pae, A.N. Investigation of molecular details of Keap1-Nrf2 inhibitors using molecular dynamics and umbrella sampling techniques. *Molecules* **2019**, *24*, 4085. [CrossRef]
47. Cloete, R.; Akurugu, W.A.; Werely, C.J.; van Helden, P.D.; Christoffels, A. Structural and functional effects of nucleotide variation on the human TB drug metabolizing enzyme arylamine N-acetyltransferase 1. *J. Mol. Graph. Model.* **2017**, *75*, 330–339. [CrossRef]
48. Farmer, L.J.; Bemis, G.; Britt, S.D.; Cochran, J.; Connors, M.; Harrington, E.M.; Hoock, T.; Markland, W.; Nanthakumar, S.; Taslimi, P.; et al. Discovery and SAR of novel 4-thiazolyl-2-phenylaminopyrimidines as potent inhibitors of spleen tyrosine kinase (SYK). *Bioorganic Med. Chem. Lett.* **2008**, *18*, 6231–6235. [CrossRef]
49. Huang, Y.; Zhang, Y.; Fan, K.; Dong, G.; Li, B.; Zhang, W.; Li, J.; Sheng, C. Discovery of new SYK inhibitors through structure-based virtual screening. *Bioorganic Med. Chem. Lett.* **2017**, *27*, 1776–1779. [CrossRef]
50. Banerjee, P.; Eckert, A.O.; Schrey, A.K.; Preissner, R. ProTox-II: A webserver for the prediction of toxicity of chemicals. *Nucleic Acids Res.* **2018**, *46*, W257–W263. [CrossRef]

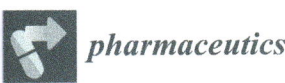

Article

Combining Human Genetics of Multiple Sclerosis with Oxidative Stress Phenotype for Drug Repositioning

Stefania Olla [1,*,†], Maristella Steri [1,†], Alessia Formato [2], Michael B. Whalen [3], Silvia Corbisiero [2] and Cristina Agresti [2,*]

1. Istituto di Ricerca Genetica e Biomedica, Consiglio Nazionale delle Ricerche, 09042 Monserrato, Italy; maristella.steri@irgb.cnr.it
2. Department of Neuroscience, Istituto Superiore di Sanità, 00161 Rome, Italy; alessia.formato@iss.it (A.F.); silvia.corbisiero@iss.it (S.C.)
3. Istituto di Biofisica, Consiglio Nazionale delle Ricerche (CNR), 38123 Trento, Italy; michaelbernard.whalen@ibf.cnr.it
* Correspondence: stefania.olla@irgb.cnr.it (S.O.); cristina.agresti@iss.it (C.A.)
† These authors contributed equally to this work.

Abstract: In multiple sclerosis (MS), oxidative stress (OS) is implicated in the neurodegenerative processes that occur from the beginning of the disease. Unchecked OS initiates a vicious circle caused by its crosstalk with inflammation, leading to demyelination, axonal damage and neuronal loss. The failure of MS antioxidant therapies relying on the use of endogenous and natural compounds drives the application of novel approaches to assess target relevance to the disease prior to preclinical testing of new drug candidates. To identify drugs that can act as regulators of intracellular oxidative homeostasis, we applied an in silico approach that links genome-wide MS associations and molecular quantitative trait loci (QTLs) to proteins of the OS pathway. We found 10 drugs with both central nervous system and oral bioavailability, targeting five out of the 21 top-scoring hits, including arginine methyltransferase (CARM1), which was first linked to MS. In particular, the direction of brain expression QTLs for CARM1 and protein kinase MAPK1 enabled us to select BIIB021 and PEITC drugs with the required target modulation. Our study highlights OS-related molecules regulated by functional MS variants that could be targeted by existing drugs as a supplement to the approved disease-modifying treatments.

Keywords: GWAS; multiple sclerosis; oxidative stress; repurposing; ADME-Tox

1. Introduction

Multiple sclerosis (MS) is the most common chronic inflammatory and progressively disabling disease of the central nervous system (CNS), affecting young adults and leading to demyelination and neuronal degeneration [1]. It is found worldwide, with the highest prevalence (>100 cases per hundred thousand) in the populations of Western Europe, North America and Australasia, with considerably lower prevalence (<30 cases per hundred thousand) in populations that live nearer to the equator [2]. MS is likely the result of an interaction between genetic and environmental factors, but its etiology remains unknown. Although approved immunomodulatory therapies are effective in the early stages of the disease, they have little or no benefit in terms of preventing the transition to a more steadily progressive phase, characterized by accumulation of neuronal injury and loss. Thus, the search for agents that slow neurodegeneration and disability progression in MS is urgent.

Neuroinflammation is recognized as a key player in MS pathogenesis. It is present in all stages of the disease and involves adaptive and innate immune responses. Histopathological studies of MS indicate that demyelination and neurodegeneration are associated with the production of inflammatory molecules by both blood-derived immune cells recruited to the CNS and activated resident microglia [3]. Prolonged or chronic generation of

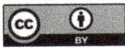

cytokines, chemokines, reactive oxygen species (ROS) and reactive nitrogen species (RNS) creates a self-perpetuating loop that provokes CNS damage and is considered to play a key role in the onset and progression of the disease [4].

ROS and RNS, including superoxide ions, hydrogen peroxide, nitric oxide and peroxynitrite, are generated by NADPH oxidase and nitric oxide synthase during normal cellular metabolism. However, these molecules are deleterious if overproduced because they can damage lipids, proteins and nucleic acids, eventually leading to cell death. Significant evidence indicates that the sustained inflammatory phase of MS creates an imbalance between ROS/RNS generation and the antioxidant defense systems, causing oxidative/nitrosative stress which has a role in CNS tissue damage [5]. Antioxidant defense is normally achieved with enzymes, such as superoxide dismutase, catalases and peroxiredoxins, as well as systems of antioxidant production, like the thioredoxin and glutathione systems. In addition, reactive species directly interact with critical signaling molecules, such as the transcription factors nuclear factor-erythroid 2-related factor 2 (Nrf2) and nuclear factor κB (NfkB) and mitogen activated kinases (MAPK) [6–8] which regulate antioxidant gene expression and cell survival. A recent gene expression study of MS brain areas adjacent to perivascular inflammatory cell infiltrates showed a significant induction of antioxidant genes in actively demyelinating and chronically active white matter lesions as part of a counter-regulatory response aimed at containing inflammation and limiting tissue damage [9]. Hence, the identification of drugs able to effectively support the maintenance of redox homeostasis represents a rational approach to limit MS-associated neurodegenerative processes.

Among current MS drugs, only dimethyl fumarate has been linked to the induction of antioxidant pathways, specifically through direct activation of Nrf2, a transcription factor with a crucial role in the regulation of the antioxidant defense response [10]. In addition, the clinical efficacy of natalizumab and fingolimod could in part be explained by their ability to increase antioxidant molecules and reduce oxidative stress (OS) biomarkers in MS patients [11,12], even though the mechanism responsible for these effects has not yet been established. Nevertheless, most complementary antioxidant therapies relying on endogenous and natural compounds have been previously investigated without overcoming MS clinical evaluation [13]. A possible explanation of this oversight is that the rationale behind the use of small molecules acting as scavengers was based on misconceptions linked to an incomplete understanding of antioxidant defense processes during disease development [14]. Hence, novel approaches should be used to assess the disease relevance of antioxidant targets prior to preclinical testing of new drug candidates.

It is now widely accepted that the selection of targets based on genetics significantly increases the success rates of clinical development programs [15,16]. The idea is to identify targets involved in disease processes that can be therapeutically modulated [17,18]. Over the past fifteen years, genome-wide association studies (GWAS), in increasingly larger sample sets, have succeeded in identifying more than 200 susceptibility loci for MS outside the major histocompatibility complex (MHC) [19]. In parallel, new functional genomic techniques assessing molecular quantitative trait loci (QTLs), such as chromatin interactions, protein level and gene expression regulation, have proven to be useful for the systematic identification of genes through which trait-association variants act, improving the clinical impact of GWAS [20]. Computational searches for existing drugs that modulate the molecular targets identified by genetic studies offer the advantage of repositioning, reducing the costs and timescales of drug development. In addition, in silico approaches are currently being used for the prediction of physicochemical properties, such as the blood–brain barrier (BBB) permeability and oral bioavailability of drugs, further reducing the risk of failure [21].

Here, we designed and applied an integrated approach that combines MS GWAS, molecular QTLs and in silico techniques of drug discovery, providing support for single drug candidates known to act as modulators of genes and/or gene products that are linked to OS pathways (Figure 1).

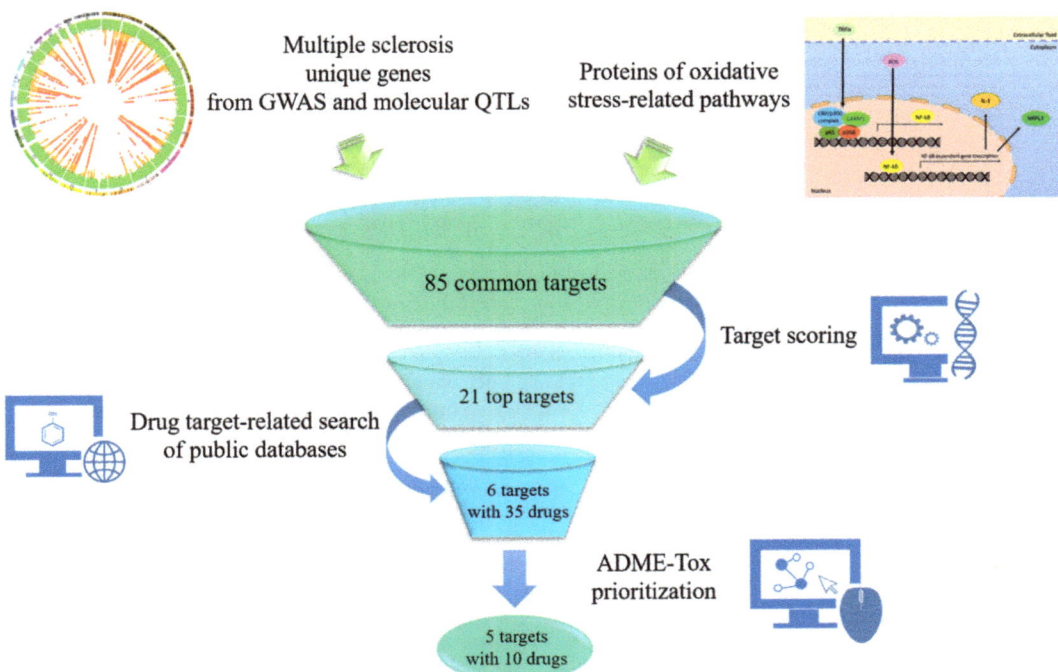

Figure 1. Schematic illustration of the in silico workflow. Multiple sclerosis (MS) genetic variants were collected from the Genome-Wide Association Studies (GWAS) Catalog and molecular Quantitative Trait Loci (QTLs) were exploited for each hit in the LinDA browser to identify gene targets. In parallel, all proteins from 22 oxidative stress-related pathways were retrieved from the Reactome database. The overlap of these data allowed for the identification of 85 common targets which were then prioritized through score assignment. Query of public drug databases for the 21 top targets enabled the selection of 35 drugs either already approved or in clinical trials that bind to six MS molecular targets. Absorption, Distribution, Metabolism, Excretion and Toxicity (ADME-Tox) selection highlighted 10 drugs with CNS localization and oral bioavailability for repurposing in MS.

2. Materials and Methods

2.1. Data Collection

MS GWAS summary statistics were extracted from the GWAS Catalog [22,23]. The selected genetic variants represent the most associated signal (top variant) in each genomic region (locus) given a significance threshold of p-value $< 1 \times 10^{-5}$. All variants have been annotated by their rsID in dbSNP154, when available, or by chromosome and genomic positions encoded in the Genome Assembly GRCh38/hg38. To assign the most reliable gene target to each associated variant, molecular QTLs were searched for each hit in a large manually curated QTL resource, the LinDA browser [24,25]. Data from protein QTLs (pQTLs), expression QTLs (eQTLs), splicing QTLs (sQTLs), polyadenylation QTLs (polyQTLs) and methylation QTLs (mQTLs) were collected. The genomic positions in the LinDA browser being encoded in the Genome Assembly GRCh37/hg19, genomic coordinates were converted from GRCh38/hg38 to GRCh37/hg19 using the LiftOver tool in the UCSC Genome Browser [26,27].

Top variants were searched for molecular QTLs, including all variants showing a linkage disequilibrium (LD) r2 > 0.7 with the top variants (proxies) in the European population. LD was calculated using the –ld option in the plink v.1.9 software [28,29] on data from the 1000 Genome Project reference panel [30].

The functional role of each tested variant was further evaluated by the Variant Effect Predictor (VEP) tool [31], and missense or more deleterious variants with a deleteriousness score (combined annotation dependent depletion, CADD-Phred) > 15 were prioritized [32].

Genes regulated at the RNA or protein level by a hit variant (or by a variant in strong LD with a hit variant) or tagged by a functionally relevant variant were flagged as "gene targets".

The direction of the effect of each disease risk variant on the target product was calculated to establish the direction of the gene target modulation by therapy. To this end, the disease risk alleles available from the GWAS Catalog were coupled with the molecular QTLs alleles by applying the Plink –ld option to the European ancestry genotypes encoded in the 1000 Genome Project reference panel [30]. The direction of the effect of the disease risk allele on the molecular QTL was thus indicated as positive if the coupled molecular QTL allele showed a positive effect, and negative otherwise.

In parallel, 22 pathways related to OS were identified by Reactome [33,34], and all proteins belonging to the pathways were extracted.

Genes and/or proteins obtained by the overlapping between the MS-related genes and the OS-related proteins were recorded as "targets".

For each target, a prioritization score was defined by leveraging the gene-level information derived from GWAS and from LD. In particular, for each target, all top variants, together with their molecular QTL proxies pointing to the same gene, were collected. A score was attributed to the target for each of the following criteria met by at least one collected variant:

Top hit significantly associated with MS (p-value $< 5 \times 10^{-8}$: score = 5, if lying in the MHC region (chr6:27–33 mb in GRCh37): score = 2);

Top hit having a high effect on the disease compared to all top hit effects (odds ratio, OR > 1.2), with a decreasing score depending on the LD with gene-level molecular QTLs (LD $\geq$ 0.99: score = 4; LD range (0.95–0.99): score = 3; LD range (0.90–0.95): score = 2; LD range (0.80–0.90): score = 1);

eQTL available (score = 10; if the eQTL acts in the brain: additional score = 5);

LD level between the top hit and the eQTL (LD $\geq$ 0.99: score = 5; LD range (0.95–0.99): score = 3; LD range (0.90–0.95): score = 2; LD range (0.80–0.90): score = 1);

QTL (except eQTL) with LD $\geq$ 0.99 with top hit: score = 3.

An overall score was calculated as the sum of the partial scores and the top 25% targets were then prioritized.

2.2. g:Profiler Analysis

To perform functional enrichment analysis, g:Profiler e94_eg41_p11_9f195a1 was used [35,36]. The parameters for the enrichment analysis were as follows. A specific organism was chosen: *H. sapiens* (human). Gene Ontology (GO) analyses, GO molecular function (GO:MF), GO cellular component (GO:CC) and GO biological process (GO:BP) were carried out sequentially. The biological pathways used were the Kyoto encyclopedia of genes and genomes (KEGG), Reactome (REAC) and WikiPathways (WP) databases. The protein databases used were the Human Protein Atlas and CORUM databases. The statistical domain scope was used only for annotated genes. The significance threshold was the g:SCS threshold. The user threshold was 0.05.

2.3. Drug Searching

Four different databases, OpenTarget [37,38], SuperTarget [39], DrugBank [40,41] and DGIdb [42,43] were used to search for drugs related to the targets of interest.

2.4. In Silico Prediction of Physicochemical Properties of Drugs

The Absorption, Distribution, Metabolism, Excretion and Toxicity (ADME-Tox) profile of the investigated compounds was predicted using the Schrodinger QikProp tool (Small-Molecule Drug Discovery Suite 2021–1, Schrodinger, LLC, New York, NY, USA). QikProp uses several indicators to estimate the activity in the CNS and thus also the ability of a compound to cross the BBB. The three most important are: (i) LogBB, which represents the blood–brain partition coefficient; (ii) the Madin–Darby dog kidney cell model (apparent MDCK permeability), which estimates the penetration of the substances through a layer of these cells, measured in nm/sec; (iii) the predictor of activity in the CNS. The indicators used to evaluate oral absorption include Human Oral Absorption, Percent Human Absorption and apparent Caco2 permeability, Caco2 being a human colon carcinoma cell line used to predict human intestinal permeability and to investigate drug efflux.

3. Results

3.1. Genetic-Driven Identification of Targets Linked to Oxidative Pathways in MS

We systematically collected GWAS data for MS from the GWAS Catalog (Methods), identifying 698 different genetic variants (hits; Table S1, Supplementary Materials). We then examined molecular QTLs to identify gene targets by searching each hit or its proxies (with r2 > 0.7) in the LinDA browser (Table S2). This LD-based searching strategy allowed us to maximize the information collected, considering that differences in the genetic map and/or in the sample size used in each study (both on disease and molecular QTLs) could lead to the identification of different genetic variants representing the same genetic signal. In addition, we evaluated the functional role of each tested variant by VEP, focusing on missense or more deleterious variants with a CADD-Phred score >15 (Table S3). Thus, each gene regulated at RNA or protein level by a hit variant or tagged by a functionally relevant variant, excluding MHC genes, was recorded for a total of 2,085 unique gene targets (Table S4). In parallel, we extracted the proteins encoded by 931 unique targets included in 22 OS-related pathways from the Reactome database [44] (Tables S5 and S6). The overlap between the 2,085 MS-related gene targets and the 931 OS-related proteins led to the identification of 85 shared targets (Table S7), including KEAP1 and HDAC1, which are both known to be modulated by drugs currently in use for MS (dimethyl fumarate and fingolimod, respectively). Among the 85 targets, 18 are supported by molecular QTLs in the brain (ASF1A, ATP6V1G2, BBC3, BCL2L11, CAPN1, CARM1, CHAC1, CRTC3, CSNK2B, DNM2, FOXO3, HSPA1L, KEAP1, MAPK1, NUP85, POM121C, PSMB9 and TRMT112). In addition, for each variant whose risk allele effect on the gene product was available in the brain, we were able to establish the direction of action (up or down) on the transcript/protein level and, consequently, to choose drugs with the proper mode of modulation: inhibition or activation (Table S8). In particular, 10 targets were regulated by MS risk variants at some level in the brain, and among them we observed increased expression levels for seven targets (ASF1A, CAPN1, CARM1, CHAC1, NUP85, POM121C and TRMT112) and decreased levels for three targets (BBC3, MAPK1 and PSMB9).

3.2. Functional Enrichment Analysis of the Identified Targets

To obtain the enrichment information for the 85 candidate targets showing QTLs, g:Profiler analysis was performed [36]. The default analysis implemented in g:Profiler searches for pathways whose genes are significantly enriched (i.e., over-represented) in the target list of interest and compares them to all genes in the genome. Among the most significant pathways detected by REAC, "cellular response to stress" (p-value = 4.248×10^{-36}) and "cellular responses to external stimuli" (p-value = 1.326×10^{-35}) have been pointed out, consistent with OS being the investigated disease phenotype (Figure 2). "Proteasome" (p-value = 8.289×10^{-7}) and "proteasome degradation" (p-value = 9.576×10^{-7}) have been identified as the most represented pathways by KEGG and WP, respectively. The three most significant cellular functions outlined by GO were "transcription factor binding" (GO:MF, 1.942×10^{-6}), "cellular response to stress" (GO:BP, 8.022×10^{-19})

and "cytosol" (GO:CC, 1.303×10^{-19}). Table S9 gives details of all the individual targets involved in the described analyses.

Figure 2. g:Profiler analysis of 85 targets. (**A**) Graphic representation of the results. (**B**) The most significant results for Gene Ontology (GO) and pathways enrichment were shown. GO molecular function (GO:MF); GO biological process (GO:BP); GO cellular component (GO:CC); Kyoto encyclopedia of genes and genomes (KEGG); Reactome (REAC); WikiPathways (WP).

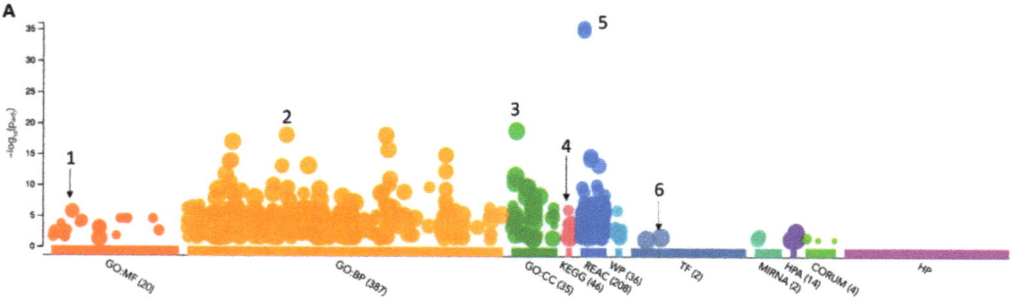

Id	Source	Term id	Term name	P-value
1	GO:MF	GO:0008134	Transcription factor binding	1.942×10^{-6}
2	GO:BP	GO:0033554	Cellular response to stress	8.022×10^{-19}
3	GO:CC	GO:0005829	Cytosol	1.303×10^{-19}
4	KEGG	KEGG:03050	Proteasome	8.289×10^{-7}
5	REAC	R-HAS-2262752	Cellular responses to stress	4.248×10^{-36}
6	WP	WP:WP183	Proteasome degradation	9.576×10^{-7}

3.3. Target Prioritization and Drug Search

To prioritize the 85 selected targets, we assigned to each of them a genetic-based score which considers the strength of association (variant effect magnitude and significance) with the disease, the presence of QTLs regulating the gene target at protein expression level, particularly in the brain, and the extent of LD supporting all the molecular information.

Based on the score distribution, we then fixed a threshold of score ≥20, which corresponds to the top 25% of the OS-related targets (Figure S1). We prioritized 21 targets (Table S10), including seven targets regulated by eQTLs in the brain for which we established the required direction of modulation (TRMT112, CAPN1, ASF1A, NUP85 and CARM1, suggested to be inhibited, and BBC3 and MAPK1, suggested to be activated).

In four different databases, we searched for modulators of the 21 top-ranking targets (Table S10), selecting only: (i) drugs approved or in clinical trials; (ii) drugs known to act directly on the specific target or as transcriptional target modulators based on established criteria (DGIdb interaction score >0.50 and published data on experimental validation); (iii) drugs having a mode of action consistent with the direction of the eQTL for the risk allele in the brain, if present. This analysis identified 35 modulators of six out of the 21 top targets (MAPK1, MAPK3, CARM1, CDK4, STAT3 and FOS), with a substantial number of drugs for each target, except for CARM1, which had only one. To increase the modulators of CARM1 and to investigate the druggability of the remaining top-ranking targets, we also looked for experimental drug trials, finding five CARM1 inhibitors and 11 compounds for two additional targets (NR1D1 and CAPN1). In addition, the presence of at least one modulator on Pharos makes the targets ASF1A, HVCN1 and YWHAQ druggable [45,46]. We then compiled a final list of 50 compounds for the next selection phase.

3.4. Pharmacokinetic Prioritization of the Selected Drugs

By QikProp, the ADME-Tox properties of 35 repurposable drugs and 15 experimental compounds associated with the eight selected targets were predicted (Table S11). Among the selection criteria, we prioritized the expected penetration into the CNS and the oral bioavailability, which are essential for maintaining drug function and potency towards the respective targets. In addition, physicochemical descriptors and other general properties related to good overall pharmacokinetics and metabolism profiles were considered. In detail, we selected compounds having (i) a value ≥ 0 for predicted CNS activity; (ii) medium–good values of logBB and MDCK apparent permeability; (iii) high values of human oral absorption and percent human oral absorption; (iv) medium–good values of Caco2 apparent permeability (Table S11). Overall, this analysis identified 10 repurposable drugs (Table 1) and seven experimental compounds. The selected drugs include: (i) the CARM1 inhibitor BIIB021 in clinical trial for breast and gastrointestinal tumors; (ii) the MAPK1 activator PEITC in clinical trial for lung and oral cancer; (iii) four CDK4 inhibitors, ABEMACICLIB approved for breast cancer, ALVOCIDIB, MILCICLIB and PHA-793887 in clinical trials for several tumors; (iv) three STAT3 modulators, ERLOTINIB approved for lung cancer, ENMD1198 and ATIPRIMOD in trial for neuroendocrine cancer and multiple myeloma; (v) PILOCARPINE approved for the treatment of presbyopia as an inducer of FOS expression. Some of the drugs that are presented in Table 1 do not directly modulate the identified targets but may act through indirect mechanisms. The MAPK1-3 inhibitors, MK8353 and LY3214996, were removed from the list since they have a mechanism of modulation not consistent with the direction of eQTLs that we identified for MAPK1 in the brain. The seven experimental compounds that exceeded the pharmacokinetics investigation comprise three CARM1 inhibitors (MS049, MS023, TP064) and four NR1D1 modulators (agonists GSK4112, SR9009 and SR9011 and antagonist SR8278) (Table S11).

Table 1. Repurposable candidates for oxidative-stress phenotype in MS. The table shows drug candidates with their mechanism of action and clinical trial status for each target. The queried databases are also reported.

Target	Drug	Mechanism of Action	Status *	Database
CARM1	BIIB021	HSP90 and CARM1 inhibitor	Phase II for breast cancer and gastrointestinal stromal tumors	DGIdb
MAPK1	PHENETHYL ISOTHIOCYANATE, (PEITC)	Bioactive compound activates ERK signal	Phase II lung cancer, tobacco use disorder and oral cancer	Super Target
CDK4	ABEMACICLIB	CDK4/6 inhibitor	Approved for breast cancer	DGIdb, DrugBank, OpenTarget
CDK4	ALVOCIDIB	CDKs inhibitor	Phase II for chronic lymphocytic leukemia; relapsed or refractory multiple myeloma; B-cell lymphoma; sarcoma; acute myeloid leukemia; prostate cancer; advanced ovarian epithelial cancer or primary peritoneal cancer; adenocarcinoma; kidney cancer; melanoma; endometrial cancer	DGIdb; DrugBank; OpenTarget

Table 1. *Cont.*

Target	Drug	Mechanism of Action	Status *	Database
CDK4	MILCICLIB	CDKs inhibitor	Phase II for malignant thymoma and hepatocellular carcinoma	DGIdb; OpenTarget
CDK4	PHA-793887	CDKs inhibitor	Phase I for advanced-metastatic solid tumors	DGIdb
STAT3	ATIPRIMOD	Blocks STAT3 activation	Phase II for neuroendocrine cancer and multiple myeloma	DGIdb
STAT3	ENMD 1198	Mitosis inhibitors; tubulin modulators; STAT3 inhibitor	Phase I for advanced cancer	DrugBank
STAT3	ERLOTINIB	EGFR inhibitor; stimulated phosphorylation and activation of STAT3	Approved for lung and pancreatic cancer	SuperTarget; DGIdb
FOS	PILOCARPINE	Muscarinic receptor agonist-induced c-fos expression	Approved for the treatment of presbyopia	DGIdb

* Only the highest phase is shown.

4. Discussion

Advanced genetic analysis in MS has identified variants that clearly influence gene expression of CNS-resident immune cells [19], highlighting potential functional consequences for dysregulation of genes involved in the generation of inflammatory and oxidative mediators that trigger neurodegenerative processes. Our purpose was to link genome-wide MS associations and the correlated molecular QTLs to targets of OS pathways, improving the prediction of drug candidates that act as regulators of intracellular oxidative homeostasis. We selected 10 drugs already in use for cancer therapies that are specific for five out of the 21 top-scoring targets involved in the interplay between oxidation–apoptosis–autophagy–inflammation. Of these, MAPK1, STAT3, CDK4 and FOS targets have been indicated in previous MS GWAS [19,47–49], while the potential genetic link of CARM1 with MS is novel. However, drugs with CNS and oral bioavailability have not been predicted for any of these targets.

GWAS-associated genes have already resulted in candidate targets for drug discovery and repositioning in both complex and monogenic diseases [50]. Concerning MS, several studies have outlined the functional consequences of a set of disease variants [47] but these findings have not yet been translated into clinical practice. Moreover, the crosstalk between OS, neurodegeneration and neuroinflammation has a central role in the pathogenesis of MS [51].

In this study, we correlated MS susceptibility loci to OS pathways, finding those alleles (outside the MHC) that influence risk for this relevant disease phenotype. Notably, 85 shared targets were identified and ranked by assigning a score to each genetic outcome available. The reliability of our results is supported by the high score for KEAP1 and HDAC1, known targets of two drugs currently in use for MS, the antioxidant dimethyl fumarate and the immunomodulator fingolimod, respectively. As expected, our selected targets are linked with OS at different levels, in line with the dynamic outline of this process, which accounts for various interrelated events occurring in different cellular compartments. Our list includes: NCF4, a component of the NADPH oxidase system, and the proton channel HVCN1, which are involved in ROS generation [52]; MAPK1, MAPK3, STAT3 and FOS, inflammatory signaling molecules directly activated by ROS [53,54]; the arginine methyltransferase CARM1, a transcriptional co-activator known to regulate NFkB-dependent gene expression [55] and to be involved in cellular processes, such as autophagy, control of the cell cycle and differentiation [56]; the kinase CDK4, which promotes cellular growth by stimulation of mitochondrial biogenesis and concomitantly increases ROS generation [57]; the circadian gene NR1D1, which improves cellular bioenergetics and is regulated by OS and inflammation [58,59]. Interestingly, targets involved in complex regulatory mechanisms have recently attracted interest in the treatment of multifactorial diseases, such as neurodegenerative diseases, in which several biochemical events and molecular targets operate simultaneously [60].

Our approach of genetic-driven target identification is based on the integration of GWAS with eQTLs, especially those measured in brain tissues, to assess genes whose expression levels are modulated by non-coding disease-related variants [49]. The fact that 80% of the genetic variants identified by GWAS map in non-coding regions highlights the potential of functional genomic tools [50,61]. The use in this pipeline of different MS GWAS datasets, including those not containing complete whole-genome results, increased the number of potential candidate targets. Moreover, when the correspondence between a disease-risk variant and an eQTL allele has been derived, we were able to obtain important information about the direction of drug target modulation to be considered.

Query of public databases, combined with in silico pharmacokinetics, allowed for the selection of 10 drugs acting as modulators of five targets associated with oxidative pathways in MS. The direction of brain eQTLs for CARM1 and MAPK1 enabled us to identify two drugs with the required target modulation, prioritizing BIIB021 and PEITC over modulators of targets without the direction of their allelic effect. In particular, BIIB021 is a CARM1 and HSP90 inhibitor currently in clinical trials for treating hematopoietic malignancies and solid tumors (NCT01004081, NCT00618319 and NCT00344786) which easily crosses the BBB and can be administered orally. The drug mechanism responsible for CARM1 inhibition has not yet been defined, and there is the possibility that it acts indirectly via the inhibition of HSP90, which was identified as a CARM1 interactor (EP 3 208 615 B1). In addition, we also indicated highly selective inhibitors of CARM1, recently developed and tested in experimental models [62–64]. PEITC is an organosulfur bioactive compound, known as an MAPK1 activator, that is currently in trial for lung cancer and leukemia treatment (NCT00691132 and NCT00968461). Notably, the anti-inflammatory and antioxidant activity of PEITC has been extensively demonstrated in both in vitro and in vivo models. [65,66]. Of note, our in silico ADME analysis confirmed previous data on the BBB permeability of this drug [67].

Lack of data on the direction of the effects of MS risk variants in the modulation of STAT3, CDK4 and FOS in the brain does not allow the selection of drugs with adequate therapeutic modulation (activation or inhibition). Previous studies based on genetic variants and QTLs have suggested drugs for repurposing without exploiting the direction of effects [49,68], further supporting the potential relevance of our results.

In our study, we exclusively selected drugs that had passed clinical phase I and which therefore should be free of serious side effects regardless of their selectivity. Nevertheless, some drugs, including the CDKs inhibitor Alvocidib, present dose-dependent adverse effects that might be evaluated in the disease of interest by a risk–benefit analysis. As shown for CARM1, small molecules with a higher selectivity can be found among compounds active in preclinical studies but, by definition, these are not currently repurposable compounds.

The knowledge about targets relevant to OS in MS for which no approved modulators are currently available could be exploited in future drug discovery studies. Our search for experimental modulators of these targets led to the identification of NR1D1 agonists and antagonists [69], thus proving the druggability of an additional target.

A major limitation of our in silico approach concerns the finding that only about 22% of protein-coding genes are druggable [70], which is consistent with the low proportion of top-identified targets engaged by approved or in clinical trial drugs. A more stringent selection of genes strongly associated with disease may result in the loss of relevant targets showing small effect sizes [71]. In addition, the smaller number of QTLs assessed in the brain compared to other tissues and the lack of protein-QTLs significantly reduce the number of candidate genes to be matched with the selected disease phenotype. It should also be kept in mind that public databases for GWAS, drug targets and pathways make available data that are usually not uniform, often incomplete and frequently not up-to-date, and these represent important constraints for the achievement of a comprehensive analysis.

5. Conclusions

This study highlights the support of genetics in identifying targets which can potentially result in an unbalance of OS-related pathways in MS and existing drugs that can be repositioned to aim at these targets. We showed for the first time an increased expression of CARM1 genetically linked to MS. This finding agrees with the emerging dysregulation of methylation pathways in MS, which may impact immune and neurological processes [72]. Notably, several links between arginine methylation and neurodegenerative diseases, such as amyotrophic lateral sclerosis, Alzheimer's and Huntington's disease, have been established over the last few years [73]. However, preclinical studies will be necessary to validate the best drug candidates in cellular or animal models before their therapeutic application. A network pharmacology analysis could be helpful in identifying combinations of drugs targeting different unbalanced signaling pathways consistent with omics data integration and a multitarget drug development approach [74].

Supplementary Materials: The following are available online at https://www.mdpi.com/article/10.3390/pharmaceutics13122064/s1, Table S1: Genome-wide association results for multiple sclerosis; Table S2: Molecular QTLs related to MS variants; Table S3: Genes tagged by functional relevant MS-related variants; Table S4: MS-related gene targets derived from GWAS and molecular QTLs; Table S5: OS-related pathways; Table S6: Unique proteins related to oxidative stress; Table S7: List of the 85 OS-related targets; Table S8: Direction of effects of MS variants on molecular gene features; Table S9: G-profiler analysis of 85 OS-related targets; Figure S1: Prioritization score distribution; Table S10: Prioritization score; Table S11: In silico ADME studies.

Author Contributions: Conceptualization, C.A., S.O. and M.S.; methodology, S.O. and M.S.; software, S.O., M.S., A.F. and S.C.; data analysis, S.O. and M.S.; investigation, C.A., S.O., A.F. and S.C.; writing—original draft preparation, C.A., S.O. and M.S.; writing—review and editing, C.A., S.O., M.S., M.B.W., A.F. and S.C.; supervision, C.A.; funding acquisition C.A. and S.O. All authors have read and agreed to the published version of the manuscript.

Funding: This study was supported by Progressive MS Alliance (collaborative research network PA-1604-08492-BRAVEinMS) to S.O. and C.A.

Institutional Review Board Statement: Not applicable.

Informed Consent Statement: Not applicable.

Data Availability Statement: Not applicable.

Acknowledgments: We thank Francesca Aloisi, Caterina Veroni and Andrea Angius for help with the manuscript revision and Michele Marongiu for technical support.

Conflicts of Interest: The authors declare no conflict of interest.

References

1. Reich, D.S.; Lucchinetti, C.F.; Calabresi, P.A. Multiple Sclerosis. *N. Engl. J. Med.* **2018**, *378*, 169–180. [CrossRef] [PubMed]
2. Hauser, S.L.; Cree, B.A.C. Treatment of Multiple Sclerosis: A Review. *Am. J. Med.* **2020**, *133*, 1380–1390. [CrossRef] [PubMed]
3. Lassmann, H. Pathogenic Mechanisms Associated with Different Clinical Courses of Multiple Sclerosis. *Front. Immunol.* **2019**, *9*, 3116. [CrossRef] [PubMed]
4. Pegoretti, V.; Swanson, K.A.; Bethea, J.R.; Probert, L.; Eisel, U.L.M.; Fischer, R. Inflammation and Oxidative Stress in Multiple Sclerosis: Consequences for Therapy Development. *Oxidative Med. Cell. Longev.* **2020**, *2020*, 1–19. [CrossRef] [PubMed]
5. Zhang, S.-Y.; Gui, L.-N.; Liu, Y.-Y.; Shi, S.; Cheng, Y. Oxidative Stress Marker Aberrations in Multiple Sclerosis: A Meta-Analysis Study. *Front. Neurosci.* **2020**, *14*, 823. [CrossRef] [PubMed]
6. Nguyen, T.; Nioi, P.; Pickett, C.B. The Nrf2-Antioxidant Response Element Signaling Pathway and Its Activation by Oxidative Stress. *J. Biol. Chem.* **2009**, *284*, 13291–13295. [CrossRef] [PubMed]

7. Morgan, M.J.; Liu, Z.G. Crosstalk of reactive oxygen species and NF-κB signaling. *Cell Res.* **2011**, *21*, 103–115. [CrossRef]
8. Takata, T.; Araki, S.; Tsuchiya, Y.; Watanabe, Y. Oxidative Stress Orchestrates MAPK and Nitric-Oxide Synthase Signal. *Int. J. Mol. Sci.* **2020**, *21*, 8750. [CrossRef]
9. Veroni, C.; Serafini, B.; Rosicarelli, B.; Fagnani, C.; Aloisi, F.; Agresti, C. Connecting Immune Cell Infiltration to the Multitasking Microglia Response and TNF Receptor 2 Induction in the Multiple Sclerosis Brain. *Front. Cell. Neurosci.* **2020**, *14*, 190. [CrossRef]
10. Gopal, S.; Mikulskis, A.; Gold, R.; Fox, R.J.; Dawson, K.T.; Amaravadi, L. Evidence of activation of the Nrf2 pathway in multiple sclerosis patients treated with delayed-release dimethyl fumarate in the Phase 3 DEFINE and CONFIRM studies. *Mult. Scler. J.* **2017**, *23*, 1875–1883. [CrossRef]
11. Yevgi, R.; Demir, R. Oxidative stress activity of fingolimod in multiple sclerosis. *Clin. Neurol. Neurosurg.* **2021**, *202*, 106500. [CrossRef]
12. Adamczyk, B.; Wawrzyniak, S.; Kasperczyk, S.; Adamczyk-Sowa, M. The Evaluation of Oxidative Stress Parameters in Serum Patients with Relapsing-Remitting Multiple Sclerosis Treated with II-Line Immunomodulatory Therapy. *Oxidative Med. Cell. Longev.* **2017**, *2017*, 1–12. [CrossRef]
13. Miller, E.D.; Dziedzic, A.; Saluk-Bijak, J.; Bijak, M. A Review of Various Antioxidant Compounds and their Potential Utility as Complementary Therapy in Multiple Sclerosis. *Nutrients* **2019**, *11*, 1528. [CrossRef]
14. Forman, H.J.; Zhang, H. Targeting oxidative stress in disease: Promise and limitations of antioxidant therapy. *Nat. Rev. Drug Discov.* **2021**, *20*, 689–709, Erratum in **2021**, *20*, 652. [CrossRef]
15. Cook, D.; Brown, D.; Alexander, R.; March, R.; Morgan, P.; Satterthwaite, G.; Pangalos, M.N. Lessons learned from the fate of AstraZeneca's drug pipeline: A five-dimensional framework. *Nat. Rev. Drug Discov.* **2014**, *13*, 419–431. [CrossRef]
16. Nelson, M.R.; Tipney, H.; Painter, J.L.; Shen, J.; Nicoletti, P.; Shen, Y.; Floratos, A.; Sham, P.C.; Li, M.J.; Wang, J.; et al. The support of human genetic evidence for approved drug indications. *Nat. Genet.* **2015**, *47*, 856–860. [CrossRef]
17. Plenge, R.M.; Scolnick, E.M.; Altshuler, D. Validating therapeutic targets through human genetics. *Nat. Rev. Drug Discov.* **2013**, *12*, 581–594. [CrossRef]
18. Floris, M.; Olla, S.; Schlessinger, D.; Cucca, F. Genetic-Driven Druggable Target Identification and Validation. *Trends Genet.* **2018**, *34*, 558–570. [CrossRef]
19. International Multiple Sclerosis Genetics Consortium. Multiple sclerosis genomic map implicates peripheral immune cells and microglia in susceptibility. *Science* **2019**, *365*, eaav7188. [CrossRef]
20. Cano-Gamez, E.; Trynka, G. From GWAS to Function: Using Functional Genomics to Identify the Mechanisms Underlying Complex Diseases. *Front. Genet.* **2020**, *11*, 424. [CrossRef]
21. Eddershaw, P.J.; Beresford, A.P.; Bayliss, M.K. ADME/PK as part of a rational approach to drug discovery. *Drug Discov. Today* **2000**, *5*, 409–414. [CrossRef]
22. GWAS Catalog (downloaded file: Gwas_catalog_v1.0.2-associations_e98_r2021-03-01.tsv). Available online: https://www.ebi.ac.uk/gwas/home (accessed on 1 March 2021).
23. Buniello, A.; MacArthur, J.A.L.; Cerezo, M.; Harris, L.W.; Hayhurst, J.; Malangone, C.; McMahon, A.; Morales, J.; Mountjoy, E.; Sollis, E.; et al. The NHGRI-EBI GWAS Catalog of published genome-wide association studies, targeted arrays and summary statistics 2019. *Nucleic Acids Res.* **2019**, *47*, D1005–D1012. [CrossRef] [PubMed]
24. LinDA. Available online: http://linda.irgb.cnr.it/ (accessed on 16 March 2021).
25. Onano, S.; Cucca, F.; Pala, M. P18.25A The eQTLs Catalog and LinDA browser: A platform for prioritising target genes of GWAS variants. Abstracts from the 51st European Society of Human Genetics Conference: Oral Presentations. *Eur. J. Hum. Genet.* **2019**, *27*, 748–869. [CrossRef]
26. Lift Genome Annotations. Available online: https://www.genome.ucsc.edu/cgi-bin/hgLiftOver (accessed on 15 March 2021).
27. Kent, W.J.; Sugnet, C.W.; Furey, T.S.; Roskin, K.M.; Pringle, T.H.; Zahler, A.M.; Haussler, D. The Human Genome Browser at UCSC. *Genome Res.* **2002**, *12*, 996–1006. [CrossRef]
28. Purcell, S.; Neale, B.; Todd-Brown, K.; Thomas, L.; Ferreira, M.A.; Bender, D.; Maller, J.; Sklar, P.; de Bakker, P.I.; Daly, M.J.; et al. PLINK: A Tool Set for Whole-Genome Association and Population-Based Linkage Analyses. *Am. J. Hum. Genet.* **2007**, *81*, 559–575. [CrossRef]
29. Plink v.1.9 Software. Available online: http://pngu.mgh.harvard.edu/purcell/plink/ (accessed on 18 March 2021).
30. Genomes Project Consortium; Auton, A.; Brooks, L.D.; Durbin, R.M.; Garrison, E.P.; Kang, H.M.; Korbel, J.O.; Marchini, J.L.; McCarthy, S.; McVean, G.A.; et al. A global reference for human genetic variation. *Nature* **2015**, *526*, 68–74. [CrossRef]
31. VEP. Available online: https://grch37.ensembl.org/Tools/VEP (accessed on 16 March 2021).
32. Kircher, M.; Witten, D.M.; Jain, P.; O'Roak, B.J.; Cooper, G.M.; Shendure, J. A general framework for estimating the relative pathogenicity of human genetic variants. *Nat. Genet.* **2014**, *46*, 310–315. [CrossRef]
33. Reactome. Available online: https://reactome.org/ (accessed on 1 March 2021).
34. Fabregat, A.; Sidiropoulos, K.; Viteri, G.; Marin-Garcia, P.; Ping, P.; Stein, L.; D'Eustachio, P.; Hermjakob, H. Reactome diagram viewer: Data structures and strategies to boost performance. *Bioinformatics* **2018**, *34*, 1208–1214. [CrossRef]
35. g:Profiler (version e94_eg41_p11_9f195a1). Available online: https://biit.cs.ut.ee/gprofiler/gost (accessed on 24 March 2021).
36. Raudvere, U.; Kolberg, L.; Kuzmin, I.; Arak, T.; Adler, P.; Peterson, H.; Vilo, J. g:Profiler: A web server for functional enrichment analysis and conversions of gene lists (2019 update). *Nucleic Acids Res.* **2019**, *47*, W191–W198. [CrossRef]

37. Open Targets Platform. Available online: https://platform.opentargets.org/ (accessed on 29 March 2021).
38. Ochoa, D.; Hercules, A.; Carmona, M.; Suveges, D.; Gonzalez-Uriarte, A.; Malangone, C.; Miranda, A.; Fumis, L.; Carvalho-Silva, D.; Spitzer, M.; et al. Open Targets Platform: Supporting systematic drug–target identification and prioritisation. *Nucleic Acids Res.* **2021**, *49*, D1302–D1310. [CrossRef]
39. Hecker, N.; Ahmed, J.; Von Eichborn, J.; Dunkel, M.; Macha, K.; Eckert, A.; Gilson, M.K.; Bourne, P.E.; Preissner, R. SuperTarget goes quantitative: Update on drug-target interactions. *Nucleic Acids Res.* **2012**, *40*, D1113–D1117. [CrossRef]
40. DrugBank. Available online: https://go.drugbank.com/ (accessed on 29 March 2021).
41. Wishart, D.S.; Feunang, Y.D.; Guo, A.C.; Lo, E.J.; Marcu, A.; Grant, J.R.; Sajed, T.; Johnson, D.; Li, C.; Sayeeda, Z.; et al. DrugBank 5.0: A Major Update to the DrugBank Database for 2018. *Nucleic Acids Res.* **2018**, *46*, D1074–D1082. [CrossRef]
42. DGIdb. Available online: https://www.dgidb.org/ (accessed on 5 April 2021).
43. Freshour, S.L.; Kiwala, S.; Cotto, K.C.; Coffman, A.C.; McMichael, J.F.; Song, J.J.; Griffith, M.; Griffith, O.L.; Wagner, A.H. Integration of the Drug-Gene Interaction Database (DGIdb 4.0) with open crowdsource efforts. *Nucleic Acids Res.* **2021**, *49*, D1144–D1151. [CrossRef]
44. Jassal, B.; Matthews, L.; Viteri, G.; Gong, C.; Lorente, P.; Fabregat, A.; Gillespie, M.; Stephan, R.; Milacic, M.; Rothfels, K.; et al. The reactome pathway knowledgebase. *Nucleic Acids Res.* **2020**, *4*, D498–D503. [CrossRef]
45. Pharos. Available online: https://pharos.nih.gov/ (accessed on 14 June 2021).
46. Sheils, T.K.; Mathias, S.L.; Kelleher, K.J.; Siramshetty, V.B.; Nguyen, D.-T.; Bologa, C.G.; Jensen, L.J.; Vidović, D.; Koleti, A.; Schürer, S.C.; et al. TCRD and Pharos 2021: Mining the human proteome for disease biology. *Nucleic Acids Res.* **2020**, *49*, D1334–D1346. [CrossRef]
47. International Multiple Sclerosis Genetics Consortium (IMSGC); Beecham, A.H.; Patsopoulos, N.A.; Xifara, D.K.; Davis, M.F.; Kemppinen, A.; Cotsapas, C.; Shah, T.S.; Spencer, C.; Booth, D.; et al. Analysis of immune-related loci identifies 48 new susceptibility variants for multiple sclerosis. *Nat. Genet.* **2013**, *45*, 1353–1360. [CrossRef]
48. International Multiple Sclerosis Genetics Consortium; Wellcome Trust Case Control Consortium 2; Sawcer, S.; Hellenthal, G.; Pirinen, M.; Spencer, C.C.; Patsopoulos, N.A.; Moutsianas, L.; Dilthey, A.; Su, Z.; et al. Genetic risk and a primary role for cell-mediated immune mechanisms in multiple sclerosis. *Nature* **2011**, *476*, 214–219. [CrossRef]
49. Manuel, A.M.; Dai, Y.; Freeman, L.A.; Jia, P.; Zhao, Z. An integrative study of genetic variants with brain tissue expression identifies viral etiology and potential drug targets of multiple sclerosis. *Mol. Cell. Neurosci.* **2021**, *115*, 103656. [CrossRef]
50. Nabirotchkin, S.; Peluffo, A.E.; Rinaudo, P.; Yu, J.; Hajj, R.; Cohen, D. Next-generation drug repurposing using human genetics and network biology. *Curr. Opin. Pharmacol.* **2020**, *51*, 78–92. [CrossRef]
51. Adamczyk, B.; Adamczyk-Sowa, M. New Insights into the Role of Oxidative Stress Mechanisms in the Pathophysiology and Treatment of Multiple Sclerosis. *Oxidative Med. Cell. Longev.* **2016**, *2016*, 1–18. [CrossRef]
52. Kawai, T.; Okochi, Y.; Ozaki, T.; Imura, Y.; Koizumi, S.; Yamazaki, M.; Abe, M.; Sakimura, K.; Yamashita, T.; Okamura, Y. Unconventional role of voltage-gated proton channels (VSOP/Hv1) in regulation of microglial ROS production. *J. Neurochem.* **2017**, *142*, 686–699. [CrossRef] [PubMed]
53. Liu, W.H.; Chang, L.S. Arachidonic acid induces Fas and FasL upregulation in human leukemia U937 cells via Ca2+/ROS-mediated suppression of ERK/c-Fos pathway and activation of p38 MAPK/ATF-2 pathway. *Toxicol Lett.* **2009**, *191*, 140–148. [CrossRef] [PubMed]
54. Xu, F.; Xu, J.; Xiong, X.; Deng, Y. Salidroside inhibits MAPK, NF-κB, and STAT3 pathways in psoriasis-associated oxidative stress via SIRT1 activation. *Redox Rep.* **2019**, *24*, 70–74. [CrossRef] [PubMed]
55. Covic, M.; Hassa, P.O.; Saccani, S.; Buerki, C.; Meier, N.I.; Lombardi, C.; Imhof, R.; Bedford, M.T.; Natoli, G.; Hottiger, M.O. Arginine methyltransferase CARM1 is a promoter-specific regulator of NF-kappaB-dependent gene expression. *EMBO J.* **2005**, *24*, 85–96. [CrossRef]
56. Suresh, S.; Huard, S.; Dubois, T. CARM1/PRMT4: Making Its Mark beyond Its Function as a Transcriptional Coactivator. *Trends Cell Biol.* **2021**, *31*, 402–417. [CrossRef]
57. Schmitz, M.L.; Kracht, M. Cyclin-Dependent Kinases as Coregulators of Inflammatory Gene Expression. *Trends Pharmacol. Sci.* **2016**, *37*, 101–113. [CrossRef]
58. Yang, G.; Wright, C.J.; Hinson, M.D.; Fernando, A.P.; Sengupta, S.; Biswas, C.; La, P.; Dennery, P.A. Oxidative stress and inflammation modulate Rev-erbα signaling in the neonatal lung and affect circadian rhythmicity. *Antioxid. Redox Signal.* **2014**, *21*, 17–32. [CrossRef]
59. Griffin, P.; Dimitry, J.M.; Sheehan, P.W.; Lananna, B.V.; Guo, C.; Robinette, M.L.; Hayes, M.E.; Cedeño, M.R.; Nadarajah, C.; Ezerskiy, L.A.; et al. Circadian clock protein Rev-erbα regulates neuroinflammation. *Proc. Natl. Acad. Sci. USA* **2019**, *116*, 5102–5107. [CrossRef]
60. Makhoba, X.H.; Viegas, C., Jr.; Mosa, R.A.; Viegas, F.P.D.; Pooe, O.J. Potential Impact of the Multi-Target Drug Approach in the Treatment of Some Complex Diseases. *Drug Des. Devel. Ther.* **2020**, *14*, 3235–3249. [CrossRef]
61. Telenti, A.; di Iulio, J. Regulatory genome variants in human susceptibility to infection. *Hum Genet.* **2020**, *139*, 759–768. [CrossRef]
62. Drew, A.E.; Moradei, O.; Jacques, S.L.; Rioux, N.; Boriack-Sjodin, A.P.; Allain, C.; Scott, M.P.; Jin, L.; Raimondi, A.; Handler, J.L.; et al. Identification of a CARM1 Inhibitor with Potent In Vitro and In Vivo Activity in Preclinical Models of Multiple Myeloma. *Sci. Rep.* **2017**, *7*, 17993. [CrossRef]

63. Zhang, Y.; de Boer, M.; van der Wel, E.J.; Van Eck, M.; Hoekstra, M. PRMT4 inhibitor TP-064 inhibits the pro-inflammatory macrophage lipopolysaccharide response in vitro and ex vivo and induces peritonitis-associated neutrophilia in vivo. *Biochim. Biophys. Acta (BBA) Mol. Basis Dis.* **2021**, *1867*, 166212. [CrossRef]
64. Hwang, J.W.; Cho, Y.; Bae, G.-U.; Kim, S.-N.; Kim, Y.K. Protein arginine methyltransferases: Promising targets for cancer therapy. *Exp. Mol. Med.* **2021**, *53*, 788–808. [CrossRef]
65. Rose, P.; Won, Y.K.; Ong, C.N.; Whiteman, M. β-Phenylethyl and 8-methylsulphinyloctyl isothiocyanates, constituents of watercress, suppress LPS induced production of nitric oxide and prostaglandin E2 in RAW 264.7 macrophages. *Nitric Oxide* **2005**, *12*, 237–243. [CrossRef]
66. Dey, M.; Ribnicky, D.; Kurmukov, A.G.; Raskin, I. In Vitro and in Vivo Anti-Inflammatory Activity of a Seed Preparation Containing Phenethylisothiocyanate. *J. Pharmacol. Exp. Ther.* **2006**, *317*, 326–333. [CrossRef]
67. Gupta, P.; Adkins, C.; Lockman, P.; Srivastava, S.K. Metastasis of Breast Tumor Cells to Brain Is Suppressed by Phenethyl Isothiocyanate in a Novel In Vivo Metastasis Model. *PLoS ONE* **2013**, *8*, e67278. [CrossRef]
68. Vitali, F.; Berghout, J.; Fan, J.; Li, J.; Li, Q.; Li, H.; Lussier, Y.A. Precision drug repurposing via convergent eQTL-based molecules and pathway targeting independent disease-associated polymorphisms. *Pac. Symp. Biocomput.* **2019**, *24*, 308–319.
69. Cho, H.; Zhao, X.; Hatori, M.; Yu, R.T.; Barish, G.D.; Lam, M.T.; Chong, L.W.; Di Tacchio, L.; Atkins, A.R.; Glass, C.K.; et al. Regulation of circadian behaviour and metabolism by REV-ERB-α and REV-ERB-β. *Nature* **2012**, *485*, 123–127. [CrossRef]
70. Finan, C.; Gaulton, A.; Kruger, F.A.; Lumbers, R.T.; Shah, T.; Engmann, J.; Galver, L.; Kelley, R.; Karlsson, A.; Santos, R.; et al. The druggable genome and support for target identification and validation in drug development. *Sci. Transl. Med.* **2017**, *9*, eaag1166. [CrossRef]
71. Lau, A.; So, H.-C. Turning genome-wide association study findings into opportunities for drug repositioning. *Comput. Struct. Biotechnol. J.* **2020**, *18*, 1639–1650. [CrossRef]
72. Webb, L.M.; Guerau-De-Arellano, M. Emerging Role for Methylation in Multiple Sclerosis: Beyond DNA. *Trends Mol. Med.* **2017**, *23*, 546–562. [CrossRef] [PubMed]
73. Blanc, R.S.; Richard, S. Arginine Methylation: The Coming of Age. *Mol. Cell* **2017**, *65*, 8–24. [CrossRef] [PubMed]
74. Chandran, U.; Mehendale, N.; Patil, S.; Chaguturu, R.; Patwardhan, B. Network pharmacology. In *Innovative Approaches in Drug Discovery*; Elsevier: Amsterdam, The Netherlands, 2017; pp. 1127–1164. [CrossRef]

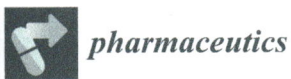

Article

Drug Repurposing Using Modularity Clustering in Drug-Drug Similarity Networks Based on Drug–Gene Interactions

Vlad Groza [1], Mihai Udrescu [1,*], Alexandru Bozdog [1] and Lucreția Udrescu [2]

1 Department of Computer and Information Technology, University Politehnica of Timișoara, 300223 Timișoara, Romania; vlad.groza@student.upt.ro (V.G.); alexandru.bozdog@cs.upt.ro (A.B.)
2 Department I—Drug Analysis, "Victor Babeș" University of Medicine and Pharmacy Timișoara, 300041 Timișoara, Romania; udrescu.lucretia@umft.ro
* Correspondence: mihai.udrescu@cs.upt.ro

Abstract: Drug repurposing is a valuable alternative to traditional drug design based on the assumption that medicines have multiple functions. Computer-based techniques use ever-growing drug databases to uncover new drug repurposing hints, which require further validation with in vitro and in vivo experiments. Indeed, such a scientific undertaking can be particularly effective in the case of rare diseases (resources for developing new drugs are scarce) and new diseases such as COVID-19 (designing new drugs require too much time). This paper introduces a new, completely automated computational drug repurposing pipeline based on drug–gene interaction data. We obtained drug–gene interaction data from an earlier version of DrugBank, built a drug–gene interaction network, and projected it as a drug–drug similarity network (DDSN). We then clustered DDSN by optimizing modularity resolution, used the ATC codes distribution within each cluster to identify potential drug repurposing candidates, and verified repurposing hints with the latest DrugBank ATC codes. Finally, using the best modularity resolution found with our method, we applied our pipeline to the latest DrugBank drug–gene interaction data to generate a comprehensive drug repurposing hint list.

Keywords: bioinformatics; drug repurposing; complex network analysis; modularity clustering; ATC code

1. Introduction

The growth in the number of newly approved pharmaceutical substances has stagnated despite the ever-growing resources that the industry allocates [1–4]. Designing, developing, and testing new medicines is an expensive, long, and cumbersome process [5], which becomes explicitly bothersome for new rare diseases—because funds are limited—and new pathogen epidemics—stopping the disease spread requires a rapid therapeutic solution [6,7]. One convenient alternative to the pharmaceutic industry's productivity challenges is drug repurposing, underpinned by the R&D in the pharmaceutical industry, as well as the observations and long-time experience indicating the favorable polypharmacological profile of drugs (in other words, most pharmaceutical substances tend to have multiple functions) [8–10]. The trend that calls for drug repurposing techniques is in sync with the recent expansion of Big Data and machine learning in genetics, biology, and medicine; therefore, we witnessed the development of a wide array of computer-based methodologies to uncover new drug repurposing [11–13].

A significant area in computational repurposing (or repositioning) relies on the complex network representations of various drug interaction/relationship types, e.g., drug–drug [14], drug–target [15–17], drug–side effect [18], drug–gene. The networks consist of nodes/edges—representing drugs, targets, genes, or side effects—and links/edges—representing interactions or other types of relationships [19]. The network of specific drug interactions allows for the characterization of a complex biological system under therapy; therefore, researchers can use computational techniques and network science principles to explore the interplay between microscale interactions and macroscale behavior [14]. An important area in network science is community/cluster detection and analysis [20,21]. The assumption is that nodes from a distinct cluster have similar topological properties and, thus, share a common feature; this results in drug repurposing opportunities [6]. (If most drugs in a cluster have a particular therapeutic function, then it is reasonable to assume that the function also exists at least in some of the other drugs in the cluster). Many network-based computational drug repurposing methods use topological network features, such as centralities (topological indicators/measures of a node's importance in the network) and modularity, to identify potential repositioning [22,23].

All computational drug repositioning methods produce lists of hints or predictions that require testing or confirmation in silico (e.g., molecular docking) [24], in vitro, and in vivo [25]. One can also indirectly prove the effectiveness of the computational technique by applying it on an earlier database version and testing the predictions on the latest data [14,22]. The existing computational pipelines predicted several important drug repurposings. Moreover, the crisis generated by the COVID-19 pandemic called for drug repurposing solutions to counter SARS-CoV-2 infections.

In our prior study, we also approached the problem of drug repositioning by building a drug–drug interaction network [14] and a drug–drug similarity network based on drug–target interactions [22]; we used the corresponding drug–drug and drug–target interaction data from DrugBank 4.1 and 4.2, respectively. In [14], we used community detection with energy-based layouts and fixed modularity; in [22], we also used energy-based layouts and fixed modularity, as well as ranking nodes by network centralities; in both previous approaches, we labeled the clusters and confirmed predictions with expert analysis.

In this paper, we also use a method based on network community detection and analysis. To this end, we build a drug–drug similarity network, because similarity networks are better suited for community detection: Nodes in the same community are more likely to be similar. Indeed, many other computational drug repurposing methods operate on similarity networks [26,27], with similarity defined on various criteria—from drug–target interactions [22] to adverse effects [18]. We find inspiration in the diseasome project [28,29] based on processing a disease–gene bipartite network (i.e., with two types of nodes, namely, genes and diseases); the processing of the disease–gene network projects it as either a gene–gene similarity or a disease–disease similarity network. In the gene–gene network, a link between two genes exists if there is at least one common disease with which they interact; in the disease–disease network, a link between two diseases exists if at least one gene is responsible for both diseases.

Our method builds a drug–gene interaction network with drug–gene interaction data from the earlier DrugBank 5.0.9 version, then projects it as a drug–drug similarity network; this is the first drug repurposing method derived from a gene-based drug–drug similarity network to the best of our knowledge. Our drug–drug similarity network is weighted—the weight of the link between two nodes/drugs represents the number of genes with which the two drugs interact in the same manner. We then use modularity-based network clustering to identify drug communities/clusters. We adopt the same assumption as in the case of the diseasome analysis in [30] that nodes inside the same community most probably share a common function or property. In this manner, if a drug inside one community does not have the ATC code level 1 of the majority, then we hypothesize that the drug can be repurposed accordingly. Nonetheless, we improve the efficiency of the approach by providing an automated procedure for tuning modularity resolution [31] by comparing the ATC code level 1 predicted with our method applied to DrugBank 5.0.9 [32] with the level 1 ATC codes of the drug in the latest DrugBank version 5.1.8 [33]. Finally, we apply our pipeline—with the optimized modularity resolution—to the latest DrugBank data to generate a new list of repurposing hints, which we support by existing literature findings. Refer to the overview of our proposed methodology in Figure 1. We only considered drugs listed as *approved* in DrugBank.

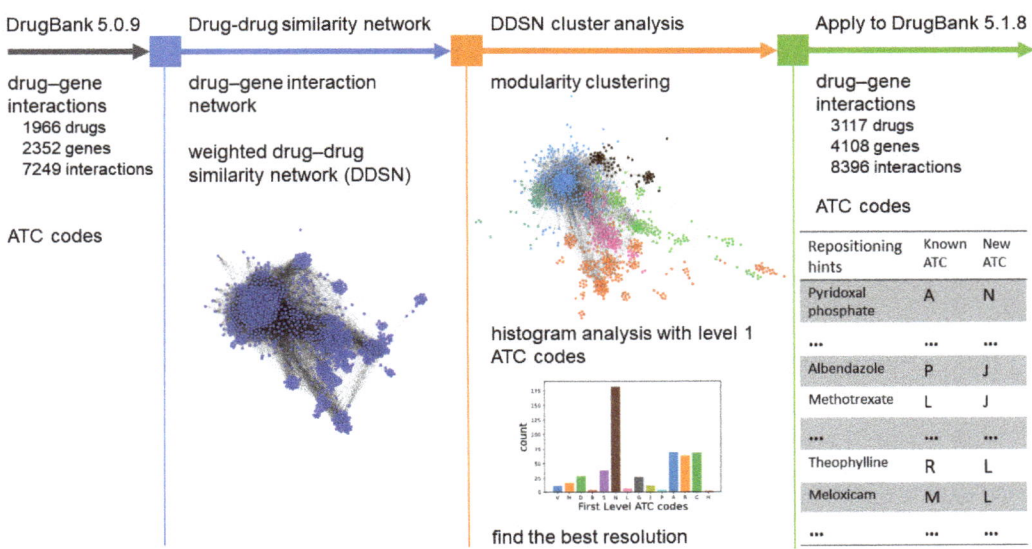

Figure 1. The overview of our proposed computational drug repurposing pipeline. In the first step, we use drug–gene interaction information from DrugBank 5.0.9 to build the (bipartite) drug–gene interaction network, which we then projected as a drug–drug similarity network (DDSN). In the second step, we used modularity class network clustering to identify drug communities with shared properties, analyzed the DrugBank 5.0.9 first-level ATC code histograms in each community to predict new drug properties, and checked these predictions against the latest DrugBank 5.1.8 level 1 ATC codes. The procedure in the second step allows maximizing the number of confirmed repositionings by adjusting modularity resolution. The third step uses our method with the optimized resolution value determined in the second step to generate a repurposing hints list according to DrugBank 5.1.8.

Three arguments support the novelty of the research presented in this paper. First, this manuscript is—to the best of our knowledge—the first to build and process a DDSN based on drug–gene interaction data. Second, we present a novel method (based on level 1 ATC codes) that labels clusters and generates repositioning hints automatically. Third, we tuned modularity resolution algorithmically and automatically confirmed repositioning hints by comparing two chronologically distinct DrugBank versions.

From a pharmacological perspective, our overarching contribution is to develop, for the first time, and promote the drug–gene interaction networks as a valuable analytical, screening, and visualization tool in drug repositioning. Our method can complement existing computational repositioning pipelines; therefore, it can be integrated into more sophisticated ensemble methods.

2. Materials and Methods

In this section, we present the conceptual description of our algorithmic drug repositioning method from Figure 1. The thorough technical implementation and description are provided on our GitHub page https://github.com/GrozaVlad/Drug-repurposing-using-DDSNs-and-modularity-clustering (last commit on 21 October 2021). We used *Nodejs* with packets *xml-js* (for parsing the DrugBank xml files) and *pg* (for interacting with the *PostgreSQL* database), and *Docker* and *Docker-compose* for containerized databases [34]. For building and clustering DDSN, we used the *Python* packages *Psycopg2*, *Pandas* [35], *NetworkX* [36], and *Cdlib* [37]; for visualizing the networks, we used *Gephi* [38]. The hardware platform for running this project was a MacBook Pro, Intel Core i9—2400 MHz with 16 GB RAM, GPU Radeon Pro 560× 4 GB.

2.1. Databases

In order to facilitate an automated procedure of validating our drug repurposing pipeline, we used the earlier DrugBank version 5.0.9 to generate repurposing predictions in one of the anatomical or pharmacological groups described by the first-level ATC codes, then we validated the predictions with the ATC codes with the latest DrugBank version 5.1.8 (last accessed on 30 September 2021).

In DrugBank version 5.0.9, there are 1966 drugs, 2352 genes, and 7249 drug–gene interactions; the interaction types are part of the set I_e = {inhibitor, agonist, antagonist, other/unknown, ligand, partial agonist, inducer, other, suppressor, binder, antibody, modulator, allosteric modulator, potentiator, neutralizer, stimulator, activator, component of, substrate, inactivator, blocker, antisense oligonucleotide}. In the latest DrugBank version 5.1.8, there are 3117 drugs, 4108 genes, and 8396 drug–gene interactions with interaction types part of the set I_l = {inhibitor, agonist, antagonist, other/unknown, antibody, substrate, ligand, partial agonist, inducer, other, suppressor, binder, potentiator, modulator, activator, cofactor, degradation, positive allosteric modulator, incorporation into and destabilization, allosteric modulator, neutralizer, stimulator, binding, inactivator, inverse agonist, blocker, chaperone, inhibition of synthesis, antisense oligonucleotide, gene replacement, regulator}. Refer to Section 4.1 for explanations.

We chose DrugBank [33] because it is a comprehensive, versioned, and scientifically curated (i.e., robust) database with consistent support for in silico drug design and repositioning space exploration [32].

2.2. Building the Drug–Drug Similarity Network

The bipartite drug–gene interaction network is a graph $\mathcal{G} = (V, E)$, where V is the set of vertices or nodes, and E is the set of edges. The network $\mathcal{G}$ is bipartite because $V = V_D \cup V_G$, where V_D is the set of drugs and V_G is the set of genes. The edges $e_{ij} \in E$ represent interactions between a drug $D_i \in V_D$ and a gene $G_j \in V_G$ (the interaction is of the type $T_k \in I$, with I defined in Section 2.1). An example of such a drug–gene bipartite graph is presented in Figure 2a, with 4 drugs, 3 genes, and 3 types of drug–gene interactions.

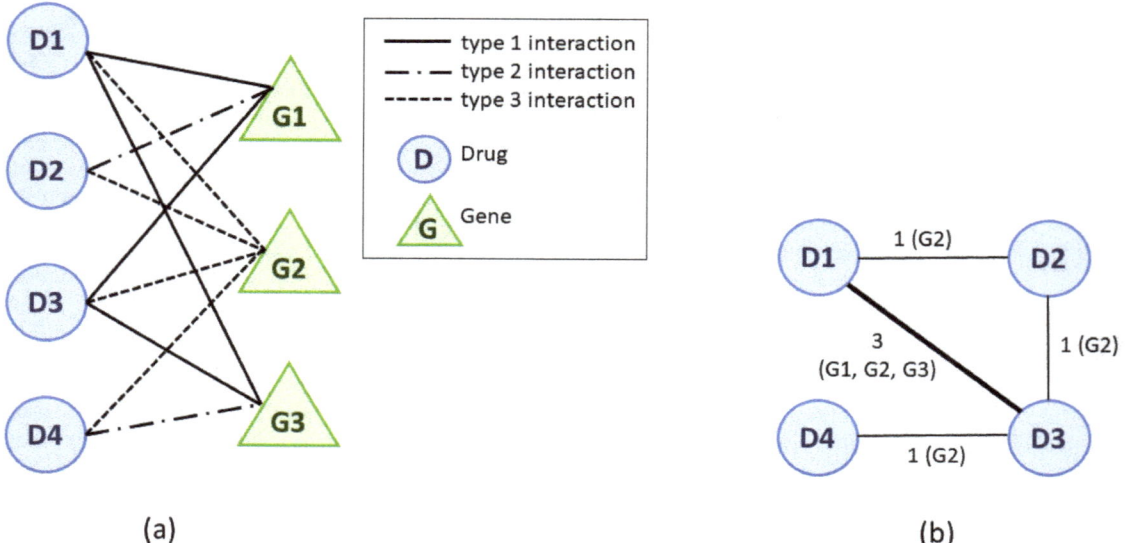

Figure 2. An illustrative example of projecting the bipartite drug–gene interaction graph $\mathcal{G}$ (a) into a weighted drug–drug similarity network $\mathcal{W}$ (b). In our example, $\mathcal{G}$ has 4 drugs (D_1, D_2, D_3, and D_4), 3 genes (G_1, G_2, and G_3), and 3 types of drug–gene interactions. In the drug–drug similarity network from panel (b), nodes are drugs, and links between two drugs represent the number of genes with which the drugs interact in the same manner. For instance, as shown, the link $w_{1,3}$ between nodes/drugs D_1 and D_3 has a weight of 3 because D_1 and D_3 have the same type of interaction with genes G_1, G_2, and G_3.

From the drug–gene bipartite network $\mathcal{G}$, we generated the weighted drug–drug similarity network $\mathcal{W} = (V_D, W)$ using network projection [39]. In the DDSN, the nodes represent drugs, and a link between two nodes exists if there is at least one gene with which the two drugs interact in the same manner (i.e., the interactions are of the same type $T_k \in I$). In Figure 2b, we present the DDSN projection of the drug–gene example network in Figure 2. The network is weighted because two drugs D_i and D_j can have the same type of interactions with m genes; therefore, the weight of edge $w_{ij} \in W$ is m.

2.3. Network Clustering Analysis

The clustering of network $\mathcal{G} = (V, E)$ is the process of classifying all nodes $v_i \in V$ in one of the n (disjoint) subsets C_j, with $V = \bigcup_{j=1}^{n} C_j$, according to their topological properties. In this paper, we use modularity-based clustering because of its proven effectiveness in drug network analysis [14,22,23]. As defined in [40], the modularity of a clustering $\mathcal{C}$ in a weighted network such as our DDSN—represented as $\mathcal{W}$—is defined as follows.

$$M = \frac{1}{2a} \sum_{ij} \left(w_{ij} - \frac{k_i k_j}{2a} \right) p(C_i, C_j). \tag{1}$$

In Equation (1), $a = \frac{1}{2} \sum_{ij} w_{ij}$; i and j are the indexes of nodes $v_i, v_j \in V_D$; k_i and k_j are the node degrees (i.e., the sums of weights of incident edges) for nodes $v_i, v_j \in V_D$; w_{ij} is the adjacency matrix of nodes in $\mathcal{W}$; C_i and C_j are the communities that include nodes $v_i, v_j \in V_D$, respectively; and p is a function $p(x, y)$ that returns 1 if $x = y$ and 0 otherwise. (In our DDSN, nodes v_i and v_j are drugs D_i and D_j, respectively).

The modularity of clustering $\mathcal{C}$ is a value $M_\mathcal{C} \in [-1, 1]$, representing the edge density within the clusters with respect to the edge density between clusters. The clustering algorithms are based on modularity search for the best partitioning $\mathcal{C}$ of the node-set such that the value of M is maximized. The problem is that an exhaustive search for the best modularity entails large computational burden. Consequently, in practice, heuristic algorithms approximate optimal modularity clustering. However, if the network is very large, such approximations cannot identify small-size clusters—even if the density of internal edges is high and the density of edges between these small clusters and the rest of the network is low.

In this paper, we use the modularity-based clustering algorithm from [41], which controls the resolution of the clustering using a recursive procedure that starts with each node being a cluster and then moving nodes v_i (i.e., D_i in our DDSN) to a different cluster C_j if this generates a positive modularity gain expressed as follows.

$$\Delta M = \left[\frac{K_{C_j}^* + K_i^{C_j}}{2a} - \left(\frac{K_{C_j} + K_i}{2a} \right)^2 \right] - \left[\frac{K_{C_j}^*}{2a} - \left(\frac{K_{C_j}}{2a} \right)^2 - \left(\frac{K_i}{2a} \right)^2 \right]. \tag{2}$$

In Equation (2), $K_{C_j}^*$ is the sum of the weights of all edges within cluster C_j; K_{C_j} is the sum of the weights of all edges incident to nodes in cluster C_j; K_i is the sum of the weights of all edges incident to node v_i (D_i in DDSN); and $K_i^{C_j}$ is the sum of the weights of links from v_i to all nodes in cluster C_j. The algorithm controls the clustering resolution using the value of $\lambda = \Delta M$—a lower λ determines a higher number of clusters.

2.4. Tuning Resolution λ

Using Algorithm 1, we tune the modularity resolution to achieve efficiency in predicting new drug properties. To this end, we try λ values in the $[0.1, 5]$ interval, with a step of 0.1, generate the modularity clustering $\mathcal{C}$ for each resolution value (Clustering($\mathcal{G}, \lambda$)), and determine the dominant property $\mathcal{P}_i$ in each cluster $C_i \in \mathcal{C}$. The dominant property $\mathcal{P}_i$ corresponds to the level 1 ATC code of the majority of drugs in cluster i, $D_j \in C_j$, as resulting from the level 1 ATC code histogram of C_i, and denoted $\mathcal{A}^1(C_i)$. Then, for each drug D_j in each cluster C_i, we checked the list of first level ATC codes for drug D_j (denoted $\mathcal{A}^1(D_j)$) against the drug's cluster dominant property $\mathcal{P}_i$. If $\mathcal{P}_i$ is not in the list of DrugBank 5.0.9 level 1 ATC codes for D_j (i.e., $\mathcal{A}^1(D_j)$), but it is present in the list of DrugBank 5.1.8 level 1 ATC codes (i.e., $\mathcal{A}_c^1(D_j)$), then we consider this as a confirmed repositioning of D_j to property $\mathcal{P}_i$. As such, we will add drug D_j to the list of repositionings confirmed with DrugBank 5.1.8 level 1 ATC codes, $\mathcal{R}^c$. Value λ_{max} corresponds to $\mathcal{R}^c$ with the biggest number of elements, namely $\max\{|\mathcal{R}^c|\}$.

Algorithm 1 Find the parameter λ, such that the clustering $\mathcal{C}$ of nodes/drugs D_i in $\mathcal{G}$ with modularity resolution λ (i.e., Clustering$(\mathcal{G}, \lambda)$) produces the biggest number of repositionings confirmed with the level 1 ATC codes in DrugBank 5.1.8.

Input: Drug-drug similarity network $\mathcal{G} = (V_D, E)$ based on drug-gene interaction data from DrugBank 5.0.9., ATC codes for drugs in DrugBank versions 5.0.9 and 5.1.8

Output: The λ value that generates the highest number of confirmed repositionings.

1: **for** λ in range (0.1 to 5), with 0.1 steps **do**
2:   $\mathcal{C} \Leftarrow$ Clustering$(\mathcal{G}, \lambda)$
3:   **for all** $C_i \in \mathcal{C}$ **do**
4:     $\mathcal{P}_i \Leftarrow \mathcal{A}^1(C_i)$
5:     $\mathcal{R}_i^c \Leftarrow \emptyset$
6:     **for all** $D_j \in C_i$ **do**
7:       **if then** $\mathcal{P}_i \notin \mathcal{A}^1(D_j)$ & $\mathcal{P}_i \in \mathcal{A}_c^1(D_j)$
8:         $\mathcal{R}_i^c \Leftarrow \mathcal{R}_i^c \cup \{D_j\}$
9:       **end if**
10:    **end for**
11:   **end for**
12:   $\mathcal{R}^c = \Leftarrow \bigcup_i \mathcal{R}_i^c$
13: **end for**
14: **Return** the value of λ_{max} corresponding to $\max\{|{\prime}R^c|\}$

2.5. Generating New Repurposing Hints

We generated a list of new repositioning hints using the modularity clustering with the resolution value determined by Algorithm 1 in Section 2.4. Algorithm 2 presents the method we follow: Cluster the DDSN built with drug–gene interaction information from DrugBank 5.1.8 using the tuned resolution λ_{max} ($\mathcal{C} =$ Clustering$(\mathcal{G}, \lambda_{max})$); determine the dominant property $\mathcal{P}_i$ of each cluster $C_i \in \mathcal{C}$ as resulted from C_i's level 1 ATC code histogram (denoted $\mathcal{A}^1(C_i)$); and check for each drug D_j in each cluster C_i the list of first level ATC codes of D_j (denoted $\mathcal{A}^1(D_j)$) against its cluster's dominant property $\mathcal{P}_i$. If the cluster's dominant property $\mathcal{P}_i$ is not in $\mathcal{A}^1(D_j)$ (the list of D_j level 1 ATC codes), we hint that D_j can be repositioned to $\mathcal{P}_i$. Consequently, we add these repositioning cases as drug–predicted property pairs $(D_j, \mathcal{P}_i)$ to the repositioning hints list $\mathcal{N}$.

Algorithm 2 Generate the list of drug repurposing hints by clustering the DDSN $\mathcal{G}$ with the tuned modularity resolution.

Input: Drug–drug similarity network $\mathcal{G} = (V_D, E)$ based on drug–gene interaction data from DrugBank 5.1.8, λ_{max}, and the ATC codes for drugs in DrugBank 5.1.8.
Output: The repositioning hints $\mathcal{N}$ as a list of drug–predicted property pairs, $(D_j, \mathcal{A}^1(C_i))$.

1: $\mathcal{C} \Leftarrow \text{Clustering}(\mathcal{G}, \lambda_{max})$
2: $\mathcal{N} \Leftarrow \emptyset$
3: **for all** $C_i \in \mathcal{C}$ **do**
4:     $\mathcal{P}_i \Leftarrow \mathcal{A}^1(C_i)$
5:     **for all** $D_j \in C_i$ **do**
6:         **if** $\mathcal{P}_i \notin \mathcal{A}^1(D_j)$ **then**
7:             $\mathcal{N} \Leftarrow \mathcal{N} \cup \{(D_j, \mathcal{P}_i)\}$
8:         **end if**
9:     **end for**
10: **end for**
11: **Return** the list of drug repositionings $\mathcal{N}$ as drug–predicted property pairs

3. Results

3.1. DDSN Using Drug–Gene Interactions from DrugBang 5.0.9

Following the algorithmic approach presented in Figure 1, according to the methods described in Sections 2.2–2.5, we employ cluster-based network analysis on the drug–drug similarity network (DDSN) built with drug–gene interaction information from DrugBank 5.0.9 to search for the most effective modularity resolution λ_{max}—in other words, the modularity resolution that produces the highest number of drug repositionings confirmed with level 1 ATC codes from DrugBank 5.1.8. Figure 3 presents the result of running Algorithm 1 from Section 2.4; the best results correspond to resolutions 1.9 and 2.0 (the same nine confirmed repositionings in both cases). Henceforth, we will consider $\lambda_{max} = 2.0$.

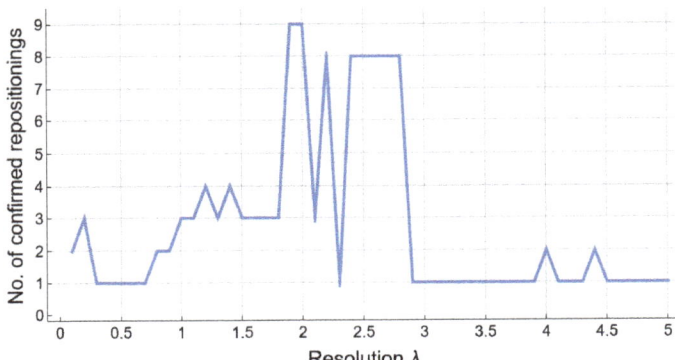

Figure 3. The number of confirmed repositionings $\mathcal{R}^c$ for resolution λ values in the $[0.1, 5]$ interval, with a step of 0.1, after running Algorithm 1 on the DDSN $\mathcal{G}$ built with drug–gene interaction information from DrugBank 5.0.9. The highest number of repositionings confirmed with level 1 ATC codes from DrugBank 5.1.8 (i.e., 9) corresponds to resolutions 1.9 and 2.0.

Figure 4 presents the largest connected component of the DDSN, constructed with drug–gene interaction data from DrugBank 5.0.9 and clustered with modularity resolution $\lambda_{max} = 2.0$; the text indicates the topological coordinates of repositionings confirmed with DrugBank 5.1.8 data.

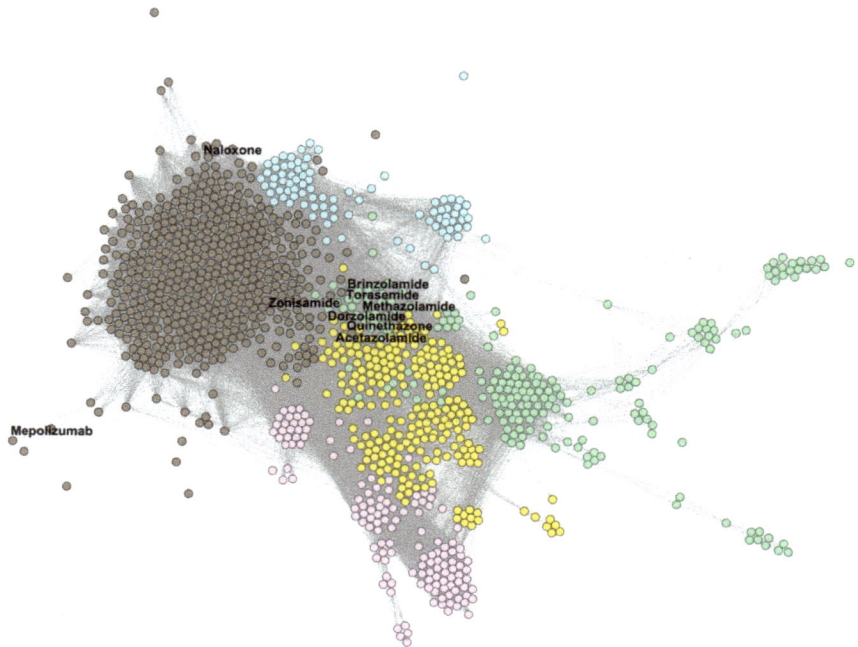

Figure 4. Drug–drug similarity network (DDSN) built with drug–gene interaction data from DrugBank 5.0.9, clustered using modularity classes for resolution $\lambda_{max} = 2.0$. We indicate the position of drugs repositioned and confirmed (with level 1 ATC codes from DrugBank 5.1.8) them by labeling the corresponding nodes with their names. The brown nodes represent drugs in cluster C_0 (512 drugs), yellow nodes represent drugs in cluster C_1 (238 drugs), green nodes represent drugs in cluster C_2 (197 drugs), pink nodes represent drugs in cluster C_3 (143 drugs), and light blue nodes represent drugs in cluster C_4 (88 drugs).

In Figure 4, nodes represent drugs, and links represent similarity relationships based on drug–gene interactions, as described in Section 2.2; node colors correspond to specific clusters, as determined by the modularity class, and all links are represented with grey lines.

In Appendix A.1, Figures A1–A3, present zoomed details of DDSN from Figure 4 in the vicinity of nine confirmed repositionings corresponding to $\lambda_{max} = 2.0$. The repositionings come from cluster C_0–brown and cluster C_2–green nodes. We indicated the drug repositionings confirmed with DrugBank 5.1.8 data with red arrows ($\rightarrow$) in Figures A1 and A2; in Figure A3, we have many confirmed repurposed drugs and a high density of nodes; hence, red diamonds ($\diamond$) were used instead of arrows.

The zoomed details provided by Figures A1 and A2 show that mepolizumab and naloxone are within cluster C_0 (brown nodes), where the dominant property is given by the level 1 ATC code N–*Nervous system*, followed by code R–*Respiratory system*. As such, our method automatically predicts that mepolizumab (listed as L–*Antineoplastic and immunomodulatory drugs* in DrugBank 5.0.9) acts as a drug with level 1 ATC code R. (In Appendix A.2, Figure A4 shows that in cluster C_0—in addition to the dominant level 1 ATC codes N—we also have many subcluster drugs with level 1 ATC codes A–*Alimentary tract and metabolism*; R–*Respiratory system*; and C–*Cardiovascular system*). Our method predicts that naloxone (an opioid overdose antidote in DrugBank 5.0.9) also acts on the nervous system (first level ATC N). The more recent DrugBank 5.1.8 confirms the predictions, listing mepolizumab with first level ATC code R and naloxone with N (see more details in Section 3.3.1).

In Appendix A.1, Figure A3, we zoom in to the region in DrugBank 5.0.9 DDSN with the confirmed repositionings in cluster C_2 (green nodes), with the dominant level

1 ATC code G–*Genitourinary system and sex hormones* (see the histogram in Appendix A.2 Figure A4). The confirmed repositionings in cluster C_2 are torasemide (ATC level 1 code C, cardiovascular system), quinetazone (C), methazolamide (S, sensory organs), acetazolamide (S), dorzolamide (S), and brinzolamide (S). Zonisamide (N, nervous system) is a brown node (cluster C_0) but in the close vicinity of cluster C_2; therefore, one can expect functional overlappings [14]. Our method automatically predicts that all these drugs have genitourinary system properties, and DrugBank 5.1.8 confirms the predictions (see the detailed description in in Section 3.3.1).

Using ATC codes as references for drug repurposing is already used in the state-of-the-art contexts, although confirmations based on ATC codes are very conservative (i.e., the World Health Organization assigns new ATCs after a long and thorough process) [25,42]. Confirming the predicted drug repositionings by performing a research literature review will reveal many more confirmations [25,43]. By this logic, our analysis of DrugBank 5.0.9 does not reveal many confirmed repurposings, yet it helps tune the modularity resolution λ.

3.2. DDSN Using Drug–Gene Interactions from DrugBang 5.1.8

According to the algorithmic approach presented in Figure 1, we generated the DDSN based on the drug–gene interactions reported in DrugBank 5.1.8 and clustered DDSN using the modularity classes obtained for resolution λ_{max} (by employing Algorithm 1 with the results presented in Section 3.1). We display the largest connected component of the DrugBank 5.1.8 DDSN in Figure 5, with cluster C_0 (brown nodes) having the dominant level 1 ATC code N–*Nervous system*; clusters C_1 and C_2 (green and orange nodes) J–*Anti-infectives for systemic use*; cluster C_3 (light blue nodes) L–*Antineoplastic and immunomodulating agents*; and cluster C_4 (pink nodes) A–*Alimentary tract and metabolism*.

By running Algorithm 2 on the DDSN built with DrugBank 5.1.8 data and clustered with modularity classes at resolution λ_{max}, we generated lists of drug repurposing hints for each drug cluster. In the Supplementary Materials Table S1 file *DDSN-results.xls*, tab *DB 5.1.8 resolution 2.0*, we present the first 10 drug clusters and the entire list of drug repurposing candidates generated with Algorithm 2 (759 candidates).

Generating a list of 759 drug repurposing candidates with the latest DrugBank data and experimental confirmation is beyond the focus of our paper, and we select the first 10 drugs in each cluster in terms of betweenness/degree centrality (the methodology used in [22]) and checked them with the state-of-the-art scientific literature. For checking repositioning hints, we searched for articles in PubMed. The terms we used to search the literature were the name of the drug and the words/pharmacological terms that form level 1 of the ATC code. For example, our methodology predicted for methotrexate ATC code with level 1 J–*Anti infectives for systemic use*; we searched for the confirmation of this prediction by using keywords *methotrexate anti-infective*, as well as keywords representing therapeutic groups included in class J (i.e., *methotrexate antiviral*, *methotrexate antibacterial*, or *methotrexate antimycotic*). The confirmation results of our extensive literature check are presented in Table 1, showing the drug name, cluster number, current level 1 ATC code, predicted level 1 ATC code, and confirmation references. We also added a detailed discussion of the repurposing hints from Table 1 in Section 3.2.

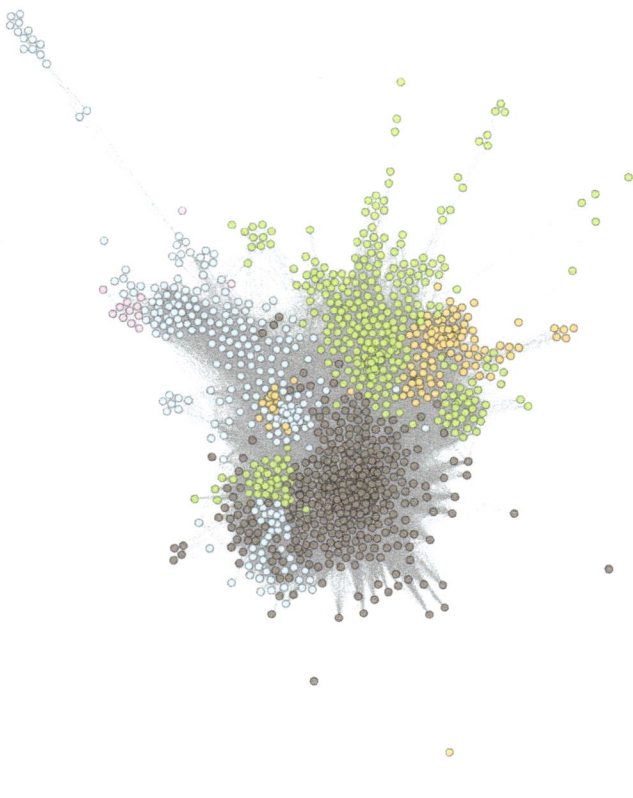

Figure 5. Drug–drug similarity network (DDSN) built with drug–gene interaction data from Drug-Bank 5.1.8, clustered using modularity classes for resolution $\lambda_{max} = 2.0$. The brown nodes represent drugs in cluster C_0 (479 drugs), green nodes represent drugs in cluster C_1 (346 drugs), light blue nodes represent drugs in cluster C_2 (270 drugs), orange nodes represent drugs in cluster C_3 (129 drugs), and pink nodes represent drugs in cluster C_4 (12 nodes).

We present the topological DDSN placement of Pyridoxal phosphate—predicted repositioning from cluster C_0—in Figure 6, where a red diamond ($\diamond$) marks the exact position.

In Figure 7, we illustrate the position of albendazole and methotrexate in the DDSN built with DrugBank 5.0.8 data as predicted drug repositionings from cluster C_1. Other drug repurposing candidates from cluster C_1 (presented in Table 1) are shown in Appendix B.1 and Figure A5: simvastatin, fluvastatin, lovastatin, and atorvastatin.

Figure 8 displays the DrugBank 5.0.8 DDSN placement of cholecalciferol, ergocalciferol, and calcifediol—drug repurposing candidates from cluster C_2. In Appendix B.1, Figures A6–A8, we identify the topological positions of the other drug repurposing canditates in cluster C_2 (Table 1): meloxicam, theophylline, and chloroquine.

Table 1. The list of drug repurposing candidates generated with our methodology in Figure 1 on data from DrugBank 5.1.8, and confirmed with scientific literature. The rows correspond to drugs or drug classes (for example, simvastatin, fluvastatin, lovastatin, and atorvastatin are statins). The columns indicate—from left to right—the name, the cluster, the current level 1 ATC code in DrugBank 5.1.8, the predicted level 1 ATC code, and the confirmation references for the drug (or drug class) in each row.

Drug	Cluster	Current Level 1 ATC	Predicted Level 1 ATC	References
Pyridoxal phosphate	C_0	A	H	[44,45]
Albendazole	C_1	P	J	[46,47]
Methotrexate	C_1	L	J	[48–50]
Simvastatin Fluvastatin Lovastatin Atorvastatin	C_1	C	J	[51,52]
Theophylline	C_2	R	L	[14,53]
Meloxicam	C_2	M	L	[54–56]
Cholecalciferol Ergocalciferol Calcifediol	C_2	M, A	L	[57,58]
Chloroquine	C_2	P	L	[59–63]
Mecasermin Mecasermin rinfabate	C_4	H	A	[64–66]
Ornithine	C_{25}	A	N	[67]

We also show the placement of drug repurposing candidates mecasermin and mecasermin rinfabate (in Figure 9, in cluster C_4, with red diamonds ◊) and ornithine (in Figure 10, in cluster C_{25}, with a red arrow →).

The histograms showing the dominant properties (as level 1 ATC codes) in clusters C_0, C_1, C_2, and C_4 are presented in Appendix B.2, Figure A9.

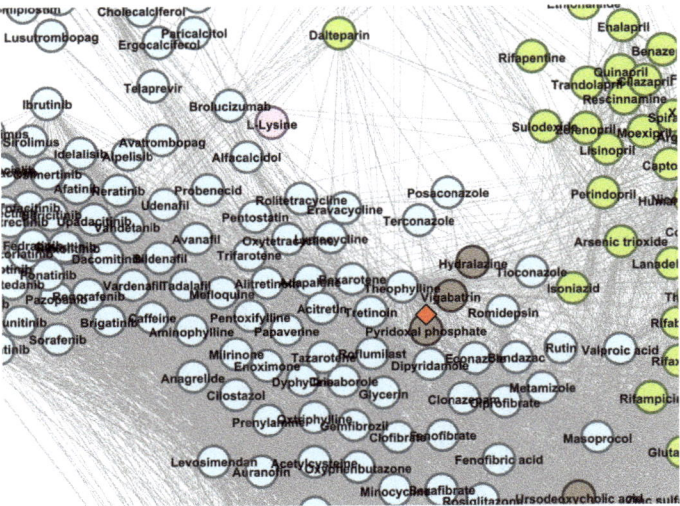

Figure 6. The DrugBank 5.1.8 DDSN network's zoomed detail shows the repositioning within cluster C_0 (brown nodes) with a red diamond (◊). Our repositioning pipeline predicts that pyridoxal phosphate (currently at ATC level 1 code A–*Alimentary tract and metabolism*) has properties described by the level 1 ATC code N—*Nervous system*.

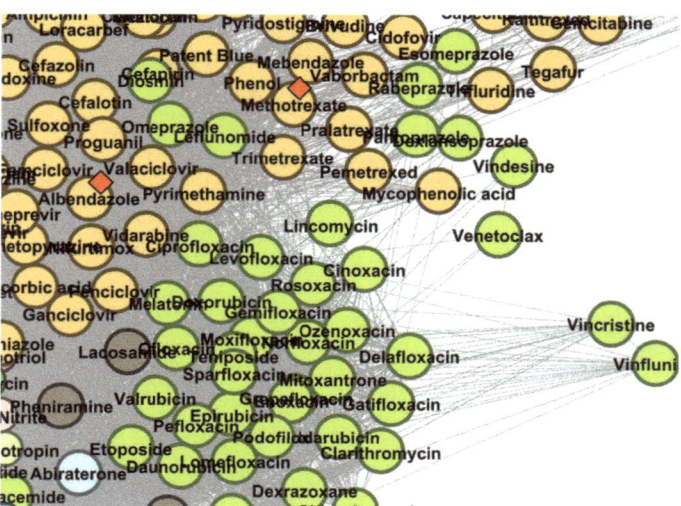

Figure 7. The DrugBank 5.1.8 DDSN network's zoomed detail shows two repositionings within cluster C_1 (green nodes) with a red diamond (◊). Our repositioning pipeline predicts that albendazole and methotrexate (currently at ATC level 1 codes P–*Antiparasitic products, insecticides, and repellents* and L–*Antineoplastic and immunomodulating agents*, respectively) have properties described by the level 1 ATC code J–*Anti infectives for systemic use*.

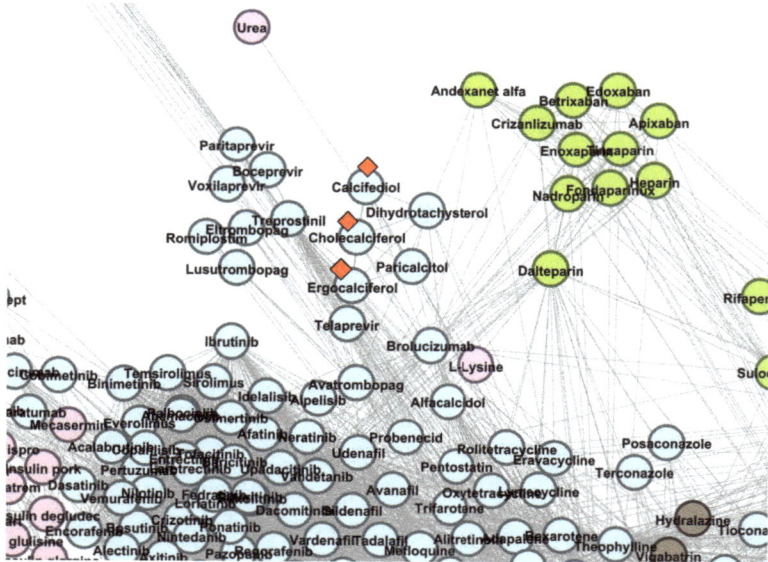

Figure 8. The DrugBank 5.1.8 DDSN network's zoomed detail shows three repositionings (vitamin D derivatives) within cluster C_2 (light blue nodes) with a red diamond (◊). Our repositioning pipeline predicts that cholecalciferol, ergocalciferol, and calcifediol (currently at ATC level 1 codes A–*Alimentary tract and metabolism* and M–*Musculo-skeletal system*) have properties described by the level 1 ATC code L–*Antineoplastic and immunomodulating agents*.

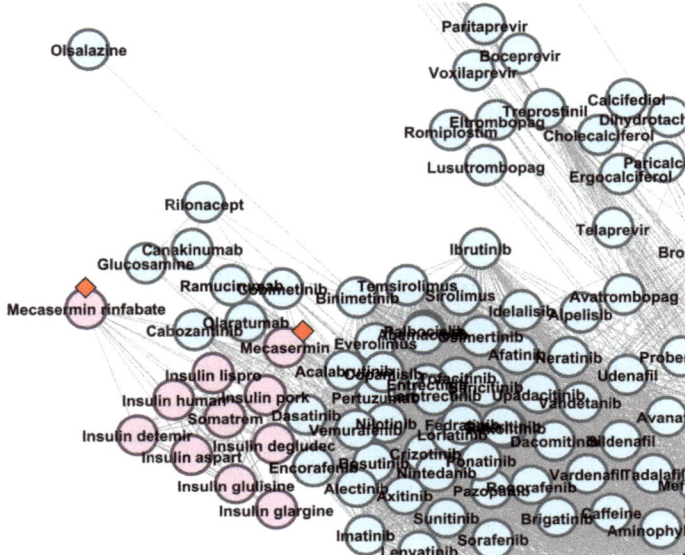

Figure 9. The DrugBank 5.1.8 DDSN network's zoomed detail shows two repositionings within cluster C_4 (pink nodes) with a red diamond (◇). Our repositioning pipeline predicts that mecasermin and mecasermin rinfabate (currently at ATC level 1 codes H–*Systemic hormonal preparations, excluding sex hormones and insulins*) have properties described by the level 1 ATC code A–*Alimentary tract and metabolism*.

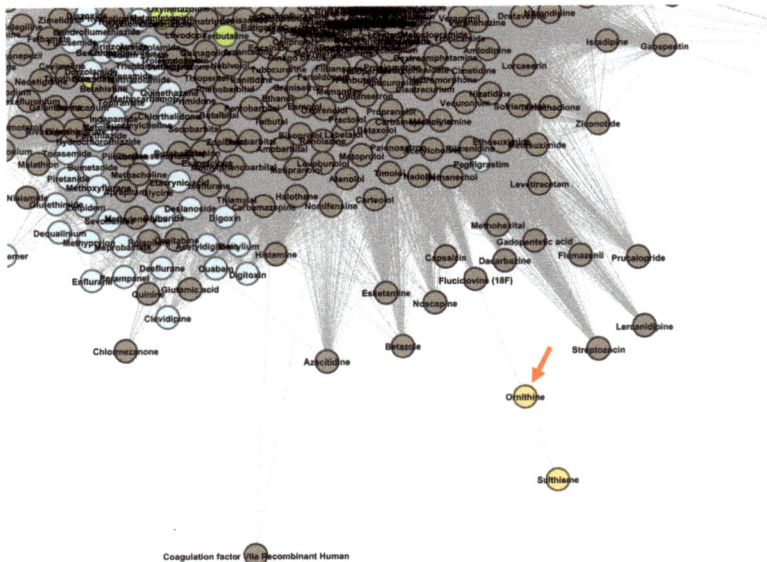

Figure 10. The DrugBank 5.1.8 DDSN network's zoomed detail shows a repositioning within cluster C_{25} (light orange) with a red arrow (→). Our method predicts that ornithine (currently at ATC level 1 code A–*Alimentary tract and metabolism*) has properties described by the level 1 ATC code N–*Nervous system*.

3.3. Repositioning Confirmations

3.3.1. Confirmed Drug Repositionings in DrugBank 5.0.9

This section discusses the drug repositioning hits generated with our methodology in DrugBank 5.0.9 and confirmed with the level 1 ATC codes in DrugBank 5.1.8. Our procedure confirmed the predicted hints in modularity classes 0 and 2.

Modularity Cluster C_0

In modularity cluster C_0, DrugBank 5.1.8 confirms mepolizumab and naloxone (see Figures A1 and A2). Naloxone (ATC code V03AB15) is a μ-opioid receptor antagonist indicated in the treatment of opioid overdose. In DrugBank 5.0.9, naloxone's first level ATC is V–*Various*; its level 4 (V03AB) means naloxone is in the *Antidotes* category.

Our methodology predicts naloxone's level 1 ATC as N–*Nervous system*; the latest DrugBank 5.1.8 adds two N level 1 ATC codes to naloxone (level 4 ATC category *Natural opium alkaloids* for the combinations with hydromorphone and oxycodone), thus confirming our prediction.

Mepolizumab (ATC code L04AC06) is a monoclonal antibody acting as an antagonist of interleukin-5, included in the L–*Antineoplastic and immunomodulating agents* level 1 ATC category by DrugBank 5.0.9.

DrugBank 5.1.8 does not list the L04AC06 code anymore for mepolizumab; instead, it uses the level 1 ATC code R–*Respiratory system* (the level 4 ATC is R03DX, which includes *other systemic drugs for obstructive airways diseases*, as mepolizumab is indicated in severe eosinophilic asthma).

Modularity Cluster C_2

In modularity cluster C_2, DrugBank 5.1.8 confirms torasemide, methazolamide, acetazolamide, dorzolamide, brinzolamide, zonisamide, and quinetazone (see Figure A3).

Torasemide, quinetazone, methazolamide, acetazolamide, dorzolamide, and zonisamide, brinzolamide (ATC codes: C03CA04, C03BA02/C03BB02, S01EC05, S01EC01, S01EC03, N03AX15, S01EC04/S01EC54) are sulfonamide compounds with various pharmacodynamic effects. According to DrugBank 5.0.9, torasemide and quinetazone are diuretics used as antihypertensive drugs, included in the C–*Cardiovascular system* level 1 ATC category. Zonisamide is an antiepileptic drug (level 1 ATC N–*Nervous system*). Methazolamide, acetazolamide, dorzolamide, and brinzolamide are carbonic anhydrase inhibitors used in glaucoma (level 1 ATC S–*Sensory organs*).

Our methodology predicts G–*Genito urinary system and sex hormones* as the level 1 ATC code for torasemide, quinetazone, methazolamide, acetazolamide, dorzolamide zonisamide, and brinzolamide. Indeed, the latest DrugBank 5.1.8 version includes all these drugs in the G level 1 ATC category—more precisely, in the G01AE level 4 ATC category of *Anti-infective and antiseptics* having a sulfonamide-based chemical structure.

3.3.2. Drug Repositioning Hints in DrugBank 5.1.8

This section discusses the validity of some drug repositioning hints generated with our methodology in DrugBank 5.1.8; as this is the latest database version, we cannot use the same confirmation procedure based on ATC codes. Consequently, we provide evidence found in the state-of-the-art literature as confirmation clues. However, as both the number of clusters and their size prohibit an exhaustive literature search, we focus on the clusters with confirmed drug repurposing candidates—clusters C_0, C_1, C_2, C_4, and C_{25}.

Pyridoxal phosphate (cluster C_0, ATC code A11HA06) is the active form of vitamin B6 and belongs to the A–*Alimentary tract and metabolism* level 1 ATC category, along with the rest of water-soluble and fat-soluble vitamins. Our method predicts pyridoxal phosphate as level 1 ATC code N–*Nervous system* (see Figure 6); H-S Wang et al. reported that pyridoxal phosphate controls idiopathic intractable epilepsy in children [44]. P.B. Mills and team identified two groups of patients with neonatal epileptic encephalopathy (determined by PNPO mutations) that respond to pyridoxal phosphate [45].

Albendazole (cluster C_1, ATC code P02CA03) is an antiparasitic drug (first level ATC P–*Antiparasitic products, insecticides and repellents*) efficient in various helminthic infections. Our methodology predicts J as level 1 ATC code, suggesting potential systemic anti-infective effects (see Figure 7). Of note, ATC lists drug classes such as antivirals, antibacterials, antimycotics, and vaccines in the J–*Anti-infectives for systemic use* category. In vitro results show that albendazole exerts antifungal activity against *Aspergillus* spp. [46]; moreover, experiments on mice revealed antifungal effects against *Pneumocystis carinii* [47], confirming the new potential antifungal medical use of albendazole.

Methotrexate (cluster C_1, ATC codes L04AX03, L01BA01) is an anticancer and immunosuppressant agent; therefore, the level 1 ATC is L–*Antineoplastic and immunomodulating agents*. We predict the first level J–*Anti infectives for systemic use* (see Figure 7). The literature survey reveals several papers reporting in vitro antiviral effects of methotrexate in a dose-dependent manner on SARS-CoV-2 [48] and Zika virus replication [49]; methotrexate also prevents the replication of human cytomegalovirus and inhibits viral DNA synthesis [50].

Simvastatin, fluvastatin, lovastatin, and atorvastatin (cluster C_1, ATC codes A10BH51/ C10AA01/C10BX04/C10BA02/C10BX01/C10BA04, C10AA04, C10AA02/C10BA01, and C10BX15/C10AA05/C10BX03/C10BA05/C10BX11/C10BX08/C10BX06/C10BX12) are HMG-CoA reductase inhibitors (also called statins) that lower serum lipid levels, reducing the risk of cardiovascular events caused by hyperlipidemia; they are in the level 1 ATC C–*Cardiovascular system* class. The first level of their ATC code, as predicted by our method, is J–*Anti infectives for systemic use* (see Figure A5), confirmed by literature; as such, simvastatin exhibits in vitro antimicrobial effect on methicillin-susceptible Staphylococcus aureus [51]. S.P. Parihar et al. [52] review the literature reporting preclinical and clinical evidence of statins effects in viral, parasitic, fungal, and bacterial infections, pointing out the factors that influence the response to statins, such as human polymorphism, metabolism, and drug interactions; this review includes data on all mentioned statins. Our algorithm predicts that all statins in cluster C_1 are potential anti-infective agents. As shown, for the statins we highlighted in Figure A5, we found literature confirming our prediction; for the other statins, new experiments and studies may provide confirmation.

Theophylline (cluster C_2, ATC codes R03DA54, R03DA74, R03DA20, R03DA04, and R03DB04) is a methylxanthine derivative used to treat obstructive respiratory conditions, such as asthma and COPD, hence having R–*Respiratory system* as first level ATC code. Our methodology indicates theophylline's *Anticancer and immunomodulating properties*, as reflected by the predicted ATC first level L (see Figure A7), thus further confirming the repositioning proposed by our previous research [14]. Indeed, recent literature demonstrates the anticancer properties of theophylline in breast and cervical cell lines [53].

Meloxicam (cluster C_2, ATC codes M01AC56 and M01AC06) is an oxicam derivative with anti-inflammatory and antirheumatic properties of the M–*Musculo-skeletal system* ATC category. Our network-based methodology predicts L as the first level of the ATC code (see Figure A6). The literature confirms our prediction of the anticancer properties of meloxicam: Meloxicam inhibits tumor growth in COX-2 positive colorectal cancer [54]. Tsubouchi et al. report that COX-2 plays a significant role in the pathogenesis and progression of non-small cell lung cancer (NSCLC), demonstrating the inhibitory effect of meloxicam on the NSCLC growth by preferentially inhibiting COX-2 [55]. Reference [56] shows that meloxicam is efficient in osteosarcoma in both COX-2-dependent and independent inhibitory manners.

Cholecalciferol, ergocalciferol, and calcifediol (cluster C_2, ATC codes M05BB09/ M05BX53/M05BB07/M05BB08/A11CC55/M05BB05/A11CC05/M05BB03/M05BB04, A11CC01, and A11CC06) are vitamin D analogs. Cholecalciferol (vitamin D3) is a fat-soluble vitamin (ATC level 1 A–*Alimentary tract and metabolism*, a category which includes hydro-soluble and lipo-soluble vitamins) with a well-established role in bone mineralization (ATC second level M05–*Musculo-skeletal system, drugs for treatment of bone diseases*). Ergocalciferol and calcifediol are also grouped in A–*Alimentary tract and metabolism* level 1 ATC. We predict these drugs as targeting diseases at level 1 ATC code

L–*Antineoplastic and immunomodulating agents* (see Figure 8).There is extensive literature reporting the beneficial effects of vitamin D analogs in different cancers and highlighting the epidemiological, preclinical, and clinical results; all these back up their evolution as prophylactic and curative anticancer drugs [57,58].

Chloroquine (cluster C_2, ATC code P01BA01) is an antimalarial drug; consequently, it belongs to the P–*Antiparasitic products, insecticides and repellents* level 1 ATC category. According to our results, the predicted first-level ATC is L–*Antineoplastic and immunomodulating agents* for chloroquine (dominant in cluster C_1, see Figure A8). Multiple research reviews report in vitro, in vivo, and clinical trials testing chloroquine's anticancer effect in glioblastoma [59] and other types of cancers [60–63], hence supporting the potential repositioning of chloroquine as an anticancer drug, as uncovered by our methodology.

Mecasermin and mecasermin rinfabate (cluster C_4, ATC codes H01AC03, H01AC05) are recombinant insulin-like growth factor-1 drugs indicated in growth failure in children with primary IGF-1 deficiency and, hence, are included in the H–*Systemic hormonal preparations, excluding sex hormones and insulins*. Literature and medicine regulatory authorities reports present the secondary pharmacologic actions of mecasermin and mecasermin rinfabate, including the anabolic and insulin-like effects (i.e., hypoglycemia) [64–66]; these pharmacologic effects could place the drugs in the A–*Alimentary tract and metabolism* level 1 ATC, as predicted by our methodology (see Figure 9).

Ornithine (cluster C_{25}, ATC code A05BA06) is a non-essential amino acid indicated as nutritional supplementation and for a good liver function and included in the A–*Alimentary tract and metabolism* level 1 ATC. M. Miyake et al. suggest that L-ornithine may interfere with the Central Nervous System, following a randomized, double-blind controlled trial that demonstrated that L-ornithine relieved stress and improved sleep quality in humans compared to the placebo group [67]. Indeed, we predicted ornithine at level 1 ATC N–*Nervous system* (see Figure 10).

4. Discussion

In this section, we discuss the particularities of our method, namely the data we use, the limitations of our method and its validation with ATC codes, and the way to integrate it into an ensemble drug repositioning framework.

4.1. Drug–Gene Interactions

The method we propose in this paper uses drug–gene interaction data from DrugBank versions 5.0.9 and 5.1.8. Table 2 presents examples of drug–gene interactions and their corresponding types, as defined by DrugBank 5.1.8 (see a detailed list of drug–gene interaction types in the Supplementary Materials Table S1 file *DDSN-results.xls* and how to retrieve such drug–gene interactions from DrugBank in the GitHub page https://github.com/GrozaVlad/Drug-repurposing-using-DDSNs-and-modularity-clustering (last commit on 21 October 2021)).

4.2. Method Limitations

The mechanisms that influence the polypharmacological profile of drugs are highly complex. Indeed, the medicinal compound interacts with a complex system represented by the human organism. Complex systems are context-dependent; in other words, any detail at the micro-scale influences the macroscale behavior. As such, many factors can be considered when analyzing the functions of any pharmaceutical substance: from the chemical structure to various types of relationships and interactions, as well as pharmacokinetics and pharmacodynamics. By this logic, our approach is limited to considering a narrow informational angle, namely drug–gene interactions. Nonetheless, considering many mechanisms and types of data simultaneously within the same model would be prohibitively complex, and the networks would become much too dense for any centrality of community analysis. Even considering one type of information has become significantly complex; for instance, the drug–drug interaction networks in DrugBank 3.0 had an average degree of $\sim$20, and in DrugBank 5.1.8 the average DDI network degree is ~600). Recent literature [68–70] advances the so-called ensemble methods to address this new situation of being confronted with an overabundance rather than scarcity of data (see Section 4.4).

Table 2. Examples of drug–gene interactions listed in DrugBank.

Drug Name	Gene Name	Interaction Type
Alteplase	PLG	activator
Hydromorphone	OPRK1	agonist
Varenicline	CHRNB2	partial agonist
Prazosin	ADRA1B	antagonist
Ascorbic acid	EGLN1	chaperone
Pyridoxal phosphate	GAD1	cofactor
Vardenafil	PDE6G	allosteric modulator
Trastuzumab	ERBB2	antibody
Nusinersen	SMN2	antisense oligonucleotide
Methysergide	HTR1F	binder
Tiapride	DRD2	blocker
Carvedilol	KCNJ4	inhibitor
Clobetasol propionate	ANXA1	inducer
Clofazimine	PPARG	modulator
Cerliponase alfa	IGF2R	ligand
Filgrastim	CSF3R	stimulator
Dalteparin	SERPINC1	potentiator
Vitamin A	RDH13	substrate
Nedocromil	CYSLTR1	suppressor
Belimumab	TNFSF13B	neutralizer
Esmirtazapine	HRH1	inverse agonist
Procainamide	DNMT1	other
Haloperidol	HTR2A	other/unknown

4.3. Labeling and Validation with ATC Codes

Employing computational methods (i.e., data mining and machine learning) in drug repositioning is generally hampered because we do not a have robust ground truth. Indeed, databases such as DrugBank record positive information about the drugs' known properties and functions, yet the absence of evidence is not evidence of absence (some drug properties may be hidden, and only future experiments can fully reveal them). That is why performance evaluation and validation of computational drug repositioning models are still an open issue; therefore, researchers adopt ad hoc, particular strategies, which are hard to compare [71]. Consequently, we resorted to making predictions with an older database version and then validating them with the latest version. However, even the latest database still cannot contain exhaustive information about drug functions. Furthermore, the negative information on drug functions/effects (stating what properties a drug does not have) will help prune the vast search space in drug repositioning. Unfortunately, negative information is scarce and scattered throughout the literature; to the best of our knowledge, no comprehensive dataset contains such data based on experimental results. As such, the existing negative information cannot be used algorithmically/automatically. As explained, one feasible method for filtering the noise and navigating the search space affected by uncertainty—an approach supported by recent research—is to integrate tools (such as the one we propose here) in ensemble methods.

Many computational drug repositioning methods based on complex networks rely on community detection and community labeling. However, labeling can be cumbersome and subjective; thus, we decided to use ATC codes, since this system is the standard for classifying medicines accepted by the WHO. Furthermore, the automated approach is fostered because the ATC code aggregates all information about a drug in a combination of letters and numbers, which are easier to process algorithmically. The ATC code classifies drugs on five levels considering three criteria simultaneously: anatomical (A)—the first level; therapeutic (T)–levels 2 and 3; and chemical (C)—levels 4 and 5. The anatomical criterion indicates the anatomical level or the physiological organ systems on which a specific drug acts. Each anatomical level is indicated in the ATC code by a letter (e.g., A–*Alimentary tract and metabolism*, C–*Cardiovascular system*, M–*Musculoskeletal system*, or R–*Respiratory system*); the ATC system contains 14 anatomical groups. Level 2 represents the therapeutic classification criterion and is encoded by two digits. Level 3 (encoded by a letter) indicates the particular pharmacological group of the drug. Level 4 (encoded by a letter) indicates the chemical class of the drug. Level 5 is encoded by two digits the chemical structure of the drug. This paper only used the first-level ATC codes for labeling and validation of prediction, although drug function is more precisely expressed by levels 1–3; we opted perform this because the sophisticated hierarchical clustering algorithms entailed by such an approach would have unnecessarily intensified the computational character of our study.

4.4. Method Application

When the problem at hand is too complex to solve by employing a single model, machine learning uses an ensemble strategy [72], which trains several models on the same set of data to operate collectively for solving the problem. This strategy is already used in bioinformatics to approach complex problems such as motif discovery in ChIP-Seq data [73]. The problem of drug repositioning is also very complex; however, prediction accuracy is not the primary indicator of success (the benefit of correctly predicting even a few drug repositionings is more significant than the cost of experiments entailed by testing the wrong predictions [74].) As such, very recent literature advances the idea of using ensemble methods for drug repositioning [69,70].

In this context, considering that—as explained in Section 4.2—our method uses drug–gene interaction data that partially describes the behavior of drugs, we indicate the ensemble strategy as ta method to use our method. As shown in Figure 11, drug repositioning prediction based on drug–gene interaction data may be Method$i$ from the group of machine learning methods based on distinct models $\{Method1, Method2, \ldots Methodm\}$. The repositioning hints list i is aggregated (i.e., via voting, averaging, or other procedures) to produce a final drug repositioning hints list. The aggregation process may use pharmacological expertise, e.g., to adjust the weights of a weighted average. However, implementing the ensemble strategy is beyond the scope of this paper, which aims to analyze and promote—for the first time—the beneficial role of drug–gene interaction networks for computational drug repositioning.

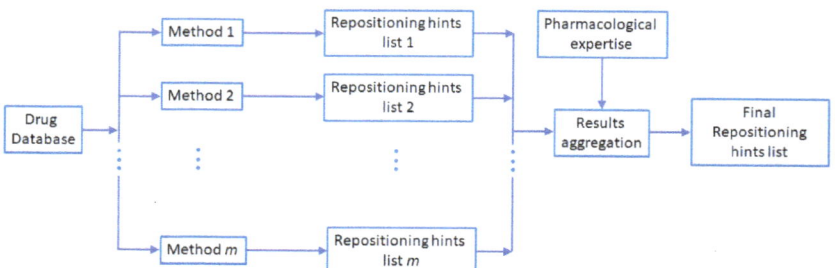

Figure 11. Overview of the ensemble strategy in drug repositioning. A group of machine learning and data mining methods $\{Method1, Method2, \ldots Methodm\}$, implementing various models and using distinct features (e.g., drug–drug interactions, drug–target interactions, drug–gene interactions, drug–adverse reactions relationships, pharmacokinetic properties) from the same comprehensive dataset and predicting a list of drug repositioning hints. Each method Method$i$ generates its repositioning hints list, and an aggregation process assembles all lists in the final repurposing hints list.

5. Conclusions

In this paper, we propose a new drug repurposing methodology based on algorithmic complex network analysis. To this end, we introduce an original method of building the Drug–Drug Similarity Network (DDSN) using drug–gene interactions from DrugBank, clustering DDSN with modularity classes, and labeling each cluster with the dominant first level ATC code of drugs within the cluster. The assumption that results in drug repurposing hints is that drugs in a cluster share the dominant property of the cluster. We use an automated procedure to tune modularity resolution, to apply our methodology on a DDSN built with data from DrugBank 5.0.9, to generate the list of drug repurposing hints (i.e., drugs for which the first level ATC does not match the dominant cluster label), and to check it against ATC codes in DrugBank 5.1.8.

By running our method on the DrugBank 5.1.8 DDSN, we generated a consistent list of drug repositioning candidates; we select the top betweenness/degree drugs in each cluster and perform a preliminary validation with state-of-the-art experimental results reported in the literature. Due to the fact that we collected many literature confirmations of our method's predictions, we argue that our fully automated pipeline, based on Big Data and unsupervised machine learning, is a practical tool that can substantially narrow the enormous search space in drug repositioning.

To summarize, the overarching methodological contributions of our paper are listed as follows:

(i) A new method to build weighted drug–drug similarity networks based on drug–gene interactions;

(ii) An automated procedure to optimize the modularity resolution such that network clustering maximizes the number of identified drug repurposings. A known/confirmed drug repurposing is a drug with more level 1 ATC codes in the latest drug database, compared with the earlier database—used to generate the drug–drug similarity network;

(iii) A new drug repurposing list was generated with our pipeline from the latest DrugBank 5.1.8 by analyzing the three most representative clusters.

In the present context, affected by the COVID-19 pandemic, we believe that the most promising findings/results presented in our paper are the anti-infective effects of statins, especially their potential antiviral effects. Indeed, the very recent comprehensive study [6] also finds, following in vitro screening, that fluvastatin presents what the authors call "strong effect" against SARS-CoV-2.

Considering all aspects presented in Section 4.2, we will extend our research on drug–gene interaction networks by implementing hierarchical clustering to predict ATC codes on levels 1–3, developing a dedicated cluster overlapping algorithm as a drug repositioning prediction strategy (i.e., one would reasonably expect that drugs in the overlapping zone would inherit the dominant properties of the respective clusters) and integrating the drug–gene network method into an ensemble strategy. These future objectives require substantial reliance on developing bioinformatic tools, entailing algorithm design, machine learning, and Big Data analytics.

Supplementary Materials: The following are available online at https://www.mdpi.com/article/10.3390/pharmaceutics13122117/s1, Table S1: DDSN-results.

Author Contributions: Conceptualization, M.U. and L.U.; methodology, V.G., M.U., A.B. and L.U.; software, V.G. and A.B.; validation, V.G., A.B. and L.U.; formal analysis, M.U.; investigation, V.G. and A.B.; resources, M.U. and L.U.; data curation, V.G. and L.U.; writing—original draft preparation, M.U. and L.U.; writing—review and editing, V.G., A.B. and L.U.; visualization, V.G., M.U. and L.U.; supervision, M.U. and L.U.; project administration, M.U. and L.U.; funding acquisition, L.U. All authors have read and agreed to the published version of the manuscript.

Funding: This study was supported by a grant of the Romanian Ministry of Education and Research, CCCDI-UEFISCDI, project number PN-III-P2-2.1-PED-2019-2842, within PNCDI III.

Institutional Review Board Statement: Not applicable.

Informed Consent Statement: Not applicable.

Data Availability Statement: This study uses only public database data.

Conflicts of Interest: The authors declare no conflicts of interest.

Abbreviations

The following abbreviations are used in this manuscript:

ATC	Anatomical Therapeutic Chemical;
COPD	Chronic Obstructive Pulmonary Disease;
COX-2	Cyclooxygenase-2;
DDSN	Drug–Drug Similarity Network;
NSCLC	Non-Small Cell Lung Cancer.

Appendix A. Repositionings and Statistics for DrugBank 5.0.9 DDSN

Appendix A.1. DDSN Zoomed Details

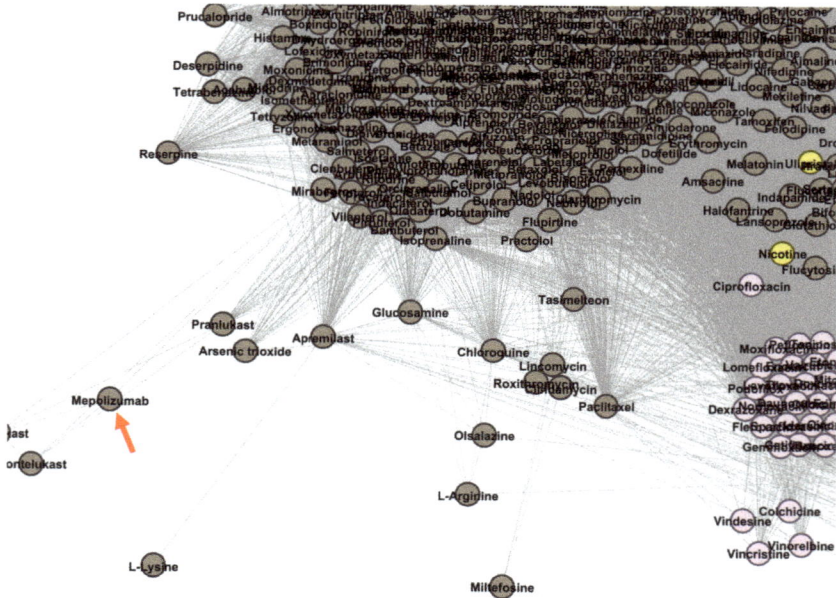

Figure A1. The zoomed detail of the DDSN network built with drug–gene interaction data from DrugBank 5.0.9, which shows the relative position of mepolizumab within cluster C_0 (brown nodes) with a red arrow (→). Our repositioning pipeline predicts that mepolizumab—listed as antineoplastic in DrugBank 5.0.9—also acts as a drug with level 1 ATC code R (*Respiratory system*), confirmed by the more recent DrugBank version 5.1.8.

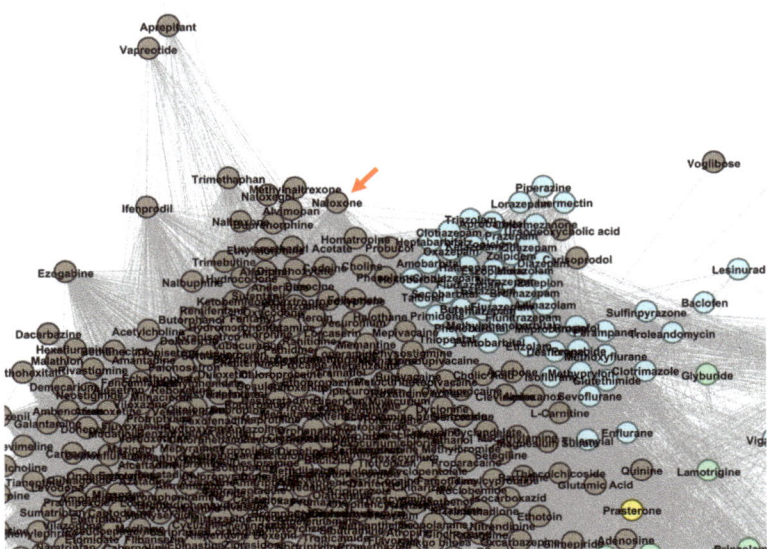

Figure A2. The zoomed detail of the DrugBank 5.0.9 DDSN network showing the relative position of naloxone within cluster C_0 (brown nodes) with a red arrow (→). Our repositioning pipeline predicts that naloxone—listed as opioid overdose antidote in DrugBank 5.0.9—also acts as a drug with level 1 ATC code N (*Nervous system*), confirmed by the more recent DrugBank version 5.1.8.

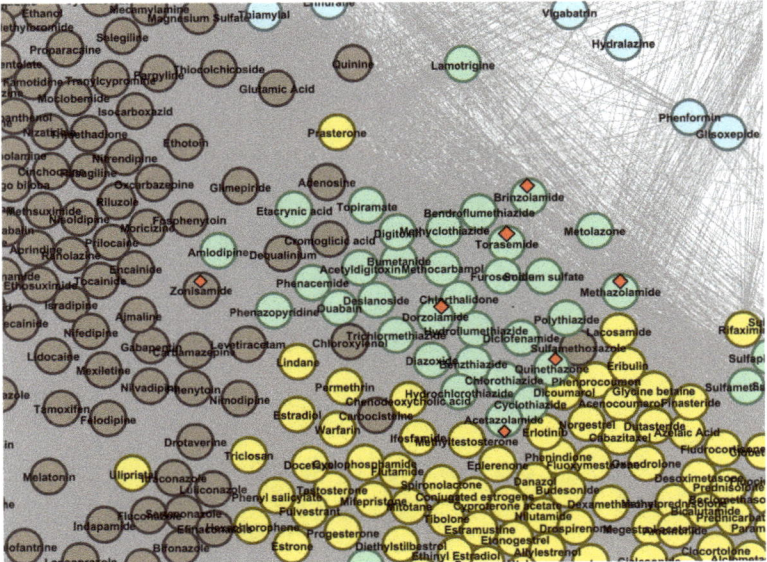

Figure A3. The DrugBank 5.0.9 DDSN network's zoomed detail shows the confirmed repositionings within cluster C_2 (green nodes) with red diamonds (◇). Our repositioning pipeline predicts that torasemide and quinetazone (both with ATC level 1 code C–*Cardiovascular system* in DrugBank 5.0.9), methazolamide, acetazolamide, dorzolamide, and brinzolamide (all with ATC level 1 code S–*Sensory organs* in DrugBank 5.0.9) are *Genito urinary system and sex hormones* drugs (first level ATC G). Zonisamide (N–*Nervous system*) is a brown node (cluster C_0) but in the close vicinity of cluster C_2; therefore, they are also predicted at level 1 ATC code G.

Appendix A.2. DDSN Cluster Histograms

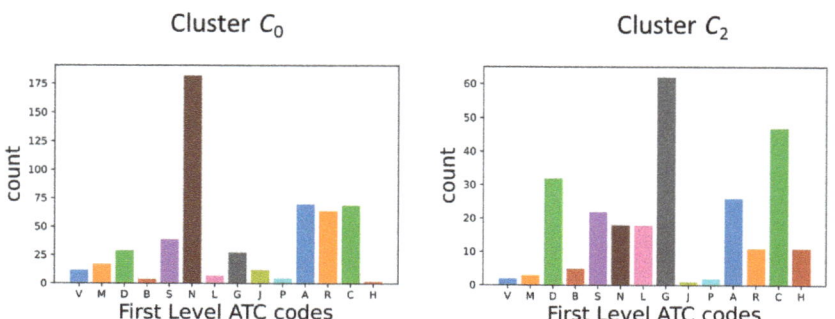

Figure A4. Histograms of level 1 ATC codes in the DrugBank 5.0.9 DDSN clusters holding drug repositionings confirmed by DrugBank 5.1.8: cluster C_0 (brown nodes) in the left panel and cluster C_2 (green nodes) in the right panel. The dominant property in cluster C_0 is N–*Nervous system*, with many subcluster drugs with level 1 ATC codes A, R, and C (*Alimentary tract and metabolism, Respiratory system,* and *Cardiovascular system,* respectively). The dominant properties in cluster C_2 are G, C, and D (*Genito urinary system and sex hormones, Cardiovascular system,* and *Dermatologicals,* respectively).

Appendix B. Repositionings and Statistics for DrugBank 5.1.8 DDSN

Appendix B.1. DDSN Zoomed Details

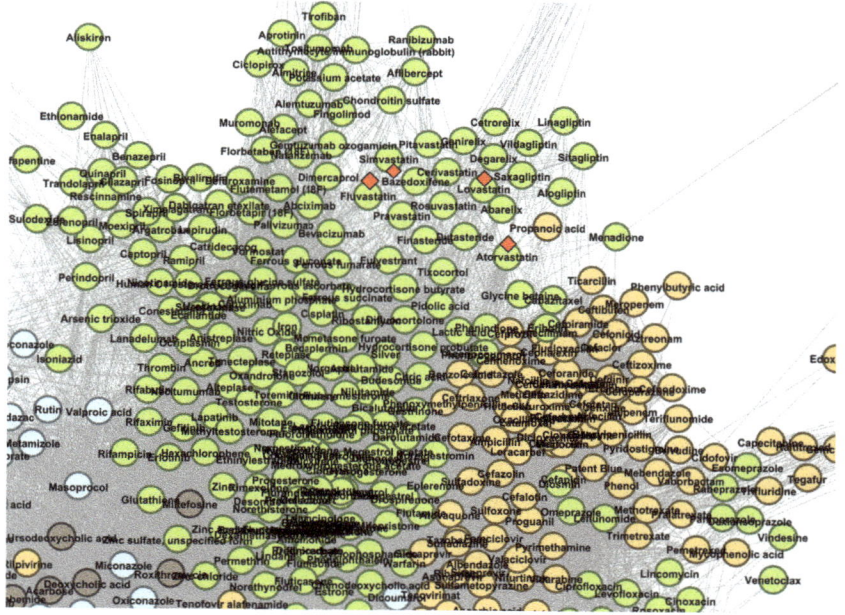

Figure A5. The DrugBank 5.1.8 DDSN network's zoomed detail shows four repositionings within cluster C_1 (green nodes) with a red diamond (◊). Our repositioning pipeline predicts that simvastatin, fluvastatin, lovastatin, and atorvastatin (currently at ATC level 1 codes C–*Cardiovascular system*) have properties described by the level 1 ATC code J–*Anti infectives for systemic use*.

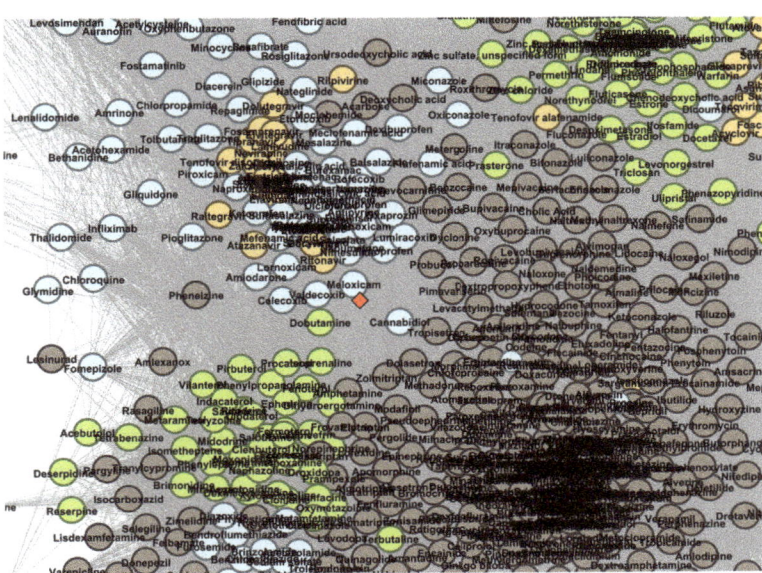

Figure A6. The DrugBank 5.1.8 DDSN network's zoomed detail shows a repositionings within cluster C_2 (light blue nodes) with a red diamond (◊). Our repositioning pipeline predicts that meloxicam (currently at ATC level 1 code M–*Musculo-skeletal system*) has properties described by the level 1 ATC code L–*Antineoplastic and immunomodulating agents*.

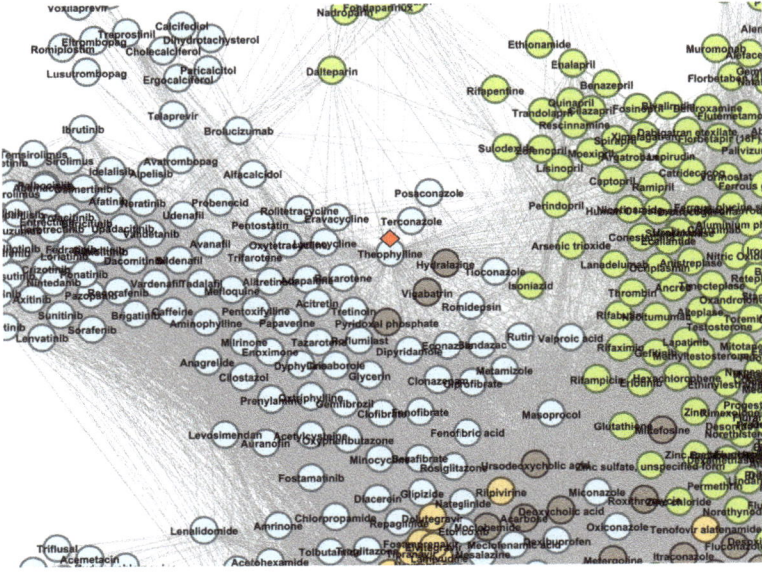

Figure A7. The DrugBank 5.1.8 DDSN network's zoomed detail shows a repositioning within cluster C_2 (light blue nodes) with a red diamond (◊). Our repositioning pipeline predicts that theophylline (currently at ATC level 1 code R–*Respiratory system*) has properties described by the level 1 ATC code L–*Antineoplastic and immunomodulating agents*.

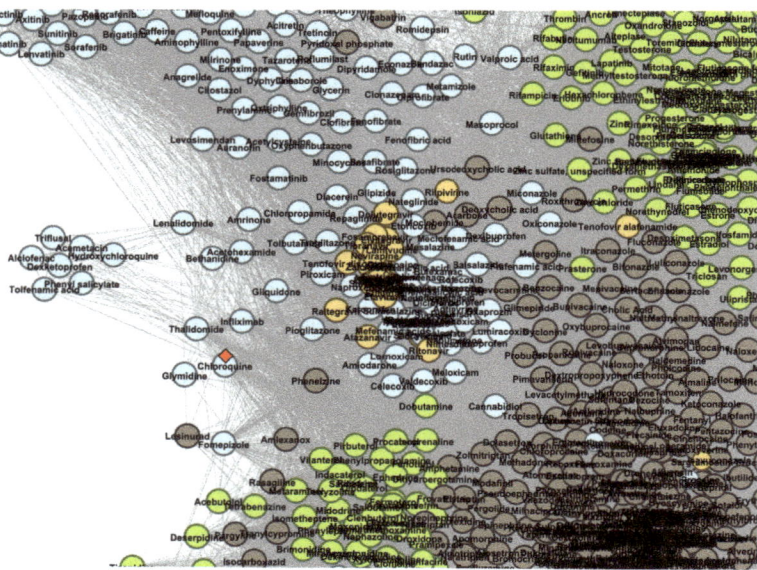

Figure A8. The DrugBank 5.1.8 DDSN network's zoomed detail shows repositioning within cluster C_2 (light blue nodes) with a red diamond (◇). Our repositioning pipeline predicts that chloroquine (currently at ATC level 1 code P–*Antiparasitic products, insecticides and repellents*) has properties described by the level 1 ATC code L–*Antineoplastic and immunomodulating agents*.

Appendix B.2. DDSN Cluster Histograms

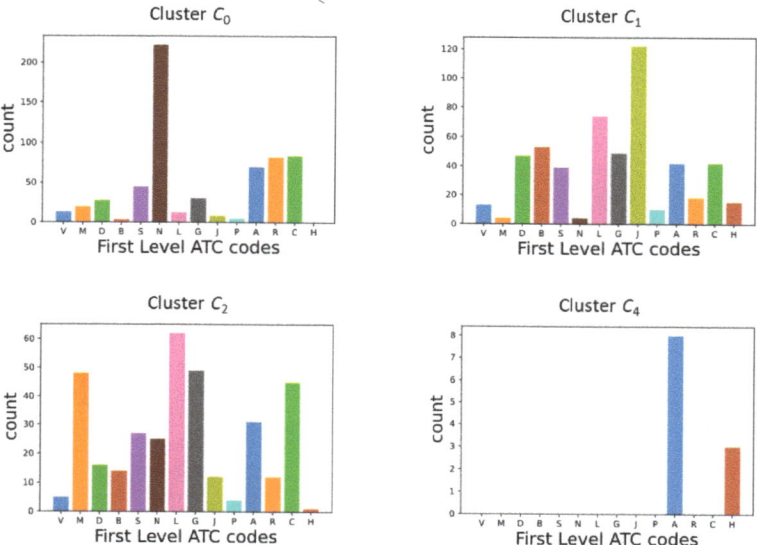

Figure A9. Histograms of level 1 ATC codes in the DrugBank 5.1.8 DDSN clusters holding drug repositionings confirmed by literature review: cluster C_0 (brown nodes), cluster C_1 (green nodes), cluster C_2 (light blue nodes), and cluster C_4 (pink nodes). The dominant property in cluster C_0 is N–*Nervous System*, J–*Anti-infectives for systemic use* in cluster C_1, L–*Antineoplastic and immunomodulating agents* in cluster C_2, and A–*Alimentary Tract and Metabolism* in cluster C_4.

References

1. Munos, B. Lessons from 60 years of pharmaceutical innovation. *Nat. Rev. Drug Discov.* **2009**, *8*, 959–968. [CrossRef] [PubMed]
2. Dickson, M.; Gagnon, J.P. The cost of new drug discovery and development. *Discov. Med.* **2009**, *4*, 172–179.
3. Chen, X.Q.; Antman, M.D.; Gesenberg, C.; Gudmundsson, O.S. Discovery pharmaceutics—Challenges and opportunities. *AAPS J.* **2006**, *8*, E402–E408. [CrossRef]
4. Pammolli, F.; Magazzini, L.; Riccaboni, M. The productivity crisis in pharmaceutical R&D. *Nat. Rev. Drug Discov.* **2011**, *10*, 428–438. [PubMed]
5. Lombardino, J.G.; Lowe, J.A. The role of the medicinal chemist in drug discovery—Then and now. *Nat. Rev. Drug Discov.* **2004**, *3*, 853–862. [CrossRef]
6. Gysi, D.M.; Do Valle, Í.; Zitnik, M.; Ameli, A.; Gan, X.; Varol, O.; Ghiassian, S.D.; Patten, J.; Davey, R.A.; Loscalzo, J.; et al. Network medicine framework for identifying drug-repurposing opportunities for COVID-19. *Proc. Natl. Acad. Sci. USA* **2021**, *118*, e2025581118
7. Meganck, R.M.; Baric, R.S. Developing therapeutic approaches for twenty-first-century emerging infectious viral diseases. *Nat. Med.* **2021**, *27*, 401–410. [CrossRef] [PubMed]
8. Ashburn, T.T.; Thor, K.B. Drug repositioning: Identifying and developing new uses for existing drugs. *Nat. Rev. Drug Discov.* **2004**, *3*, 673–683. [CrossRef] [PubMed]
9. Reddy, A.S.; Zhang, S. Polypharmacology: Drug discovery for the future. *Expert Rev. Clin. Pharmacol.* **2013**, *6*, 41–47. [CrossRef]
10. Pinzi, L.; Tinivella, A.; Caporuscio, F.; Rastelli, G. Drug repurposing and polypharmacology to fight SARS-CoV-2 through inhibition of the main protease. *Front. Pharmacol.* **2021**, *12*, 84. [CrossRef]
11. Aliper, A.; Plis, S.; Artemov, A.; Ulloa, A.; Mamoshina, P.; Zhavoronkov, A. Deep learning applications for predicting pharmacological properties of drugs and drug repurposing using transcriptomic data. *Mol. Pharm.* **2016**, *13*, 2524–2530. [CrossRef] [PubMed]
12. Zhou, Y.; Wang, F.; Tang, J.; Nussinov, R.; Cheng, F. Artificial intelligence in COVID-19 drug repurposing. *Lancet Dig. Health* **2020**, *2*, e667–e676. [CrossRef]
13. Pushpakom, S.; Iorio, F.; Eyers, P.A.; Escott, K.J.; Hopper, S.; Wells, A.; Doig, A.; Guilliams, T.; Latimer, J.; McNamee, C.; et al. Drug repurposing: Progress, challenges and recommendations. *Nat. Rev. Drug Discov.* **2019**, *18*, 41–58. [CrossRef] [PubMed]
14. Udrescu, L.; Sbârcea, L.; Topîrceanu, A.; Iovanovici, A.; Kurunczi, L.; Bogdan, P.; Udrescu, M. Clustering drug-drug interaction networks with energy model layouts: community analysis and drug repurposing. *Sci. Rep.* **2016**, *6*, 1–10. [CrossRef] [PubMed]
15. Cheng, F.; Desai, R.J.; Handy, D.E.; Wang, R.; Schneeweiss, S.; Barabasi, A.L.; Loscalzo, J. Network-based approach to prediction and population-based validation of in silico drug repurposing. *Nat. Commun.* **2018**, *9*, 1–12. [CrossRef]
16. Luo, Y.; Zhao, X.; Zhou, J.; Yang, J.; Zhang, Y.; Kuang, W.; Peng, J.; Chen, L.; Zeng, J. A network integration approach for drug-target interaction prediction and computational drug repositioning from heterogeneous information. *Nat. Commun.* **2017**, *8*, 1–13. [CrossRef] [PubMed]
17. AY, M.; Goh, K.I.; Cusick, M.E.; Barabasi, A.L.; Vidal, M. Drug–target network. *Nat. Biotechnol.* **2007**, *25*, 1119–1127.
18. Ye, H.; Liu, Q.; Wei, J. Construction of drug network based on side effects and its application for drug repositioning. *PLoS ONE* **2014**, *9*, e87864. [CrossRef]
19. Lotfi Shahreza, M.; Ghadiri, N.; Mousavi, S.R.; Varshosaz, J.; Green, J.R. A review of network-based approaches to drug repositioning. *Brief. Bioinf.* **2018**, *19*, 878–892. [CrossRef]
20. de Oliveira, T.B.; Zhao, L.; Faceli, K.; de Carvalho, A.C. Data clustering based on complex network community detection. In Proceedings of the 2008 IEEE Congress on Evolutionary Computation (IEEE World Congress on Computational Intelligence), Hong Kong, China, 1–6 June 2008; pp. 2121–2126.
21. Yang, Z.; Algesheimer, R.; Tessone, C.J. A comparative analysis of community detection algorithms on artificial networks. *Sci. Rep.* **2016**, *6*, 1–18.
22. Udrescu, L.; Bogdan, P.; Chiş, A.; Sîrbu, I.O.; Topîrceanu, A.; Văruţ, R.M.; Udrescu, M. Uncovering New Drug Properties in Target-Based Drug-Drug Similarity Networks. *Pharmaceutics* **2020**, *12*, 879. [CrossRef] [PubMed]
23. Badkas, A.; De Landtsheer, S.; Sauter, T. Topological network measures for drug repositioning. *Brief. Bioinf.* **2021**, *22*, bbaa357. [CrossRef] [PubMed]
24. Pérez-Moraga, R.; Forés-Martos, J.; Suay-García, B.; Duval, J.L.; Falcó, A.; Climent, J. A COVID-19 Drug Repurposing Strategy through Quantitative Homological Similarities Using a Topological Data Analysis-Based Framework. *Pharmaceutics* **2021**, *13*, 488. [CrossRef] [PubMed]
25. Iorio, F.; Bosotti, R.; Scacheri, E.; Belcastro, V.; Mithbaokar, P.; Ferriero, R.; Murino, L.; Tagliaferri, R.; Brunetti-Pierri, N.; Isacchi, A.; et al. Discovery of drug mode of action and drug repositioning from transcriptional responses. *Proc. Natl. Acad. Sci. USA* **2010**, *107*, 14621–14626. [CrossRef] [PubMed]
26. Cheng, F.; Li, W.; Wu, Z.; Wang, X.; Zhang, C.; Li, J.; Liu, G.; Tang, Y. Prediction of polypharmacological profiles of drugs by the integration of chemical, side effect, and therapeutic space. *J. Chem. Inf. Model.* **2013**, *53*, 753–762. [CrossRef]
27. Gottlieb, A.; Stein, G.Y.; Ruppin, E.; Sharan, R. PREDICT: A method for inferring novel drug indications with application to personalized medicine. *Mol. Syst. Biol.* **2011**, *7*, 496. [CrossRef] [PubMed]

28. Langhauser, F.; Casas, A.I.; Guney, E.; Menche, J.; Geuss, E.; Kleikers, P.W.; López, M.G.; Barabási, A.L.; Kleinschnitz, C.; Schmidt, H.H.; et al. A diseasome cluster-based drug repurposing of soluble guanylate cyclase activators from smooth muscle relaxation to direct neuroprotection. *NPJ Syst. Biol. Appl.* **2018**, *4*, 1–13. [CrossRef] [PubMed]
29. Goh, K.I.; Choi, I.G. Exploring the human diseasome: The human disease network. *Brief. Funct. Gen.* **2012**, *11*, 533–542. [CrossRef] [PubMed]
30. Goh, K.I.; Cusick, M.E.; Valle, D.; Childs, B.; Vidal, M.; Barabási, A.L. The human disease network. *Proc. Natl. Acad. Sci. USA* **2007**, *104*, 8685–8690. [CrossRef] [PubMed]
31. Lancichinetti, A.; Fortunato, S. Limits of modularity maximization in community detection. *Phys. Rev. E* **2011**, *84*, 066122. [CrossRef] [PubMed]
32. Wishart, D.S.; Knox, C.; Guo, A.C.; Shrivastava, S.; Hassanali, M.; Stothard, P.; Chang, Z.; Woolsey, J. DrugBank: A comprehensive resource for in silico drug discovery and exploration. *Nucl. Acids Res.* **2006**, *34*, D668–D672. [CrossRef]
33. Wishart, D.S.; Feunang, Y.D.; Guo, A.C.; Lo, E.J.; Marcu, A.; Grant, J.R.; Sajed, T.; Johnson, D.; Li, C.; Sayeeda, Z.; et al. DrugBank 5.0: A major update to the DrugBank database for 2018. *Nucl. Acids Res.* **2018**, *46*, D1074–D1082. [CrossRef]
34. Merkel, D. Docker: Lightweight linux containers for consistent development and deployment. *Linux J.* **2014**, *2014*, 2.
35. McKinney, W. Pandas: A foundational Python library for data analysis and statistics. *Python High Perform. Sci. Comput.* **2011**, *14*, 1–9.
36. Hagberg, A.; Swart, P.; Chult, D.S. *Exploring Network Structure, Dynamics, and Function Using NetworkX*; Technical report; Los Alamos National Lab. (LANL): Los Alamos, NM, USA, 2008.
37. Rossetti, G.; Milli, L.; Cazabet, R. CDLIB: A python library to extract, compare and evaluate communities from complex networks. *Appl. Netw. Sci.* **2019**, *4*, 1–26. [CrossRef]
38. Bastian, M.; Heymann, S.; Jacomy, M. Gephi: An open source software for exploring and manipulating networks. In Proceedings of the Third international AAAI Conference on Weblogs and Social Media, San Jose, CA, USA, 17–20 May 2009.
39. Zhou, T.; Ren, J.; Medo, M.; Zhang, Y.C. Bipartite network projection and personal recommendation. *Phys. Rev. E* **2007**, *76*, 046115. [CrossRef]
40. Girvan, M.; Newman, M.E. Community structure in social and biological networks. *Proc. Natl. Acad. Sci. USA* **2002**, *99*, 7821–7826. [CrossRef] [PubMed]
41. Blondel, V.D.; Guillaume, J.L.; Lambiotte, R.; Lefebvre, E. Fast unfolding of communities in large networks. *J. Stat. Mech. Theory Exp.* **2008**, *2008*, P10008. [CrossRef]
42. Peng, Y.; Wang, M.; Xu, Y.; Wu, Z.; Wang, J.; Zhang, C.; Liu, G.; Li, W.; Li, J.; Tang, Y. Drug repositioning by prediction of drug's anatomical therapeutic chemical code via network-based inference approaches. *Brief. Bioinf.* **2021**, *22*, 2058–2072. [CrossRef]
43. Tan, F.; Yang, R.; Xu, X.; Chen, X.; Wang, Y.; Ma, H.; Liu, X.; Wu, X.; Chen, Y.; Liu, L.; et al. Drug repositioning by applying 'expression profiles' generated by integrating chemical structure similarity and gene semantic similarity. *Mol. BioSyst.* **2014**, *10*, 1126–1138. [CrossRef]
44. Wang, H.; Kuo, M.; Chou, M.; Hung, P.; Lin, K.; Hsieh, M.; Chang, M. Pyridoxal phosphate is better than pyridoxine for controlling idiopathic intractable epilepsy. *Arch. Dis. Child.* **2005**, *90*, 512–515. [CrossRef]
45. Mills, P.B.; Camuzeaux, S.S.; Footitt, E.J.; Mills, K.A.; Gissen, P.; Fisher, L.; Das, K.B.; Varadkar, S.M.; Zuberi, S.; McWilliam, R.; et al. Epilepsy due to PNPO mutations: genotype, environment and treatment affect presentation and outcome. *Brain* **2014**, *137*, 1350–1360. [CrossRef] [PubMed]
46. Berthet, N.; Faure, O.; Bakri, A.; Ambroise-Thomas, P.; Grillot, R.; Brugere, J.F. In vitro susceptibility of *Aspergillus* spp. clinical isolates to albendazole. *J. Antimicrob. Chemother.* **2003**, *51*, 1419–1422. [CrossRef] [PubMed]
47. Bartlett, M.S.; Edlind, T.D.; Lee, C.H.; Dean, R.; Queener, S.F.; Shaw, M.M.; Smith, J.W. Albendazole inhibits Pneumocystis carinii proliferation in inoculated immunosuppressed mice. *Antimicrob. Agents Chemother.* **1994**, *38*, 1834–1837. [CrossRef]
48. Caruso, A.; Caccuri, F.; Bugatti, A.; Zani, A.; Vanoni, M.; Bonfanti, P.; Cazzaniga, M.E.; Perno, C.F.; Messa, C.; Alberghina, L. Methotrexate inhibits SARS-CoV-2 virus replication "in vitro". *J. Med. Virol.* **2021**, *93*, 1780–1785. [CrossRef] [PubMed]
49. Beck, S.; Zhu, Z.; Oliveira, M.F.; Smith, D.M.; Rich, J.N.; Bernatchez, J.A.; Siqueira-Neto, J.L. Mechanism of action of methotrexate against Zika virus. *Viruses* **2019**, *11*, 338. [CrossRef]
50. Lembo, D.; Gribaudo, G.; Cavallo, R.; Riera, L.; Angeretti, A.; Hertel, L.; Landolfo, S. Human cytomegalovirus stimulates cellular dihydrofolate reductase activity in quiescent cells. *Intervirology* **1999**, *42*, 30–36. [CrossRef]
51. Jerwood, S.; Cohen, J. Unexpected antimicrobial effect of statins. *J. Antimicrob. Chemother.* **2008**, *61*, 362–364. [CrossRef] [PubMed]
52. Parihar, S.P.; Guler, R.; Brombacher, F. Statins: A viable candidate for host-directed therapy against infectious diseases. *Nat. Rev. Immunol.* **2019**, *19*, 104–117. [CrossRef]
53. Chang, Y.L.; Hsu, Y.J.; Chen, Y.; Wang, Y.W.; Huang, S.M. Theophylline exhibits anti-cancer activity via suppressing SRSF3 in cervical and breast cancer cell lines. *Oncotarget* **2017**, *8*, 101461. [CrossRef]
54. Goldman, A.P.; Williams, C.S.; Sheng, H.; Lamps, L.W.; Williams, V.P.; Pairet, M.; Morrow, J.D.; DuBois, R.N. Meloxicam inhibits the growth of colorectal cancer cells. *Carcinogenesis* **1998**, *19*, 2195–2199. [CrossRef] [PubMed]
55. Tsubouchi, Y.; Mukai, S.; Kawahito, Y.; Yamada, R.; Kohno, M.; Inoue, K.; Sano, H. Meloxicam inhibits the growth of non-small cell lung cancer. *Anticancer Res.* **2000**, *20*, 2867–2872. [PubMed]
56. Naruse, T.; Nishida, Y.; Hosono, K.; Ishiguro, N. Meloxicam inhibits osteosarcoma growth, invasiveness and metastasis by COX-2-dependent and independent routes. *Carcinogenesis* **2006**, *27*, 584–592. [CrossRef]

57. Deeb, K.K.; Trump, D.L.; Johnson, C.S. Vitamin D signalling pathways in cancer: potential for anticancer therapeutics. *Nat. Rev. Cancer* **2007**, *7*, 684–700. [CrossRef]
58. Chiang, K.C.; Chen, T.C. The anti-cancer actions of vitamin D. In *Anti-Cancer Agents in Medicinal Chemistry (Formerly Current Medicinal Chemistry—Anti-Cancer Agents)*; Bentham Science Publishers: Sharjah, United Arab Emirates, 2013; Volume 13, pp. 126–139.
59. Weyerhäuser, P.; Kantelhardt, S.R.; Kim, E.L. Re-purposing chloroquine for glioblastoma: potential merits and confounding variables. *Front. Oncol.* **2018**, *8*, 335. [CrossRef] [PubMed]
60. Verbaanderd, C.; Maes, H.; Schaaf, M.B.; Sukhatme, V.P.; Pantziarka, P.; Sukhatme, V.; Agostinis, P.; Bouche, G. Repurposing Drugs in Oncology (ReDO)—Chloroquine and hydroxychloroquine as anti-cancer agents. *ecancermedicalscience* **2017**, *11*, 781. [CrossRef] [PubMed]
61. Dolgin, E. Anticancer autophagy inhibitors attract 'resurgent' interest. *Nat. Rev. Drug Discov.* **2019**, *18*, 408–410. [CrossRef] [PubMed]
62. Varisli, L.; Cen, O.; Vlahopoulos, S. Dissecting pharmacological effects of chloroquine in cancer treatment: Interference with inflammatory signaling pathways. *Immunology* **2020**, *159*, 257–278. [CrossRef]
63. Zhou, W.; Wang, H.; Yang, Y.; Chen, Z.S.; Zou, C.; Zhang, J. Chloroquine against malaria, cancers and viral diseases. *Drug Discov. Today* **2020**, 2012–2022. [CrossRef]
64. Kemp, S.F.; Thrailkill, K.M. Mecasermin rinfabate for severe insulin-like growth factor-I deficiency. *Clin. Pract.* **2007**, *4*, 133. [CrossRef]
65. IPLEX™ (Mecasermin Rinfabate [rDNA Origin] Injection). Available online: https://www.accessdata.fda.gov/drugsatfda_docs/label/2007/021884s001lbl.pdf (accessed on 21 October 2021).
66. INCRELEX, INN: Mecasermin. Scientific Discussion. Available online: https://www.ema.europa.eu/en/documents/scientific-discussion/increlex-epar-scientific-discussion_en.pdf (accessed on 21 October 2021).
67. Miyake, M.; Kirisako, T.; Kokubo, T.; Miura, Y.; Morishita, K.; Okamura, H.; Tsuda, A. Randomised controlled trial of the effects of L-ornithine on stress markers and sleep quality in healthy workers. *Nutr. J.* **2014**, *13*, 1–8. [CrossRef]
68. Zhou, X.; Wang, M.; Katsyv, I.; Irie, H.; Zhang, B. EMUDRA: Ensemble of multiple drug repositioning approaches to improve prediction accuracy. *Bioinformatics* **2018**, *34*, 3151–3159. [CrossRef] [PubMed]
69. Wang, J.; Wang, W.; Yan, C.; Luo, J.; Zhang, G. Predicting Drug-Disease Association Based on Ensemble Strategy. *Front. Genet.* **2021**, *12*, 548. [CrossRef] [PubMed]
70. Ghorbanali, Z.; Zare-Mirakabad, F.; Mohammadpour, B. DRP-VEM: Drug repositioning prediction using voting ensemble. *arXiv* **2021**, arXiv:2110.01403.
71. Jarada, T.N.; Rokne, J.G.; Alhajj, R. A review of computational drug repositioning: strategies, approaches, opportunities, challenges, and directions. *J. Cheminf.* **2020**, *12*, 1–23. [CrossRef] [PubMed]
72. Sagi, O.; Rokach, L. Ensemble learning: A survey. *Wiley Interdiscip. Rev. Data Min. Knowl. Discov.* **2018**, *8*, e1249. [CrossRef]
73. Lihu, A.; Holban, Ș. A review of ensemble methods for de novo motif discovery in ChIP-Seq data. *Brief. Bioinf.* **2015**, *16*, 964–973. [CrossRef] [PubMed]
74. Xue, H.; Li, J.; Xie, H.; Wang, Y. Review of drug repositioning approaches and resources. *Int. J. Biol. Sci.* **2018**, *14*, 1232. [CrossRef]

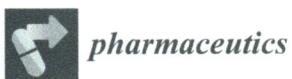

Article

In Silico Screening of Available Drugs Targeting Non-Small Cell Lung Cancer Targets: A Drug Repurposing Approach

Muthu Kumar Thirunavukkarasu [1], Utid Suriya [2], Thanyada Rungrotmongkol [3,4,*] and Ramanathan Karuppasamy [1,*]

1. Department of Biotechnology, School of Bio Sciences and Technology, Vellore Institute of Technology, Vellore 632014, India; muthukumar.t@vit.ac.in
2. Program in Biotechnology, Faculty of Science, Chulalongkorn University, Bangkok 10330, Thailand; noteutidii@gmail.com
3. Biocatalyst and Environmental Biotechnology Research Unit, Department of Biochemistry, Faculty of Science, Chulalongkorn University, Bangkok 10330, Thailand
4. Program in Bioinformatics and Computational Biology, Graduate School, Chulalongkorn University, Bangkok 10330, Thailand
* Correspondence: thanyada.r@chula.ac.th (T.R.); kramanathan@vit.ac.in (R.K.)

Abstract: The RAS–RAF–MEK–ERK pathway plays a key role in malevolent cell progression in many tumors. The high structural complexity in the upstream kinases limits the treatment progress. Thus, MEK inhibition is a promising strategy since it is easy to inhibit and is a gatekeeper for the many malignant effects of its downstream effector. Even though MEK inhibitors are under investigation in many cancers, drug resistance continues to be the principal limiting factor to achieving cures in patients with cancer. Hence, we accomplished a high-throughput virtual screening to overcome this bottleneck by the discovery of dual-targeting therapy in cancer treatment. Here, a total of 11,808 DrugBank molecules were assessed through high-throughput virtual screening for their activity against MEK. Further, the Glide docking, MLSF and prime-MM/GBSA methods were implemented to extract the potential lead compounds from the database. Two compounds, DB012661 and DB07642, were outperformed in all the screening analyses. Further, the study results reveal that the lead compounds also have a significant binding capability with the co-target PIM1. Finally, the SIE-based free energy calculation reveals that the binding of compounds was majorly affected by the van der Waals interactions with MEK receptor. Overall, the in silico binding efficacy of these lead compounds against both MEK and PIM1 could be of significant therapeutic interest to overcome drug resistance in the near future.

Keywords: drug-repositioning; MEK inhibitor; MM/GBSA; Glide docking; MD simulation; MM/PBSA

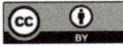

1. Introduction

Lung cancer accounts for about a quarter of all cancer deaths, among them 82% of deaths were being caused by intentionally smoking cigarettes. The development of advanced therapies for the management of the early and metastatic stages of lung cancer were not yet discovered over the past 40 years. Although some treatment measures are available to control the earlier stages of lung cancer, poor outcomes reduce the overall patient survival rates. One of the common clinical symptoms of lung cancer is frequently coughing for a particular period. For example, patients in the United States who had been coughing for three weeks were finally identified with lung cancer [1]. In the United Kingdom, smoking is responsible for 71% of lung cancer deaths, whereas 1% of the deaths of passive smokers were reported. The Canadian researchers reports that the lung cancer deaths in smokers were 15% higher than in non-smokers. In India, 9.3% of the cancer deaths were associated with lung cancer, containing both male and female patients [2]. The low lung cancer survival rates reflect the high number of patients diagnosed with metastatic disease (57%). Currently, surgery, radiation therapy, chemotherapy and targeted therapies were used to treat the lung cancer patients. Among these methods, targeted therapies demonstrated better outcome during the cancer treatment [3,4]. Genetic expression and mutational studies were certainly used to identify the definitive target for lung cancer. The incidence of particular mutations varies depending on ethnicity and location. The EGFR mutations that were reported in Caucasians were found to be 10%, whereas 60% of the mutational rates were reported in Asian people [5]. Ultimately, the tyrosine kinase pathway plays a major role in the tremendous increase in lung cancer deaths. Mitogen-activated protein kinase (MAPK) is one of the promising growth signaling pathways. The aberrant activation of this pathway's intermediates leads to uncontrolled cell growth and differentiation. In many cancer types, concomitant mutations occurred in RAS and BRAF, which is the reason for the consecutive activation of ERK, which is responsible for the activation of many transcription factors [6]. Hence, targeting the pathway receptors using checkpoint inhibitors leads to effective therapy in most cancers. However, a strong association between RAS and GTP impedes the direct inhibition of RAS. The lack of understanding regarding the allosteric sites is also a hindrance to the development of RAS targeting inhibitors [7]. The next intermediate RAF is another important target when there is an existence of BRAFV^{600} mutations. Nevertheless, the acquired resistance in RAF selective inhibitors is the reason for the constant activation of the MAPK pathway in many cancers [8]. Therefore, it is possible to affirm a downstream cut-off of the MAPK pathway at a protein kinase called MEK. The MEK receptor is a key node in the MAPK pathway, which is the only known substrate of its downstream effector, ERK. In the recent decade, hundreds of MEK inhibitors were discovered to target the allosteric binding site of MEK [9]. Although these selective inhibitors were effective at the allosteric site, a poor cytotoxicity profile limits their treatment progress. For instance, the most potent kinase inhibitors, such as binimetinib, selumetinib, cobimetinib and rafametinib, caused diarrhea, elevated lipase levels and rashes as adverse effects [10,11]. It is important to note that a recently approved MEK selective inhibitor trametinib showed the most efficacy in the BRAF mutant tumors in combination with dabrafenib [12,13]. However, trametinib alone showed additional side effects during the treatment period in non-small cell lung cancer patients. For instance, trametinib specifically affects the ocular region of the patients. Moreover, a severe complication in the ocular region may lead to permanent vision loss in the patients [14]. In addition to their toxic effects, several MEK inhibitors were resistant to the BRAF mutations through the activation of adjutant signaling pathway receptors. The initial solution to the problem of resistance to therapy is the dual inhibition of crucial targets with the administration of a single therapy. It is also interesting to note that the inhibition of multiple kinases will produce better outcomes during clinical trials. For instance, the combination of MEK and JAK2/STAT3 pathway inhibition reduces the potential impact on drug resistance in colon cancer [15]. Similarly, a combination of MEK and PI3K inhibitors is a powerful treatment option for NSCLC patients who have developed resistance to EGFR–TKIs [16]. Note that dual inhibitors will produce more beneficial effects than the combined inhibitors in terms of cost and time taken for the approval. Note also that PIM1 is a critical effector facilitating cross-talk across several neighboring pathways, in particular to the MAPK pathway. Recent studies highlight that MEK inhibitors lead to the increased expression of PIM1, thereby increasing cancer cell growth [17,18]. Keeping this in mind, we framed an in silico-based drug repurposing workflow to screen the potential inhibitors that act against both MEK and PIM1.

Drug repurposing has become one of the most popular ways for increasing the efficiency and cost-effectiveness of drug development. Importantly, the discoveries of the novel indications of existing drugs were the major applications in drug repurposing strategies. In recent years, almost 30% of the FDA-approved drugs and vaccines were discovered by in silico approaches. For instance, the discovery of zanamivir was made possible using a computer-aided drug design technique based on the crystal structure of influenza virus neuraminidase [19]. Adding together the implementation of machine learning principles and virtual screening would certainly enhance the accuracy of screening results. Machine-learning-based approaches produce more reliable results and provide faster outcomes by learning existing experimental data [20]. Hence, we incorporated machine-learning-based scoring functions (MLSF) to screen the potential compounds against the MEK receptor since they have attained a plateau in their performance during the binding affinity prediction [21]. We are certain that the outcome of this study is of immense importance for the experimental biologist involved in the screening of MEK inhibitors.

2. Methodology

2.1. Dataset

Structural information of proteins and ligand molecules were retrieved from the protein data bank (PDB) and DrugBank database, respectively. The 3D structure of two protein molecules, such as MEK1 (PDB ID:3W8Q) and PIM1 (PDB ID: 5KZI), were downloaded in the PDB format [22,23]. Eventually, the DrugBank molecules were downloaded as three subsets containing FDA (Food and Drug Administration)-approved drugs (n = 3085), experimental drugs (n = 5689) and investigational drugs (n = 3034) for screening application.

2.2. Protein and Ligand Preparation

Preparation of the receptor molecules was carried out using protein preparation wizard present in the maestro workspace. The four major pre-processing steps that were carried out include: (i) bond order assignment, (ii) addition of missing hydrogen atoms, (iii) creation of zero-order bond for the metal atoms and (iv) di-disulfide bond creation. The pre-processed proteins were then subjected to a hydrogen bond optimization process. During the optimization, the protonation state of each amino acid residue was calculated, and the pH was adjusted to 7 ± 0.5 using the predicted pKa values. The predicted and adjusted pKa values of amino acid residues of the proteins were presented in Supplementary Materials Table S1. If the predicted pKa was less than pH value, the amino acid functional groups were protonated during the optimization process. On the other hand, if the pKa was greater than pH value, the deprotonation process took place in those amino acid functional groups. Note that, if the pKa and pH values were equal, 50% protonation and 50% deprotonation took place. Subsequently, the excess water molecules were removed because of the higher occupancy at the receptor binding pocket. Finally, the heavy atoms were converged at the RMSD (root-mean-square deviation) value of 0.30 Å using restrained minimization process [24].

The ligand molecules were processed using LigPrep module in the maestro workspace. Initially, all the ligand molecules were subjected to energy minimization using OPLS_2005 (optimized potentials for liquid simulations) force field at pH 7.0 ± 2. To avoid stereoisomer formation, the chiral centers of all the ligand molecules were chosen to preserve their original state. Notably, all the ligand molecules were allowed to generate only one structural conformation.

2.3. Binding Site Analysis and Grid Generation

Binding site prediction and pocket druggability analysis are the few important perquisites in drug repurposing strategy [25,26]. Here, we used the sitemap algorithm to predict the binding as well as druggable pockets present is the target receptor. Sitemap predicts the hot spots based on the number of hydrogen bond donors and acceptors, hydrophobic atoms and the concave sites present in the receptor [27]. Later, the grid generation was executed by using receptor grid generation wizard. The grid box was generated around the predicted hot spot residues with the partial charge cut-off of 0.25 and a scaling factor of 1.

2.4. Glide Docking and MM/GBSA Analysis

All prepared ligand molecules were screened through the high-throughput virtual screening (HTVS) method followed by being docked into the predicted binding sites using Glide XP (Extra-precision) protocols. We have utilized a flexible docking method with the van der Waals radii scaling factor of 1 Å to soften the receptor binding site. The atoms of the protein with partial charges less than or equal to 0.25 were scaled with a van der Waals scale factor of 0.8 [28]. Later, the ligand interaction diagram was visualized for the in-depth understanding of ligand contacts with the target receptor. Further, the docking score was revalidated by the binding free energy calculations using Prime-MM/GBSA (molecular mechanics with generalized born surface area) analysis. XP docked complexes were further subjected to minimization at the local optimization feature with the force field of OPLS_2005. Prime estimates the binding free energy by comparing the energy of the complex state to the energy of the individual protein and ligand molecules [29].

2.5. Scoring Functions

2.5.1. RF-Score Analysis

The MLSF analyzes the molecular docking outputs of the existing protein–ligand complex to predict the binding affinity of unknown compounds [30]. Here, we used RF-Score-VS, which uses a random forest algorithm to predict the binding affinity of the molecules. It is a standalone program (https://github.com/oddt/rfscorevs, accessed on 3 June 2021) that was implemented using the ubuntu terminal. In this tool, a random forest model was robustly set to generate a maximum number of 500 trees. It is worth noting that random forest model used in this study implicitly captures binding effects that are hard to model explicitly. Protein and ligand molecules were supplied in sdf and pdb format, respectively, for the RF score calculation.

2.5.2. Tanimoto Coefficient Calculation

Tanimoto coefficient is one of the most important similarity measures during the virtual screening process [31]. BulkTanimotoSimilarity() function in the RDKit package gets a fingerprint query and a collection of fingerprints to display the list of similarity results for each fingerprint target. This metric estimates the proportion of the common bits in the range of 0 to 1 between the chemical fingerprints. In this section, the Tanimoto resemblances of all DrugBank compounds were tested against the fingerprints generated by the trametinib.

2.6. Molecular Dynamics (MD) Simulations

The complex structures of two focused compounds and the known drug from molecular docking were dynamically simulated by the near-physiological-motion MD simulations. The AMBER ff14SB force field and generalized AMBER force field version 2 (GAFF2) were employed to treat bonded and non-bonded interaction parameters of all simulated complexes [32]. The TIP3P water model [33] was used to solvate the system with minimum padding of 10.0 Å between the protein surface and the solvation box edge. Then, either sodium or chloride ions were randomly added to neutralize the overall charge of the molecular system. Minimization of the hydrogen atoms and water molecules was performed by using 500 steps of steepest descent (SD) followed by 1500 steps of conjugated gradient (CG) methods. All studied systems were proceeded to run under the periodic boundary condition with the isothermal–isobaric (NPT) scheme according to the previous studies [34–38]. The electrostatic interactions were treated by the particle mesh Ewald summation method [39], whereas The SHAKE algorithm [40] was used to constrain all covalently connected hydrogen atoms. The temperature was controlled by the Langevin thermostat [41] with a collision frequency of 2 ps^{-1} and gradually increased from 10 to 310 K. In addition, Berendsen barostat [42] was employed to control pressure with a relaxation time of 1 ps. Each simulated system was subsequently simulated under the NPT ensemble (310 K, 1 atm) until reaching 100 ns. The MD production for all systems was set to 100 ns by the 2-fs increment of a time step. The root-mean-square displacement (RMSD) and hydrogen bond (H-bond) occupations were calculated through the cpptraj module, while per-residue decomposition energy ($\Delta G_{binding}^{residue}$) was estimated by MM/PBSA.py implemented in AMBER16.

2.7. End-Point Binding Free Energy Calculations

To evaluate the ligand-binding capability, the total binding free energy ($\Delta G_{binding}$) of each complex was estimated based upon the solvated interaction energy (SIE) approach [43]. In theory, ΔG_{bind} can be estimated as the summation of the van der Waals (E_{vdW}), electrostatic ($E_{ele}(D_{in})$), reaction field ($\Delta G_{RF}(\rho,D_{in})$), cavity ($\gamma\Delta SA(\rho)$), and a constant ($C$) value, which was expressed as the following equation

$$\Delta G_{bind}\ (\rho, D_{in}, \alpha, \gamma, C) = \alpha[E_{vdW} + E_{ele}(D_{in}) + \Delta G_{RF}(\rho, D_{in}) + \gamma\Delta SA(\rho)] + constant$$

where D_{in} is the solute interior dielectric constant. E_{vdW} and E_{ele} are denoted as intermolecular van der Waals and Coulombic interaction energies in the bound state, respectively. ΔG_{RF} is the electrostatic polarization component of the solvation free energy to binding, and ΔG_{cavity} ($\gamma\Delta SA$) represents the nonpolar contribution of the solvation free energy to the binding. The coefficients set to every calculation are $\alpha = 0.105$, $\gamma = 0.013$ and $C = -2.89$.

3. Result and Discussion

3.1. Binding Site Prediction

The identification and characterization of the druggable binding pocket of the MEK1 receptor were identified by employing the sitemap module. The best five binding sites of MEK1 and their physiological characteristics predicted by the sitemap were tabulated in Table 1. The larger quantity of hydrophobic residues at the top three sites shows improved pocket adaptation for the ligand binding. Notably, the druggability score of each pocket was in the range of 0.6 to 1. Sites 4 and 5 have a Dscore less than 0.7, which implies the poor druggability of those pockets. Whereas, sites 1, 2 and 3 have resulted in a Dscore of ~1, which indicates that these sites highly encourage the binding of drug-like molecules on their pocket residues [44]. Although the enclosure of site 3 (0.673) is lower, the higher Dscore (1.005) and sitescore (0.974) make the pocket suitable for molecule binding. The top three sites that displayed significant physiological characteristics for the binding of drug-like molecules are shown in Figure 1. Among these three binding sites, site 1 encompasses the end of the activation loop region where the substrate ERK binds to MEK. In addition, site 1 comprises the important amino acid residues for the activation of the MEK receptor and DGF motif, which is an important motif involved in the MEK phosphorylation process. In addition, site 1 comprises amino acid residues, such as VAL 127, SER212, LYS97, VAL211 and ATP binding site [45]. Since site 1 comprises the crucial pockets, we have utilized the results obtained from site 1 during the validation step and other analyses.

Table 1. The top five binding sites of MEK1 receptor predicted by sitemap.

Sites	Site Score	Dscore	Binding Pocket Region
1	1.067	0.995	LEU74, GLY75, ALA76, GLY77, ASN78, GLY79, GLY80, VAL82, ALA95, LYS97, ILE99, VAL127, MET143, GLU144, HIS145, MET146, GLY149, SER150, ASP152, GLN153, LYS192, SER194, ASN195, LEU197, CYS207, ASP208, PHE209, GLY210, VAL211, SER212
2	1.028	1.05	GLU39, GLN45, GLN46, ARG49, LEU50, ALA52, PHE53, LEU54, GLN56, LYS57, LEU92, VAL93, HIS119, GLU120, CYS121, ASN122, SER123, PRO124, TYR125, ILE126, VAL127, GLY128, PHE129, TYR130, GLU144, HIS145, MET146, ASP147, LYS168, ILE171, ALA172, LYS175, ASN199, ARG201, GLY202, GLU203, ILE204, LYS205, ASP365, VAL369, ASP370, PHE371, ALA372
3	0.974	1.005	GLU39, LEU40, GLU41, LEU42, GLN46, ASN122, SER123, PRO124, TYR125, ILE174, LYS175, THR178, TYR179, ARG181, GLU182, LYS183, VAL242, LEU352, LYS353, MET356
4	0.819	0.782	LEU118, HIS119, ILE126, LEU180, HIS184, LYS185, ILE186, MET187, HIS188, ARG189, ASP208, PHE209, GLY210, GLY213, GLN214, ASP217
5	0.702	0.673	VAL254, VAL258, PRO262, PRO265, PRO266, LEU271, PRO321, PRO322, PRO323, LYS324, LEU325, PRO326, SER327, GLN335, ASN339

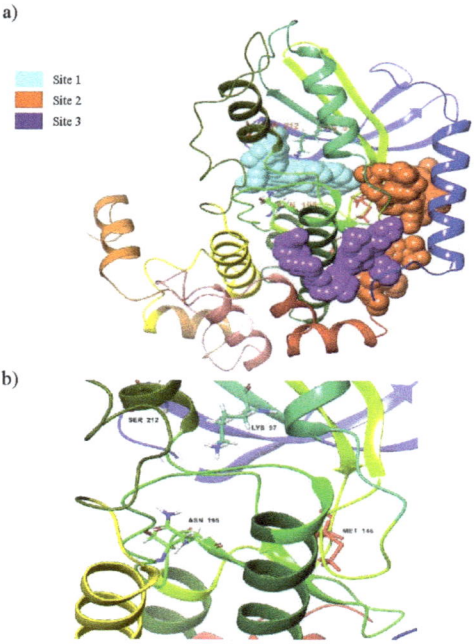

Figure 1. (a) Schematic representation of top three predicted binding sites. (b) Functionally important residues in site 1.

3.2. Validation of Molecular Docking

The validation of Glide XP docking and RF-Score-VS were accomplished by using external datasets (Table S2). The dataset consists of 25 active compounds and 75 decoy compounds against mitogen-activated protein kinase, which were randomly sampled from the Database of Useful Decoys-Enhanced (DUD-E) using the 'sample()' function in pandas to validate the docking and RF-Score-VS analysis. The results were incorporated into the maestro workspace for enrichment analysis [46]. The 'enrichment calculator' tool was used here to evaluate the screening process. On both of the screening analyses, the compounds were sorted by the respective scoring functions, for instance, the Glide XP score and RF-Score-VS_v2 for molecular docking and RF-Score-VS analysis, respectively. Later, the effectiveness of the screening methodologies to differentiate between the actives in the decoy set of compounds was tested by producing a receiver operating curve (ROC) (Figure S1). A total of 11 decoys were outranked during the screening process using RF-Score-VS. On the other hand, seven decoys were outranked during the molecular docking analysis. The smaller number of outranked compounds indicates the effectiveness of these screening algorithms. Further, these measures were evaluated using receiver operating characteristic curve (ROC) analysis. Importantly, the ROC value of docking and RF-Score-VS were 0.902 and 0.850, respectively. Moreover, the area under the curve (AUC) was calculated as 0.801 and 0.762 for molecular docking and RF-Score-VS, respectively. Since the AUC value of docking and RF-Score-VS are above 0.7, we believe that both algorithms have the potential to discriminate the active compounds from the target database. Further, we have accessed Pearson's and Spearman's correlations between the docking score and experimentally determined binding affinity of the 25 active compounds. It is worth noting that Pearson's and Spearman's correlation values of 0.758 and 0.818, respectively, were observed. All of these findings indicate that the lead compounds produced through these screening approaches may potentially be effective towards further experimental works.

3.3. Virtual Screening

A total of 11,808 molecules from the three subsets of Drugbank were screened through the HTVS docking method. Later, the screened hit molecules (n = 7075) were docked into the best predicted binding site, such as site 1, using the Glide XP method. Note that trametinib was used as a reference compound in all the analyses. The XP docking score of reference compound −3.423 kcal/mol in site 1 was then used as a threshold for further screening of hit molecules. Subsequently, the top 50% of the molecules resulting from the XP docking on site 1 were redocked to site 2 and site 3. A total of 3125 and 2813 compounds were predicted to bind better than the reference compound on site 2 and site 3, respectively. The results from the docking study were then integrated to eliminate the false positive compounds. The results indicate that 2468 compounds were able to bind tightly with all three binding sites predicted by the algorithm.

Recently, machine-learning-based scoring functions evolved to measure the binding affinity of the compounds with their multiple characteristic features. In particular, RF-Score-VS obtains a remarkable hit rate up to 88.6% throughout the DUD-E targets [21]. Hence, we analyzed the binding ability of all the screened hit compounds using RF-Score-VS. It is notable that the reference compound trametinib showed an RF-score of 6.565. Fortunately, a total of 5152 compounds were ranked better than the reference compound in RF-Score-VS analysis. The comparison of the docking study and RF-Score calculation yielded a total of 1654 compounds. These compounds were screened through the Tanimoto coefficient calculation using the rdkit package. All the compounds' fingerprints were generated and tested for structural similarity against the reference compound. The calculations of the Tanimoto coefficients of the screened hit compounds were tabulated in Table S3. Here, we chose a Tanimoto coefficient of 0.6 as a threshold value for screening the compounds [47]. Overall, 368 compounds gained a Tanimoto coefficient value above 0.6, which will be taken for further screening studies.

3.4. MM/GBSA Analysis

Recent literature studies highlight that the total binding free energy values predicted during the MM/GBSA calculation correlate well with the experimentally measured biological activity [48]. Thus, Prime-MM/GBSA was implemented as a post-scoring process for the validation of the screened hit molecules. The pose viewer file generated during the Glide XP docking on site 1 was considered as an input file for this analysis. The results of the MM/PBSA studies on the top 15 hit compounds and their associated energy values were represented in Table 2. Moreover, the replicability of the binding affinity by Glide docking was evaluated through three-fold validation of XP docking on 15 hit compounds. The binding free energy values obtained during the three iterations were represented in Table S4. It is evident from the table that the 14 hit compounds were able to display a better docking score than the reference compound in all three docking processes. Although the docking score slightly differs during each docking simulation, the compounds ranking was most likely the same as the initial docking simulation. These results demonstrate the excellent consistency of the compounds ranking during the docking simulation. It is evident from Table 2 that the binding free energy values of the compounds varied from −46 to −87 kcal/mol. The available literature information depicts that lipophilicity and van der Waals energy were key factors for the proper binding of the ligand molecules with the target receptor [49,50]. It is evident from the table that the lipophilicity of the compounds DB12661, DB07642, DB01771 and DB07177 were highly favorable for the ligand binding. Although two compounds, DB01711 and DB07177, showed better lipophilicity, the minimal van der Waals interaction limits the total binding free energy of these compounds.

It should be noted that, except DB02849 and DB04841, most compounds in terms of binding have been highly favored by van der Waals interaction energy. In particular, the compounds DB12661 and DB07642 displayed a massive van der Waals interaction energy value of −57.476 and −55.062 kcal/mol, respectively. Although these compounds show limited coulombic potential, the maximum contribution of van der Waals interaction energy is responsible for the tight binding of these compounds with the MEK1 receptor. Moreover, the total binding free energy values of these compounds, DB012661 and DB07642, were much higher (>−80 kcal/mol), which is also higher than the other compounds investigated in this analysis. Hence, we believe that the compounds DB012661 and DB07642 may more tightly bind with the MEK1 receptor than the other compounds screened in our analysis.

Table 2. Molecular docking and binding free energy calculations of hit compounds against MEK1 receptor.

Compound ID	Docking Score (kcal/mol)	ΔG_{bind} (kcal/mol)	ΔG_{bind} Coulomb	ΔG_{bind} Lipophilic	ΔG_{bind} Solv GB	ΔG_{bind} vdW	Ligand Strain Energy
Reference	−3.423	−46.137	−13.639	−32.888	32.888	−43.528	24.43
DB12661	−7.051	−87.013	−16.84	−46.647	31.692	−57.476	5.29
DB07642	−6.174	−83.845	−20.352	−42.431	28.151	−55.062	8.453
DB02366	−7.427	−76.925	−34.282	−36.488	39.865	−47.657	7.09
DB08251	−11.98	−75.956	−34.186	−24.74	27.909	−44.926	3.995
DB01771	−7.775	−75.093	−28.532	−45.543	38.739	−46.271	10.615
DB12847	−6.716	−66.948	−29.293	−28.799	31.254	−41.632	4.669
DB07177	−6.989	−65.876	−14.264	−51.153	31.763	−39.082	18.693
DB13174	−9.287	−64.939	−22.947	−21.409	20.618	−42.359	2.315
DB07125	−8.416	−63.963	−20.194	−26.628	25.206	−42.305	8.554
DB07773	−9.256	−61.255	−31.925	−29.541	32.325	−36.44	7.628
DB07546	−6.456	−61.064	−24.4	−37.67	35.031	−36.04	9.162
DB02849	−8.72	−59.793	−49.808	−16.914	42.084	−35.493	5.028
DB02709	−7.091	−59.576	−21.878	−29.309	21.114	−32.041	3.817
DB04241	−8.469	−57.965	−46.177	−23.207	30.706	−27.2	10.366

3.5. Structural Properties of Hit Compounds

The similarity between the ligand molecules was evaluated by mapping the pharmacophoric structure of the hit compounds. Here, we have used "2D structure alignment" utility present in the maestro workspace to align the structure of the compound. Moreover, we have predicted the ADME/T properties of the hit compounds using the QikProp module available in the Schrödinger package. These results were incorporated in Table 3. Note that these structures were aligned against the reference compound trametinib. Interestingly, four hit compounds, such as trametinib, DB08251, DB02849, DB04241 and DB12847, had pyridine as a common scaffold in their structures. Pyridine is an essential pharmacophore and an extraordinary heterocyclic system in the realm of anti-cancer drug development [51]. It is also noted that the hit compounds displayed acceptable ADME/T values during the QikProp analysis. The central nervous system activity prediction is one of the main properties during the ADME/T prediction [52]. All the compounds except DB12661 and DB07642 were exhibited at the in-active state, which is indicated by a CNS value of −2. Moreover, the other properties, such as stars (acceptable range: 0–5) and HOA (acceptable range: 1–3), were in the acceptable range in all the hit compounds.

Table 3. 2D structure of hit compounds with their predicted ADME properties.

DrugBank ID	2D Strucure	Stars [a]	CNS [b]	QPlogS [c]	HOA [d]
Reference		1	−2	−8.042	1

Table 3. Cont.

DrugBank ID	2D Strucure	Stars [a]	CNS [b]	QPlogS [c]	HOA [d]
DB08251		1	−2	−3.274	1
DB13174		0	−2	−2.449	2
DB07773		0	−2	−1.457	1
DB02849		1	−2	−2.647	2
DB04241		0	−2	−3.902	2
DB07125		0	−2	−1.666	1
DB01771		0	−2	−2.794	3
DB02366		0	−2	−5.171	3

Table 3. Cont.

DrugBank ID	2D Strucure	Stars [a]	CNS [b]	QPlogS [c]	HOA [d]
DB02709		0	−2	−0.905	2
DB12661		0	0	−5.177	3
DB07177		0	−2	−4.861	3
DB12847		0	−2	−3.52	2
DB07546		0	−2	−5.71	3
DB07642		0	−1	−3.874	3

[a]—The number of attributes or descriptor values that are beyond the 95% range of similar values for identified drugs; [b]—predicted central nervous system activity; [c]—predicted aqueous solubility; [d]—Human Oral Absorption; pink color indications in the 2D structure represent the 2D structure alignment of the compounds against the reference compound.

3.6. Binding Mode Analysis

The binding frequencies of the top 14 compounds on the three different binding sites were represented in Figure S2. It is notable that the binding positions of the compounds at each binding site were more or less the same in site 1 and site 3. Since the binding site residues were dispersed larger in site 2, a few compounds, such as DB12661, DB02709, DB12847 and DB08251, were positioned differently from the other compounds. Most of the ligand molecules were bound tightly in site 1, as indicated by the better docking score in Table S3. Hence, the ligand binding conformations of the top hit compounds in site 1 were analyzed (Figure 2). It is evident from the figure that all the hit compounds exhibited two hydrogen bond interactions with the MEK1 receptor, while the reference compound displayed three hydrogen bond interactions with the binding site of MEK1. The iodoalinine moiety of trametinib produces a hydrogen bond interaction with SER 194 of the MEK1 receptor. On the other hand, the cyclopropyl moiety of trametinib makes two hydrogen bond interactions with SER 194 and ASN 195 of the MEK1 receptor. Surprisingly, the quinazoline moiety of the compound DB07642 and methoxy phenyl group DB012661 were producing interactions with LYS 97, which is also an important catalytic residue present in the rooftop of the MEK1 binding pocket. It is also noted that LYS 97 located in the β strand is responsible for the pairing of ATP phosphate to GLU 114 on an adjacent alpha helix [45]. Moreover, the oxygen atom linked with the pyrimidine group of DB12661 makes a hydrogen bond interaction with MET 146, a hinge residue that connects the N and C lobes in the MEK1 receptor [53]. Most importantly, the quinazoline moiety of DB07642 forms an additional hydrogen bond interaction with activation loop residue, such as SER 212, which plays a major role in the phosphorylation of MEK1. It is evident from the literature that most of the MEK 1/2 ligands generate strong interactions with SER 212 [54]. It is important to note that both the lead compounds are bound on the same pattern where the known MEK inhibitors bind. For instance, rafemetinib and RO4987655 interacted with the amino acid residues LYS97 and SER212 of the MEK receptor. On the other hand, CI-1040, PD-0325901, cobimetinib, TAK-733 and GDC-0623 were successfully involved in contact with SER212 of the MEK receptor [6,45]. Based on these pieces of evidence, we are certain that compounds such as DB07642 and DB12661 make strong contact with the functionally important amino acid residues of MEK.

In general, the compound DB012661, also known as urapidil, acts as an antihypertensive drug that inhibits the activity of α-adrenoceptor. It is worth noting that the compound urapidil also resulted in substantial inhibitory activity in several cancer cell lines [55]. On the other hand, the compound DB07642 (5-[1-(2-Fluorobenzyl)piperidin-4-yl]methoxyquinazoline-2,4-diamine) contains crucial pharmacophores. For instance, piperidine, a heterocyclic pharmacophore, has immense importance in the field of drug development. The piperidine derivatives effectively block the several kinase targets (ERK 2, VEGFR 2 and Alb 1) during the in vitro assessment in the liver cancer cell line (HepG2) [56]. Quinazoline is another important pharmacophore that is present in the many approved anticancer drugs, such as erlotinib and vandetanib [57]. Overall, we believe that these compounds may potentially block the activation of MEK, thereby reducing the risk of many malignant effects.

3.7. Binding Analysis of Lead Compounds with PIM1

The binding abilities of the lead compounds were also tested on the PIM1 receptor, which is frequently cross-talked with the MAPK pathway. Molecular docking and prime-MM/GBSA analysis of the lead compounds tested against PIM1 were tabulated in Table S5. It is notable that the recently identified dual inhibitor (MEK1 and PIM1) KZ-02 was used as the reference compound in this analysis. The compound KZ-02 obtained a docking score of −4.892 kcal/mol and a binding free energy value of −50.61 kcal/mol. It is notable that both lead compounds displayed better docking scores and binding free energy values than the PIM1 reference compound. The interactions of the lead compounds with the PIM1 receptor were represented in Figure S3. Interestingly, the compound DB07642 displayed three hydrogen bond interactions and 2 pi-pi stacking with the PIM1 receptor. This implies the greater binding potential of the compound DB07642 with the PIM1 receptor. Altogether, we hypothesize that the lead compounds specified in this study may significantly inhibit the activation of both MEK1 and PIM1.

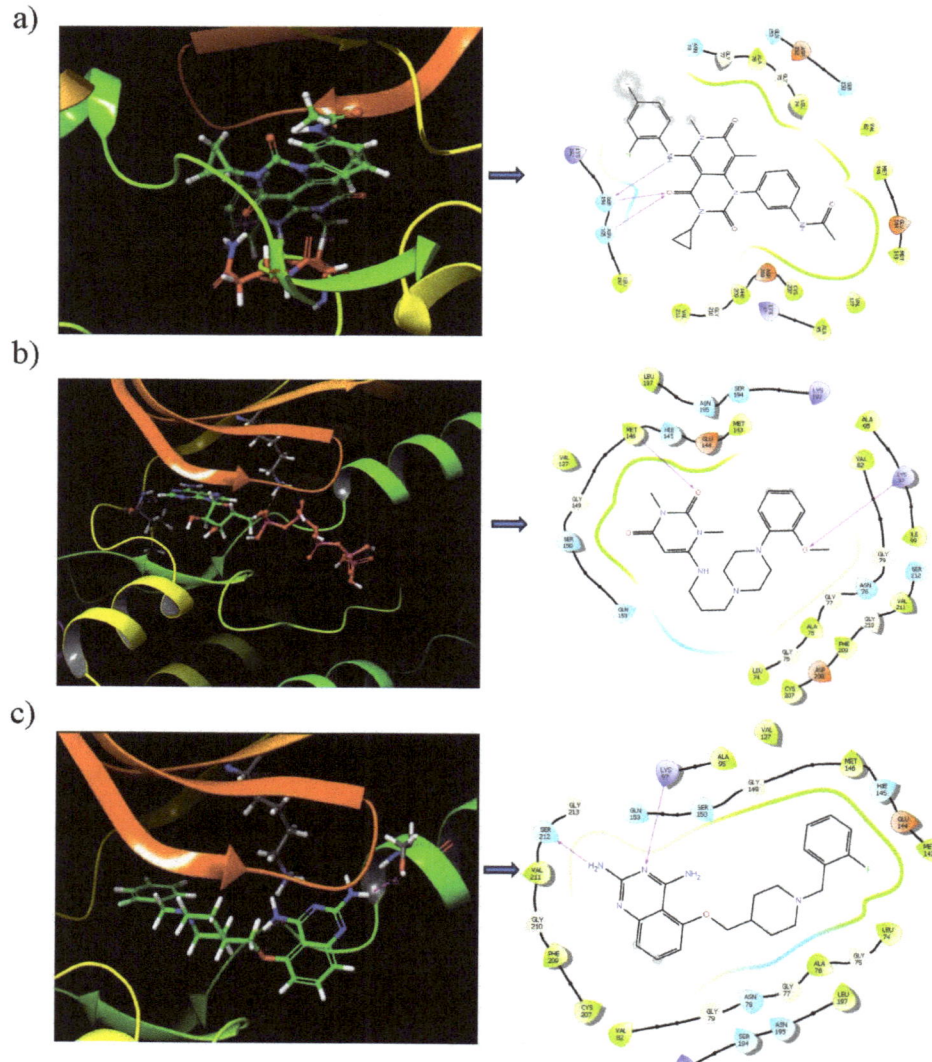

Figure 2. Ligand interaction diagram of the hit compounds. (**a**) Reference; (**b**) DB12661; (**c**) DB07642 with MEK1 receptor.

3.8. SIE-Based Free Energy of Binding

Since molecular recognition and drug binding have been recognized as dynamic processes, it is thus particularly important to elaborate on the protein–ligand binding capabilities in a presumed dynamic system. To this end, the free energy of binding (ΔG_{bind}) calculations based on the solvated interaction energy (SIE) were applied and theoretically used to predict the inhibitory activity as it is directly proportional to an experimental inhibitory parameter, K_d ($\Delta G_{bind} = -RT\ln 1/Kd$) [58]. Here, the ΔG_{bind} values of two focused compounds extracted from the last 10 ns (90–100 ns) snapshots, which were considered to be reaching their equilibrated state (Figure S4), were listed in Table 4 in comparison to the trametinib. The calculated molecular mechanics calculations showed that

Van der Waal (vdW) is the main interactive force contributing to the process of molecular complexation of all the focused compounds as well as trametinib (>five to six-fold than electrostatic interaction energy), which corresponds to the molecular docking study by Glide XP. Apart from that, the average ΔG_{bind} values of the focused compounds and a reference drug were nearly the same, within the range of −8.4 to −7.5 kcal/mol. In particular, DB12661 possessed a slightly lower ΔG_{bind} when compared to the trametinib (ΔG_{bind} of −8.41 and −8.17 kcal/mol, respectively), suggesting a minutely higher binding strength than the known drug. On the contrary, compound DB07642 exhibited a slightly higher ΔG_{bind} value (ΔG_{bind} of −7.52 kcal/mol), which may imply a slight reduction in the ligand binding capability. However, we believed that these two screened compounds could be thermodynamically able to bind to the MEK1 at the ATP-binding site, and both are of particular interest to be subjected to next-step experimental studies, for which DB12661 and DB07642 were rationally considered as a priority and a second top, accordingly.

Table 4. Average ΔG_{bind} values (kcal/mol) of focused compounds as well as trametinib in complex with MEK1 calculated by the SIE method using α = 0.105, γ = 0.013 and C = −2.89, respectively.

Compounds	Energy Components				
	E_{vdW}	E_{ele}	Reaction Field	Cavity	ΔG_{bind}
Trametinib	−51.05 ± 0.34	−9.58 ± 0.20	19.25 ± 0.26	−9.05 ± 0.07	−8.17 ± 0.04
DB12661	−52.08 ± 0.32	−4.29 ± 0.17	12.18 ± 0.24	−8.52 ± 0.05	−8.41 ± 0.04
DB07642	−43.91 ± 0.37	−6.90 ± 0.21	14.62 ± 0.36	−8.02 ± 0.06	−7.52 ± 0.04

3.9. Key Binding Residues

In order to elucidate the key binding amino acid residues within the ATP-binding pocket located at the ATPase domain of MEK1, the decomposition free energy ($\Delta G_{residue}^{bind}$) based upon the MM/GBSA method was computationally predicted, and the total contribution of each amino acid of the known drug and focused complexes was plotted, in which the negative and positive decomposition free energy values manifested the ligand stabilization and destabilization, respectively, as illustrated in Figure 3. It was found that the contributing amino acid residues observed in all the complexes were mainly stabilized through van der Waals (vdW) interactions rather than electrostatic force. This indicates that these two candidate compounds may rely on a mechanism of inhibitory action similar to trametinib. In particular, the amino acids that largely contributed towards the trametinib's binding ($\Delta G < -1.0$ kcal/mol) include ASN78, VAL82, LYS97, SER150, SER194, ASN195, LEU197 and ASP208, of which the SER194 and ASN195 were also found from the docking pose. Among these, ASN78, LYS97 and ASN195 played a pivotal role in the complex stabilization ($\Delta G < -2.0$ kcal/mol). In the case of the candidate compounds, it was found that the key amino acid residues contributing to the DB07642 binding are mostly the same residues responsible for trametinib's binding (ASN78, VAL82, LYS97 and ASN195); one additional residue, M143, was observed. Apart from that, compound DB12661 was primarily stabilized through hydrophobic residue of VAL82 ($\Delta G_{bind} = -2.73$ kcal/mol), while seven other residues (LEU74, GLY80, VAL81, LYS97, HIS145, MET146 and LEU197) were also found in the stabilization of the complex via vdW interactions with $\Delta G_{residue}^{bind}$ in the range of −2.0 to −1.0 kcal/mol. Nevertheless, one negatively charged residue, ASP208, was found to be slightly destabilized; that was probably due to the charge–charge repulsion in the complex system. To sum up, with a higher number of residues largely contributing to DB12661 binding, this compound, as expected, possessed the lowest vdW interactive and total binding free energy (Table 4), where the set of vdW interactions became the main driving force towards the complex formation. On the contrary, some contributing amino acid residues (observed in both trametinib and DB12661) may be somewhat lost during the MEK1–DB07642 complex formation, resulting in the slightly lower ΔG_{bind} when compared to the trametinib. We noted that these results are correlated well with the calculated SIE-based ΔG_{bind} and each energy component, as listed in Table 4.

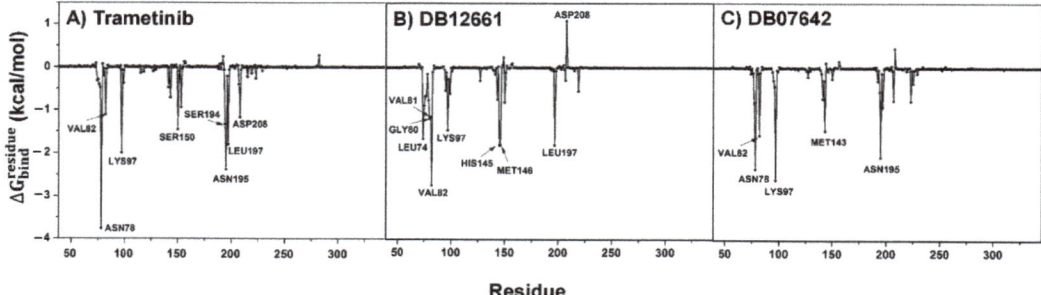

Figure 3. Per-residue decomposition free energy ($\Delta G^{bind}_{residue}$) of the ATPase pocket of MEK1 for the binding of the (**A**,**B**) two screened compounds and (**C**) the known drug, trametinib.

3.10. Ligand–Protein Hydrogen Bonding

Hydrogen bonding is one of the non-covalent interactions observed in the formation of protein–ligand complexes and could influence the ligand binding strength. Hence, the intermolecular hydrogen bond interactions were investigated in terms of the percentage of occupations and plotted in Figure 4. As expected, a few strong hydrogen bonds could be observed in the screened compounds and even the trametinib since they are intrinsically hydrophobic ligands. The reference drug trametinib created a strong hydrogen bond with ASN195 (65%), which was also observed by the docking pose (Figure 2). In addition, ALA76 and ASN78 moderately stabilized the drug through 45% and 44.5% of the hydrogen bond occupations, while ASN78 could additionally interact with the drug through 35% of it. For the MEK1–DB12661 complex, we found that the H atom in the backbone (-NH$_2$) of MET146 exhibited a very strong hydrogen bond, while the polar H atom in the imidazole ring of HIS145 showed a moderate level. In the case of DB07642, there are three amino acid residues stabilizing the DB07642 binding, which include ASN195, ASP208 and SER194. Among these, the H atom in the amino side chain of ASN195 displayed the highest chance of hydrogen bond occurrence with percentage occupations of 26%, while the other two residues merely exhibited a weak hydrogen bond ($\approx$17%). Altogether, these obtained results suggested that the intermolecular hydrogen bond interactions did not play a major role responsible for the complex stabilization observed in all the studied compounds, including the trametinib. On the other hand, the ligand binding within the ATP-binding pocket of MEK1 was predominantly contributed by vdW interactions, as discussed previously.

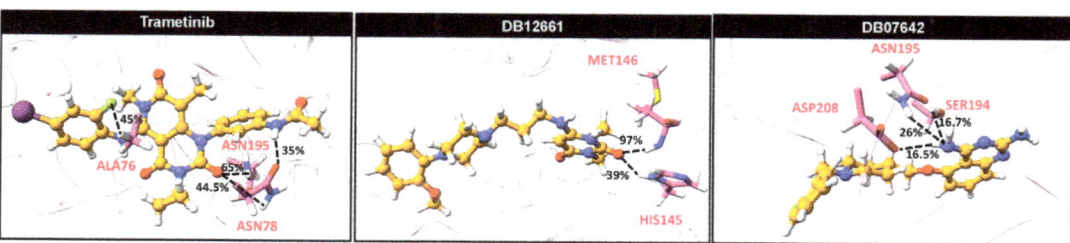

Figure 4. Percentage of hydrogen bond occupations contributing to the binding of two screened compounds (DB12661 and DB07642) and the trametinib within the ATPase domain of MEK1 using two criteria involving the distance and angle between the hydrogen bond donor (HD) and hydrogen acceptor (HA) of $\leq$3.5 Å for the distance and $\geq$120° for the angle, respectively.

4. Conclusions

In conclusion, the DrugBank compounds were screened through the different computational approaches to discover the potential MEK inhibitors. Initially, molecular docking and various scoring functions were implemented to screen the active molecules against the MEK protein. Overall, the screening demonstrated that compounds such as DB07642 and DB12661 were able to tightly bind with the MEK receptor. Notably, the presence of crucial pharmacophore moieties in the hit compounds gives additional support to their inhibitory activity. In addition, the modes of action of these compounds were comprehended through the connection of the ligand with the MEK active segment residues. Most importantly, the compounds' inhibitory activity was also examined with the PIM1 receptor since it upregulated during the action of several MEK inhibitors. Further, the MD simulation and end-point free energy calculation validated the binding mode of the lead compounds with the MEK receptor. Thus, we hypothesize that further experimental validation of our research findings will help to level up the cancer treatment in the near future.

Supplementary Materials: The following supporting information can be downloaded at: https://www.mdpi.com/article/10.3390/pharmaceutics14010059/s1. Table S1: Predicted pKa values of each amino acid residues at different conditions. Table S2: Compounds used for validation of docking and RF-Score-VS. Table S3: Multiple screening analysis of the compounds against MEK1. Table S4: Three-fold validation on glide docking analysis of hit compounds. Table S5: Molecular docking and binding free energy calculations of top hit compounds against PIM1 receptor. Figure S1: ROC analysis of screening methods. (a) Docking; (b) RF-Score-VS. Figure S2: Binding frequency of the ligand molecules on top three predicted binding sites. The coloured dots represent the binding sites: site 1 (red), site 2 (orange), and site 3 (yellow). The coloured chemical structures depict ligand molecules binding positions on various binding sites. Ligand bound in site 1 (purple); site 2 (green); site 3 (sky blue). Figure S3: Ligand interaction diagram of hit compounds (a) KZ-02 (Reference); (b) DB012661; (c) DB07642 with PIM1 receptor. Figure S4: Root-mean-square displacement (RMSD) plot for the backbone amino acid residues within a 5-Å sphere around the ligand. The data were derived from the three independent runs with different initial velocities.

Author Contributions: M.K.T. performed the data collection, preparation and virtual screening. U.S. performed the molecular dynamic simulation and binding free energy analysis. M.K.T. and U.S. performed the result analysis and wrote the initial version of manuscript. R.K. and T.R. conceived this study and are responsible for the overall design, interpretation, manuscript preparation, and communication. All authors have read and agreed to the published version of the manuscript.

Funding: T.R. acknowledge the supports from the Thailand Research Fund (grant number RSA6280085).

Institutional Review Board Statement: Not applicable.

Informed Consent Statement: Not applicable.

Data Availability Statement: Not applicable.

Acknowledgments: The authors (M.K.T. and R.K.) thank the management of Vellore Institute of Technology. The author (U.S. and T.R) would like to thank the Science Achievement Scholarship (SAST) of Thailand for the Ph.D. scholarship, the 90th Anniversary of Chulalongkorn University Fund (Ratchadaphiseksomphot), and the Overseas Presentations of Graduate Level Academic Thesis from Graduate School.

Conflicts of Interest: The authors declare that they have no conflict of interest.

References

1. Bradley, S.H.; Kennedy, M.P.T.; Neal, R.D. Recognising lung cancer in primary care. *Adv. Ther.* **2019**, *36*, 19–30. [CrossRef] [PubMed]
2. Malik, P.S.; Raina, V. Lung cancer: Prevalent trends & emerging concepts. *Indian J. Med. Res.* **2015**, *141*, 5–7. [PubMed]
3. Li, S.; Xu, S.; Liang, X.; Xue, Y.; Mei, J.; Ma, Y.; Liu, Y.; Liu, Y. Nanotechnology: Breaking the current treatment limits of lung cancer. *Adv. Healthc. Mater.* **2021**, *10*, 2100078. [CrossRef]
4. Yuan, M.; Huang, L.-L.; Chen, J.-H.; Wu, J.; Xu, Q. The emerging treatment landscape of targeted therapy in non-small-cell lung cancer. *Signal Transduct. Target.* **2019**, *4*, 61. [CrossRef]

5. Sharma, S.V.; Bell, D.W.; Settleman, J.; Haber, D.A. Epidermal growth factor receptor mutations in lung cancer. *Nat. Rev. Cancer* 2007, *7*, 169–181. [CrossRef] [PubMed]
6. Han, J.; Liu, Y.; Yang, S.; Wu, X.; Li, H.; Wang, Q. Mek inhibitors for the treatment of non-small cell lung cancer. *J. Hematol. Oncol.* 2021, *14*, 1. [CrossRef]
7. Ostrem, J.M.; Peters, U.; Sos, M.L.; Wells, J.A.; Shokat, K.M. K-RAS (G12C) inhibitors allosterically control GTP affinity and effector interactions. *Nature* 2013, *503*, 548–551. [CrossRef]
8. Yaeger, R.; Corcoran, R.B. Targeting alterations in the RAF–MEK pathway. *Cancer Discov.* 2019, *9*, 329–341. [CrossRef] [PubMed]
9. Hegedüs, L.; Okumus, Ö.; Livingstone, E.; Baranyi, M.; Kovács, I.; Döme, B.; Tóvári, J.; Bánkfalvi, Á.; Schadendorf, D.; Aigner, C. Allosteric and ATP-competitive MEK-inhibition in a novel spitzoid melanoma model with a RAF-and phosphorylation-independent mutation. *Cancers* 2021, *13*, 829. [CrossRef]
10. Heigener, D.F.; Gandara, D.R.; Reck, M. Targeting of MEK in lung cancer therapeutics. *Lancet Respir. Med.* 2015, *3*, 319–327. [CrossRef]
11. Zhao, Y.; Adjei, A.A. The clinical development of MEK inhibitors. *Nat. Rev. Clin. Oncol.* 2014, *11*, 385–400. [CrossRef]
12. Menzies, A.M.; Long, G.V. Dabrafenib and trametinib, alone and in combination for BRAF-mutant metastatic melanoma. *Clin. Cancer Res.* 2014, *20*, 2035–2043. [CrossRef]
13. Odogwu, L.; Mathieu, L.; Blumenthal, G.; Larkins, E.; Goldberg, K.B.; Griffin, N.; Bijwaard, K.; Lee, E.Y.; Philip, R.; Jiang, X. Fda approval summary: Dabrafenib and trametinib for the treatment of metastatic non-small cell lung cancers harboring BRAF V600E mutations. *Oncologist* 2018, *23*, 740. [CrossRef]
14. Renouf, D.J.; Velazquez-Martin, J.P.; Simpson, R.; Siu, L.L.; Bedard, P.L. Ocular toxicity of targeted therapies. *J. Clin. Oncol.* 2012, *30*, 3277–3286. [CrossRef]
15. Jin, J.; Guo, Q.; Xie, J.; Jin, D.; Zhu, Y. Combination of MEK inhibitor and the JAK2-STAT3 pathway inhibition for the therapy of colon cancer. *Pathol. Oncol. Res.* 2019, *25*, 769–775. [CrossRef]
16. Sato, H.; Yamamoto, H.; Sakaguchi, M.; Shien, K.; Tomida, S.; Shien, T.; Ikeda, H.; Hatono, M.; Torigoe, H.; Namba, K.; et al. Combined inhibition of MEK and PI3K pathways overcomes acquired resistance to EGFR-TKIs in non-small cell lung cancer. *Cancer Sci.* 2018, *109*, 3183–3196. [CrossRef]
17. Cortes, J.; Tamura, K.; DeAngelo, D.J.; De Bono, J.; Lorente, D.; Minden, M.; Uy, G.L.; Kantarjian, H.; Chen, L.S.; Gandhi, V. Phase I studies of azd1208, a proviral integration moloney virus kinase inhibitor in solid and haematological cancers. *Br. J. Cancer* 2018, *118*, 1425–1433. [CrossRef] [PubMed]
18. Le, X.; Antony, R.; Razavi, P.; Treacy, D.J.; Luo, F.; Ghandi, M.; Castel, P.; Scaltriti, M.; Baselga, J.; Garraway, L.A. Systematic functional characterization of resistance to PI3K inhibition in breast cancer. *Cancer Discov.* 2016, *6*, 1134–1147. [CrossRef] [PubMed]
19. Swinney, D.C.; Anthony, J. How were new medicines discovered? *Nat. Rev. Drug Discov.* 2011, *10*, 507–519. [CrossRef]
20. Sohraby, F.; Bagheri, M.; Aryapour, H. Performing an in silico repurposing of existing drugs by combining virtual screening and molecular dynamics simulation. In *Computational Methods for Drug Repurposing*; Springer: Cham, Switzerland, 2019; pp. 23–43.
21. Wójcikowski, M.; Ballester, P.J.; Siedlecki, P. Performance of machine-learning scoring functions in structure-based virtual screening. *Sci. Rep.* 2017, *7*, 46710. [CrossRef] [PubMed]
22. Wurz, R.P.; Sastri, C.; D'Amico, D.C.; Herberich, B.; Jackson, C.L.; Pettus, L.H.; Tasker, A.S.; Wu, B.; Guerrero, N.; Lipford, J.R. Discovery of imidazopyridazines as potent PIM-1/2 kinase inhibitors. *Bioorg. Med. Chem. Lett.* 2016, *26*, 5580–5590. [CrossRef]
23. Protein Data Bank; Nakae, S.; Kitamura, M.; Shirai, T.; Tada, T. Structure of the Human Mitogen-Activated Protein Kinase Kinase 1 (MEK1). 2014. Available online: https://datamed.org/display-item.php?repository=0002&id=5952ebec5152c64c3b126f08&query=MAP2K1 (accessed on 3 May 2021).
24. Rohini, K.; Ramanathan, K.; Shanthi, V. Multi-dimensional screening strategy for drug repurposing with statistical framework—A new road to influenza drug discovery. *Cell Biochem. Biophys.* 2019, *77*, 319–333. [CrossRef] [PubMed]
25. Halgren, T.A. Identifying and characterizing binding sites and assessing druggability. *J. Chem. Inf. Model.* 2009, *49*, 377–389. [CrossRef] [PubMed]
26. Patschull, A.O.; Gooptu, B.; Ashford, P.; Daviter, T.; Nobeli, I. In silico assessment of potential druggable pockets on the surface of α1-antitrypsin conformers. *PLoS ONE* 2012, *7*, e36612. [CrossRef] [PubMed]
27. Schrödinger. *Sitemap, Schrödinger Release-2020*; Schrödinger: New York, NY, USA, 2020.
28. Zhou, H.; Wang, C.; Deng, T.; Tao, R.; Li, W. Novel urushiol derivatives as HDAC8 inhibitors: Rational design, virtual screening, molecular docking and molecular dynamics studies. *J. Biomol. Struct. Dyn.* 2018, *36*, 1966–1978. [CrossRef]
29. Borkotoky, S.; Meena, C.K.; Murali, A. Interaction analysis of T7 RNA polymerase with heparin and its low molecular weight derivatives—An in silico approach. *Bioinform. Biol. Insights* 2016, *10*, 155–166. [CrossRef]
30. Ballester, P.J.; Mitchell, J.B. A machine learning approach to predicting protein–ligand binding affinity with applications to molecular docking. *Bioinformatics* 2010, *26*, 1169–1175. [CrossRef]
31. Williams, C. Reverse fingerprinting, similarity searching by group fusion and fingerprint bit importance. *Mol. Divers.* 2006, *10*, 311–332. [CrossRef]
32. Wang, J.; Wolf, R.M.; Caldwell, J.W.; Kollman, P.A.; Case, D.A. Development and testing of a general amber force field. *J. Comput. Chem.* 2004, *25*, 1157–1174. [CrossRef]
33. Jorgensen, W.L.; Chandrasekhar, J.; Madura, J.D.; Impey, R.W.; Klein, M.L. Comparison of simple potential functions for simulating liquid water. *J. Chem. Phys.* 1983, *79*, 926–935. [CrossRef]

34. Kammarabutr, J.; Mahalapbutr, P.; Nutho, B.; Kungwan, N.; Rungrotmongkol, T. Low susceptibility of asunaprevir towards R155K and D168A point mutations in HCV NS3/4A protease: A molecular dynamics simulation. *J. Mol. Graph.* **2019**, *89*, 122–130. [CrossRef] [PubMed]
35. Mahalapbutr, P.; Wonganan, P.; Chavasiri, W.; Rungrotmongkol, T. Butoxy mansonone G inhibits STAT3 and AKT signaling pathways in non-small cell lung cancers: Combined experimental and theoretical investigations. *Cancers* **2019**, *11*, 437. [CrossRef]
36. Meeprasert, A.; Hannongbua, S.; Rungrotmongkol, T. Key binding and susceptibility of NS3/4A serine protease inhibitors against hepatitis C virus. *J. Chem. Inf. Model.* **2014**, *54*, 1208–1217. [CrossRef] [PubMed]
37. Nutho, B.; Mahalapbutr, P.; Hengphasatporn, K.; Pattaranggoon, N.C.; Simanon, N.; Shigeta, Y.; Hannongbua, S.; Rungrotmongkol, T. Why are lopinavir and ritonavir effective against the newly emerged coronavirus 2019? Atomistic insights into the inhibitory mechanisms. *Biochemistry* **2020**, *59*, 1769–1779. [CrossRef] [PubMed]
38. Nutho, B.; Rungrotmongkol, T. Binding recognition of substrates in NS2B/NS3 serine protease of zika virus revealed by molecular dynamics simulations. *J. Mol. Graph. Model.* **2019**, *92*, 227–235. [CrossRef]
39. Darden, T.; York, D.; Pedersen, L. Particle mesh ewald: An N·log(N) method for ewald sums in large systems. *J. Chem. Phys.* **1993**, *98*, 10089–10092. [CrossRef]
40. Ryckaert, J.-P.; Ciccotti, G.; Berendsen, H.J.C. Numerical integration of the cartesian equations of motion of a system with constraints: Molecular dynamics of n-alkanes. *J. Comput. Phys.* **1977**, *23*, 327–341. [CrossRef]
41. Uberuaga, B.P.; Anghel, M.; Voter, A.F. Synchronization of trajectories in canonical molecular-dynamics simulations: Observation, explanation, and exploitation. *J. Chem. Phys.* **2004**, *120*, 6363–6374. [CrossRef]
42. Berendsen, H.J.; Postma, J.V.; van Gunsteren, W.F.; DiNola, A.R.H.J.; Haak, J.R. Molecular dynamics with coupling to an external bath. *J. Chem. Phys.* **1984**, *81*, 3684–3690. [CrossRef]
43. Naïm, M.; Bhat, S.; Rankin, K.N.; Dennis, S.; Chowdhury, S.F.; Siddiqi, I.; Drabik, P.; Sulea, T.; Bayly, C.I.; Jakalian, A.; et al. Solvated interaction energy (SIE) for scoring protein−ligand binding affinities. 1. Exploring the parameter space. *J. Chem. Inf. Model.* **2007**, *47*, 122–133. [CrossRef]
44. Ghattas, M.A.; Raslan, N.; Sadeq, A.; Al Sorkhy, M.; Atwater, N. Druggability analysis and classification of protein tyrosine phosphatase active sites. *Drug Des. Dev. Ther.* **2016**, *10*, 3197. [CrossRef] [PubMed]
45. Wu, P.-K.; Park, J.-I. Mek1/2 inhibitors: Molecular activity and resistance mechanisms. *Semin. Oncol.* **2015**, *42*, 849–862. [CrossRef]
46. Gentile, F.; Agrawal, V.; Hsing, M.; Ton, A.-T.; Ban, F.; Norinder, U.; Gleave, M.E.; Cherkasov, A. Deep docking: A deep learning platform for augmentation of structure based drug discovery. *ACS Cent. Sci.* **2020**, *6*, 939–949. [CrossRef]
47. Backman, T.W.; Cao, Y.; Girke, T. Chemmine tools: An online service for analyzing and clustering small molecules. *Nucleic Acids Res.* **2011**, *39*, W486–W491. [CrossRef]
48. Tripathi, S.K.; Muttineni, R.; Singh, S.K. Extra precision docking, free energy calculation and molecular dynamics simulation studies of CDK2 inhibitors. *J. Theor. Biol.* **2013**, *334*, 87–100. [CrossRef]
49. Abdel-Hamid, M.K.; McCluskey, A. In silico docking, molecular dynamics and binding energy insights into the bolinaquinone-clathrin terminal domain binding site. *Molecules* **2014**, *19*, 6609–6622. [CrossRef]
50. Singh, K.D.; Muthusamy, K. Molecular modeling, quantum polarized ligand docking and structure-based 3D-QSAR analysis of the imidazole series as dual AT1 and ETa receptor antagonists. *Acta Pharmacol. Sin.* **2013**, *34*, 1592–1606. [CrossRef] [PubMed]
51. Sahu, R.; Mishra, R.; Kumar, R.; Mazumder, A.; Kumar, A. Pyridine moiety: Recent advances in cancer treatment. *Indian J. Pharm. Sci.* **2021**, *83*, 162–185. [CrossRef]
52. Miles, J.A.; Ng, J.H.; Sreenivas, B.Y.; Courageux, C.; Igert, A.; Dias, J.; McGeary, R.P.; Brazzolotto, X.; Ross, B.P. Discovery of drug-like acetylcholinesterase inhibitors by rapid virtual screening of a 6.9 million compound database. *Chem. Biol. Drug Des.* **2021**, *97*, 1048–1058. [CrossRef]
53. Roskoski, R., Jr. MEK1/2 dual-specificity protein kinases: Structure and regulation. *Biochem. Biophys. Res. Commun.* **2012**, *417*, 5–10. [CrossRef] [PubMed]
54. Zhao, Z.; Xie, L.; Bourne, P.E. Insights into the binding mode of MEK Type-III inhibitors. A step towards discovering and designing allosteric kinase inhibitors across the human kinome. *PLoS ONE* **2017**, *12*, e0179936. [CrossRef]
55. Varalda, M.; Antona, A.; Bettio, V.; Roy, K.; Vachamaram, A.; Yellenki, V.; Massarotti, A.; Baldanzi, G.; Capello, D. Psychotropic drugs show anticancer activity by disrupting mitochondrial and lysosomal function. *Front. Oncol.* **2020**, *10*, 2148. [CrossRef]
56. Jin, F.; Gao, D.; Wu, Q.; Liu, F.; Chen, Y.; Tan, C.; Jiang, Y. Exploration of N-(2-aminoethyl) piperidine-4-carboxamide as a potential scaffold for development of VEGFR-2, ERK-2 and ABL-1 multikinase inhibitor. *Bioorg. Med. Chem.* **2013**, *21*, 5694–5706. [CrossRef] [PubMed]
57. Ahmad, I. An insight into the therapeutic potential of quinazoline derivatives as anticancer agents. *MedChemComm* **2017**, *8*, 871–885.
58. Du, X.; Li, Y.; Xia, Y.L.; Ai, S.M.; Liang, J.; Sang, P.; Ji, X.L.; Liu, S.Q. Insights into protein-ligand interactions: Mechanisms, models, and methods. *Int. J. Mol. Sci.* **2016**, *17*, 144. [CrossRef] [PubMed]

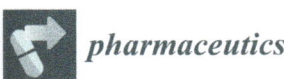

Article

A Single-Cell Network-Based Drug Repositioning Strategy for Post-COVID-19 Pulmonary Fibrosis

Albert Li [1], Jhih-Yu Chen [1], Chia-Lang Hsu [2,3], Yen-Jen Oyang [1], Hsuan-Cheng Huang [4,*] and Hsueh-Fen Juan [1,5,6,*]

1 Graduate Institute of Biomedical Electronics and Bioinformatics, National Taiwan University, Taipei 106, Taiwan; albert0325162@gmail.com (A.L.); a402250025@gmail.com (J.-Y.C.); yjoyang@csie.ntu.edu.tw (Y.-J.O.)
2 Department of Medical Research, National Taiwan University Hospital, Taipei 106, Taiwan; chialanghsu@ntuh.gov.tw
3 Graduate Institute of Medical Genomics and Proteomics, National Taiwan University, Taipei 106, Taiwan
4 Institute of Biomedical Informatics, National Yang Ming Chiao Tung University, Taipei 112, Taiwan
5 Department of Life Science, National Taiwan University, Taipei 106, Taiwan
6 Center for Computational and Systems Biology, National Taiwan University, Taipei 106, Taiwan
* Correspondence: hsuancheng@nycu.edu.tw (H.-C.H.); yukijuan@ntu.edu.tw (H.-F.J.)

Abstract: Post-COVID-19 pulmonary fibrosis (PCPF) is a long-term complication that appears in some COVID-19 survivors. However, there are currently limited options for treating PCPF patients. To address this problem, we investigated COVID-19 patients' transcriptome at single-cell resolution and combined biological network analyses to repurpose the drugs treating PCPF. We revealed a novel gene signature of PCPF. The signature is functionally associated with the viral infection and lung fibrosis. Further, the signature has good performance in diagnosing and assessing pulmonary fibrosis. Next, we applied a network-based drug repurposing method to explore novel treatments for PCPF. By quantifying the proximity between the drug targets and the signature in the interactome, we identified several potential candidates and provided a drug list ranked by their proximity. Taken together, we revealed a novel gene expression signature as a theragnostic biomarker for PCPF by integrating different computational approaches. Moreover, we showed that network-based proximity could be used as a framework to repurpose drugs for PCPF.

Keywords: single-cell RNA sequencing; COVID-19; pulmonary fibrosis; biological networks; drug repurposing

1. Introduction

Since 2019, the outbreak of the COVID-19 pandemic has caused millions of infections globally. Some patients may suffer from sequelae of the viral infection [1]. Post-COVID-19 pulmonary fibrosis (PCPF) is one of the long-term complications being emphasized recently [1]. Considering the medical treatments for this disease are limited, it is crucial to leverage pharmacogenomic data to repurpose drugs treating this disease. In this study, we combine single-cell analysis, machine learning, and network biology to identify a novel transcriptomic signature. We show that this signature is promising in assessing the disease and surveying drugs that can potentially treat pulmonary fibrosis.

Previously, network-based methods have successfully repurposed drugs treating several diseases [2–5]. Based on the property of biological networks, drugs with smaller proximity tend to be more effective than those with larger proximity [3]. However, since the choice of disease-related genes will largely impact results and inferences [6], whether the network-based approach can be applied to PCPF needs further verification.

Single-cell RNA-sequencing analysis (scRNA-seq) has been used to investigate the host response in severe COVID-19 cases [7]. Melms et al. discovered that two cell types,

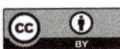

pathological and intermediate-pathological fibroblasts, are associated with the pathogenesis of pulmonary fibrosis; these cells strongly express markers of pathological fibroblasts (*CTHRC1*) and pathological extracellular matrix (*COL1A1* and *COL3A1*) [7]. They also revealed a clear relationship between fibrosis score and mortality, highlighting the importance of pulmonary fibrosis in patients' survival. Although the roles of pathological fibroblasts have been elucidated, whether these cells are applicable in clinical diagnosis, severity assessment, and treatment still needs further investigation.

Here, we aim to reveal a novel signature of PCPF by interrogating scRNA-seq data. We showed that the signature could be used to diagnose and assess pulmonary fibrosis. Further, this signature can also be used to repurpose and prioritize potentially effective drugs treating PCPF.

2. Materials and Methods

2.1. Construction and Evaluation of the PCPF Signature

The preprocessed single-cell gene expression profile underwent linearly dimensional reduction by principal component analysis (PCA). We used the Louvain algorithm to cluster the cells on the K-nearest neighbors (KNN) graph, which was constructed on the principal component (PC) space. We referred to the cell (sub)type information provided by Melms et al. [7]. We annotated each cell cluster based on the majority of the cell subtype in each cluster. Next, we made a case-control comparison to calculate the proportion difference in different cell clusters. To identify the characters of the cluster with the greatest proportional changes, we conducted differential gene expression analysis to compare the gene expression profiles of the cases and controls. We selected the top 200 up-regulated differentially expressed genes (DEGs) as the PCPF signature. We defined the signature score as the mean of the signature gene expression. We implemented the single-cell analysis with Scanpy [8].

We used DAVID (Available online: https://david.ncifcrf.gov/; (accessed on July 2021)) [9] to infer the signature-related biological functions. We selected the Benjamini–Hochberg procedure for the adjustment of multiple hypothesis testing.

2.2. Support Vector Machine (SVM)

Samples from GSE32537 underwent a random selection where 80% of samples were used for model training and the remainder for testing. A non-linear decision boundary, radial kernel function, was used to maximize the margin M that delineates two different classes (i.e., cases and controls). Ten-fold cross-validation was used to select optimal tuning parameters C and γ, where C determines the tolerance of violation to the margin and γ defines how far the support vectors should be taken. We compared the SVM values between cases and controls in the testing dataset (Wilcoxon rank-sum test). The procedure was implemented with the R package e1071.

2.3. Principal Component Regression

Observations from GSE32537 underwent random sampling where 2/3 of samples were used for model training, and the remaining samples were used for testing. Expression levels of genes within the signature were dimensionally reduced to PCs. We used PCs as features to predict DLCO and FVC. Suppose there are m observations, $\mathbf{y}$ represents the response vector in $\mathcal{R}^m$, and n is the total number of PCs. We composed a design matrix $\mathbf{P}_{m \times (k+1)}$ with a constant column and the first k PCs, and fitted a linear regression model as:

$$y = P\beta + \epsilon \tag{1}$$

With the lowest loss (mean square error, MSE), where $\beta \in \mathcal{R}^{k+1}$ is the coefficient vector, $\epsilon \in \mathcal{R}^m$ is the error vector, and $k \in [1, n]$. Ten-fold cross-validation was used to assess the models for different k. Since the cut-offs of abnormal DLCO and FVC (% predicted) are typically set at 75% and 80% [10], respectively, we filtered out samples beyond those thresholds. The testing dataset was used to predict clinical traits (DLCO and

FVC). Correlation analysis (Pearson's r) was conducted to assess the association between predicted and observed values. We implemented the procedure with the R package *pls* [11].

2.4. Calculation of Network-Based Proximity

Proximity is the shortest path length between two sets of nodes (drug targets and disease-related proteins) in the interactome. Suppose that T is the set of protein target(s) of a drug, D is the set of proteins relating to the disease, and $l(t, d)$ is the shortest path length between node t and d. Therefore, the shortest proximity (ds) is defined as follows:

$$\text{ds} = \frac{1}{\|T\|} \sum_{t \in T} \frac{1}{\|D\|} \sum_{d \in D} l(t,d) \; \forall \, t \in T, \, d \in D \quad (2)$$

To reduce the degree effect in proximity, we calculated the relative proximity Zds by stratifying the nodes according to their degrees. Specifically, nodes in the interactome were firstly arranged according to node degree and assigned to bins sequentially, where each bin can at most contain 100 nodes. Here, nodes in each bin will have similar, if not identical, degrees. Second, we randomly selected nodes from the same bin as nodes in the set T and D, then computed their shortest proximity. The procedure was iterated 100 times to obtain the mean (μds) and standard deviation (σds) of ds. The relative proximity (Zds) is defined as:

$$\text{Zds} = \frac{\text{ds} - \mu \text{ds}}{\sigma \text{ds}} \quad (3)$$

3. Results

3.1. An Overview of the Analytical Pipeline

The aims of this study are to discover a novel PCPF signature and leverage the network-based drug repurposing method to explore medications treating PCPF. The analytical pipeline is shown in Figure 1. We first identify the cell (sub)types and annotate cell clusters. We next construct the PCPF signature and evaluate its roles in diagnosing and assessing pulmonary fibrosis. Finally, we use a network-based method to explore effective treatment for PCPF.

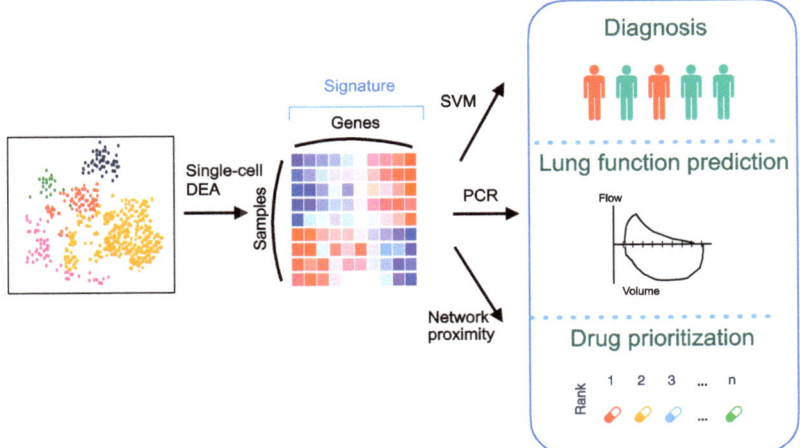

Figure 1. An overall analytical pipeline of this study. Schematic representation of the scRNA-seq analysis, signature construction, and application of the signature by integrating various computational methods. DEA: differential expression analysis; PCR: principal component regression; SVM: support vector machine.

3.2. Identifying PCPF-Related Cell Clusters at the Single-Cell Level

To explore cell clusters contributing to PCPF, we first investigated lung tissues on the dimensionally-reduced 2D plane (Figure 2A). To discover which cell cluster is mainly associated with PCPF, we conducted a case-control comparison on each cell cluster to compare their proportional differences (Figure 2B). We then noticed that cluster 12, pathological fibroblasts (PFBs), has the most considerable difference (Figure 2C). Therefore, we posited that PFBs play crucial roles in PCPF pathogenesis and further explored their clinical impact.

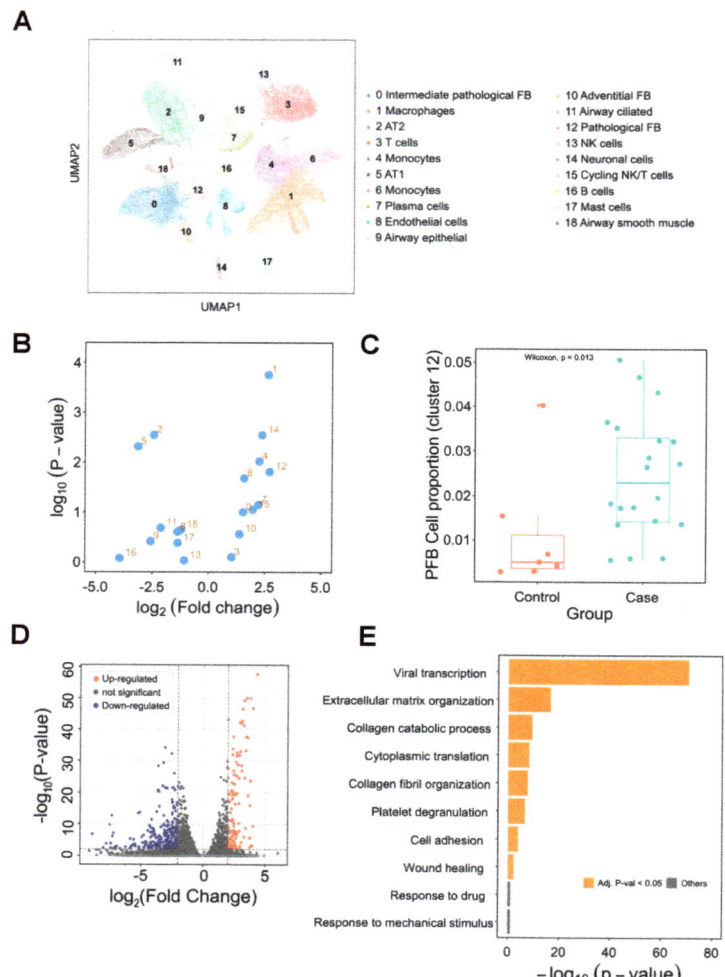

Figure 2. Single-cell transcriptome analysis of the lung tissues in COVID-19 cases. (**A**) Single-cell analysis of 116,314 cells from lung tissues. Nineteen cell clusters were identified and annotated based on the cell (sub)types provided by the literature [7]. (**B**) Visualization of the proportional difference of cells between COVID-19 patients and healthy controls. (**C**) Comparison of cluster 12 (PFBs) proportion between COVID-19 patients and healthy controls. (**D**) Differentially expressed gene analysis of cluster 12. Up-regulated and down-regulated genes are highlighted in red and blue, respectively. (**E**) Functional enrichment analysis of the differentially expressed genes. Enriched biological processes are shown in a bar plot. pFB: pathological fibroblast. PCPF: post-COVID-19 pulmonary fibrosis.

3.3. Comparison of Pathological Fibroblasts (PFBs) to Other Cell Types

To deduce the roles of PFBs in PCPF, we compared the gene expression profile between PFBs and other cells (Figure 2D and Supplementary Figure S1). To infer the biological functions in which DEGs are involved, we performed a functional enrichment analysis to identify the enriched biological processes (BP) in PFBs (Figure 2E). We found that viral transcription is the most enriched term, followed by fibrosis formation (e.g., extracellular matrix organization and collagen fibril organization). The DEGs derived from PFBs show meaningful and related biological functions, suggesting that PFBs may contribute to PCPF pathogenesis. Therefore, we constructed a transcriptome signature (Supplementary Table S1) to represent the distinct expression profile of these PFBs and further explored the roles of the signature on pulmonary fibrosis patients' outcomes.

3.4. Difference in PFB Signature between the Patients and Healthy Controls

To further discover the signature derived from the scRNA-seq of COVID-19 samples, we externally validated the PFB signature in another cohort, comprising 119 idiopathic pulmonary fibrosis (IPF) patients and 50 healthy controls [12]. IPF patients and healthy people have a distinct signature pattern (Figure 3A,B). Next, we examined whether patients' symptoms (SGRQ) and lung function (FVC and DLCO) could be clearly visualized within the two main PCs as well. DLCO and FVC show an increasing trend from the top left to the bottom in the first two principal component dimensions (Figure 3C,D), suggesting that patients with different IPF severity are dissimilar in terms of their signature. Although not as clear as that in lung function, the SGRQ trend is also similar, where more severe patients appeared in the top left, and less impaired patients appeared in the bottom right (Figure 3E).

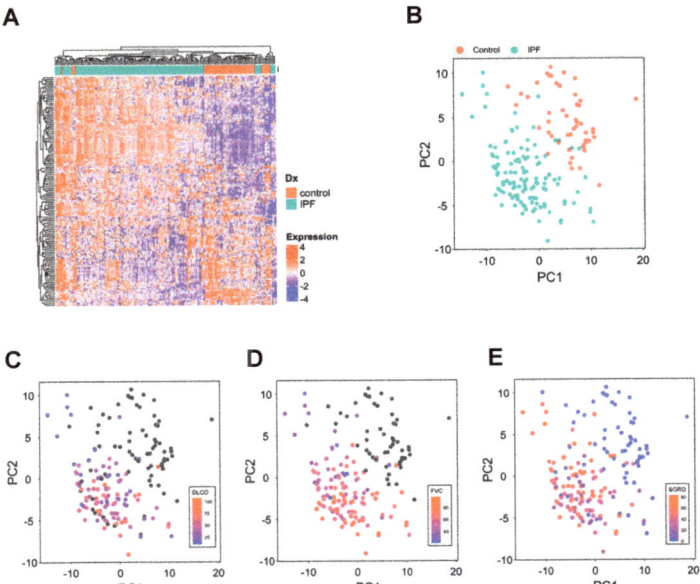

Figure 3. Discovery of distinct expression of the signature in pulmonary fibrosis patients. (**A**) Hierarchical clustering of samples based on the signature expression. Heatmap values are the scaled gene expression. (**B**) Visualization of patients and controls in the two main principal components. (**C–E**) Visualization of DLCO (**C**), FVC (**D**), and SGRQ (**E**) in the two main principal components. DLCO: diffusing capacity for carbon monoxide; FVC: forced vital capacity; SGRQ: St. George's Respiratory Questionnaire.

3.5. The Signature Can Be Used in the Diagnosis and Severity Assessment of Pulmonary Fibrosis

Current genetic tools for the diagnosis and assessment of pulmonary fibrosis are limited. Therefore, we explored whether the signature can be applied to these clinical challenges. We first revealed that FVC, DLCO, and SGRQ are significantly correlated with the signature score (Figure 4A–C). Moreover, as a potential confounder of clinical traits, age has a very weak correlation with SGRQ, FVC, and DLCO (Supplementary Figure S2). Next, we compared signature scores between IPF patients and healthy people and found IPF patients have significantly higher scores compared to the controls (Figure 4D).

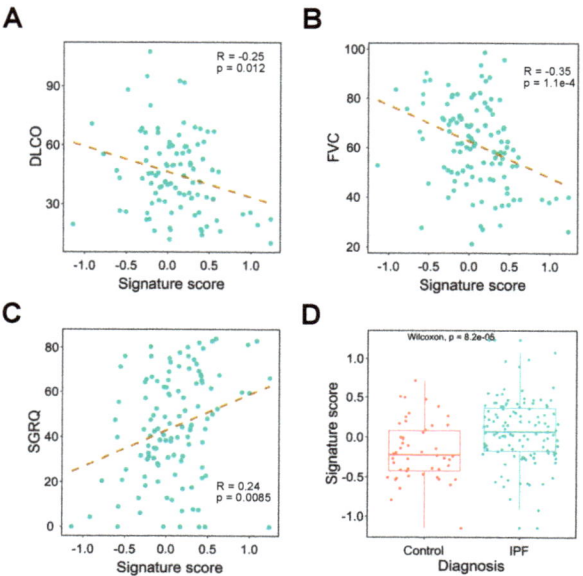

Figure 4. Investigating the association between signature expression and lung functions. (**A–C**) Correlation analysis of signature score and DLCO (**A**), FVC (**B**), and SGRQ (**C**). The dashed line represents the linear regression line. (**D**) Comparison of signature expression between IPF patients and healthy controls. DLCO: diffusing capacity for carbon monoxide; FVC: forced vital capacity; IPF: idiopathic pulmonary fibrosis; SGRQ: St. George's Respiratory Questionnaire.

Considering the correlation between gene signature and traits, we next used the signature to train machine learning models to predict clinical outcomes of pulmonary fibrosis patients. We found that an SVM could perfectly differentiate pulmonary fibrosis patients from healthy controls (Figure 5A,B) without adding extra clinical features. We next explored whether the signature could predict patients' lung function test results (% of predicted DLCO and FVC). PC regression was used to fit the training data. The correlation coefficients between the predicted and observed DLCO and FVC are 0.61 ($p = 2.91 \times 10^{-4}$) and 0.77 ($p = 2.52 \times 10^{-6}$) respectively (Figure 5C,D).

Altogether, the signature has high confidence in classifying pulmonary fibrosis patients and predicting lung function test results; this implies its potential applicability in clinical diagnosis and severity assessment.

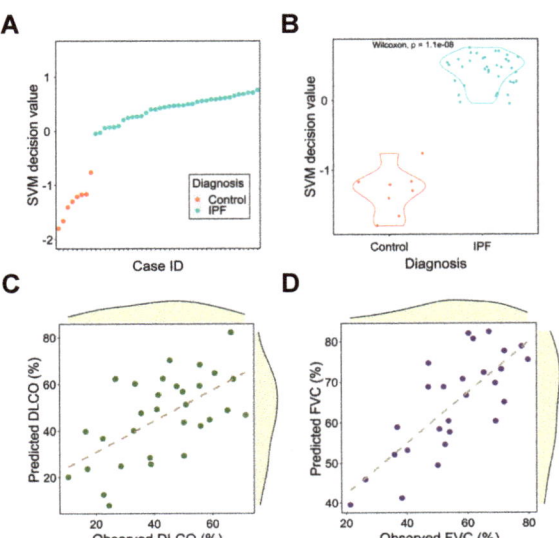

Figure 5. Signature as a diagnosis and assessment tool for pulmonary fibrosis using machine learning models. (**A**) The SVM scores for IPF patients and healthy controls. (**B**) Comparison of SVM decision value between IPF patients and healthy controls. (**C,D**) Correlation analysis between observed and predicted DLCO (**C**) and FVC (**D**). The dashed line represents the linear regression line. DLCO: diffusing capacity for carbon monoxide; FVC: forced vital capacity; IPF: idiopathic pulmonary fibrosis; SVM: support vector machine.

3.6. The Network-Based Proximity between Anti-Pulmonary Fibrosis Drugs and the Signature

Considering the roles of the signature in the diagnosis and assessment of pulmonary fibrosis, we defined the top-20 genes in the signature as the disease-related genes. Since the network proximity has been used to evaluate drugs for various diseases [3,4], we postulated that this method could also prioritize and repurpose the anti-PCPF drugs. In this case, anti-pulmonary fibrosis drugs should have closer proximity than the drugs with unknown anti-pulmonary fibrosis effects.

We calculated the shortest proximity (d_s) between drug targets and PCPF-related proteins on the interactome (Figure 6A). Since our hypothesis is that shorter proximity is associated with therapeutic effects, it is necessary to examine other factors that simultaneously affect proximity. In particular, node degree has been known to be anti-correlated with proximity [3], defined here as degree effect. Degree effect can lead to a biased interpretation of proximity in drug repurposing analyses. For instance, the cytotoxic agents typically have lower proximity than other drug categories because anti-cancer drugs' targets tend to have higher node degrees [2]. In this study, we also observed this phenomenon (Supplementary Figure S3A,B). We then calculated the relative proximity (Z_{ds}) by randomly selecting the degree-stratifying nodes on the interactome (Figure 6B). It is clear that the degree effect is less prominent in Z_{ds} (Supplementary Figure S3C,D). Next, to prove that the known-effect (anti-pulmonary fibrosis) drugs have smaller proximity than the unknown-effect drugs, we compared Z_{ds} between these two categories. We found that the known-effect drugs have significantly lower proximity (Figure 6C), with predictive performance AUC equal to 0.672 (Figure 6D). To further validate the results, we used another set of anti-fibrosis drugs (not restricted to pulmonary fibrosis) [13] and found identical trends (Supplementary Figure S4A,B). Based on the above results, Z_{ds} can be used as a predictor to assess anti-pulmonary fibrosis effects. Therefore, we summarized the drugs with high repurposing potential in Table 1. The full drug list and their proximity information can be found in Supplementary Table S2.

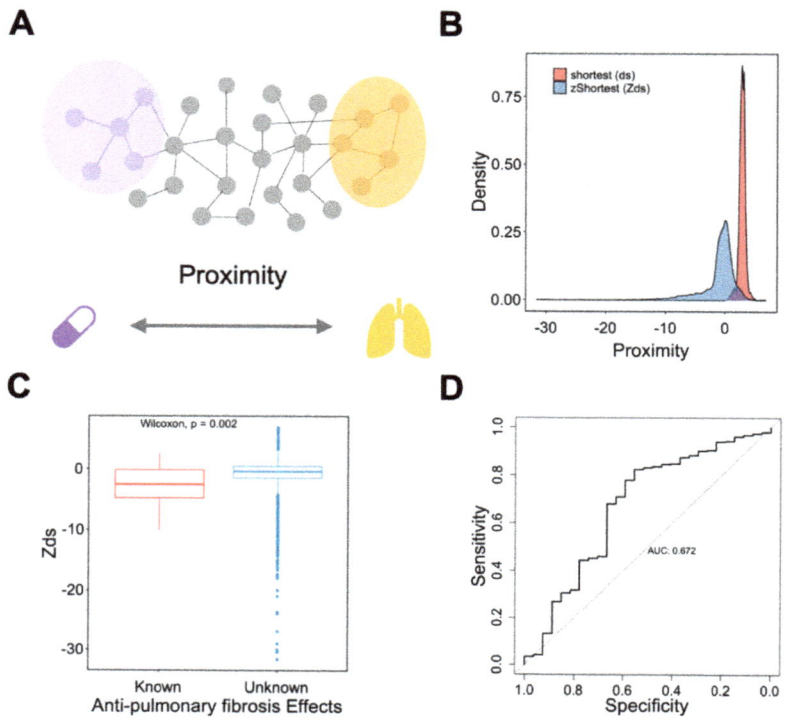

Figure 6. Characterizing the roles of proximity on drug repurposing for anti-pulmonary fibrosis drugs. (**A**) Schematic representation of the method. (**B**) Distribution of different proximity measures. (**C**) Comparison of proximity, Zds, between drugs with known and unknown anti-pulmonary fibrosis effects. (**D**) Analysis of the predictive performance of Zds on anti-pulmonary fibrosis effects using the ROC curve.

Table 1. Selected top-ranked drugs with highly anti-pulmonary fibrosis potential.

Name	Z-Shortest Proximity (Zds)	Shortest Proximity (ds)	Structure	Reference
Benzoic Acid	−17.91	0.726		[14,15]
Artenimol	−14.18	2.019		[16]
Quercetin	−12.48	2.060		[17]

Table 1. *Cont.*

Name	Z-Shortest Proximity (Zds)	Shortest Proximity (ds)	Structure	Reference
Tauroursodeoxycholic acid	−11.73	0.783		[18]
Atorvastatin	−10.51	2.323		[19,20]
Dinoprostone	−10.45	2.376		[21]
Emodin	−10.25	1.238		[22]
Valproic Acid	−10.11	2.373		[23]
Fluvastatin	−10.03	2.379		[20]
Cerulenin	−10.03	0.688		[24]
Naringenin	−9.40	2.204		[25]
Fisetin	−9.18	1.325		[26]

Table 1. Cont.

Name	Z-Shortest Proximity (Zds)	Shortest Proximity (ds)	Structure	Reference
Vitamin D	−9.18	1.690		[27]

4. Discussion

This study integrates various computational approaches to reveal a crucial theragnostic signature in PCPF. We show that the signature is associated with viral infections, pulmonary fibrosis, and clinical outcomes. Moreover, we demonstrate that the machine learning models trained with the signature show decent performance in diagnosing pulmonary fibrosis and predicting patients' lung function. Lastly, we prove that drugs with known anti-pulmonary fibrosis effects have closer proximity than those with unknown effects, suggesting that a network-based framework can also be applied to prioritize and repurpose drugs in PCPF.

Considering the design of this study was for PCPF, we notice that the viral infection-related GO term is the most enriched (Figure 2E). This phenomenon also appears in the network-based analysis, where drugs with strong anti-COVID-19 effects have significantly closer (smaller) proximity than drugs with weak or no-effect (Supplementary Figure S3D). This observation suggests that the signature may be associated with two events: COVID-19 viral infection and pulmonary fibrosis. Although pulmonary fibroblasts are less well known as target cells of the virus, recent studies revealed that alveolar fibroblasts could also be infected by the virus due to their expression of ACE2 receptors [28]. Aloufi et al. found that IPF fibroblasts have an even higher expression of ACE2 receptor, highlighting the roles of pathological fibroblasts in COVID-19 infection [29].

We also observe some medical procedure-related terms (e.g., response to mechanical stimulus). Although these terms are not significantly enriched (Figure 2E), they still imply that patients may undergo specific medication therapies or receive mechanical ventilation during hospital treatment.

One of the advantages of performing scRNA-seq on clinical samples is the high-resolution mapping of each cell. However, a deeper inspection may imply a smaller patient sample size because the number of patients enrolled can rarely be as large as that in bulk RNA analysis. There are 26 cases in the scRNA-seq dataset; it is reasonable to challenge any inference made from only 26 persons. Therefore, externally validating the results derived from scRNA-seq in a broader population can generate more confidence in the results. Nonetheless, it is undeniable that some facts exist such that the results from scRNA-seq may not be fully in concordance with bulk RNA analysis. Zero inflation, for instance, can lead to the underestimation of the low-expressed genes [30]. Another challenge is that the result in one patient cohort may not be reproducible in another simply due to numerous uncontrollable factors between the two cohorts. However, in our study, the signature derived from scRNA-seq also play a vital role in another bulk-sample patient cohort, suggesting that the signature is reproducible and can be externally validated.

There are limitations to this study. First, we applied the signature derived from PCPF to IPF patients. It is undeniable that the etiologies of PCPF and IPF are less likely to be identical. The causes of PCPF may include the viral infection and the host immune response; on the other hand, the causes of IPF remain unclear, even though there are several studies revealed the genetic predispositions or causal variants of IPF using genome-wide association studies with fine-mapping [31] or polygenic risk score [32]. However, regardless of the causes, PCPF and IPF are fibrogenesis and fibrosis in the lung tissue. Considering the limited clinical information on PCPF, we used IPF as a surrogate to investigate the potential impacts and clinical insights of this PCPF signature, in particular the application in drug repurposing. We understand that population structure and other bassline demographic characteristics could influence the performance of the gene signature score, and thus the signature score should be carefully interpreted when applying to other ethnic groups, such as Asians. Another limitation is the lack of lung function test results in the single-cell cohort. This makes it harder to compare the baseline characteristics of the IPF and PCPF patients.

The rationale for the network-based drug repurposing approach is that a drug may still be effective when its target proteins are 'close' to the disease-related protein(s) in the interactome [3,33,34]. If this argument is true, drugs with known effects on disease should have closer proximity compared to the unknown-effect drugs. Accordingly, this requires identifying a significant difference in proximity between known-effect and unknown-effect drugs. However, in some diseases, medical treatment options are very limited, such as IPF [35,36]. There are, in fact, only two FDA-approved drugs, nintedanib, and pirfenidone, that seem to be associated with a slower progression of IPF [36]. Therefore, if we simply assign drugs to either known or unknown effects based on current clinical knowledge, hypothesis testing between the two drug categories (known vs. unknown effect) can hardly be conducted due to highly unbalanced sample sizes. To address this problem, we searched the published literature which conducted drug repurposing for pulmonary fibrosis [37] and pan-fibrosis [13] and used the repurposed drugs as the known-effect drugs.

Previous studies have applied the network-based drug repurposing framework to various diseases [3,38]. Nonetheless, due to the complexity of disease mechanisms, validating this method is necessary when dealing with different conditions. For instance, previously, we found that, in lung adenocarcinoma, the closest proximity on the weighted interactome shows the best performance in identifying promising drugs [2]. In this study, however, we noticed that z-transformed shortest proximity, Zds, has better performance. This observation implies that the performance of proximity metrics may be context-dependent.

Although proximity may be associated with drug effectiveness, we urge caution when interpreting the ranked drug list, as proximity is not the only factor contributing to drug effectiveness. For instance, we found that nintedanib, one of the two currently approved drugs for IPF, has small proximity (Zds = -3.22; rank = 798/5643). However, the other approved anti-IPF agent, pirfenidone, has large proximity (Zds = 1.45; rank = 5115/5643). Therefore, this observation suggests that drugs with distant proximity could still be effective, as proximity may be only one of the many factors affecting drug effectiveness. Other crucial factors, such as binding affinity, also matter.

Within the top-ranked repurposed drugs (top 3% of the drugs in Supplementary Table S2), we found some drugs belonging to antibiotic or antiviral agent categories, which may be related to pneumonia treatment [39], acute exacerbation of pulmonary fibrosis [40], or other morbidities, such as pneumonitis, opportunistic infection, or tissue inflammation [41]. They may not truly show strong anti-fibrosis effects. On the other hand, we noticed that many top-ranked candidates on this list show promising anti-pulmonary fibrosis effects. Artenimol (Zds = -14.18; rank = 28/5643) (also known as dihydroartemisinin), for instance, can reduce lung fibrosis by suppressing the Notch signaling pathway [42] and pro-fibrotic pathways [43]. Another example is dinoprostone (also known as prostaglandin E2). It was reported that inhaling liposomal prostaglandin E2 can treat pulmonary fibrosis by restricting inflammation and fibrotic injury in the lungs [21].

Another interesting drug category is statins, a well-known class of lipid-lowering agents. A retrospective study surveying 323 IPF patients found that statin-users have a slower annual decline in DLCO and FVC than non-users [20]. We then searched our drug list for the types of the statin used in this study [20] and found that all of them have very small Zds: atorvastatin (Zds = -10.5), fluvastatin (Zds = -10.03), rosuvastatin (Zds = -8.37), pravastatin (Zds = -6.73), and simvastatin (Zds = -4.43).

5. Conclusions

We reveal a novel theragnostic signature for PCPF and provide a prioritized drug list based on network-based proximity, Zds. Our study shows the applicability of integrating various computational methods when analyzing biomedical data and, importantly, provides useful information for diagnosing, assessing, and treating PCPF.

Supplementary Materials: The following are available online at https://www.mdpi.com/article/10.3390/pharmaceutics14050971/s1, Figure S1: The expression of DEGs in PCPF patients and the controls, Figure S2: The correlation analysis between age and other clinical features, Figure S3: The degree effect on proximity, Figure S4: Characterizing the roles of proximity on the repurposing of anti-fibrosis drugs, Table S1: The transcriptome signature of pathological fibroblasts in PCPF, Table S2: The full list with 5644 drugs and their proximity (Zds).

Author Contributions: Conceptualization, A.L., H.-C.H. and H.-F.J.; methodology, A.L., C.-L.H., Y.-J.O., H.-C.H. and H.-F.J.; validation, A.L. and J.-Y.C.; data analysis, A.L. and J.-Y.C.; investigation, A.L., C.-L.H., H.-C.H. and H.-F.J.; data curation, A.L., J.-Y.C., H.-C.H. and H.-F.J.; writing—original draft preparation, A.L., H.-C.H. and H.-F.J.; writing—review and editing, H.-C.H. and H.-F.J.; visualization, A.L. and J.-Y.C.; supervision, H.-C.H. and H.-F.J.; project administration, H.-C.H. and H.-F.J.; funding acquisition, H.-C.H. and H.-F.J. All authors have read and agreed to the published version of the manuscript.

Funding: This research was funded by the Ministry of Science and Technology (MOST 109-2221-E-002-161-MY3, MOST 109-2221-E-010-012-MY3, MOST 109-2327-B-002-009, MOST 111-2321-B-002-017). The Higher Education Sprout Project (NTU-110L8808 and NTU-CC-109L104702-2). Emerging Infectious and Major Disease Research Program and Taiwan Biotech Innovation Academy (AS-KPQ-110-EIMD).

Institutional Review Board Statement: Not applicable.

Informed Consent Statement: Not applicable.

Data Availability Statement: The COVID-19 scRNA-seq dataset was derived from Melms et al. [7]. It contains autopsy lung tissues from 26 patients, containing 116,314 cells. The pulmonary fibrosis cohort was downloaded from GEO (GSE32537) [12], which provided the gene expression profiles and clinical traits of 119 idiopathic pulmonary fibrosis (IPF) patients and 50 healthy controls. The clinical traits include St. George's Respiratory Questionnaire (SGRQ) and lung function test results (diffusing capacity for carbon monoxide (DLCO) and forced vital capacity (FVC)). For the proximity calculations, we adapted human protein–protein interaction data from Guney et al. [3], which comprises 140,637 interactions among 13,101 proteins. We retrieved and adapted drug-related information, including drug targets and their anti-SARS-CoV-2 effects, from the Drugbank database [44] and Gysi et al. [4], respectively.

Acknowledgments: We would like to appreciate Chen-Hao Huang for his help and suggestion to this study.

Conflicts of Interest: The authors declare no conflict of interest.

References

1. Fraser, E. Long term respiratory complications of COVID-19. *BMJ* **2020**, *370*, m3001. [CrossRef] [PubMed]
2. Li, A.; Huang, H.T.; Huang, H.C.; Juan, H.F. LncTx: A network-based method to repurpose drugs acting on the survival-related lncRNAs in lung cancer. *Comput. Struct. Biotechnol. J.* **2021**, *19*, 3990–4002. [CrossRef] [PubMed]
3. Guney, E.; Menche, J.; Vidal, M.; Barábasi, A.L. Network-based in silico drug efficacy screening. *Nat. Commun.* **2016**, *7*, 10331. [CrossRef] [PubMed]
4. Morselli Gysi, D.; do Valle, Í.; Zitnik, M.; Ameli, A.; Gan, X.; Varol, O.; Ghiassian, S.D.; Patten, J.J.; Davey, R.A.; Loscalzo, J.; et al. Network medicine framework for identifying drug-repurposing opportunities for COVID-19. *Proc. Natl. Acad. Sci. USA* **2021**, *118*, e2025581118. [CrossRef]
5. Zhou, Y.; Hou, Y.; Shen, J.; Huang, Y.; Martin, W.; Cheng, F. Network-based drug repurposing for novel coronavirus 2019-nCoV/SARS-CoV-2. *Cell Discov.* **2020**, *6*, 14. [CrossRef] [PubMed]
6. Sharma, A.; Menche, J.; Huang, C.C.; Ort, T.; Zhou, X.; Kitsak, M.; Sahni, N.; Thibault, D.; Voung, L.; Guo, F.; et al. A disease module in the interactome explains disease heterogeneity, drug response and captures novel pathways and genes in asthma. *Hum. Mol. Genet.* **2015**, *24*, 3005–3020. [CrossRef]
7. Melms, J.C.; Biermann, J.; Huang, H.; Wang, Y.; Nair, A.; Tagore, S.; Katsyv, I.; Rendeiro, A.F.; Amin, A.D.; Schapiro, D.; et al. A molecular single-cell lung atlas of lethal COVID-19. *Nature* **2021**, *595*, 114–119. [CrossRef]
8. Wolf, F.A.; Angerer, P.; Theis, F.J. SCANPY: Large-scale single-cell gene expression data analysis. *Genome Biol.* **2018**, *19*, 15. [CrossRef]

9. Huang, D.W.; Sherman, B.T.; Lempicki, R.A. Systematic and integrative analysis of large gene lists using DAVID bioinformatics resources. *Nat. Protoc.* **2009**, *4*, 44–57. [CrossRef]
10. Vandevoorde, J.; Verbanck, S.; Schuermans, D.; Broekaert, L.; Devroey, D.; Kartounian, J.; Vincken, W. Forced vital capacity and forced expiratory volume in six seconds as predictors of reduced total lung capacity. *Eur. Respir. J.* **2008**, *31*, 391–395. [CrossRef]
11. Mevik, B.-H.; Wehrens, R. The pls Package: Principal Component and Partial Least Squares Regression in R. *J. Stat. Softw.* **2007**, *18*, 1–23. [CrossRef]
12. Yang, I.V.; Coldren, C.D.; Leach, S.M.; Seibold, M.A.; Murphy, E.; Lin, J.; Rosen, R.; Neidermyer, A.J.; McKean, D.F.; Groshong, S.D.; et al. Expression of cilium-associated genes defines novel molecular subtypes of idiopathic pulmonary fibrosis. *Thorax* **2013**, *68*, 1114–1121. [CrossRef] [PubMed]
13. Wu, D.; Gao, W.; Li, X.; Tian, C.; Jiao, N.; Fang, S.; Xiao, J.; Xu, Z.; Zhu, L.; Zhang, G.; et al. Dr AFC: Drug repositioning through anti-fibrosis characteristic. *Brief. Bioinform.* **2021**, *22*, bbaa115. [CrossRef] [PubMed]
14. Venkatadri, R.; Iyer, A.K.; Ramesh, V.; Wright, C.; Castro, C.A.; Yakisich, J.S.; Azad, N. MnTBAP Inhibits Bleomycin-Induced Pulmonary Fibrosis by Regulating VEGF and Wnt Signaling. *J. Cell. Physiol.* **2017**, *232*, 506–516. [CrossRef] [PubMed]
15. Oury, T.D.; Thakker, K.; Menache, M.; Chang, L.Y.; Crapo, J.D.; Day, B.J. Attenuation of bleomycin-induced pulmonary fibrosis by a catalytic antioxidant metalloporphyrin. *Am. J. Respir. Cell Mol. Biol.* **2001**, *25*, 164–169. [CrossRef]
16. Dolivo, D.; Weathers, P.; Dominko, T. Artemisinin and artemisinin derivatives as anti-fibrotic therapeutics. *Acta Pharm. Sin. B* **2021**, *11*, 322–339. [CrossRef]
17. Sellarés, J.; Rojas, M. Quercetin in Idiopathic Pulmonary Fibrosis: Another Brick in the Senolytic Wall. *Am. J. Respir. Cell Mol. Biol.* **2019**, *60*, 3–4. [CrossRef]
18. Tong, B.; Fu, L.; Hu, B.; Zhang, Z.C.; Tan, Z.X.; Li, S.R.; Chen, Y.H.; Zhang, C.; Wang, H.; Xu, D.X.; et al. Tauroursodeoxycholic acid alleviates pulmonary endoplasmic reticulum stress and epithelial-mesenchymal transition in bleomycin-induced lung fibrosis. *BMC Pulm. Med.* **2021**, *21*, 149. [CrossRef]
19. Kreuter, M.; Costabel, U.; Richeldi, L.; Cottin, V.; Wijsenbeek, M.; Bonella, F.; Bendstrup, E.; Maher, T.M.; Wachtlin, D.; Stowasser, S.; et al. Statin Therapy and Outcomes in Trials of Nintedanib in Idiopathic Pulmonary Fibrosis. *Respiration* **2018**, *95*, 317–326. [CrossRef]
20. Lambert, E.M.; Wuyts, W.A.; Yserbyt, J.; De Sadeleer, L.J. Statins: Cause of fibrosis or the opposite? Effect of cardiovascular drugs in idiopathic pulmonary fibrosis. *Respir. Med.* **2021**, *176*, 106259. [CrossRef]
21. Ivanova, V.; Garbuzenko, O.B.; Reuhl, K.R.; Reimer, D.C.; Pozharov, V.P.; Minko, T. Inhalation treatment of pulmonary fibrosis by liposomal prostaglandin E2. *Eur. J. Pharm. Biopharm.* **2013**, *84*, 335–344. [CrossRef] [PubMed]
22. Guan, R.; Wang, X.; Zhao, X.; Song, N.; Zhu, J.; Wang, J.; Wang, J.; Xia, C.; Chen, Y.; Zhu, D.; et al. Emodin ameliorates bleomycin-induced pulmonary fibrosis in rats by suppressing epithelial-mesenchymal transition and fibroblast activation. *Sci. Rep.* **2016**, *6*, 35696. [CrossRef] [PubMed]
23. Chen, L.; Alam, A.; Pac-Soo, A.; Chen, Q.; Shang, Y.; Zhao, H.; Yao, S.; Ma, D. Pretreatment with valproic acid alleviates pulmonary fibrosis through epithelial–mesenchymal transition inhibition in vitro and in vivo. *Lab. Investig.* **2021**, *101*, 1166–1175. [CrossRef] [PubMed]
24. Jung, M.-Y.; Kang, J.-H.; Hernandez, D.M.; Yin, X.; Andrianifahanana, M.; Wang, Y.; Gonzalez-Guerrico, A.; Limper, A.H.; Lupu, R.; Leof, E.B. Fatty acid synthase is required for profibrotic TGF-β signaling. *FASEB J.* **2018**, *32*, 3803–3815. [CrossRef] [PubMed]
25. Du, G.; Jin, L.; Han, X.; Song, Z.; Zhang, H.; Liang, W. Naringenin: A Potential Immunomodulator for Inhibiting Lung Fibrosis and Metastasis. *Cancer Res.* **2009**, *69*, 3205–3212. [CrossRef] [PubMed]
26. Zhang, L.; Tong, X.; Huang, J.; Wu, M.; Zhang, S.; Wang, D.; Liu, S.; Fan, H. Fisetin Alleviated Bleomycin-Induced Pulmonary Fibrosis Partly by Rescuing Alveolar Epithelial Cells From Senescence. *Front. Pharmacol.* **2020**, *11*, 553690. [CrossRef]
27. Tzilas, V.; Bouros, E.; Barbayianni, I.; Karampitsakos, T.; Kourtidou, S.; Ntassiou, M.; Ninou, I.; Aidinis, V.; Bouros, D.; Tzouvelekis, A. Vitamin D prevents experimental lung fibrosis and predicts survival in patients with idiopathic pulmonary fibrosis. *Pulm. Pharmacol. Ther.* **2019**, *55*, 17–24. [CrossRef]
28. Sahin, M.; Akkus, E. Fibroblast function in COVID-19. *Pathol. Res. Pract.* **2021**, *219*, 153353. [CrossRef]
29. Aloufi, N.; Traboulsi, H.; Ding, J.; Fonseca, G.J.; Nair, P.; Huang, S.K.; Hussain, S.N.A.; Eidelman, D.H.; Baglole, C.J. Angiotensin-converting enzyme 2 expression in COPD and IPF fibroblasts: The forgotten cell in COVID-19. *Am. J. Physiol. Lung Cell. Mol. Physiol.* **2021**, *320*, L152–L157. [CrossRef]
30. Lähnemann, D.; Köster, J.; Szczurek, E.; McCarthy, D.J.; Hicks, S.C.; Robinson, M.D.; Vallejos, C.A.; Campbell, K.R.; Beerenwinkel, N.; Mahfouz, A.; et al. Eleven grand challenges in single-cell data science. *Genome Biol.* **2020**, *21*, 31. [CrossRef]
31. Seibold, M.A.; Wise, A.L.; Speer, M.C.; Steele, M.P.; Brown, K.K.; Loyd, J.E.; Fingerlin, T.E.; Zhang, W.; Gudmundsson, G.; Groshong, S.D.; et al. A common MUC5B promoter polymorphism and pulmonary fibrosis. *N. Engl. J. Med.* **2011**, *364*, 1503–1512. [CrossRef] [PubMed]
32. Duckworth, A.; Gibbons, M.A.; Allen, R.J.; Almond, H.; Beaumont, R.N.; Wood, A.R.; Lunnon, K.; Lindsay, M.A.; Wain, L.V.; Tyrrell, J.; et al. Telomere length and risk of idiopathic pulmonary fibrosis and chronic obstructive pulmonary disease: A mendelian randomisation study. *Lancet Respir. Med.* **2021**, *9*, 285–294. [CrossRef]
33. Barabási, A.L.; Gulbahce, N.; Loscalzo, J. Network medicine: A network-based approach to human disease. *Nat. Rev. Genet.* **2011**, *12*, 56–68. [CrossRef]

34. Fotis, C.; Antoranz, A.; Hatziavramidis, D.; Sakellaropoulos, T.; Alexopoulos, L.G. Network-based technologies for early drug discovery. *Drug Discov. Today* **2018**, *23*, 626–635. [CrossRef] [PubMed]
35. Raghu, G.; Rochwerg, B.; Zhang, Y.; Garcia, C.A.; Azuma, A.; Behr, J.; Brozek, J.L.; Collard, H.R.; Cunningham, W.; Homma, S.; et al. An Official ATS/ERS/JRS/ALAT Clinical Practice Guideline: Treatment of Idiopathic Pulmonary Fibrosis. An Update of the 2011 Clinical Practice Guideline. *Am. J. Respir. Crit. Care Med.* **2015**, *192*, e3–e19. [CrossRef] [PubMed]
36. Canestaro, W.J.; Forrester, S.H.; Raghu, G.; Ho, L.; Devine, B.E. Drug Treatment of Idiopathic Pulmonary Fibrosis: Systematic Review and Network Meta-Analysis. *Chest* **2016**, *149*, 756–766. [CrossRef]
37. Karatzas, E.; Kakouri, A.C.; Kolios, G.; Delis, A.; Spyrou, G.M. Fibrotic expression profile analysis reveals repurposed drugs with potential anti-fibrotic mode of action. *PLoS ONE* **2021**, *16*, e0249687. [CrossRef]
38. Cheng, F.; Kovács, I.A.; Barabási, A.L. Network-based prediction of drug combinations. *Nat. Commun.* **2019**, *10*, 1197. [CrossRef]
39. Sieswerda, E.; de Boer, M.G.J.; Bonten, M.M.J.; Boersma, W.G.; Jonkers, R.E.; Aleva, R.M.; Kullberg, B.-J.; Schouten, J.A.; van de Garde, E.M.W.; Verheij, T.J.; et al. Recommendations for antibacterial therapy in adults with COVID-19—An evidence based guideline. *Clin. Microbiol. Infect.* **2021**, *27*, 61–66. [CrossRef]
40. Molyneaux, P.L.; Maher, T.M. The role of infection in the pathogenesis of idiopathic pulmonary fibrosis. *Eur. Respir. Rev.* **2013**, *22*, 376–381. [CrossRef]
41. Wuyts, W.A.; Willems, S.; Vos, R.; Vanaudenaerde, B.M.; De Vleeschauwer, S.I.; Rinaldi, M.; Vanhooren, H.M.; Geudens, N.; Verleden, S.E.; Demedts, M.G.; et al. Azithromycin reduces pulmonary fibrosis in a bleomycin mouse model. *Exp. Lung Res.* **2010**, *36*, 602–614. [CrossRef] [PubMed]
42. Liu, Y.; Huang, G.; Mo, B.; Wang, C. Artesunate ameliorates lung fibrosis via inhibiting the Notch signaling pathway. *Exp. Ther. Med.* **2017**, *14*, 561–566. [CrossRef] [PubMed]
43. Yang, D.; Yuan, W.; Lv, C.; Li, N.; Liu, T.; Wang, L.; Sun, Y.; Qiu, X.; Fu, Q. Dihydroartemisinin supresses inflammation and fibrosis in bleomycine-induced pulmonary fibrosis in rats. *Int. J. Clin. Exp. Pathol.* **2015**, *8*, 1270–1281. [PubMed]
44. Wishart, D.S.; Knox, C.; Guo, A.C.; Shrivastava, S.; Hassanali, M.; Stothard, P.; Chang, Z.; Woolsey, J. DrugBank: A comprehensive resource for in silico drug discovery and exploration. *Nucleic Acids Res.* **2006**, *34*, D668–D672. [CrossRef] [PubMed]

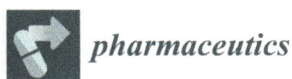

Article

Integration of In Silico Strategies for Drug Repositioning towards P38α Mitogen-Activated Protein Kinase (MAPK) at the Allosteric Site

Utid Suriya [1], Panupong Mahalapbutr [2] and Thanyada Rungrotmongkol [3,4,*]

1. Program in Biotechnology, Faculty of Science, Chulalongkorn University, Bangkok 10330, Thailand; noteutidii@gmail.com
2. Department of Biochemistry, Center for Translational Medicine, Faculty of Medicine, Khon Kaen University, Khan Kaen 40002, Thailand; panupma@kku.ac.th
3. Center of Excellence in Structural and Computational Biology, Department of Biochemistry, Chulalongkorn University, Bangkok 10330, Thailand
4. Ph.D. Program in Bioinformatics and Computational Biology, Graduate School, Chulalongkorn University, Bangkok 10330, Thailand
* Correspondence: thanyada.r@chula.ac.th

Abstract: P38α mitogen-activated protein kinase (p38α MAPK), one of the p38 MAPK isoforms participating in a signaling cascade, has been identified for its pivotal role in the regulation of physiological processes such as cell proliferation, differentiation, survival, and death. Herein, by shedding light on docking- and 100-ns dynamic-based screening from 3210 FDA-approved drugs, we found that lomitapide (a lipid-lowering agent) and nilotinib (a Bcr-Abl fusion protein inhibitor) could alternatively inhibit phosphorylation of p38α MAPK at the allosteric site. All-atom molecular dynamics simulations and free energy calculations including end-point and QM-based ONIOM methods revealed that the binding affinity of the two screened drugs exhibited a comparable level as the known p38α MAPK inhibitor (BIRB796), suggesting the high potential of being a novel p38α MAPK inhibitor. In addition, noncovalent contacts and the number of hydrogen bonds were found to be corresponding with the great binding recognition. Key influential amino acids were mostly hydrophobic residues, while the two charged residues including E71 and D168 were considered crucial ones due to their ability to form very strong H-bonds with the focused drugs. Altogether, our contributions obtained here could be theoretical guidance for further conducting experimental-based preclinical studies necessary for developing therapeutic agents targeting p38α MAPK.

Keywords: drug repositioning; p38α MAPK; molecular docking; MD simulation; allosteric inhibitors; in silico screening; computer-aided drug discovery

1. Introduction

Mitogen-activated protein kinase (MAPK) signaling pathways are a cascade comprising three kinases including extracellular signal-regulated kinase (ERK), c-Jun NH$_2$-terminal kinase (JNK), and p38, in which the upstream kinase (MAPKKK) responds to various extra- and intracellular signals and activates the middle kinase (MAPKK) by direct phosphorylation [1]. Then, MAPKKs phosphorylate and activate a MAPK, resulting in cell-specific physiological phenomena such as cell proliferation, differentiation, survival, and death [2]. MAPKs are known to be able to react with a wide range of input signals including hormones, cytokines, and growth factors, as well as endogenous stress and environmental factors. To this end, they were classified into two distinct responsive MAPKs; mitogen activated (ERK) and stress activated kinases (JNK and p38) [3]. Substantial studies revealed that the p38 pathway is a key player in response to environmental stress signals and inflammatory stimuli as well as being responsible for the production of some inflammatory cytokines such as tumor necrosis factor-α (TNF-α), interleukin-1β, interleukin-6, and interleukin-12 in response to proinflammatory signaling [4,5]. Furthermore, p38 can be a restraint in cancer tumorigenesis (e.g., breast, lung, colon, and liver cancer), which induces a p38-mediated proapoptotic mechanism and the killing of incipient tumor cells by a mechanism involved in the production of reactive oxygen species (ROS) [6]. However, p38 activity functions conversely once a tumor has already been established by supporting its growth [7]. Experimental evidence indicates that tumor cells need to modulate the level of p38 MAPK activity in order to perform metastases, and this signaling occurs in a variety of diseases [8]. To this end, inhibition of the p38 pathway has attracted much attention for the reason that it could be a promising strategy in the management of cancer, neurodegeneration, inflammation, and even the newly emerged pandemic, COVID-19 [9].

Structurally, there are four homologues of p38 MAPK including p38α, p38β, p38γ, and p38δ [3]. Among these, p38α is the best characterized and seems to be the most physiologically related protein involved in inflammatory responses [4,10]. According to the site of the ligand modulation, there are two different generations of p38α MAPK inhibitors, including type I and type II inhibitors, which modulate the activity of the enzyme at the ATP-binding and the allosteric site, respectively. However, targeting an ATP-binding site has limited the clinical use due to a high level of sequence and structural similarity among kinase enzymes [2], which could result in non- or low selective behavior and cause undesirable side effects and toxicities [11]. In order to overcome this issue, recent research has been focusing on utilizing a novel allosteric regulatory site, which is distinct from the ATP pocket at about 60° spatially, and there is no structural overlap between compounds bound to the allosteric site and ATP [12]. The conserved residues Asp-Phe-Gly (DFG) motif in the active site were conformationally altered, which is often known as DFG-out conformation and seems to be more stable in protein Tyr kinases [12]. To date, even though a number of clinical p38 MAPK inhibitors have emerged for inflammatory disease indications such as rheumatoid arthritis, there have been no approved agents [13,14] due to the lack of target modulation, adverse events, toxicities, and poor pharmacokinetics [4,14]. Some toxicities reported by clinical studies of well-known p38 MAPK inhibitors, BIRB796 (doramapimod), VX-745 (Vertex), and SCIO-469 (talmapimod) included hepatotoxic elevation of liver transaminases, skin rash, and so forth [15–17]. Accordingly, searching for novel compounds capable of impeding p38 MAPK has still been necessarily important to provide bottom-up preclinical information, guiding the development of therapeutic agents disrupting the MAPK signaling pathway.

Herein, by shedding light on the advancement of computational biology partly contributed to a preclinical stage of drug discovery and development, we aimed to search for novel agents capable of binding to p38α MAPK at the allosteric site by a drug repositioning approach. Bioinformatic databases and in silico methods including docking-based virtual screening, molecular dynamics (MD) simulations, and free energy calculations were employed to guide the discovery of hit compounds that may present a significant potential for further optimization. All the results obtained here provide some useful information and may outline the next steps governing experimental studies for drug discovery and development against p38α MAPK.

2. Materials and Methods
2.1. Preparation of the 3D Structure of P38α MAPK and Ligands

The three-dimensional structure of p38α MAPK in complex with a known inhibitor, BIRB796, was retrieved from the RCSB Protein Data Bank (PDB ID: 1KV2). The missing residues (170–184) of p38α MAPK were constructed by means of the homology model implemented in the SWISS-MODEL server [18]. The newly generated structure was consequently validated by plotting the Ramachandran diagram (Figure S1), using PROCHECK [19]. The protonation states of all ionizable amino acids were predicted based on their pKa value by using the PROPKA 3.0 web interface [20], and were then set into the modeled complex structure before performing molecular docking and MD simulations.

Partial atomic charges of BIRB796 were calculated for their geometry and then assigned for the electrostatic potential (ESP) charges via the Gaussian 09W program (G09) using the Hartree–Fock method and 6-31G(d) level of theory [21]. Its structure was then assigned for atom type, and we generated its topology file using the Antechamber program [22]. Converting from the 'mol2' file into a 'pdbqt' format was achieved by AutoDockTools (ADT). For the virtual screening studies, all focused compounds were obtained from the 3210 FDA-approved drugs available in the ZINC database (http://zinc.docking.org, accessed on 12 November 2019). These ligands were also subsequently converted from the 'mol2' format into a 'pdbqt' format using ADT.

2.2. Molecular Docking and Visual Inspection

Docking calculations were carried out on a Linux operating system using AutoDock VinaXB, which provides a new empirical halogen bond scoring function [23]. Three docking parameters, including exhaustiveness, num_modes, and energy_range, were set to 20, 50, and 5 kcal/mol, respectively. For system validation, the crystallized ligand was redocked into the same binding site (Figure S2), and the verified grid box was then employed for all ligands in virtual screening. Predicted binding affinity ($E_{binding}$, kcal/mol) of the most likely occurring conformation was a parameter used to rank the studied compounds, and the structure coordinate was employed to be the initial structure for the MD run.

To reduce the chance of false-positive scoring, a visual inspection of the intermolecular interactions between each ligand and amino-acid residues lining in the focused allosteric site was carried out by specifically examining (i) hydrogen bonding with E71, M109, and D168 as well as (ii) hydrophobic interactions with V38, A51, K53, R67, L75, I84, L104, L108, A157, L167, and F169, which were derived from the binding mode observed in the inhibitor prototype, BIRB796. For this purpose, compounds sharing features of intermolecular interactions with BIRB796 greater than five interactions were then selected.

2.3. Molecular Dynamics (MD) Simulations

The protein-ligand complex coordinates of the two screened drugs and the inhibitor prototype from molecular docking were dynamically modeled under the periodic boundary condition with the isothermal-isobaric (NPT) scheme [24–28]. The AMBER ff14SB and generalized AMBER force field version 2 (GAFF2) [29] were selected for a force field governing bonded and nonbonded interaction parameters. Electrostatic interactions were treated by the particle mesh Ewald summation method [30] with a cutoff distance for nonbonded interactions of 10 Å. The SHAKE algorithm [31] was retrieved to constrain hydrogen atoms. The temperature was controlled by the Langevin thermostat [32] and set to 310 K by increasing from 10 to 310 K. Controlling the pressure was achieved by the Berendsen barostat [33] with a relaxation time of 1 ps. Moreover, the TIP3P water model [34] was used to solvate the system with minimum padding of 10.0 Å between the protein surface and the solvation box edge. The overall charge of the molecular system was neutralized by randomly adding either sodium or chloride ions. Minimization of the added hydrogen atoms and water molecules was carried out using 500 steps of steepest descent (SD) followed by 1500 steps of conjugated gradient (CG) methods before running the MD simulations with constrained solvent molecules. The whole complex was then fully minimized using the same procedure. For MD production, all systems were set to 100 ns (2-fs increment). The root-mean-square displacement (RMSD), the numbers of hydrogen bond (H-bond), and the contact atoms were calculated through the cpptraj module whilst the per-residue decomposition energy ($\Delta G_{binding}^{residue}$) was estimated by MM/PBSA.py implemented in AMBER16.

2.4. End-Point Binding Energy Calculations

To observe the ligand-binding affinity, the end-point binding free energy (ΔG_{bind}) of each system was predicted by the solvated interaction energy (SIE) approach [35]. ΔG_{bind} can be estimated by the summation of the van der Waals (E_{vdW}), electrostatic (E_{ele}), reaction field (G_{RF}), cavity ($\gamma\Delta SA(\rho)$), and a constant (C) value. The mathematical equation can be expressed as follow:

$$\Delta G_{bind}\ (\rho, D_{in}, \alpha, \gamma, C) = \alpha[E_{vdW} + E_{ele}(D_{in}) + \Delta G_{RF}(\rho,D_{in}) + \gamma\Delta SA(\rho)] + C$$

where D_{in} denotes the solute dielectric value. E_{vdW} and E_{ele} represent intermolecular van der Waals and Coulombic interaction energies in the bound state, respectively. ΔG_{RF} is the alteration of the reaction field energy between the bound and free states, ΔG_{cavity} ($\gamma\Delta SA$) denotes the change in the non-electrostatic solvation free energy between the bound and free forms, and C is the constant value. The coefficients were set as α = 0.105, γ = 0.013, and C = −2.89.

2.5. QM-Based ONIOM Binding Energy Calculations

A quantum mechanics (QM)-based Our Own N-layered Integrated Molecular Orbital and Molecular mechanics (ONIOM) [36,37] was carried out to additionally observe the binding strength between BIRB796 and the screened drug candidate(s). Before calculating the binding energy, the constructed complexes were optimized using the Hartree−Fock method and a mechanical parameter (HF/6-31G(d):UFF). After optimization, two-layered ONIOM calculations (B3LYP/6-31G(d,):PM6) were applied to determine and compare the binding energies of the three systems. The residues lining within the 5 Å from the ligand, which include Y35, V38, A51, V52, K53, L55, R67, T68, R70, E71, L74, L75, I84, L86, L104, V105, T106, H107, M109, H148, R149, L167, D168, F169, G107, and L171, were selected to represent an allosteric site of p38α MAPK and separated into a low-level layer, while each screened drug was set to a high-level layer. Then, the selected amino acid residues and the ligand were again simulated individually with the B3LYP/6-31G(d) basis set and the PM6 method, respectively. The polarizable continuum model (PCM) was applied to observe the effect of water solvent on the binding energy. All calculations were performed by using the GAUSSIAN16 software package [38], and the binding energy was estimated using the equation below [39].

$$E_{binding}^{solvation} = E_{complex}^{PCM} - E_{residues}^{PCM} - E_{ligand}^{PCM}$$

where $E_{binding}^{solvation}$ is the binding energy of the drug-receptor in the solvation system, $E_{complex}^{PCM}$ is the extrapolated ONIOM energy of the complex, $E_{residues}^{PCM}$ is the potential energy of residues lining within the 5 Å from the ligand, and E_{ligand}^{PCM} is the potential energy of the studied ligand.

3. Results and Discussion

3.1. Docking-Based Screening and Visual Inspection

Finding the existing drugs that can offer inhibition towards novel targets is a great challenge. To this end, 3210 compounds retrieved from the FDA-approved drugs available in the ZINC database were docked into the allosteric site of the p38α MAPK where its 3D-structure and the inhibitor binding site are illustrated in Figure 1. The compounds were selected and ranked according to their binding affinity ($E_{binding}$) predicted by the scoring function of the Autodock XB software package. By considering their binding affinity, it was found that, among the 3210 compounds, only ZINC27990463 exhibited higher binding affinity ($E_{binding}$ = −12.10 kcal/mol) when compared to the ligand reference, BIRB796 ($E_{binding}$ = −11.9 kcal/mol). However, to reduce false-negative selection, compounds exhibiting $E_{binding}$ lower than −10.00 kcal/mol were also clustered, which were totally filtered into 22 compounds. Note that the in silico filtering scheme and the plot of binding affinity of the selected first-round screened compounds were illustrated in Figures 2 and 3, respectively. All these first-round screened compounds were then inspected for intermolecular interactions inside the cleft of the allosteric site, which is commonly known as "visual inspection". This method has been widely used in the decision-making step for a great number of drug discovery campaigns [40].

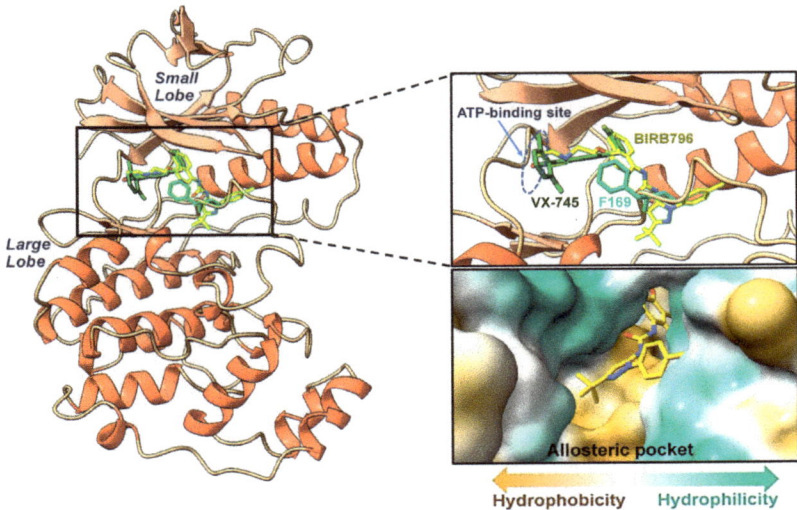

Figure 1. The ribbon representation of the 3D structure of p38α MAPK (PDB ID: 1KV2). The close-up regions illustrate two common inhibitors including VX-745 (green) and BIBR796 (yellow), indicating the ATP-binding site and allosteric pocket, which is distinct from each other at about 60° spatially. An orientation of F169 exhibiting the unique DFG-out conformation is also shown. Additionally, the hydrophobic nature (obtained via UCSF ChimeraX 1.4, Resource for Biocomputing, Visualization, and Informatics (RBVI), San Francisco, CA, USA.) within the focused allosteric cleft is depicted in a close-up view.

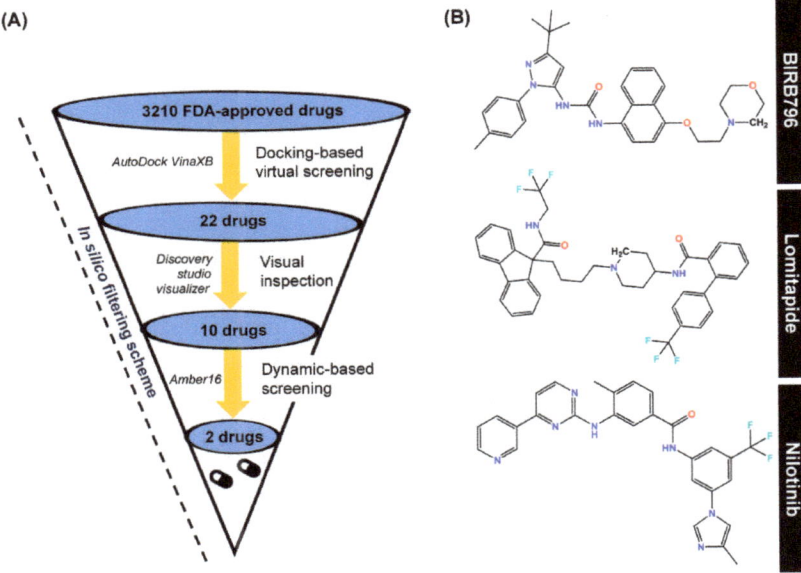

Figure 2. (**A**) In silico filtering scheme, which includes first-round docking-based screening, visual inspection, and SIE-based dynamic screening as well as the program used during each step. (**B**) Chemical structures of a well-known p38α MAPK allosteric inhibitor (BIRB796), lomitapide and nilotinib, obtained via this computational platform.

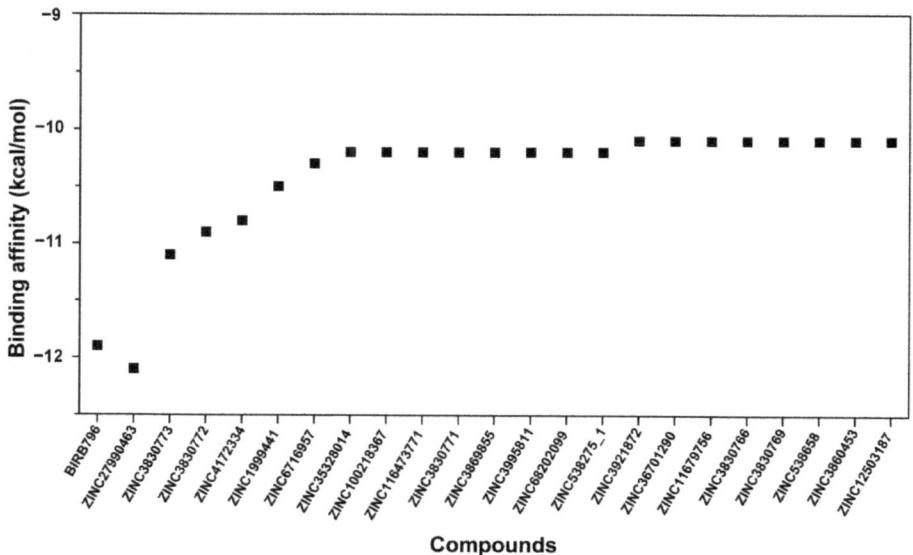

Figure 3. Binding affinity in kcal/mol of selected first-round screened compounds that were successfully docked into the focused allosteric site of p38α MAPK compared to BIRB796. Note that the prediction was based upon the scoring function implemented in the Autodock VinaXB, Sirimulla Research Group at the University of Texas at El Paso, TX, USA.

It is obviously known that noncovalent interactions are essentially responsible for ligand binding. Compounds showing sufficient interactions in both qualitative and quantitative manners tend to exhibit greater binding capability and could form a more stable complex. Thus, an inspection of intermolecular interactions between each ligand and amino-acid residues lining in the focused allosteric site was visually carried out by specifically examining (i) hydrogen bonding with E71, M109, and D168, as well as (ii) hydrophobic interactions with V38, A51, K53, R67, L75, I84, L104, L108, A157, L167, and F169, which were derived from the binding mode observed in the inhibitor prototype, BIRB796. For this purpose, compounds sharing features of intermolecular interactions with BIRB796 greater than five interactions were then selected, for which the detailed information of all 22 compounds is listed in Figure 4. Thus, we could obtain 10 promising compounds (Figure 2A), which are hereinafter referred to as "hit compounds". These 10 hit compounds were subsequently subjected to second-round screening by MD simulations, and the MD output was used to compute SIE-based end-point free energy calculations.

3.2. Dynamic-Based Screening and End-Point Binding Free Energy Calculations

To observe and screen the hit compounds' binding capability in a near-physiological condition and dynamic system, the constructed protein-ligand complexes were performed to run MD simulations for 100 ns. The trajectories in the last ten nanoseconds (90–100 ns) was considered to have reached the equilibrated state (supported by the plot of root-mean-square displacement (RMSD) for the backbone amino acids within 5 Å from the ligand as shown in Figure S3) were used to calculate the binding free energy (ΔG_{bind}). This parameter was used to indicate the protein-ligand binding affinity and to employ a dynamics-based screening tool for ranking the hit compounds in the aftermath of rigid docking.

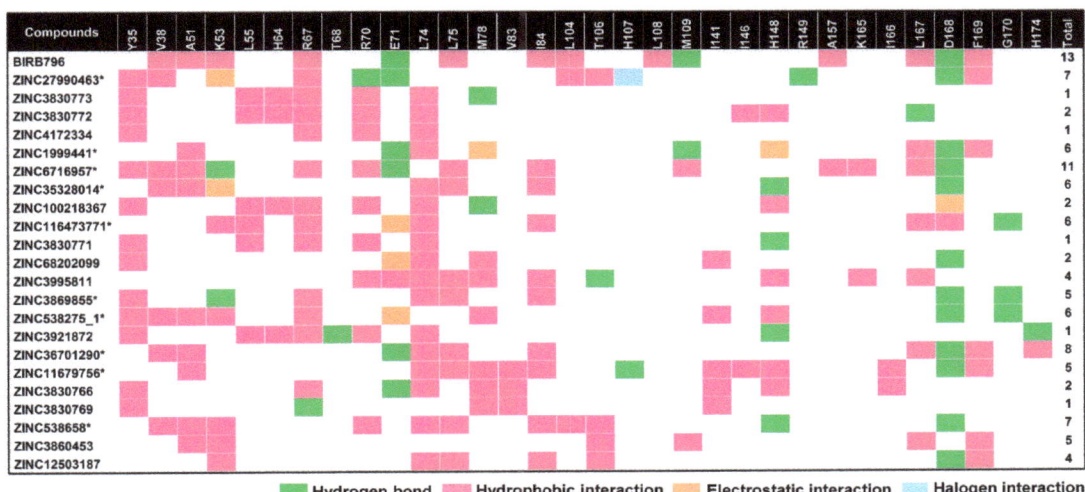

Figure 4. Map of intermolecular interactions of BIRB796 and all 22 screened compounds as well as total features sharing interactions with BIRB796. Each type of noncovalent interaction was also illustrated in different colors. It is worth noting that these occurred interactions were based upon the best docked conformation and visualized by Accelrys Discovery Studio 2.5. * The compounds selected to run MD simulations.

As listed in Table 1, the ΔG_{bind} values of all hit compounds were in the range of −11.4 to −7.2 kcal/mol, whilst the ΔG_{bind} of BIRB796 is −11.95 kcal/mol. Importantly, the predicted ΔG_{bind} of BIRB796 (−11.95 ± 0.04 kcal/mol) is close to the experimental-derived ΔG_{bind} value (−10.98 kcal/mol [41]), showing the verification of the predictive method and the reliability of the results obtained. For screening purposes, only two hit compounds, lomitapide (ΔG_{bind} = −11.39 ± 0.05 kcal/mol) and nilotinib (ΔG_{bind} = −11.21 ± 0.04 kcal/mol) displaying a similar level of binding strength to the BIRB796, were selected for further investigation and the chemical structures of these three drug candidates are illustrated in Figure 2B. For nilotinib, it was previously reported that it could be a new off-target to p38 MAPK in the myoblast cell line [42], which could support our theoretical findings. In particular, the calculated energy terms shown in Table 1 could imply the influence of specific types of noncovalent interactions responsible for drug recognition. In this case, we found that all three drugs possessed a considerably higher contribution of van der Waals interaction energies than other types of interaction energies, agreeing well with the previous study that suggested the hydrophobicity of the binding pocket [43]. Additionally, the higher contribution of vdW interaction energies might imply that the screened drugs could preferentially target the hydrophobic regions within the focused binding site, which was similarly observed in the previously reported potent inhibitors [11]. For the solvation effect, the polar solvation energies expressed as the ΔG_{RF} were in the range of 10.52 to 20.55 kcal/mol. Lomitapide showed a slightly higher ΔG_{RF} (17.01 ± 0.24) than nilotinib and BIRB796 (15.54 ± 0.19 and 15.60 ± 0.20, respectively), implying the relatively minute higher polar solvation in the lomitapide complex system. For ΔG_{cavity}, it was found that the nonpolar solvation energies were in the range of −7.13 to −14.43 kcal/mol. Among candidates, lomitapide possessed the highest contribution of ΔG_{cavity} (−14.43 ± 0.04), showing that the drug could be well-buried into the cleft of the binding site while nilotinib and BIRB796 demonstrated a slight reduction in the nonpolar solvation effect (−12.35 ± 0.03 and −13.63 ± 0.04, respectively). By including the solvation free energy, the vdW term ($\Delta E_{vdW} + \Delta G_{sol}^{nonpolar}$) was the main contribution to the total binding free energies of both drug candidates as well as BIRB796 whilst the electrostatic term ($\Delta E_{ele} + \Delta G_{sol}^{polar}$) became much less favorable to the binding (Figure S4).

Table 1. ΔG_{bind} values (kcal/mol) of the candidate compounds as well as BIRB796 in complex with p38α MAPK calculated by the SIE-based end-point method using α, γ, and constant coefficients of 0.10, 0.01, and −2.89, respectively.

Drugs (ZINC ID)	Energy Components (kcal/mol)				
	E_{VdW}	E_{coul}	ΔG_{RF}	ΔG_{cavity}	ΔG_{bind}
BIRB796	experiment				−10.98 *
	−78.53 ± 0.29	−9.93 ± 0.15	15.60 ± 0.20	−13.63 ± 0.04	−11.95 ± 0.04
Lomitapide (ZINC27990463)	−77.77 ± 0.39	−5.95 ± 0.18	17.01 ± 0.24	−14.43 ± 0.04	−11.39 ± 0.05
Nebivolol (ZINC1999441)	−49.57 ± 0.29	−12.66 ± 0.26	12.78 ± 0.21	−10.19 ± 0.03	−9.14 ± 0.03
Nilotinib (ZINC6716957)	−69.53 ± 0.35	−13.04 ± 0.17	15.54 ± 0.19	−12.35 ± 0.03	−11.21 ± 0.04
Ibrutinib (ZINC35328014)	−61.87 ± 0.29	−4.07 ± 0.17	13.21 ± 0.23	−10.81 ± 0.04	−9.55 ± 0.04
Atovaquone (ZINC116473771)	−42.15 ± 0.27	−2.43 ± 0.39	10.94 ± 0.23	−7.90 ± 0.05	−7.24 ± 0.03
Dicumarol (ZINC3869855)	−39.68 ± 0.26	−13.87 ± 0.40	20.55 ± 0.32	−7.13 ± 0.03	−7.09 ± 0.03
Raloxifene (ZINC538275)	−51.19 ± 0.44	−12.45 ± 0.50	18.50 ± 0.25	−9.90 ± 0.05	−8.66 ± 0.07
Ponatinib (ZINC36701290)	−61.66 ± 0.25	−4.92 ± 0.14	16.99 ± 0.24	−12.08 ± 0.05	−9.35 ± 0.03
Eltrombopag (ZINC11679756)	−59.44 ± 0.33	−5.39 ± 0.17	10.52 ± 0.17	−10.97 ± 0.03	−9.73 ± 0.04
Samsca (ZINC538658)	−51.69 ± 0.26	−16.63 ± 0.21	19.86 ± 0.18	−10.38 ± 0.04	−9.05 ± 0.03

* The experimental binding free energy was derived from the IC$_{50}$ of 0.018 µM [41] and was calculated by the equation $\Delta G_{bind} = RT\ln IC_{50}$.

3.3. Contact Atoms and Numbers of Hydrogen Bond Formation

Identifying the number of atoms surrounding a ligand is one of the crucial parameters implying the ability of the drug recognition within the focused allosteric target. Herein, noncovalent contacts of any atoms within the 5.0 Å from the ligand were computed, and we found that the number of surrounding atoms averaged in the last 10 nanoseconds of each focused complex was in the order of lomitapide (429 ± 17 atoms) > BIRB796 (424 ± 6 atoms) > nilotinib (405 ± 2 atoms) as illustrated in Figure 5. The number of surrounding atoms of the lomitapide complex was slightly higher than that of the BIRB796 and nilotinib complexes, suggesting that the binding pocket residues are close-packed during complexation.

Furthermore, the quantity of hydrogen bonds (H-bond), which was considered one of the strong interactions responsible for drug-receptor binding, was analyzed during 90–100 ns with three independent replicates. As shown in Figure 5, the numbers of averaged H-bond interactions in BIRB796 and nilotinib were in a vicinity of a similar level (≈3–4 bonds), while the lomitapide displayed lower numbers of this kind of interaction (≈2–3 bonds). For drug binding, this indicated that both BIRB796 and nilotinib could form more H-bonds when compared to lomitapide. This is likely to occur since the intrinsic structural characteristic of lomitapide consists of gradual lower numbers of hydrogen bond donors and acceptors when compared to BIRB796 and nilotinib, (total numbers of H-bond donors and acceptors of BIRB796, nilotinib, and lomitapide are 7, 8, and 5, respectively (analyzed by PharmaGist web interface [44] as listed in Table S1).

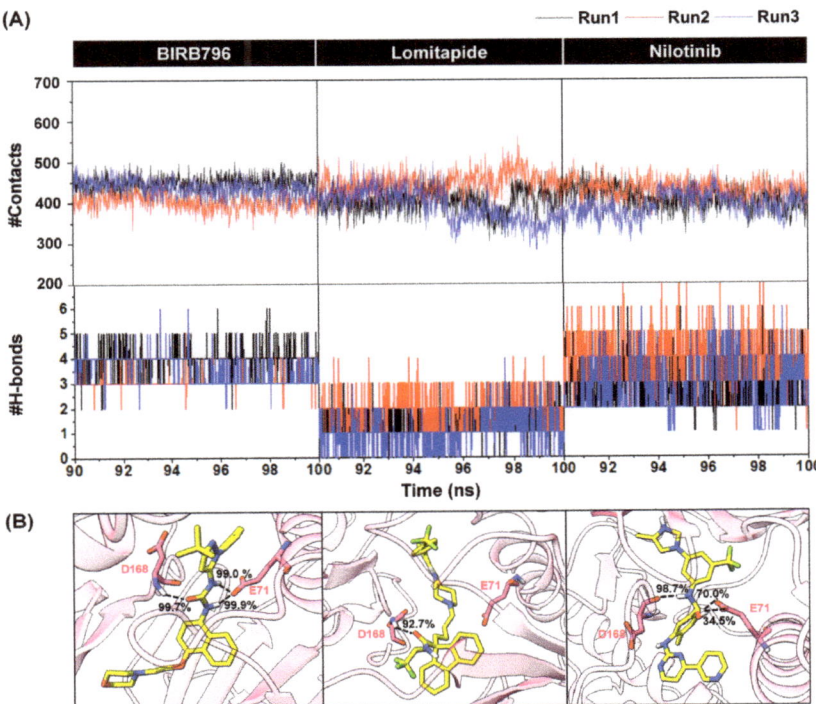

Figure 5. (**A**) Numbers of surrounding atoms counted within the 5.0 Å from the ligand and number of H-bonds within p38α MAPK-BIRB796 complex and two focused drugs at the last 10 nanoseconds (90–100 ns). The results were shown in three independent runs. (**B**) Percentage of H-bond occurrence during a complex formation of two screened drugs and the BIRB796 using two criteria as follows: (1) the distance between the hydrogen bond donor (HD) and hydrogen acceptor (HA) of ≤3.5 Å (2) the angle ≥120°.

In addition, the intermolecular H-bond interactions were observed in terms of the percentage of occupations (Figure 5B), which indicated how often the transient H-bonds could occur during the whole simulated time. As expected, a few strong hydrogen bonds could be seen in all focused drugs and even in BIRB796 since their inhibitory actions were mainly driven by hydrophobic interactions (Table 1). Obviously, all three compounds were found to have very strong H-bonds with D168 (99.7%, 92.7%, and 98.7% occupations for BIRB796, lomitapide, and nilotinib, respectively). Additionally, the BIRB796 showed an additional very strong H-bond with E71 (≈99%), while this bond was reduced to 70% and 34.5% for nilotinib. The slight loss of this interaction in nilotinib might cause a slight reduction in binding affinity when compared to BIRB796 (Table 1). Nonetheless, we could not observe the H-bond with E71 for lomitapide binding since it lacks H-bond donors at that oriented position. Hence, we hypothesized that adding functional groups containing H-bond donors (e.g., -NH$_2$) onto the carbon atom in the piperidine ring within its structure might allow it to have more additional H-bond interactions with E71. Hence, we ran MD simulations of the modified structure of lomitapide and subjected the MD output to analyze the binding energy at the last 10 ns by using the end-point SIE-based method (as the same protocol used previously with other compounds). As expected, the H-bond occupation with

E71 could be formed at 82.45% during the whole simulated time. Moreover, the binding energy was decreased from -11.39 ± 0.05 kcal/mol to -12.15 ± 0.06 kcal/mol (better binding affinity, Table S3), and slightly lower than BIRB796 (-11.95 ± 0.04 kcal/mol). This finding suggested that modification of a lomitapide's structure by permitting it to interact with E71 could improve its binding affinity, which encouraged us to investigate further.

3.4. Key Binding Residues

To elucidate the key binding amino acids responsible for the drug recognition within the allosteric pocket of p38α MAPK, the decomposition of free energy ($\Delta G_{residue}^{bind}$) based on the MM/GBSA method was computed. The negative and positive $\Delta G_{residue}^{bind}$ values indicate the ligand stabilization and destabilization, respectively. The contribution of each amino acid of the known inhibitor and two focused complexes is shown in Figure 6. Note that among residues 5–352 of p38α MAPK, only residues 5–250 are shown.

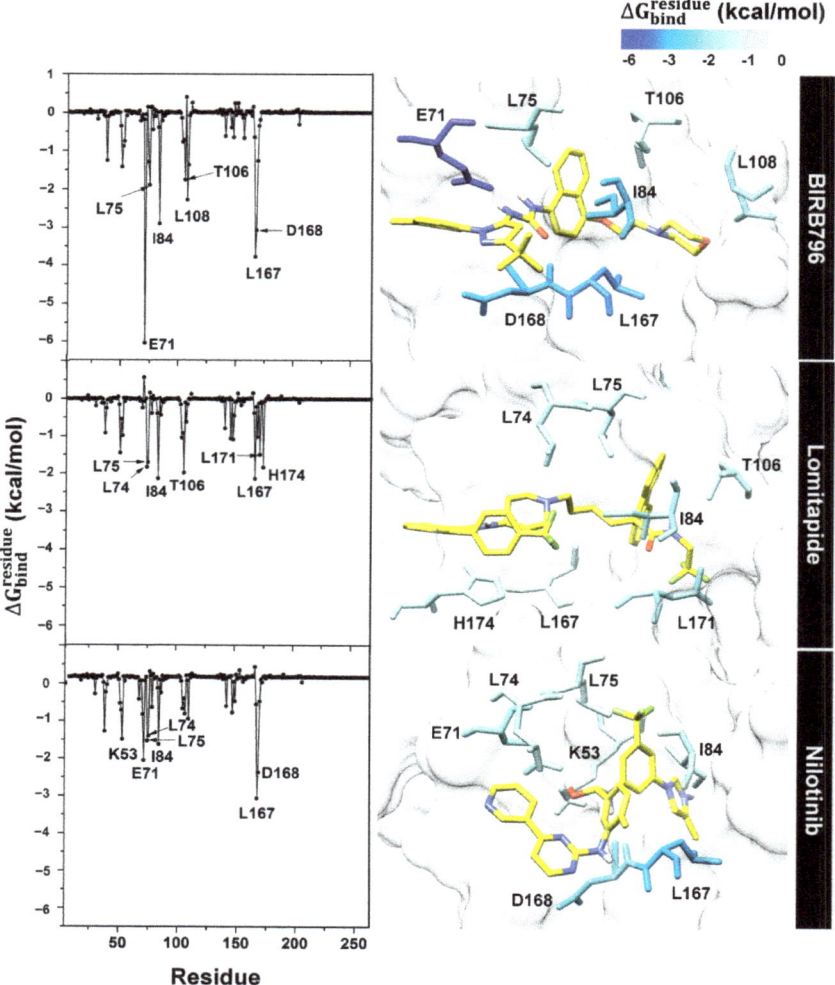

Figure 6. Per-residue free energy decomposition of amino acids involved in ligand binding where the highest to lowest $\Delta G_{residue}^{bind}$ contribution (more negative value) was shaded from dark blue to white.

For the BIRB796, it was obviously seen that E71 and D168 played a pivotal role in stabilizing the protein–ligand complex as its large $\Delta G_{residue}^{bind}$ value was observed (approximately −6 and −4 kcal/mol, respectively). In addition, four hydrophobic residues (L75, I84, L108, and L107) and one polar uncharged amino acid (T106) were found to be involved in a process of complex formation. This key-binding elucidation agreed well with the previous reports of BIRB796's binding mode analysis [11,41]. Apart from a reference ligand, the amino acids largely contributing to the lomitapide binding ($\Delta G_{residue}^{bind} < -1.5$ kcal/mol) include L74, L75, T106, L167, L171, and H174. Almost all were hydrophobic residues (except H174, a polar positively charged residue), suggesting the ensembles of hydrophobic interactions were dominant towards the binding (supported by per-residue vdW interaction energy as illustrated in Figure S4). Among these, the four residues L75, I84, T106, and L167 shared binding features in common with BIRB796. Interestingly, unlike BIRB796, lomitapide could bind to L171 and H174. Having interaction with the amino acids in the region of 170–199 attracted considerable attention, as similarly observed in a new series of benzooxadiazole-based p38 inhibitors which was granted a patent in 2014–2015 (Allinky Biopharma. Co., Madrid, Spain) [11]. In the case of nilotinib, it was found that key amino acids contributing to its binding were mostly the same residues responsible for BIRB796 binding (E71, L75, I84, L107, L108, and D168) since it belongs to the same type of inhibitor (kinase inhibitor). Among these, E71 and D168 were essentially responsible for stabilizing the complex via H-bond while the others relied on hydrophobic interactions (Figure S4). Two additional residues, K53 and L74 were also observed. We noted that these results are correlated well with the calculated SIE-based ΔG_{bind} and each energy component as listed in Table 1.

3.5. QM-Based ONIOM Binding Energy

The analysis of the ONIOM binding energies was employed to additionally observe the binding ability of the two screened drugs within the focused allosteric site of p38α MAPK. The calculations were based on the QM method, which could provide a more reliable prediction when compared to the end-point estimation [45]. As shown in Table 2, the calculated binding energy ($E_{binding}^{solvation}$) values ranged from approximately −41.0 to −48.5 kcal/mol. The $E_{binding}^{solvation}$ values displayed a similar trend to the SIE-based prediction in which the binding affinity of BIRB7996 was slightly higher than that of lomitapide and nilotinib. Even though the $E_{binding}^{solvation}$ of the two screened drugs showed as slightly lower, their predicted binding strength was still high and comparable to the reference inhibitor, BIRB796. Accordingly, we believe that lomitapide and nilotinib could be able to inhibit the phosphorylation of p38α MAPK, and the ONIOM-based method theoretically confirmed their inhibitory capability towards p38α MAPK at the allosteric site. It is worth noting that the prediction trend of binding affinity by ONIOM energy calculations was in good agreement with the SIE-based end-point method.

Table 2. Calculated binding energy ($E_{binding}^{solvation}$) in kcal/mol of two screened drugs and BIRB796 by means of ONIOM at B3LYP/6-31G(d):PM6 level of theory.

Drugs	Energy Terms			
	$E_{complex}^{PCM}$ (a.u.)	$E_{residues}^{PCM}$ (a.u.)	E_{ligand}^{PCM} (a.u.)	$E_{binding}^{solvation}$ (kcal/mol)
BIRB796	−1706.396	−3.391	−1702.927	−48.536
Lomitapide	−2425.571	−3.303	−2422.203	−41.159
Nilotinib	−1841.536	−3.240	−1838.230	−41.048

4. Conclusions

Since there have been no drugs approved as therapeutic agents for p38α MAPK, our research is considered one of the collective efforts to search for effective drugs targeting this target at the allosteric site by a drug repurposing approach. Verified docking- and dynamic-based screening revealed that lomitapide and nilotinib could alternatively impede the p38α MAPK's function with a great binding affinity and characteristics. The binding affinity estimated by both end-point and QM-based ONIOM methods revealed a comparable level to the inhibitor prototype (BIRB796), supported by the calculated numbers of atoms surrounded within the 5.0 Å from the ligand. Specifically, vdW interaction energies were the main force driving the complex formation. Moreover, all drugs could form a few H-bonds with the amino acids lining in the allosteric site, which could rank in the order of BIRB796 ≈ nilotinib > lomitapide. The two residues (E71 and D168) played a pivotal role in forming very strong H-bonds with the focused drugs. More importantly, we proposed that modifying a lomitapide's structure by allowing it to interact with E71 via H-bonds could improve its binding affinity. Altogether, our in silico study not only presented the potential inhibitors, but also provided useful information at the atomic level to shed light on rationally designing more potent inhibitors disrupting the MAPK signaling pathway. However, experiments determining the biological activities of these elucidated compounds including enzyme- and cell-based assays should be further carried out.

Supplementary Materials: The following are available online at https://www.mdpi.com/article/10.3390/pharmaceutics14071461/s1, Figure S1: Ramanchandran plot analysis of a homologically constructed protein structure, Figure S2: Alignment of the re-docked pose and available crystallized ligand (BIRB796) of p38α MAPK indicating a verified docking protocol used in this study, Figure S3: Plot of root-mean-square displacement (RMSD) for the backbone amino acids within 5 Å from the ligand, Figure S4: Analysis of per-residue VdW and electrostatic decomposition energy, Table S1: Summary of key pharmacophore features of BIRB796, lomitapide, and nilotinib detected by using the PharmaGist web interface, Table S2: The Δ_{Gbind} value (kcal/mol) in each run and the averaged Δ_{Gbind} of the two focused drug candidates and BIRB796 in complex with p38α MAPK, Table S3: The Δ_{Gbind} value (kcal/mol) of the modified structure of lomitapide in complex with p38α MAPK, calculated by using end-point SIE method.

Author Contributions: U.S. carried out the preparation, data collection, virtual screening, molecular dynamic simulations, binding free energy calculations, and wrote the initial version of the manuscript. P.M. and T.R. conceived this study and are responsible for the overall design, interpretation, manuscript preparation, and communication. All authors have read and agreed to the published version of the manuscript.

Funding: This work was financially supported by the Thailand Research Fund (grant number RSA6280085). P.M. would like to thank the Fundamental Fund of Khon Kaen University and the National Science, Research and Innovation Fund (NSRF) for the funding support.

Institutional Review Board Statement: Not applicable.

Informed Consent Statement: Not applicable.

Data Availability Statement: Not applicable.

Acknowledgments: U.S. would like to thank the Science Achievement Scholarship (SAST) of Thailand for the Ph.D. scholarship, the 90th Anniversary of Chulalongkorn University Fund (Ratchadaphiseksomphot Endowment Fund; GCUGR1125651029D), and the Overseas Presentations of Graduate Level Academic Thesis from Graduate School.

Conflicts of Interest: The authors declare no conflict of interest.

References

1. Cargnello, M.; Roux, P. Activation and function of the MAPKs and their substrates, the MAPK-activated protein kinases. *Microbiol. Mol. Biol. Rev.* **2011**, *75*, 50–83. [CrossRef] [PubMed]
2. Astolfi, A.; Manfroni, G.; Cecchetti, V.; Barreca, M. A comprehensive structural overview of p38α mitogen-activated protein kinase in complex with ATP-Site and non-ATP-site binders. *ChemMedChem* **2018**, *13*, 7–14. [CrossRef] [PubMed]
3. Lee, S.; Rauch, J.; Kolch, W. Targeting MAPK signaling in cancer: Mechanisms of drug resistance and sensitivity. *Int. J. Mol. Sci.* **2020**, *21*, 1102. [CrossRef] [PubMed]

4. Kumar, S.; Boehm, J.; Lee, J. P38 MAP kinases: Key signalling molecules as therapeutic targets for inflammatory diseases. *Nat. Rev. Drug Discov.* **2003**, *2*, 717–726. [CrossRef]
5. Schett, G.; Zwerina, J.; Firestein, G. The p38 mitogen-activated protein kinase (MAPK) pathway in rheumatoid arthritis. *Ann. Rheum. Dis.* **2008**, *67*, 909–916. [CrossRef]
6. Dolado, I.; Swat, A.; Ajenjo, N.; De Vita, G.; Cuadrado, A.; Nebreda, A. P38α MAP kinase as a sensor of reactive oxygen species in tumorigenesis. *Cancer Cell* **2007**, *11*, 191–205. [CrossRef]
7. Igea, A.; Nebreda, A. The stress kinase p38α as a target for cancer therapy. *Cancer Res.* **2015**, *75*, 3997. [CrossRef]
8. Kim, E.; Choi, E. Pathological roles of MAPK signaling pathways in human diseases. *Biochim. Biophys. Acta (BBA)—Mol. Basis Dis.* **2010**, *1802*, 396–405. [CrossRef]
9. Grimes, J.; Grimes, K. P38 MAPK inhibition: A promising therapeutic approach for COVID-19. *J. Mol. Cell. Cardiol.* **2020**, *144*, 63–65. [CrossRef]
10. Canovas, B.; Nebreda, A. Diversity and versatility of p38 kinase signalling in health and disease. *Nat. Rev. Mol. Cell Biol.* **2021**, *22*, 346–366. [CrossRef]
11. Haller, V.; Nahidino, P.; Forster, M.; Laufer, S. An updated patent review of p38 MAP kinase inhibitors (2014–2019). *Expert Opin. Ther. Pat.* **2020**, *30*, 453–466. [CrossRef] [PubMed]
12. Pargellis, C.; Tong, L.; Churchill, L.; Cirillo, P.; Gilmore, T.; Graham, A.; Grob, P.; Hickey, E.; Moss, N.; Pav, S.; et al. Inhibition of p38 MAP kinase by utilizing a novel allosteric binding site. *Nat. Struct. Biol.* **2002**, *9*, 268–272. [CrossRef] [PubMed]
13. Grant, S. Therapeutic protein kinase inhibitors. *Cell. Mol. Life Sci.* **2009**, *66*, 1163–1177. [CrossRef]
14. Schindler, J.; Monahan, J.; Smith, W. p38 pathway kinases as anti-inflammatory drug targets. *J. Dent. Res.* **2007**, *86*, 800–811. [CrossRef] [PubMed]
15. Damjanov, N.; Kauffman, R.; Spencer-Green, G. Safety and Efficacy of VX-702, a p38 MAP Kinase Inhibitor, in Rheumatoid arthritis. OP-0246 European League Against Rheumatism. In Proceedings of the Annual Congress, Paris, France, 21 September 2008; pp. 11–14.
16. Matthew, R.; Celia, D. MAP kinase p38 inhibitors: Clinical results and an intimate look at their interactions with p38alpha protein. *Curr. Med. Chem.* **2005**, *12*, 2979–2994.
17. Sweeney, S.; Firestein, G. Mitogen activated protein kinase inhibitors: Where are we now and where are we going? *Ann. Rheum. Dis.* **2006**, *65*, 83. [CrossRef]
18. Waterhouse, A.; Bertoni, M.; Bienert, S.; Studer, G.; Tauriello, G.; Gumienny, R.; Heer, F.; Beer, T.; Rempfer, C.; Bordoli, L.; et al. SWISS-MODEL: Homology modelling of protein structures and complexes. *Nucleic Acids Res.* **2018**, *46*, 296–303. [CrossRef]
19. Laskowski, R.; MacArthur, M.; Moss, D.; Thornton, J. PROCHECK: A program to check the stereochemical quality of protein structures. *J. Appl. Crystallogr.* **1993**, *26*, 283–291. [CrossRef]
20. Olsson, M.; Søndergaard, C.; Rostkowski, M.; Jensen, J. Computation, PROPKA3: Consistent treatment of internal and surface residues in empirical pKa predictions. *J. Chem. Theory Comput.* **2011**, *7*, 525–537. [CrossRef]
21. Frisch, M.J.; Trucks, G.W.; Schlegel, H.B.; Scuseria, G.E.; Robb, M.A.; Cheeseman, J.R.; Scalmani, G.; Barone, V.; Petersson, G.A.; Nakatsuji, H.; et al. Gaussian 09 Revision D. 01, Gaussian Inc. 2009. Volume 112. Available online: http://www.gaussian.com (accessed on 31 January 2020).
22. Wang, J.; Wang, W.; Kollman, P.; Case, D. ANTECHAMBER: An accessory software package for molecular mechanical calculations. *J. Chem. Inf. Comput. Sci.—JCISD* **2000**, *222*, U403.
23. Koebel, M.R.; Schmadeke, G.; Posner, R.; Sirimulla, S. AutoDock VinaXB: Implementation of XBSF, new empirical halogen bond scoring function, into AutoDock Vina. *J. Cheminform.* **2016**, *8*, 27. [CrossRef] [PubMed]
24. Sanachai, K.; Mahalapbutr, P.; Sanghiran Lee, V.; Rungrotmongkol, T.; Hannongbua, S. In silico elucidation of potent inhibitors and rational drug design against SARS-CoV-2 Papain-like protease. *J. Phys. Chem. B* **2021**, *125*, 13644–13656. [CrossRef] [PubMed]
25. Verma, K.; Mahalapbutr, P.; Suriya, U.; Somboon, T.; Aiebchun, T.; Shi, L.; Maitarad, P.; Rungrotmongkol, T. In silico screening of DNA gyrase B potent flavonoids for the treatment of clostridium difficile infection from phytoHub database. *Braz. Arch. Biol. Technol.* **2021**, *64*. [CrossRef]
26. Sripattaraphan, A.; Sanachai, K.; Chavasiri, W.; Boonyasuppayakorn, S.; Maitarad, P.; Rungrotmongkol, T. Computational screening of newly designed compounds against coxsackievirus A16 and enterovirus A71. *Molecules* **2022**, *27*, 1908. [CrossRef]
27. Thirunavukkarasu, M.; Suriya, U.; Rungrotmongkol, T.; Karuppasamy, R. In silico screening of available drugs targeting non-small cell lung cancer targets: A drug repurposing approach. *Pharmaceutics* **2022**, *14*, 59. [CrossRef] [PubMed]
28. Mahalapbutr, P.; Wonganan, P.; Chavasiri, W.; Rungrotmongkol, T. Butoxy mansonone G inhibits STAT3 and akt signaling pathways in non-small cell lung cancers: Combined experimental and theoretical investigations. *Cancers* **2019**, *11*, 437. [CrossRef]
29. Wang, J.; Wolf, R.; Caldwell, J.; Kollman, P.; Case, D. Development and testing of a general amber force field. *J. Comput. Chem.* **2004**, *25*, 1157–1174. [CrossRef]
30. Darden, T.; York, D.; Pedersen, L. Particle mesh ewald: An n· log (N) method for ewald sums in large systems. *J. Chem. Phys.* **1993**, *98*, 10089–10092. [CrossRef]
31. Ryckaert, J.; Ciccotti, G.; Berendsen, H. Numerical integration of the cartesian equations of motion of a system with constraints: Molecular dynamics of n-alkanes. *J. Comput. Phys.* **1977**, *23*, 327–341. [CrossRef]
32. Uberuaga, B.; Anghel, M.; Voter, A. Synchronization of trajectories in canonical molecular-dynamics simulations: Observation, explanation, and exploitation. *J. Chem. Phys.* **2004**, *120*, 6363–6374. [CrossRef]

33. Berendsen, H.; Postma, J.; van Gunsteren, W.; DiNola, A.; Haak, J. Molecular dynamics with coupling to an external bath. *J. Chem. Phys.* **1984**, *81*, 3684–3690. [CrossRef]
34. Jorgensen, W.; Chandrasekhar, J.; Madura, J.; Impey, R.; Klein, M. Comparison of simple potential functions for simulating liquid water. *J. Chem. Phys.* **1983**, *79*, 926–935. [CrossRef]
35. Naïm, M.; Bhat, S.; Rankin, K.N.; Dennis, S.; Chowdhury, S.; Siddiqi, I.; Drabik, P.; Sulea, T.; Bayly, C.I.; Jakalian, A.; et al. Solvated interaction energy (SIE) for scoring protein−ligand binding affinities. 1. exploring the parameter space. *J. Chem. Inf. Model.* **2007**, *47*, 122–133. [CrossRef]
36. Dapprich, S.; Komáromi, I.; Byun, K.S.; Morokuma, K.; Frisch, M.J. A new ONIOM implementation in Gaussian98. Part I. The calculation of energies, gradients, vibrational frequencies and electric field derivatives. *J. Mol. Struct. THEOCHEM* **1999**, *461–462*, 1–21. [CrossRef]
37. Vreven, T.; Morokuma, K. Chapter 3 hybrid methods: ONIOM(QM:MM) and QM/MM. In *Annual Reports in Computational Chemistry*; Elsevier: Amsterdam, The Netherlands, 2006; pp. 35–51.
38. Frisch, M.J.; Trucks, G.W.; Schlegel, H.B.; Scuseria, G.E.; Robb, M.A.; Cheeseman, J.R.; Scalmani, G.; Barone, V.; Petersson, G.A.; Nakatsuji, H.; et al. *Gaussian 16 Rev. B.01*; Gaussian, Inc.: Wallingford, CT, USA, 2016.
39. Li, Q.; Gusarov, S.; Evoy, S.; Kovalenko, A. Electronic structure, binding energy, and solvation structure of the streptavidin−biotin supramolecular complex: ONIOM and 3D-RISM study. *J. Phys. Chem. B* **2009**, *113*, 9958–9967. [CrossRef] [PubMed]
40. Fischer, A.; Smieško, M.; Sellner, M.; Lill, M. Decision making in structure-based drug discovery: Visual inspection of docking results. *J. Med. Chem.* **2021**, *64*, 2489–2500. [CrossRef]
41. Yang, Y.; Shen, Y.; Liu, H.; Yao, X. Molecular dynamics simulation and free energy calculation studies of the binding mechanism of allosteric inhibitors with p38α MAP kinase. *J. Chem. Inf. Model.* **2011**, *51*, 3235–3246. [CrossRef]
42. Contreras, O.; Villarreal, M.; Brandan, E. Nilotinib impairs skeletal myogenesis by increasing myoblast proliferation. *Skeletal Muscle* **2018**, *8*, 5. [CrossRef]
43. Chang, H.; Chung, F.; Yang, C. Molecular modeling of p38α mitogen-activated protein kinase inhibitors through 3D-QSAR and molecular dynamics simulations. *J. Chem. Inf. Model.* **2013**, *53*, 1775–1786. [CrossRef]
44. Schneidman, D.; Dror, O.; Inbar, Y.; Nussinov, R.; Wolfson, H. Pharmagist: A webserver for ligand-based pharmacophore detection. *Nucleic Acids Res.* **2008**, *36*, W223–W228. [CrossRef]
45. Maier, S.; Thapa, B.; Erickson, J.; Raghavachari, K. Comparative assessment of QM-based and MM-based models for prediction of protein–ligand binding affinity trends. *Phys. Chem. Chem. Phys.* **2022**, *24*, 14525–14537. [CrossRef] [PubMed]

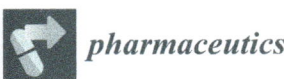

Article

Drug Repurposing Based on Protozoan Proteome: In Vitro Evaluation of In Silico Screened Compounds against *Toxoplasma gondii*

Débora Chaves Cajazeiro [1], Paula Pereira Marques Toledo [1], Natália Ferreira de Sousa [2], Marcus Tullius Scotti [2] and Juliana Quero Reimão [1,*]

[1] Laboratory of Preclinical Assays and Research of Alternative Sources of Innovative Therapy for Toxoplasmosis and Other Sicknesses (PARASITTOS), Departamento de Morfologia e Patologia Básica, Faculdade de Medicina de Jundiaí, Jundiaí 13202-550, Brazil

[2] Programa de Pós-graduação em Produtos Naturais e Sintéticos Bioativos (PgPNSB), Instituto de Pesquisa em Fármacos e Medicamentos (IPeFarM), Universidade Federal da Paraíba, Campus I, Cidade Universitária, João Pessoa 58051-900, Brazil

* Correspondence: julianareimao@g.fmj.br

Abstract: *Toxoplasma gondii* is a protozoan that infects up to a third of the world's population. This parasite can cause serious problems, especially if a woman is infected during pregnancy, when toxoplasmosis can cause miscarriage, or serious complications to the baby, or in an immunocompromised person, when the infection can possibly affect the patient's eyes or brain. To identify potential drug candidates that could counter toxoplasmosis, we selected 13 compounds which were pre-screened in silico based on the proteome of *T. gondii* to be evaluated in vitro against the parasite in a cell-based assay. Among the selected compounds, three demonstrated in vitro anti-*T. gondii* activity in the nanomolar range (almitrine, bortezomib, and fludarabine), and ten compounds demonstrated anti-*T. gondii* activity in the micromolar range (digitoxin, digoxin, doxorubicin, fusidic acid, levofloxacin, lomefloxacin, mycophenolic acid, ribavirin, trimethoprim, and valproic acid). Almitrine demonstrated a Selectivity Index (provided by the ratio between the Half Cytotoxic Concentration against human foreskin fibroblasts and the Half Effective Concentration against *T. gondii* tachyzoites) that was higher than 47, whilst being considered a lead compound against *T. gondii*. Almitrine showed interactions with the Na$^+$/K$^+$ ATPase transporter for *Homo sapiens* and *Mus musculus*, indicating a possible mechanism of action of this compound.

Keywords: bioinformatics; drug repurposing; toxoplasmosis; *Toxoplasma gondii*; in vitro screening; drug targets; drug discovery

1. Introduction

Toxoplasma gondii is an obligate intracellular protozoan parasite that belongs to Apicomplexa Phylum and is the etiological agent of toxoplasmosis [1]. The parasite diverged from closer species due to its ability to infect a wide range of hosts, re-enforced by flexible transmission pathways [2]. Because of this, it is estimated that more than 60% of the population throughout the world have been infected [3] and, in Brazil, the serologic prevalence of *T. gondii* human infection ranges from 50% to 80% [4].

Despite the importance of toxoplasmosis to public health, considering its high prevalence in the human population and the serious clinical manifestations, mainly in immunocompromised patients and in cases of congenital infection [5], there are still very few therapeutic options available, these being effective only against the acute form of the disease [6].

Ideal drugs for toxoplasmosis treatments should be effective against the chronic form of infection and be offered at an affordable price, and present low or zero toxicity [7].

Ideally, they should also not present risks of congenital malformation, allowing pregnant women to use them freely. However, several of these characteristics are not found in drugs currently used in standard toxoplasmosis therapy, which has remained unchanged since the beginning of the 1990s [7]. Since current chemotherapy is insufficiently effective, with extended treatments that vary from weeks to over a year in duration, or show high toxicity [8], alternative therapeutic options for toxoplasmosis treatment are of utmost importance.

The research and development of new drugs represent a slow and onerous process. New techniques have been proposed to speed up this process, and one of these is called 'drug repositioning'. It consists of a strategy that seeks new applications for an existing drug, which have not been previously referenced and are not currently prescribed or researched [9].

Aiming to find new uses for already known compounds, the international organization Medicines for Malaria Venture (MMV) and the Drugs for Neglected Diseases initiative (DNDi), together with researchers from the industrial and academic fields, created the Pandemic Response Box and the COVID Box. Together, these collections consist of 560 structurally diverse active compounds, all set for trial against infectious and neglected diseases. These compounds were selected from an extensive list of antibacterial, antifungal, and antiviral compounds, all of which are already being commercialized or are in the clinical development phase [10].

Malaria Box and Pathogen Box are two other collections created by MMV that gather around 800 compounds with confirmed activity against the most socio-economic relevant diseases all over the world, such as malaria, tuberculosis, sleeping sickness, leishmaniasis, schistosomiases, ancylostomiasis, toxoplasmosis, cryptosporidiosis, and dengue. These collections were used to identify new drug candidates for the treatment of many diseases, including toxoplasmosis [2,11,12].

Databases of bioactivity, such as ChEMBL and DrugBank, provide information about the interaction between compounds and proteins. Sarteriale et al. [13] have presented an approach to pre-track the entire proteome of any organism with available genomic data against known drug targets, using a combination of Ruby scripts and freely available resources. This method was used to predict inhibitors for disease-causing protozoan parasites. The authors performed the in vitro validation of the in silico results obtained, using a cell-based *Cryptosporidium parvum* growth assay, showing that the predicted inhibitors were significantly more likely than those expected randomly by chance. However, the identified compounds had not yet been evaluated against *T. gondii* in a cell-based assay until now. Here, we tested some of the inhibitors identified by Sarteriale et al. 2014 [13], aiming to confirm the in silico predicted activity against *T. gondii* in a cell-based assay.

Amongst the compounds that presented a *T. gondii* protein as their target in the virtual screening, 13 were selected for evaluation against *T. gondii* in the present work. This selection was based on the presence of these compounds in the MMV Pandemic Response Box and COVID Box collections, aiming to evaluate in vitro the predicted activity against *T. gondii* (Figure 1).

We crossed the in silico screening results achieved by Sarteriale et al. 2014 [13] with the MMV libraries, aiming to build a small enriched compound collection for in vitro drug testing.

Our objective was to test only the in silico predicted *T. gondii* inhibitors available in the Pandemic Response Box and COVID Box collections, enabling a more efficient use of laboratory resources. We obtained 100% accuracy, since all these 13 compounds showed anti-*T. gondii* activity in the micromolar or nanomolar range, this being the first report about the in vitro anti-*T. gondii* activity of almitrine, bortezomib, and fludarabine.

Drug development is a lengthy, complex, and costly process, entrenched with a high degree of uncertainty that a drug will succeed. In this context, drug repurposing—A strategy for identifying new clinical uses for existing drugs—Becomes an interesting strategy for drug discovery, as it involves potentially lower financial costs in drug development as well as shorter timelines [14].

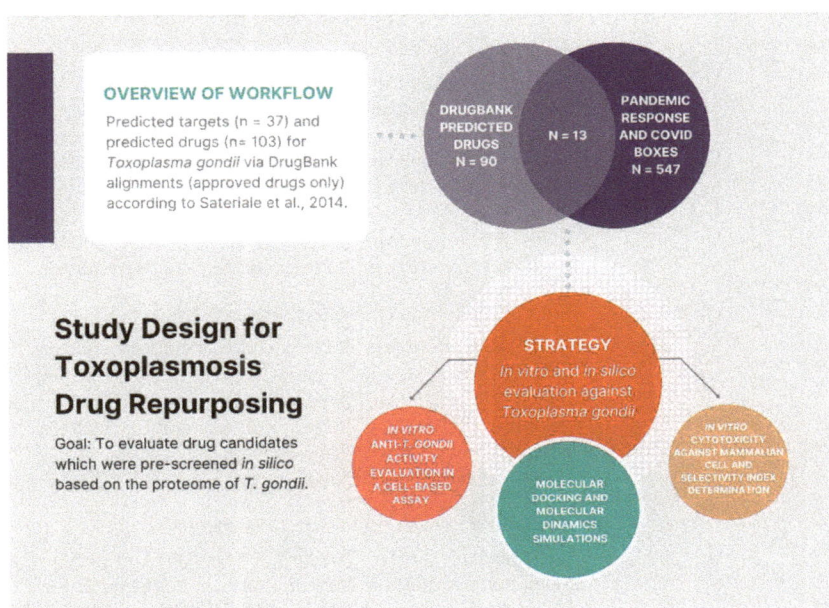

Figure 1. Study design and workflow. Following the publication of predicted drugs for *T. gondii* via DrugBank alignments by Sarteriale et al., (2014) [13], we selected 13 compounds from Pandemic Response and COVID Boxes to be in vitro evaluated against *T. gondii* and for Molecular Docking and Dinamics Simulations in the present work. Among the 13 selected compounds, three demonstrated in vitro anti-*T. gondii* activity in the nanomolar range (almitrine, bortezomib, and fludarabine), and ten compounds demonstrated anti-*T. gondii* activity in the micromolar range.

Because repurposing screens can be costly and time consuming, an in silico drug screen with the ability to identify drugs with a high likelihood of activity improves the chances of success by enabling the pre-selection of compounds to test in vitro.

Here we connected traditional drug discovery techniques with computer-based tools to deliver robust drug repurposing hints. We used a target-based pre-screen that utilized simple sequence alignment techniques to discover potential drugs [13]. Drugs' structural and physicochemical properties and the predicted drug-target interactions were explored to select potential re-positioned compounds to treat toxoplasmosis. Therefore, the contributions of this manuscript are:

- To demonstrate the in vitro anti-*T. gondii* activity of the 13 pre-screened compounds: almitrine, bortezomib, digitoxin, digoxin, doxorubicin, fludarabine, fusidic acid, levofloxacin, lomefloxacin, mycophenolic acid, ribavirin, trimethoprim, and valproic acid;
- To demonstrate the in vitro cytotoxic of almitrine, bortezomib and fludarabine against human foreskin fibroblasts;
- To investigate the mechanism of action of the 13 compounds using Molecular Docking through the binding affinity of the compound and the predicted molecular target;
- To carry out Molecular Dynamics simulations of almitrine to assess the flexibility of the transporting ATPase alpha 1 and the stability of the enzyme interactions in the presence of factors such as solvent, ions, pressure and temperature.

The goal of the present work is therefore to contribute to the discovery of new candidates for toxoplasmosis chemotherapy, using repositioned compounds. The strategy of drug repositioning allows for efficient progress in the drug discovery process since many of the compounds are clinically safe and have well established pharmacological action.

2. Materials and Methods

2.1. Drugs and Chemicals

Pyrimethamine (PYR), dimethyl sulfoxide (DMSO), chlorophenol red-β-D-galactop yranosidase (CPRG), phosphate buffer saline (PBS) and 3-[4,5-dimethylthiazol-2-yl]-2,5-diphenyltetrazolium bromide (MTT) were purchased from Sigma-Aldrich Corporation. Dulbecco's Modified Eagle's Medium (DMEM), fetal bovine serum (FBS), dithiothreitol (DTT), HEPES and sodium dodecyl sulfate (SDS) were purchased from Thermo Fisher Scientific. Pandemic Response Box (PRB) and COVID Box (CB) were kindly donated by the Medicines for Malaria Venture (MMV) foundation. Other analytical reagents were purchased from Sigma-Aldrich, unless otherwise stated.

2.2. Cell Culture and Parasite Propagation

Tachyzoites of the RH strain encoding a transgenic copy of β-galactosidase (type I, clone 2F1) [15] were continually passaged in confluent monolayers of human foreskin fibroblasts (HFF), cultured in DMEM supplemented with 2% FBS (D2 medium), L-glutamine (2 mM) and gentamycin (10 µg/mL) [16]. Fresh emerging tachyzoites were counted, diluted in a fresh culture medium, and added to 96-well plates containing HFF monolayers as described below. All HFF and parasite cultures were grown in a 37 °C incubator supplemented with 5% CO_2.

2.3. β-Galactosidase-Based Growth Inhibition Assays

Firstly, 5×10^3 HFF cells/well (in 100 µL volume) were placed in 96-well plates and incubated overnight to adhere. Afterwards, the wells were emptied and refilled with fresh D2 medium containing 5×10^3 RH-2F1 parasites (in 100 µL volume) and incubated for 3 h at 37 °C, 5% CO_2. Subsequently, compounds were serially diluted in D2 medium and added to the infected plates and incubated for 72 h at 37 °C, 5% CO_2. Each drug concentration was assessed in two replicate wells. Finally, β-galactosidase activity was evaluated as previously described [17]. Infected cells were incubated with 100 µL of lysis buffer (100 mM HEPES, 1 mM $MgSO_4$, 0.1% Triton X-100, 5 mM DTT) for 15 min. Afterwards, the lysates were mixed with 160 µL of assay buffer (100 mM phospate buffer pH 7.3, 102 mM β-mercaptoethanol, 9 mM $MgCl_2$) and, subsequently, with 40 µL of 6.25 mM CPRG. After incubating the reaction mixtures for 30 min, the β-galactosidase activity was measured at 570 nm using a microplate reader (Thermo Scientific™ Varioskan LUX). Pyrimethamine was used as a reference drug (positive control) in all assays. Data presented are representative of the results of two or more biological replicates. Dose-response inhibition curves (Log (inhibitor) vs. normalized response—Variable slope) were obtained using Skanlt Software (Thermo Scientific, Waltham, MA, USA).

2.4. Cytotoxicity in Mammalian Cells

HFF were seeded at 5×10^4 cells/well in 96-well microplates and incubated overnight to adhere to the plate. After that, the cells were incubated in the presence of increasing concentrations of the compounds for 72 h at 37 °C in a 5% CO_2 humidified incubator. The viability of the cells was determined by the MTT assay as previously described [18]. The medium in each well was replaced by PBS (100 µL/well), MTT (5 mg/mL) was added (20 µL/well), and the plate was incubated for 4 h at 37 °C. Formazan extraction was performed using 10% SDS for 18 h (80 µL/well) at room temperature, and the optical density was measured at 550 nm using a microplate reader (Thermo Scientific™ Varioskan LUX). HFF incubated in D2 without drug treatment were used as viability control. Viability of 100% was expressed based on the optical density of untreated HFF cells, after normalization. The Selectivity Index (SI) was provided by the ratio between the CC_{50} against HFF cells and the EC_{50} against *T. gondii* tachyzoites. Data presented are representative of the results of two or more biological replicates. Dose-response inhibition curves (Log (inhibitor) vs. normalized response—Variable slope) were obtained using Skanlt Software (Thermo Scientific).

2.5. Molecular Docking

Molecular Docking was used to investigate the mechanism of action of the 13 compounds included in the study that contribute to the inhibitory effect of *T. gondii* through the binding affinity of the compound and the predicted molecular target [19]. The 3D structure of the enzyme was obtained from the Protein Data Bank (PDB) (https://www.rcsb.org/pdb/home/home.do accessed on 14 March 2022) [20]. Initially, all water molecules were removed from the crystalline structure and the root mean square deviation (RMSD) was calculated from the postures, indicating the degree of reliability of the fit. RMSD provides the connection mode close to the experimental structure and is considered successful if the value is less than 2.0 Å [21]. We used two softwares—Molegro Virtual Docker v.6.0.1 (MVD) (CLC Bio Company, Aarhus, Denmark) and PYRX—Virtual Screening Tool, Source Force, 2022, Slashdot Media. The complexed ligand was used to define the active site. The compound was then imported to analyze the stability of the system through the interactions identified with the active site of the enzyme, taking as a reference the energy value of the MolDock Score [22]. The MolDock SE (Simplex Evolution) algorithm was used with the following parameters: A total of 10 runs with a maximum of 1500 iterations, using a population of 50 individuals, with 2000 minimization steps for each flexible residual and 2000 global minimization steps per run. The MolDock score (GRID) scoring function was used to calculate docking energy values. A GRID was set at 0.3 A and the search sphere was set at 15 A in radius. For the analysis of ligand energy, internal electrostatic interactions, internal hydrogen bonds and sp2-sp2 torsions were evaluated [23,24]. The PYRX—Virtual Screening Tool, Source Force, 2022, Slashdot Media features two main programs, corresponding to: Auto Dock (version 4.2.6), (Center for Computational Structural Biology, San Diego, CA, USA) which uses force fields such as AMBER in conjunction with free energy scoring functions, plus affinity maps and pre-calculated electrostatic maps for specific atoms [25,26]. The second program refers to Auto Dock Vina (version 1.2), (Center for Computational Structural Biology, San Diego, CA, USA), which corresponds to a more recent and improved version of the calculation platform. The software uses a semi-flexible docking algorithm by default. The anchoring site of the receptor being defined within the binding site of the co-crystallized ligand, identified through the coordinates of the ligand after importing and labeling the macromolecule [27,28]. The program was used with a default plug-in parameter. Furthermore, the hydrogen bonding distance (O-H) was defined at <2.50 Å between the donor and acceptor atoms with a minimum hydrogen donor-acceptor angle of 120°. Grid size was adjusted to 25 Å in each dimension. The proteins used in the study were, respectively: thymidyl synthase in complex with 2-amino-5-(phenylsulfanyl)-3,9-dihydro-4H-pyrimido[4,5-b]indol-4-one (PDB: 4KY4) [29], purine nucleoside phosphorylase in complex with 1,4-dideoxy-4-aza-1-(s)-(9-deazahypoxanthine-9-yl)-d-ribitol (PDB: 3MB8) [30], enoyl-acyl carrier protein reductase (ENR) in complex with triclosan (PDB: 2O2S) [31], and calcium dependent protein kinase 1 in complex with 5-amino-1-tert-butyl-3-(quinolin-2-yl)-1H-pyrazole-4-carboxamide (PDB: 4M84) [32]. In addition, to evaluate the specificity of the mechanism of action with Na^+/K^+-transporting ATPase alpha 1, the construction of this macromolecule was carried out for the species *Homo sapiens* and *Mus musculus* [32] with thapsigargin [33] as a positive control.

Docking Consensus

To increase the accuracy of the results obtained, a Docking consensus analysis was performed in order to provide a better selection of the compounds under study. Regarding the Molegro Virtual Docker v.6.0.1 (MVD) program (CLC Bio Company, Aarhus, Denmark), the values of the Moldock Score and PlantScore algorithms were used. Regarding the PYRX program—Virtual Screening Tool, Source Force, 2022, Slashdot Media, AutoDock Vina (version 1.2) (Center for Computational Structural Biology, San Diego, CA, USA) was used.

The determination of the affinity of the 13 compounds under study for the targets of *T. gondii* and the ATPase alpha 1 transporter was established by probability calculations. The probability was calculated by dividing the score of the molecule under study by the lowest energy score (p = composite score/minor score) (Supplementary Tables S1–S5), for each algorithm, and at the end an overall average was calculated between the algorithms to generate the enzyme average ((p) Enzyme = ((p) Moldock Score + (p) Plants Score + (p) Vina Score)/3) [33,34]. The sum of the enzyme mean and division by the number of information originated the total probability (Total P).

2.6. Alignment of Protein Sequences

The sequences of the two proteins that do not contain 3D structures in the Protein Data Bank [35] were obtained from the GenBank database [36]. These proteins were: Na^+/K^+-transporting ATPase alpha 1—*M. musculus* (NP_659149.1) and Na^+/K^+-transporting ATPase alpha 1—*H. sapiens* (NP_000695.2). A global alignment was then performed with the sequence of a protein with a known three-dimensional structure, using the Clustal Omega web tool (WMBL-EBI, 2022 https://www.ebi.ac.uk/Tools/msa/clustalo/ accessed on 14 March 2022) [37], which aligns all protein sequences entered by a user. Alignment facilitated the investigation of the active site and the determination of similarity and shared identity between proteins.

2.7. Modeling by Homology

Target sequences were obtained as amino acid sequences in FASTA format and were imported from the SWISS-MODEL website (https://swissmodel.expasy.org/ accessed on 14 March 2022) [38]. For each identified mold, the quality was predicted from alignment features such as ProMod3, QMEAN and GMQE. The stereochemical quality of the models was evaluated by the PSVS (protein structure validation software suite) web server (http://psvs-1_5-dev.nesg.org/ accessed on 14 March 2022), using PROCHECK [39]. PROCHECK generates a Ramachandran chart [34,35], which determines the allowed and disallowed regions of the amino acid backbone.

2.8. Molecular Dynamics Simulations

Molecular dynamics simulations were performed to estimate the flexibility of interactions between proteins and ligands, using GROMACS 5.0 software (European Union Horizon 2020 Program, Uppsala, Sweden) [40,41]. The protein and ligand topologies were also prepared using the GROMOS96 54a7 force field. The Molecular Dynamics simulation was performed using the SPC water model of point load, extended in a cubic box [42]. The system was neutralized by the addition of ions (Cl^- and Na^+) and minimized, to remove bad contacts between complex molecules and the solvent. The system was also balanced at 300 K, using the 100 ps V-rescale algorithm, represented by NVT (constant pressure particles and temperature), up to 100 ps. DM simulations were performed in 5,000,000 steps, at 10 ns. To determine the flexibility of the structure and whether the complex is stable close to the experimental structure, RMSD values of all Cα atoms were calculated relative to the starting structures. RMSF values were also analyzed to understand the roles played by residues near the receptor binding site. The RMSD and RMSF graphs were generated using Grace software (Grace Development Team, http://plasma-gate.weizmann.ac.il/Grace/ accessed on 23 June 2022) [43].

3. Results

3.1. In Vitro Anti-T. gondii Activity and Cytotoxicity against HFF

We tested 13 compounds that have been in silico selected against *T. gondii* from the MMV foundation's Pandemic Response Box and COVID Box. Table 1 and Figure 2 show the structures and general characteristics of the tested compounds.

Table 1. General characteristics of the 13 compounds tested against *T gondii* in vitro.

MMV Code [a]	Compound (Trivial Name)	Molecular Formula [b]	Mol wt [b]	aLogP [b]	Rule of Five [b]
MMV1804175	Almitrine	$C_{26}H_{29}F_2N_7$	477.5	6.09	3
MMV009415	Bortezomib	$C_{19}H_{25}BN_4O_4$	384.2	2.14	4
MMV002436	Digitoxin	$C_{41}H_{64}O_{13}$	764.9	3.11	2
MMV002832	Digoxin	$C_{41}H_{64}O_{14}$	780.9	2	1

Table 1. *Cont.*

MMV Code [a]	Compound (Trivial Name)	Molecular Formula [b]	Mol wt [b]	aLogP [b]	Rule of Five [b]
MMV004066	Doxorubicin	$C_{27}H_{29}NO_{11}$	543.5	−0.05	1
MMV003219	Mycophenolic acid	$C_{17}H_{20}O_6$	320.3	3.16	4
MMV001439	Ribavirin	$C_8H_{12}N_4O_5$	244.2	−2.75	4
MMV003305	Valproic acid	$C_8H_{16}O_2$	144.2	2.75	4
MMV637413	Fludarabine	$C_{10}H_{12}FN_5O_4$	285.2	−1.32	4
MMV1578575	Fusidic acid	$C_{31}H_{48}O_6$	516.7	5.1	2
MMV687798	Levofloxacin	$C_{18}H_{20}FN_3O_4$	361.4	−1.38	4
MMV002350	Lomefloxacin	$C_{17}H_{19}F_2N_3O_3$	387.8	−0.83	4
MMV000028	Trimethoprim	$C_{14}H_{18}N_4O_3$	290.3	1.55	4

[a] Compounds are named by their MMV identifier codes. [b] Molecular formula, molecular weight (Mol wt), aLogP values, and information about rule of five were obtained from the Pandemic Response Box and COVID Box supporting information.

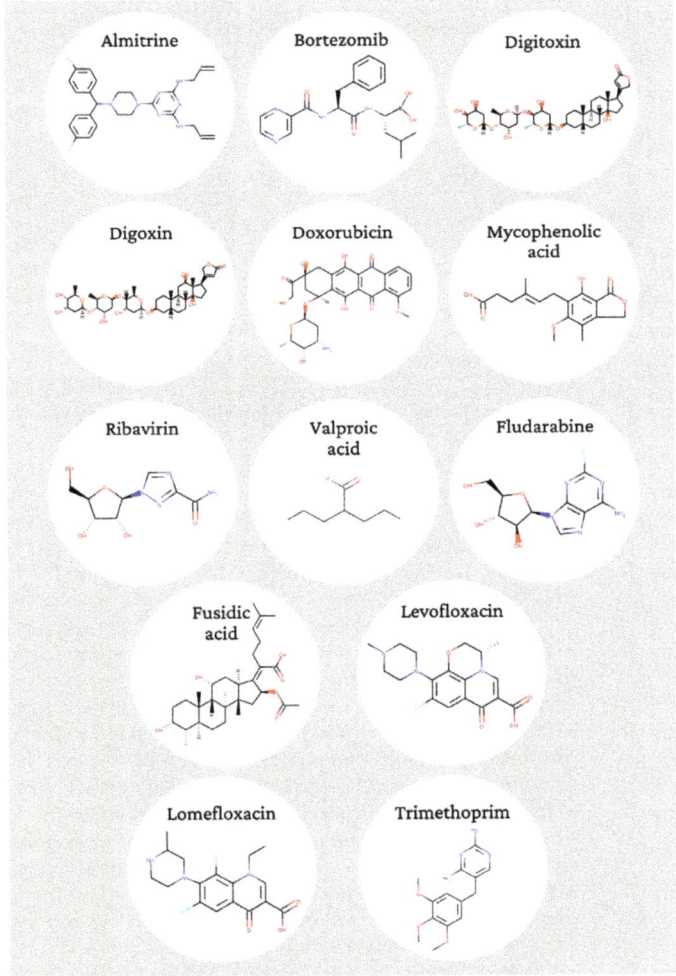

Figure 2. Structures of the 13 compounds tested against *T. gondii* in vitro. The structures were obtained from http://www.ebi.ac.uk/chembl.

We used a 96-well plate assay based on β-galactosidase expression to estimate the *T. gondii* tachyzoites' viability. From the 13 tested compounds, three demonstrated anti-*T. gondii* activity at nanomolar range, named almitrine (MMV1804175), bortezomib (MMV009415), and fludarabine (MMV637413), with activity comparable to the reference drug pyrimethamine. A total of ten compounds demonstrated EC_{50} at the micromolar range (digitoxin, digoxin, doxorubicin, fusidic acid, levofloxacin, lomefloxacin, mycophenolic acid, ribavirin, trimethoprim, and valproic acid). The cytotoxicity against mammalian cells was evaluated for the three most active compounds (almitrine, bortezomib, and fludarabine). Almitrine presented the highest selectivity (SI > 47), with a CC_{50} value greater than 20 μM (the higher tested concentration) against HFF. Results concerning the anti-*T. gondii* activity and mammalian cytotoxicity are shown in Table 2.

Table 2. In vitro activity of the selected compounds against *T. gondii*, with pyrimethamine as the reference drug.

Compound	EC_{50} (μM) [a]	CC_{50} (μM) [b]	SI [c]
Almitrine	0.424	>20	>47
Bortezomib	0.223	0.079	0.35
Digitoxin	5.66	n.d.	n.d.
Digoxin	42.59	n.d.	n.d.
Doxorubicin	2.39	n.d.	n.d.
Mycophenolic acid	8.06	n.d.	n.d.
Ribavirin	83.31	n.d.	n.d.
Valproic acid	99.61	n.d.	n.d.
Fludarabine	0.75	2.140	2.85
Fusidic acid	16.70	n.d.	n.d.
Levofloxacin	70.58	n.d.	n.d.
Lomefloxacin	7.32	n.d.	n.d.
Trimethoprim	7.36	n.d.	n.d.
Pyrimethamine	0.121	n.d.	n.d.

[a] Half Effective Concentration (EC_{50}) against *T. gondii* tachyzoites. [b] Half Cytotoxic Concentration (CC_{50}) against HFF cells. [c] Selectivity indexes (SI) were calculated based on the CC_{50} HFF cells/EC_{50} *T. gondii* ratio. n.d.: not determined.

Based on these results, almitrine was considered a promising anti-*T. gondii* drug candidate. The 13 compounds were subjected to Molecular Docking screening in four proteins for *T. gondii*, and the compound almitrine was subjected to docking simulations with the Na^+/K^+-ATPase alpha 1 transporter of *H. sapiens* and *M. musculus*.

3.2. In Silico Results

The in silico screening was carried out in two stages, the first corresponding to the evaluation of the probabilities of the compounds against the specific targets for *T. gondii* and the second referring to the screening of the compounds in the ATPase alpha 1 transporter to the species *H. sapiens* and *M. musculus*. Prior to carrying out the Molecular Docking simulations, redocking was performed, aiming to validate the enzymes used in the study. The redocking results (Supplementary Table S1) showed that all targets obtained from the PDB for the organism *T. gondii* had RMSDs below 2.0 Å, indicating that the generated poses of the co-crystallized ligand are correctly positioned at the ligand's active site.

Docking results were generated using three scoring functions (moldock score, plants score and autodock vina). In addition, the probability of activity in each of the enzymes was calculated. The obtained probability in each algorithm is shown for *T. gondii* enzymes (Supplementary Tables S2–S5) and for the ATPase alpha 1 transporter (Supplementary Tables S6 and S7). The total probability of the compound in the organism was also calculated for *T. gondii* and for the transporter ATPase alpha 1 (Supplementary Tables S8 and S9, respectively). The protein in which the compound obtained probability higher than, or close to, the values obtained by the ligand in at least one scoring function was considered active.

Therefore, the ligands selected in the study are co-crystallized in the structure obtained in the PDB library and present experimental validation for the respective enzymes.

For *T. gondii* enzymes, the compound doxorubicin achieved the highest total probability, corresponding to 0.8816 (Supplementary Table S8). Furthermore, the compounds almitrine (0.8461) and bortezomib (0.8383) presented probabilities greater than 0.80, which are close to those obtained for the PDB ligands.

Almitrine presented a significant probability for the ATPase alpha 1 transporter (*H. sapiens*) equivalent to 0.8362 (Supplementary Table S9). Furthermore, it was the most likely compound for the ATPase transporter (*M. musculus*), with $p = 0.9508$, and presented the highest total probability for the two enzymes under study (0.8935). This demonstrates a potency and affinity of this compound for this macromolecule. The molecular coupling of almitrine with transporters for the species *M. musculus* and *H. sapiens* can be seen in Supplementary Tables S4 and S5. The molecular coupling study of almitrine indicated steric, hydrophobic and hydrogen bonding interactions. In addition, it presented residues similar to the positive control tapsigargin, involved the hydrogen interactions of the Arg 551 and Asp 619 residues.

After the analysis of the potential activity of the 13 compounds under study against important *T. gondii* enzymes, Molecular Dynamics simulations were carried out with the compound almitrine to assess the flexibility of the transporting ATPase alpha 1 and the stability of the enzyme interactions in the presence of factors such as solvent, ions, pressure and temperature. This information is important since it complements the docking results and allows one to evaluate whether the compound remains strongly linked to the studied enzymes in the presence of factors that are found in the host organism. To evaluate the stability with the ATPase alpha 1 transporter, the compound almitrine was selected, as it presented the highest total probability for this transporter, taking into account the two species under study: *H. sapiens* and *M. musculus* (Supplementary Table S9). The RMSD was then calculated for the Cα atoms of the complexed enzyme and the structures of each ligand, separately.

The RMSD analysis of the transporting ATPase alpha 1 of *H. sapiens* with the compound almitrine showed conformations ranging from 0.12 to 0.15 nm in size for 10 ns, with high stability (Figure 3). The stability of this protein is essential to keep compounds bound to the active site. Furthermore, stability prevents the ligand from losing important contacts with the enzyme's active site.

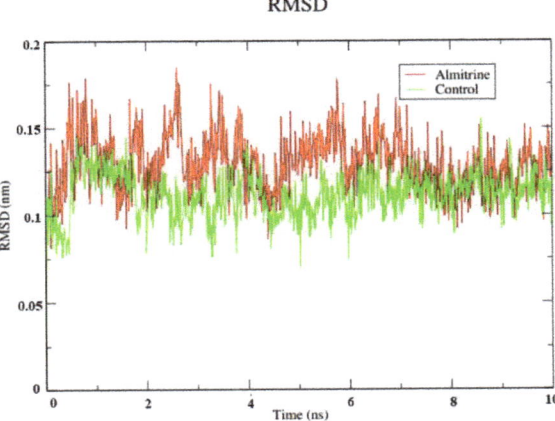

Figure 3. RMSD values of the Cα atoms of almitrine and the control (thapsigargine) with the transporting ATPase aplha 1. Legend: Green: ATPase of *H. sapiens* complexed with thapsigargine; and Red: ATPase of *H. sapiens* complexed with almitrine.

Regarding the analysis of the flexibility of the ligands through the RMSD calculations of the protein (Figure 4), the profile demonstrated by the isolated protein was similar to the result observed by the control, remaining stable up to 0.4 ns. Almitrine maintained stability up to a certain point, showing a peak in the period from 8.0 to 9.0 ns. Despite the small variation in the protein structure by the peak demonstrated, there was no interference in the structure of the ligands within the active site even if the protein changes its conformation. Therefore, in the presence of solvents, ions and other factors, almitrine was able to establish stronger bonds with the active site.

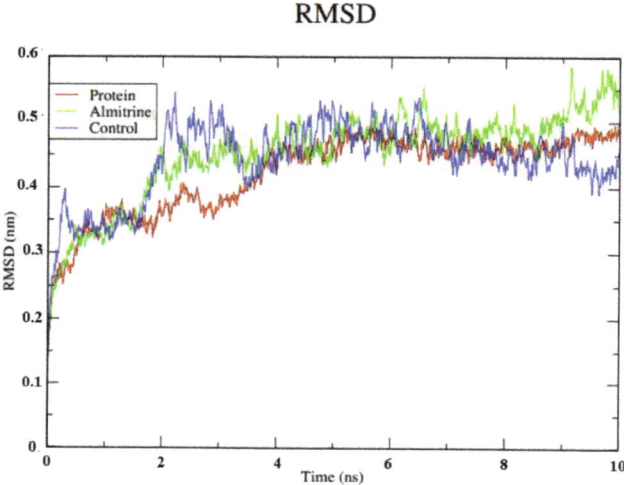

Figure 4. RMSD values for the Cα atoms of the transporting ATPase alpha 1 of *H. sapiens* complexed with almitrine and the control (thapsigargine). Legend: Green: ATPase of *H. sapiens* complexed with almitrine; Blue: ATPase of *H. sapiens* complexed with thapsigargine; and Red: *H. sapiens* transporting ATPase homologous protein.

To understand the flexibility of the residues and amino acids that contribute to the conformational changes in the transporting ATPase alpha 1 of *H. sapiens*, the mean quadratic fluctuation (RMSF) was calculated for each amino acid in each enzyme. High RMSF values suggest greater flexibility. Since amino acids with fluctuations above 0.3 nm contribute to the flexibility of the protein structure, we found that residues at positions 39, 41, 86, 122, 123, 124, 125, 275, 276, 277, 278, 497, 498, 499, 500, 564, 566, 567, 568, 570, 575, 649, 835, 1011, 1012, 1013 and 1016 contribute to conformational changes in the transporting ATPase alpha 1 of *H. sapiens* (Figure 5). We also found that none of the amino acids that affect the structural conformations identified in the transporting ATPase alpha 1 of *H. sapiens* are a component of the active site. This helps almitrine to remain in the active site.

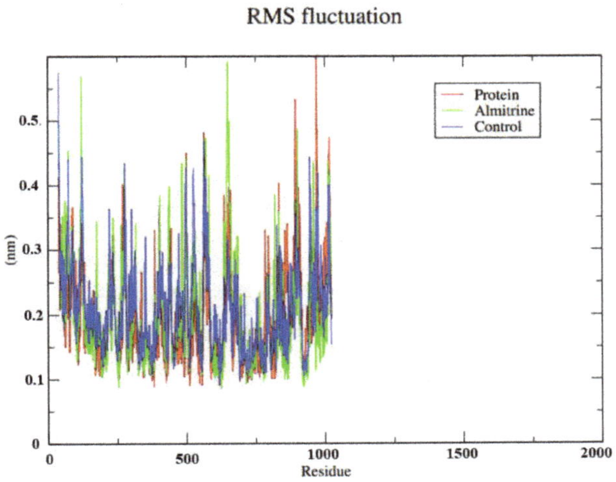

Figure 5. Root-mean-square fluctuation (RMSF) for the Cα atoms of the transporting ATPase of *H. sapiens* alpha 1 complexed with the almitrine and the control thapsigargine. Legend: Green: ATPase of *H. sapiens* complexed with almitrine; Blue: ATPase of *H. sapiens* complexed with the control thapsigargine; and Red: *H. sapiens* transporting ATPase homologous protein.

4. Discussion

Sarteriale et al., 2014 [13] performed an in silico study based on the proteome of *T. gondii* to identify potential drug candidates for toxoplasmosis therapy. Among the inhibitors previously identified, we selected 13 compounds from the MMV collections to be tested against the parasite in a cell-based assay. We found that the selected compounds were in vitro active against the parasite, with EC_{50} values ranging from 0.22 to 99.69 µM.

The obtained results indicated that this method is valuable and can be used to build enriched compound libraries for in vitro drug testing, which could enable a more efficient use of laboratory resources, as suggested by Sarteriale et al. 2014 [13], bringing the advantage of reduced speed and cost and extra broadness. We also confirmed that the compound collections from MMV are promising sources of anti-*T. gondii* agents.

In our study, diverse antitoxoplasmic compounds were identified, representing the first time that this combined set of compounds has been evaluated against *T. gondii* in vitro.

A total of three compounds showed EC_{50} values against *T. gondii* at the nanomolar range. Two of them (MMV1804175 and MMV009415) belong to the COVID Box and one of them is part of the Pandemic Response Box (MMV637413).

Compound MMV1804175, commercially named almitrine, was the most selective, with an EC_{50} value of 0.424 µM against the parasite and a CC_{50} value higher than 20 µM, the top concentration evaluated. The ratio between the CC_{50} against HFF and the EC_{50} against the parasite resulted in a selectivity index greater than 47. Almitrine is a selective pulmonary vasoconstrictor, which has been proposed as an interesting therapeutic option to manage severe hypoxemia in patients with the Coronavirus 2019 disease [44]. This is the first report about the anti-*T. gondii* activity of almitrine. Previously published work has demonstrated the in vitro activity of this drug against chloroquine-susceptible and chloroquine-resistant *P. falciparum*, with EC_{50} values ranging from 2.6 to 19.8 µM [45]. When almitrine bismesylate was administered to young subjects in single or multiple oral doses, the physiological and blood parameters indicated that the drug was safe at all doses tested, up to 400 mg per day, with symptoms of mild nausea and headache [46].

Bortezomib (MMV009415) is a proteasome inhibitor and antineoplastic agent that is used in the treatment of refractory multiple myeloma and certain lymphomas [47]. The compound was equally effective against drug-sensitive and -resistant *P. falciparum*, blocking its intraerythrocytic development prior to DNA synthesis [48]. Here, we report for the first time the anti-*T. gondii* activity of bortezomib. This compound was the most active, with an EC_{50} value of 0.223 µM against *T. gondii*. However, this compound presented low selectivity, with a CC_{50} value of 0.079 against the mammalian lineage HFF, indicating the need to design possible changes in the chemical structure, aimed at finding more selective analogues.

The purine analogue fludarabine (MMV637413) is an antineoplastic agent used in the therapy of chronic lymphocytic leukemia and in immunosuppressive regimens in preparation of hematopoietic cell transplantation. This small molecule is an analog of the antiviral agent vidarabine and acts interrupting DNA synthesis and inhibiting tumor cell growth. Fludarabine is associated with a low rate of transient serum enzyme elevations during therapy and has only rarely been implicated in cases of clinically apparent acute liver injury [49]. To the best of our knowledge, this is the first report about the anti-parasitic activity of this compound.

Among the ten compounds presenting anti-*T. gondii* activity in the micromolar range, we can highlight doxorubicin, an antibiotic isolated from *Streptomyces peucetius* var. *caesius*. The compound triggers oxidative stress causing cardiotoxicity, which compromises its clinical use as an antineoplastic agent [50]. This anti-*T. gondii* candidate also showed activity against another three parasitic protozoan species, named *C. parvum*, *Trichomonas vaginalis* and *P. falciparum* [51]. To the best of our knowledge, this is the first report about the anti *T. gondii* activity of this compound.

Antibiotics have a history of repurposing success for Apicomplexan parasites and are the conventional treatment for human toxoplasmosis, in the form of pyrimethamine + sulphadiazine, trimethoprim + sulphamethoxazole and pyrimethamine + clindamycin [52]. Other antibiotics with anti-*T. gondii* activity identified in the present work were lomefloxacin, mycophenolic acid, fusidic acid, levofloxacin, and trimethoprim. Mycophenolic acid is an antineoplastic antibiotic derived from various *Penicillium* fungal species. It was previously reported that this drug triggers *T. gondii* extracellular tachyzoites differentiation into cyst-like structures [53]. Fusidic acid, an antibiotic that inhibits the growth of bacteria by preventing the release of translation elongation factor G from the ribosome, has been shown to be effective in tissue culture against *P. falciparum* and *T. gondii* [54]. Trimethoprim is an antimicrobial used to treat and prevent toxoplasmosis and many bacterial infections [55]. Therefore, the in vitro activity of this drug against *T. gondii* is not a novelty. Lomefloxacin is used to treat bacterial infections including bronchitis and urinary tract infections [56]. Levofloxacin is an antibacterial drug with a broad spectrum of activity. This drug diffuses through the bacterial cell wall and acts by inhibiting DNA gyrase (bacterial topoisomerase II), leading to blockage of bacterial cell growth [57]. The in vitro anti-*T. gondii* activity of lomefloxacin and levofloxacin is reported here for the first time.

Digitoxin is a lipid soluble cardiac glycoside that inhibits the plasma membrane Na^+/K^+-ATPase, with anticancer effects when used at therapeutic concentrations [58]. In addition, digoxin is a cardiac glycoside long used to treat congestive heart failure and has been found more recently to show anticancer activity [59]. Ribavirin is an inhibitor of the hepatitis C virus polymerase with a broad spectrum of activity against DNA and RNA viruses [60]. To the best of our knowledge, the in vitro anti-*T. gondii* activity of digitoxin, digoxin and ribavirin is first reported here. Valproic acid, a mood-stabilizing and antipsychotic drug, presents efficacy against chronic *T. gondii* infection, as previously demonstrated [61].

Among the three compounds presenting anti-*T. gondii* activity at nanomolar range, we consider almitrine to be the most promising, since this compound showed in vitro selective anti-*T. gondii* activity and presents good oral availability and low human toxicity. The future evaluation of the efficacy of almitrine in *T. gondii*-infected animals is encouraging.

5. Conclusions

Promising anti-*T. gondii* candidates were identified and previously published in silico data was confirmed, indicating that this is a useful tool in the search for active compounds in the target-based drug development process. In addition, we suggest that almitrine represents a lead compound against *T. gondii*, which may be useful for antitoxoplasmic chemotherapy.

The 13 selected compounds showed interaction with specific enzymes of *T. gondii*, whilst the compounds almitrine, bortezomib, digoxin, digitoxin, doxorubicin, mycophenolic acid, ribavirin, fludarabine and fusidic acid presented greater affinity than the ligands under study for the selected mechanisms. Almitrine showed a lower score than the positive control tapsigargin, regarding the Na+/K+ ATPase transporter of *H. sapiens* and *M. musculus* referring to the Plantscore algorithm. In addition, almitrine showed interactions such as the positive control tapsigargin, thus indicating a possible mechanism of action of this compound.

Supplementary Materials: The following supporting information can be downloaded at: https://www.mdpi.com/article/10.3390/pharmaceutics14081634/s1. Refs. [62,63] are mentioned in Supplementary Materials.

Author Contributions: Investigation: D.C.C., P.P.M.T. and N.F.d.S.; Supervision: M.T.S. and J.Q.R. All authors have read and agreed to the published version of the manuscript.

Funding: This work was supported by the São Paulo Research Foundation (FAPESP) (grant number 2018/18954-4 and 2020/03399-5). The FAPESP process number 2022/05069-8 was also involved.

Institutional Review Board Statement: Not applicable.

Acknowledgments: We would like to thank the Medicines for Malaria Venture foundation (MMV; Switzerland) for having provided the open-access Boxes. We would also like to thank Tiago W. P. Mineo, Samuel C. Teixeira (Universidade Federal de Uberlândia), André G. Tempone and Cristina Cristina Meira-Strejevitch (Instituto Adolfo Lutz of São Paulo) for their help through their sharing of cell cultures, protocols and experience.

Conflicts of Interest: The authors declare no conflict of interest.

References

1. Kochanowsky, J.A.; Koshy, A.A. Toxoplasma Gondii. *Curr. Biol.* **2018**, *28*, R770–R771. [CrossRef] [PubMed]
2. Radke, J.B.; Burrows, J.N.; Goldberg, D.E.; Sibley, L.D. Evaluation of Current and Emerging Antimalarial Medicines for Inhibition of *Toxoplasma gondii* Growth in Vitro. *ACS Infect. Dis.* **2018**, *4*, 1264–1274. [CrossRef] [PubMed]
3. CDC. Toxoplasmosis. Available online: https://www.cdc.gov/parasites/toxoplasmosis/ (accessed on 16 March 2022).
4. Garcia Bahia-Oliveira, L.M.; Jones, J.L.; Azevedo-Silva, J.; Alves, C.C.F.; Oréfice, F.; Addiss, D.G. Highly Endemic, Waterborne Toxoplasmosis in North Rio de Janeiro State, Brazil. *Emerg. Infect. Dis.* **2003**, *9*, 55–62. [CrossRef] [PubMed]
5. Aspinall, T.V.; Joynson, D.H.M.; Guy, E.; Hyde, J.E.; Sims, P.F.G. The Molecular Basis of Sulfonamide Resistance in *Toxoplasma gondii* and Implications for the Clinical Management of Toxoplasmosis. *J. Infect. Dis.* **2002**, *185*, 1637–1643. [CrossRef]
6. Dittmar, A.J.; Drozda, A.A.; Blader, I.J. Drug Repurposing Screening Identifies Novel Compounds That Effectively Inhibit *Toxoplasma gondii* Growth. *mSphere* **2016**, *1*, e00042-15. [CrossRef]
7. Blader, I.J.; Saeij, J.P. Communication between *Toxoplasma gondii* and Its Host: Impact on Parasite Growth, Development, Immune Evasion, and Virulence. *Apmis* **2009**, *117*, 458–476. [CrossRef]
8. Alday, P.H.; Doggett, J.S. Drugs in development for toxoplasmosis: Advances, challenges, and current status. *Drug Des. Dev. Ther.* **2017**, *25*, 273–293. [CrossRef]
9. Buckle, D.R.; Erhardt, P.W.; Ganellin, C.R.; Kobayashi, T.; Perun, T.J.; Proudfoot, J.; Senn-Bilfinger, J. Glossary of Terms Used in Medicinal Chemistry Part II (IUPAC Recommendations 2013). *Annu. Rep. Med. Chem.* **2013**, *48*, 387–418. [CrossRef]
10. MMV. The Pandemic Response Box | Medicines for Malaria Venture. Available online: https://www.mmv.org/mmv-open/pandemic-response-box (accessed on 16 March 2022).
11. Duffy, S.; Sykes, M.L.; Jones, A.J.; Shelper, T.B.; Simpson, M.; Lang, R.; Poulsen, S.A.; Sleebs, B.E.; Avery, V.M. Screening the Medicines for Malaria Venture Pathogen Box across Multiple Pathogens Reclassifies Starting Points for Open-Source Drug Discovery. *Antimicrob. Agents Chemother.* **2017**, *61*, e00379-17. [CrossRef]
12. Spalenka, J.; Escotte-Binet, S.; Bakiri, A.; Hubert, J.; Renault, J.H.; Velard, F.; Duchateau, S.; Aubert, D.; Huguenin, A.; Villena, I. Discovery of New Inhibitors of *Toxoplasma gondii* via the Pathogen Box. *Antimicrob. Agents Chemother.* **2018**, *62*, e01640-17. [CrossRef]
13. Sateriale, A.; Bessoff, K.; Sarkar, I.N.; Huston, C.D. Drug Repurposing: Mining Protozoan Proteomes for Targets of Known Bioactive Compounds. *J. Am. Med. Inform. Assoc.* **2014**, *21*, 238–244. [CrossRef] [PubMed]
14. Silva, M.D.; Teixeira, C.; Gomes, P.; Borges, M. Promising Drug Targets and Compounds with Anti-*Toxoplasma gondii* Activity. *Microorganisms* **2021**, *15*, 1960. [CrossRef] [PubMed]

15. Castro, A.S.; Alves, C.M.O.S.; Angeloni, M.B.; Gomes, A.O.; Barbosa, B.F.; Franco, P.S.; Silva, D.A.O.; Martins-Filho, O.A.; Mineo, J.R.; Mineo, T.W.P.; et al. Trophoblast Cells Are Able to Regulate Monocyte Activity to Control *Toxoplasma gondii* Infection. *Placenta* **2013**, *34*, 240–247. [CrossRef]
16. Wang, Q.; Sibley, L.D. Assays for Monitoring *Toxoplasma gondii* Infectivity in the Laboratory Mouse. *Methods Mol. Biol.* **2020**, *2071*, 99–116. [CrossRef] [PubMed]
17. Chin, F.T.; Xing, W.Z.; Bogyo, M.; Carruthers, V.B. Cysteine Protease Inhibitors Block *Toxoplasma gondii* Microneme Secretion and Cell Invasion. *Antimicrob. Agents Chemother.* **2007**, *51*, 679–688. [CrossRef]
18. Reimão, J.Q.; Mesquita, J.T.; Ferreira, D.D.; Tempone, A.G. Investigation of Calcium Channel Blockers as Antiprotozoal Agents and Their Interference in the Metabolism of *Leishmania* (L.) Infantum. *Evid.-Based Complementary Altern. Med.* **2016**, *2016*, 1523691. [CrossRef] [PubMed]
19. Bernstein, F.C.; Koetzle, T.F.; Williams, G.J.B.; Meyer, E.F., Jr.; Brice, M.D.; Rodgers, J.R.; Kennard, O.; Shimanouchi, T.; Tasumi, M. NoA Computer-based Archival File for Macromolecular Structures Title. *Eur. J. Biochem.* **1977**, *112*, 535–542.
20. Yusuf, D.; Davis, A.M.; Kleywegt, G.J.; Schmitt, S. An Alternative Method for the Evaluation of Docking Performance: RSR vs. RMSD. *J. Chem. Inf. Model.* **2008**, *48*, 1411–1422. [CrossRef]
21. Thomsen, R.; Christensen, M.H. MolDock: A New Technique for High-Accuracy Molecular Docking. *J. Med. Chem.* **2006**, *49*, 3315–3321. [CrossRef]
22. Da Silva Calixto, P.; de Almeida, R.N.; Salvadori, M.G.S.S.; Dos Santos Maia, M.; Filho, J.M.B.; Scotti, M.T.; Scotti, L. In Silico Study Examining New Phenylpropanoids Targets with Antidepressant Activity. *Curr. Drug Targets* **2021**, *22*, 539–554. [CrossRef]
23. De Azevedo, W., Jr. MolDock Applied to Structure-Based Virtual Screening. *Curr. Drug Targets* **2010**, *11*, 327–334. [CrossRef] [PubMed]
24. Morris, G.M.; Goodsell, D.S.; Huey, R.; Lindstrom, W.; Hart, W.E.; Kurowski, S.; Halliday, S.; Belew, R.; Olson, A.J. AutoDock Tolls 4.2. Available online: https://onlinelibrary.wiley.com/doi/full/10.1002/jcc.21256 (accessed on 14 March 2022).
25. Solis-Vasquez, L.; Santos-Martins, D.; Koch, A.; Forli, S. Evaluating the Energy Efficiency of Opencl-Accelerated Autodock Molecular Docking. In Proceedings of the 2020 28th Euromicro International Conference on Parallel, Distributed and Network-Based Processing (PDP), IEEE, Västerås, Sweden, 11–13 March 2020; pp. 162–166.
26. Trott, O.; Olson, A.J. AutoDock Vina 1.1.1. Available online: https://pubmed.ncbi.nlm.nih.gov/19499576/ (accessed on 14 March 2022).
27. Trott, O.; Olson, A.J. Software News and Update AutoDock Vina: Improving the Speed and Accuracy of Docking with a New Scoring Function. *Effic. Optim. Multithreading* **2009**, *31*, 455–461.
28. Zaware, N.; Sharma, H.; Yang, J.; Devambatla, R.K.V.; Queener, S.F.; Anderson, K.S.; Gangjee, A. Discovery of Potent and Selective Inhibitors of *Toxoplasma gondii* Thymidylate Synthase for Opportunistic Infections. *ACS Med. Chem. Lett.* **2013**, *4*, 1148–1151. [CrossRef] [PubMed]
29. Donaldson, T.M.; Cassera, M.B.; Ho, M.C.; Zhan, C.; Merino, E.F.; Evans, G.B.; Tyler, P.C.; Almo, S.C.; Schramm, V.L.; Kim, K. Inhibition and Structure of *Toxoplasma gondii* Purine Nucleoside Phosphorylase. *Eukaryot. Cell* **2014**, *13*, 572–579. [CrossRef] [PubMed]
30. Muench, S.P.; Prigge, S.T.; McLeod, R.; Rafferty, J.B.; Kirisits, M.J.; Roberts, C.W.; Mui, E.J.; Rice, D.W. Studies of *Toxoplasma gondii* and Plasmodium Falciparum Enoyl Acyl Carrier Protein Reductase and Implications for the Development of Antiparasitic Agents. *Acta Crystallogr. Sect. D Biol. Crystallogr.* **2007**, *63*, 328–338. [CrossRef] [PubMed]
31. Zhang, Z.; Ojo, K.K.; Vidadala, R.; Huang, W.; Geiger, J.A.; Scheele, S.; Choi, R.; Reid, M.C.; Keyloun, K.R.; Rivas, K.; et al. Potent and Selective Inhibitors of CDPK1 from *T. Gondii* and *C. Parvum* Based on a 5-Aminopyrazole-4-Carboxamide Scaffold. *ACS Med. Chem. Lett.* **2014**, *5*, 40–44. [CrossRef] [PubMed]
32. Yan, C.; Liang, L.J.; Zhang, B.B.; Lou, Z.L.; Zhang, H.F.; Shen, X.; Wu, Y.Q.; Wang, Z.M.; Tang, R.X.; Fu, L.L.; et al. Prevalence and Genotyping of *Toxoplasma gondii* in Naturally-Infected Synanthropic Rats (Rattus Norvegicus) and Mice (Mus Musculus) in Eastern China. *Parasites Vectors* **2014**, *7*, 591. [CrossRef]
33. Xue, Q.; Liu, X.; Russell, P.; Li, J.; Pan, W.; Fu, J.; Zhang, A. Evaluation of the Binding Performance of Flavonoids to Estrogen Receptor Alpha by Autodock, Autodock Vina and Surflex-Dock. *Ecotoxicol. Environ. Saf.* **2022**, *233*, 113323. [CrossRef]
34. Dos Santos Maia, M.; de Sousa, N.F.; Rodrigues, G.C.S.; Monteiro, A.F.M.; Scotti, M.T.; Scotti, L. Lignans and Neolignans Anti-Tuberculosis Identified by QSAR and Molecular Modeling. *Comb. Chem. High Throughput Screen.* **2020**, *23*, 504–516. [CrossRef]
35. Mito, T.; Kuwahara, S.; Delamere, N.A. The Influence of Thapsigargin on Na,k-ATPase Activity in Cultured Nonpigmented Ciliary Epithelial Cells. *Curr. Eye Res.* **1995**, *14*, 651–657. [CrossRef]
36. RCSB. Protein Data Bank. Available online: https://www.rcsb.org/.2022 (accessed on 16 March 2022). [CrossRef]
37. Engel. NCBI. Available online: https://www.ncbi.nlm.nih.gov/ (accessed on 16 March 2022).
38. Waterhouse, A.; Bertoni, M.; Bienert, S.; Studer, G.; Tauriello, G.; Gumienny, R.; Heer, F.T.; De Beer, T.A.P.; Rempfer, C.; Bordoli, L.; et al. SWISS-MODEL: Homology Modelling of Protein Structures and Complexes. *Nucleic Acids Res.* **2018**, *46*, W296–W303. [CrossRef]
39. Laskowski, R.A.; MacArthur, M.W.; Moss, D.S.; Thornton, J.M. PROCHECK: A Program to Check the Stereochemical Quality of Protein Structures. *J. Appl. Crystallogr.* **1993**, *26*, 283–291. [CrossRef]
40. Abraham, M.J.; Murtola, T.; Schulz, R.; Páll, S.; Smith, J.C.; Hess, B.; Lindahl, E. GROMACS: High performance molecular simulations through multi-level parallelism from laptops to supercomputers. *SoftwareX* **2015**, *1–2*, 19–25. [CrossRef]
41. Berendsen, H.J.C.; van der Spoel, D.; van Drunen, R. GROMACS: A message-passing parallel molecular dynamics implementation. *Comput. Phys. Commun.* **1995**, *91*, 43–56. [CrossRef]
42. Bondi, A. Van der Waals Volumes and Radii. *J. Phys. Chem.* **1964**, *68*, 441–451. [CrossRef]

43. Pettersen, E.F.; Goddard, T.D.; Huang, C.C.; Couch, G.S.; Greenblatt, D.M.; Meng, E.C.; Ferrin, T.E. UCSF Chimera—A visualization system for exploratory research and analysis. *J. Comput. Chem.* **2004**, *25*, 1605–1612. [CrossRef]
44. Caplan, M.; Goutay, J.; Bignon, A.; Jaillette, E.; Favory, R.; Mathieu, D.; Parmentier-Decrucq, E.; Poissy, J.; Duburcq, T. Lille Intensive Care COVID-19 Group. Almitrine Infusion in Severe Acute Respiratory Syndrome Coronavirus 2-Induced Acute Respiratory Distress Syndrome: A Single-Center Observational Study. *Crit. Care Med.* **2021**, *1*, e191–e198. [CrossRef]
45. Basco, L.K.; Le Bras, J. In Vitro Activity of Mitochondrial ATP Synthetase Inhibitors Against Plasmodium Falciparum. *J. Eukaryot. Microbiol.* **1994**, *41*, 179–183. [CrossRef]
46. MacLeod, C.N.; Thomas, R.W.; Bartley, E.A.; Parkhurst, G.W.; Bachand, R.T. Effects and handling of almitrine bismesylate in healthy subjects. *Eur. J. Respir. Dis. Suppl.* **1983**, *126*, 275–289.
47. Jung, L.; Holle, L.; Dalton, W.S. Discovery, Development, and clinical applications of bortezomib. *Oncology* **2004**, *18* (14 Suppl. 11), 4–13.
48. Reynolds, J.M.; El Bissati, K.; Brandenburg, J.; Günzl, A.; Mamoun, C.B. Antimalarial Activity of the Anticancer and Proteasome Inhibitor Bortezomib and Its Analog ZL3B. *BMC Clin. Pharmacol.* **2007**, *7*, 13. [CrossRef] [PubMed]
49. *LiverTox: Clinical and Research Information on Drug-Induced Liver Injury. Fludarabine.* 1 February 2018; National Institute of Diabetes and Digestive and Kidney Diseases: Bethesda, MD, USA, 2012.
50. Octavia, Y.; Tocchetti, C.G.; Gabrielson, K.L.; Janssens, S.; Crijns, H.J.; Moens, A.L. Doxorubicin-induced cardiomyopathy: From molecular mechanisms to therapeutic strategies. *J. Mol. Cell. Cardiol.* **2012**, *52*, 1213–1225. [CrossRef] [PubMed]
51. Andrews, K.T.; Fisher, G.; Skinner-Adams, T.S. Drug repurposing and human parasitic protozoan diseases. *Int. J. Parasitol. Drugs Drug Resist.* **2014**, *4*, 95–111. [CrossRef] [PubMed]
52. Rajapakse, S.; Shivanthan, M.C.; Samaranayake, N.; Rodrigo, C.; Fernando, S.D. Antibiotics for human toxoplasmosis: A systematic review of randomized trials. *Pathog. Glob. Health* **2013**, *107*, 162–169. [CrossRef]
53. Castro-Elizalde, K.N.; Hernández-Contreras, P.; Ramírez-Flores, C.J.; González-Pozos, S.; Gómez de León, C.T.; Mondragón-Castelán, M.; Mondragón-Flores, R. Mycophenolic acid induces differentiation of *Toxoplasma gondii* RH strain tachyzoites into bradyzoites and formation of cyst-like structure in vitro. *Parasitol. Res.* **2018**, *117*, 547–563. [CrossRef] [PubMed]
54. Payne, A.J.; Neal, L.M.; Knoll, L.J. Fusidic acid is an effective treatment against *Toxoplasma gondii* and Listeria monocytogenes in vitro, but not in mice. *Parasitol. Res.* **2013**, *112*, 3859–3863. [CrossRef]
55. Kemnic, T.R.; Coleman, M. Trimethoprim Sulfamethoxazole. In *StatPearls*; StatPearls Publishing: Treasure Island, FL, USA, 2021.
56. Al-Wabli, R.I. Lomefloxacin. In *Profiles of Drug Substances, Excipients and Related Methodology*; Academic Press: Cambridge, MA, USA, 2017; Volume 42, pp. 193–240. [CrossRef]
57. Tunitskaya, V.L.; Khomutov, A.R.; Kochetkov, S.N.; Kotovskaya, S.K.; Charushin, V.N. Inhibition of DNA gyrase by levofloxacin and related fluorine-containing heterocyclic compounds. *Acta Nat.* **2011**, *3*, 94–99. [CrossRef]
58. Elbaz, H.A.; Stueckle, T.A.; Tse, W.; Rojanasakul, Y.; Dinu, C.Z. Digitoxin and its analogs as novel cancer therapeutics. *Exp. Hematol. Oncol.* **2012**, *1*, 4. [CrossRef]
59. Ren, Y.; Ribas, H.T.; Heath, K.; Wu, S.; Ren, J.; Shriwas, P.; Chen, X.; Johnson, M.E.; Cheng, X.; Burdette, J.E.; et al. Na+/K+-ATPase-Targeted Cytotoxicity of (+)-Digoxin and Several Semisynthetic Derivatives. *J. Nat. Prod.* **2020**, *83*, 638–648. [CrossRef]
60. Hofmann, W.P.; Herrmann, E.; Sarrazin, C.; Zeuzem, S. Ribavirin mode of action in chronic hepatitis C: From clinical use back to molecular mechanisms. *Liver Int.* **2008**, *28*, 1332–1343. [CrossRef]
61. Enshaeieh, M.; Saadatnia, G.; Babaie, J.; Golkar, M.; Choopani, S.; Sayyah, M. Valproic Acid Inhibits Chronic Toxoplasma Infection and Associated Brain Inflammation in Mice. *Antimicrob. Agents Chemother.* **2021**, *65*, e0100321. [CrossRef] [PubMed]
62. Lovell, S.C.; Davis, I.W.; Arendall, W.B.; De Bakker, P.I.W.; Word, J.M.; Prisant, M.G.; Richardson, J.S.; Richardson, D.C. Structure Validation by Cα Geometry: φ,ψ and Cβ Deviation. *Proteins Struct. Funct. Genet.* **2003**, *50*, 437–450. [CrossRef] [PubMed]
63. Hilge, M.; Siegal, G.; Vuister, G.W.; Güntert, P.; Gloor, S.M.; Abrahams, J.P. ATP-Induced Conformational Changes of the Nucleotide-Binding Domain of Na, K-ATPase. *Nat. Struct. Mol. Biol.* **2003**, *10*, 468–474. [CrossRef] [PubMed]

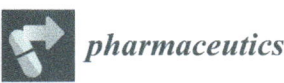

Article

Drug-Disease Severity and Target-Disease Severity Interaction Networks in COVID-19 Patients

Verena Schöning and Felix Hammann *

Clinical Pharmacology and Toxicology, Department of General Internal Medicine, Inselspital, Bern University Hospital, University of Bern, 3010 Bern, Switzerland
* Correspondence: felix.hammann@insel.ch

Abstract: Drug interactions with other drugs are a well-known phenomenon. Similarly, however, pre-existing drug therapy can alter the course of diseases for which it has not been prescribed. We performed network analysis on drugs and their respective targets to investigate whether there are drugs or targets with protective effects in COVID-19, making them candidates for repurposing. These networks of drug-disease interactions (DDSIs) and target-disease interactions (TDSIs) revealed a greater share of patients with diabetes and cardiac co-morbidities in the non-severe cohort treated with dipeptidyl peptidase-4 (DPP4) inhibitors. A possible protective effect of DPP4 inhibitors is also plausible on pathophysiological grounds, and our results support repositioning efforts of DPP4 inhibitors against SARS-CoV-2. At target level, we observed that the target location might have an influence on disease progression. This could potentially be attributed to disruption of functional membrane micro-domains (lipid rafts), which in turn could decrease viral entry and thus disease severity.

Keywords: COVID-19; network analysis; drug-disease interaction; target-disease interaction; DPP4 inhibitors; lipid rafts; drug repurposing

1. Introduction

In Switzerland, patients seen by general practitioners have a median of two chronic conditions, and receive a median of two prescribed drugs [1]. The most common conditions are cardiovascular diseases, including arterial hypertension and lipid disorders, and diabetes [2]. Not only do drug-drug interactions increase with pill burden, but also the risk for drug-disease interactions (DDSIs), where drugs that are beneficial in one disease may be harmful in another [3]. A drug's action is brought about by its interaction with molecular targets. The relationship is asymmetric, meaning that a given drug can interact with multiple targets, and one target with multiple drugs [4]. By consequence, the interaction of drugs with specific molecular targets can also influence the progression or severity of a disease, which could lead to a target-disease interaction (TDSI).

The current pandemic of coronavirus disease 2019 (COVID-19) is caused by the severe acute respiratory syndrome coronavirus 2 (SARS-CoV-2). By now, several risk factors for severe COVID-19 progression are known, such as age [5,6], male sex [7,8], or obesity [9–12]. Additionally, common co-morbidities such as diabetes [13–15], cardiac [16,17] and pulmonary diseases [18,19], or dementia [20] can influence prognosis of COVID-19. Furthermore, both the number and the combination of certain co-morbidities have been found to be predictors of severity [21]. Several studies have already been conducted to analyze the influence of specific co-medications on COVID-19 incidence and progression. For example, hypertension is a common chronic condition and a risk factor for severe COVID-19 progression [22]. Some researchers analyzed the influence of anti-hypertensive drugs acting on the renin-angiotensin-aldosterone-system (RAAS)-system [23,24]. The majority of these studies provided evidence that angiotensin converting enzyme (ACE)

Citation: Schöning, V.; Hammann, F. Drug-Disease Severity and Target-Disease Severity Interaction Networks in COVID-19 Patients. *Pharmaceutics* **2022**, *14*, 1828. https://doi.org/10.3390/pharmaceutics14091828

Academic Editors: Paul Bogdan, Lucreția Udrescu, Mihai Udrescu and Ludovic Kurunczi

Received: 16 May 2022
Accepted: 27 August 2022
Published: 30 August 2022

Publisher's Note: MDPI stays neutral with regard to jurisdictional claims in published maps and institutional affiliations.

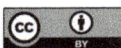

Copyright: © 2022 by the authors. Licensee MDPI, Basel, Switzerland. This article is an open access article distributed under the terms and conditions of the Creative Commons Attribution (CC BY) license (https://creativecommons.org/licenses/by/4.0/).

inhibitors and angiotensin-receptor blockers (ARBs) do not adversely affect the COVID-19 progression or may even be beneficial [22–28]. In general, studies showed that polypharmacy increases the risk for severe COVID-19 [29,30].

Network analysis is used to investigate a group of objects (e.g., friends, internet servers, patients, enzymes, or proteins) and their connection with each other. The objects are the nodes of the network, whereas the relationships are the edges connecting the nodes. One famous example is Zachary's "karate club" network, which displays the pattern of friendships amongst the members of a university karate club [31]. In recent years, network analysis has increasingly been applied in the context of pharmacology, e.g., to investigate the relationships between drugs and their respective targets [4] or the relationship between proteins and metabolites [32]. In addition, several network studies on the repurposing of drugs against SARS-CoV-2 have been conducted, mainly as drug-target, target-human, viral-human, or protein-protein-interactions, or combinations thereof [32–34]. In addition, transcriptomes of COVID-19 patients, patients with related conditions and healthy controls were compared to identify possible drugs candidates for repurposing [35].

However, none of these studies used clinical data to investigate the influence of pre-existing drug treatment on patient outcomes as measure of disease severity.

The aim of this study was to analyze the impact of DDSIs and TDSIs on COVID-19 severity using network analysis as a tool to inform drug repurposing efforts and increase drug safety. We compared drugs on admission (i.e., drugs patients were taking before or on the day of admission) and their molecular targets in patients who tested positive for SARS-CoV-2, and used severe (required critical care or died) or non-severe outcome (outpatient or never requiring critical care) as endpoint.

2. Materials and Methods

2.1. Study Population

We carried out this retrospective study at the Insel Hospital Group (IHG), a tertiary hospital network with six locations and about 860,000 patients treated per year, making it the biggest health care provider in Switzerland. The Cantonal Ethics Committee of Bern approved the protocol (2020-00973). We considered all patients who tested positive for SARS-CoV-2 by reverse-transcriptase polymerase chain reaction (RT-PCR) assay on nasopharyngeal swabs at the IHG between 1 February through 16 November 2020—covering the 'first wave' and most of the 'second wave' of COVID-19 in the region (Figure 1).

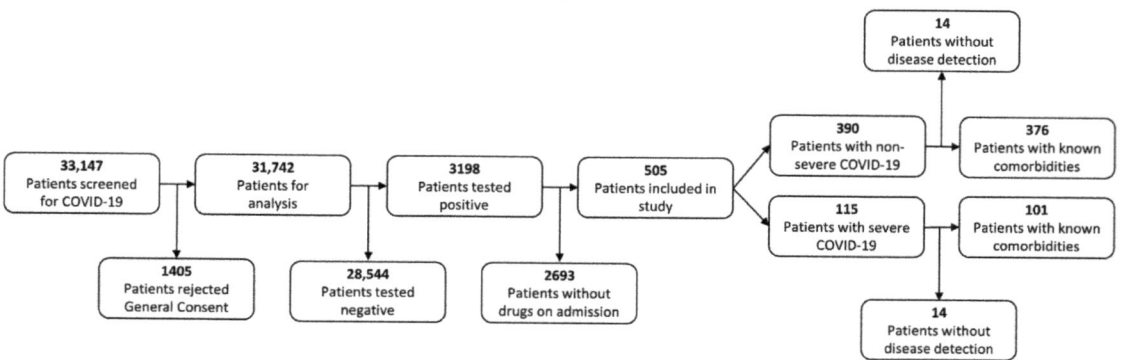

Figure 1. Flowchart of patient selection process.

For patients with no registered general research consent status, a waiver of consent was granted by the ethics committee. Objection to the general research consent of the IHG was an exclusion criterion for this study, whereas participation in other trials (including COVID-19 related treatment studies) was not. Disease progression was classified as *severe* if, for any reason, an intensive care unit (ICU) admission was required at any stage, or the patient died during the stay. All other patients were classified as *non-severe*. We selected only patients for whom drugs on admission had been recorded. Therefore, this study included 115 severe and 390 non-severe COVID-19 patients. We identified pre-existing conditions using Natural Language Processing from a previous study [36]. For a total of 28 patients (14 non-severe and 14 severe cases), we could not perform disease detection. Characteristics of the study population are provided in Table 1.

Table 1. Characteristics of study population.

General Characteristics	Non-Severe (*n* = 390)	Severe (*n* = 115)	*p* Value
Age (years) Median (Q1, Q3)	67.00 (52.00, 77.00)	70.00 (60.50, 81.00)	<0.001
Sex Female (%)	155 (39.74%)	31 (26.96%)	0.017
BMI Median (Q1, Q3)	26.05 (23.51, 29.43)	27.73 (24.74, 31.70)	<0.006
Drugs on admission Median (Q1, Q3)	7.00 (4.00, 12.00)	8.00 (4.00, 13.00)	0.403
Diseases			
Arterial hypertension (%)	182 (48.40%)	64 (63.37%)	0.011
Chronic heart failure (%)	92 (24.47%)	37 (36.63%)	0.021
Atrial fibrillation (%)	57 (15.16%)	23 (22.77%)	0.095
Coronary heart disease (%)	52 (13.83%)	32 (31.68%)	<0.002
Coronary sclerosis (%)	9 (2.39%)	6 (5.94%)	0.136
Diabetes (%)	105 (27.93%)	34 (33.66%)	0.316
Dementia (%)	39 (10.37%)	15 (14.85%)	0.278

To study the effects of co-morbidities, we created four sub-groups:

1. Cardiac conditions (chronic heart failure, atrial fibrillation, coronary heart disease, and/or coronary sclerosis) (*n* = 184)
2. Arterial hypertension (*n* = 246)
3. Diabetes (including pre-diabetes, type 1 and 2 diabetes) (*n* = 139)
4. Dementia (*n* = 54)

Note: patients can be members of more than one group, e.g., 70 patients suffered from diabetes as well as from cardiac conditions.

2.2. Network Analysis

Drugs on admission (drugs taken before admission to the IHG) were obtained from the electronic health records (EHR). As this part of the EHR was not always complete, we also considered drugs administered in-house on the day of admission. This also mitigates the effect of patients transferred from other hospitals compared to patients who were initially admitted to the IHG.

We evaluated different levels of detail in drug classification. First, we compared the fourteen main groups of the Anatomical Therapeutic Chemical (ATC) classification system [37]. Then we selected 90 pharmacological, chemical subgroups or substances, which we categorized in 30 therapeutic groups. We identified drugs in the EHR by ATC codes. By and large, the drug groups and subgroups are based on the categorization of the ATC classification, but some minor deviations are present, e.g., acetylsalicylic acid was included as antithrombotic agents, whereas in the ATC code, it is grouped with the analgesics, an uncommon indication in Switzerland. Considering the hyper-thrombotic state of COVID-19 patients [38], we considered its rheological effect to be more important than its analgesic effect. Further information on our grouping is available in the Supplements, Table S1.

Lastly, we analyzed the molecular targets of the drugs on admission. We used DrugBank [39] to map drugs to targets and their target locations.

As the two severity cohorts are imbalanced, we normalized the number of patients for network analysis in each drug (sub-)group by dividing them through the total number of patients in the respective cohort. The obtained value was used as weight in the network analysis.

A network consists of nodes connected by edges. A node's weight is determined by the number of patients receiving the drug, and an edge's weight by the number of patients receiving two drugs simultaneously. In our analysis, drugs, drug classes, and targets were represented as nodes and concurrent use or interaction was represented by connecting undirected edges. Therefore, the weights of nodes or edges are both positively correlated with drug use or target engagement.

2.3. Software and Statistical Tests

Data wrangling, analysis, and visualization were performed in GNU R (version 4.0.2, R Foundation for Statistical Computing, http://www.R-project). Statistical significance levels were defined at a p value of <0.05, and determined with the Student's t-test for continuous parameters and Chi-square test for categorical parameters using the *stats* package (version 4.0.2). Network analysis was performed using the *igraph* package (Version 1.2.6) [40]. For network visualization, we used Gephi (Version 0.9.2) [41].

3. Results

3.1. Network Metrics

The main network metrics are presented in the Supplements, Table S2. Main nodes (hubs) and main edges are defined as those with the highest weight, i.e., largest share of patients taking this drug or drug combination. All main nodes and edges are identical between the severity cohorts, except for one edge in the drug subgroups (non-severe: *other analgesics and antipyretics—heparin*; severe: *other analgesics and antipyretics—antibiotics*). The diameter of the network (maximum distance between any two nodes; or the longest shortest path), was in general larger in the severe cohort. Node betweenness centrality (betweenness, indicating how often a node lies on the shortest path between two other nodes) in the non-severe cohort was higher than in the severe cohort (43 and 24 drug subgroups, respectively). More molecular targets had a higher betweenness in the non-severe than in the severe cohort (418 and 124 molecular targets, respectively). In addition, betweenness values in the non-severe cohort were higher (median: 150 vs. 48 and mean: 225 vs. 104, respectively). In Table S2, we show nodes with the greatest differences in the betweenness between the cohorts.

3.2. DDSI Network

There are significant differences ($p < 0.05$) in all three networks (anatomical/pharmacological group, drug group, and drug subgroup) with regards to the drugs (nodes, Table 2) and drug combinations (edges, Table 3) taken on admission. In all nodes and edges with significant differences, the percentage of occurrence was higher in the cohort with severe disease progression unless stated otherwise. As an example, visualization of the anatomical/pharmacological group network is shown in Figure 2.

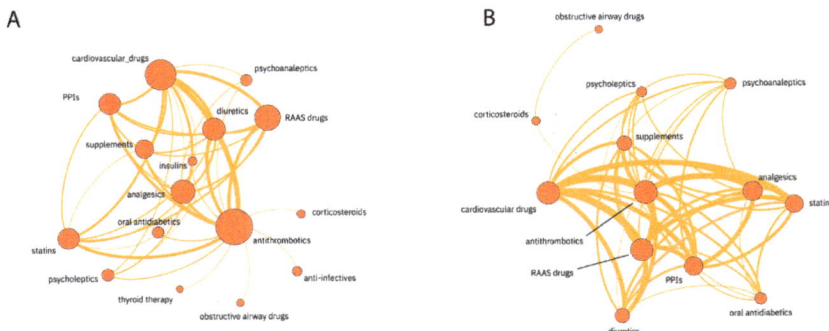

Figure 2. Drug group networks for severe (**A**) and non-severe (**B**) COVID-19 (only nodes with three or more edges are shown).

No differences can be observed in the anatomical/pharmacological group *Alimentary tract and metabolism* or any of the corresponding (sub-)groups between the severity cohorts considering all diseases. However, *anti-hyperglycemics*, specifically *dipeptidyl peptidase-4 (DPP4) inhibitors* and *sodium glucose co-transporter 2 (SGLT2) inhibitors* (only borderline significant, $p = 0.06$), were taken more often by non-severe COVID-19 patients with cardiovascular conditions or cardiovascular conditions and diabetes (see Supplements, Table S3).

In the anatomical/pharmacological group *Blood and blood forming organs*, *anti-hemorrhagics* and *anti-platelet agents* (even though only borderline significant with $p = 0.095$), and within these groups, especially *Vitamin K and other hemostatics* and *acetylsalicylic acid* (only borderline significant, $p = 0.085$), respectively, were significantly different between the severity cohorts.

In the anatomical/pharmacological group *Cardiovascular system*, which showed no cohort difference, the drug group *diuretics* and *cardiovascular drugs* had a higher percentage in severe COVID-19. In the former group, *loop diuretics* and in the latter, *beta blockers* are significant differences over all patients regardless of co-morbidity.

Table 2. Significant nodes of the DDSI network.

Anatomical/Pharmacological Group	Non-Severe COVID-19 [%]	Severe COVID-19 [%]	p Value
Blood and blood forming organs	85.64	94.78	0.014
Various	4.1	10.43	0.018
Musculo-skeletal system	21.79	13.91	0.085
Drug Groups			
Anti-hemorrhagics	0.51	3.48	0.037
Diuretics	23.08	32.17	0.064
Cardiovascular drugs	36.67	46.09	0.087
Antiplatelet agents	23.08	31.3	0.095
Drug Subgroups			
NSAID	12.56	4.35	0.020
Loop diuretics [1]	14.87	24.35	0.025
Beta blockers [1]	26.41	37.39	0.030
Vitamin K and other hemostatics	0.51	3.48	0.037
Opioids [1]	10.51	17.39	0.068
Acetylsalicylic acid	21.28	29.57	0.085

[1] Drug subgroups that were associated with death or severe COVID-19 by Iloanusi et al. and McKeigue et al. [29,30].

Table 3. Significant edges of the DDSI network.

Anatomical/Pharmacological Group Combinations		Non-Severe COVID-19 [%]	Severe COVID-19 [%]	p Value
Various	Alimentary tract and metabolism	3.85	10.43	0.012
	Nervous system	3.33	9.57	0.012
	Blood and blood forming organs	3.85	9.57	0.028
Drug Group Combinations		**Non-Severe COVID-19 [%]**	**Severe COVID-19 [%]**	**p Value**
Psycholeptics	Anti-hemorrhagics	0.26	3.48	0.011
Antiplatelet agents	Anti-infectives	7.44	15.65	0.013
Cardiovascular drugs	Diuretics	16.92	26.09	0.004
	Obstructive airway drugs	5.9	12.17	0.039
Drug Subgroup Combinations		**Non-Severe COVID-19 [%]**	**Severe COVID-19 [%]**	**p Value**
Antipsychotics [1]	Loop diuretics [1]	1.28	7.83	<0.001
	Opioids [1]	1.03	6.09	0.004
	Adrenergic inhalants	0.51	4.35	0.008
	Beta blockers [1]	2.82	8.7	0.012
	Proton pump inhibitors [1]	3.59	8.7	0.044
	Other analgesics	5.38	11.30	0.044
Heparin [1]	Direct Xa inhibitors [1]	0.51	4.35	0.008
	Loop diuretics [1]	4.62	10.43	0.036
Platelet inhibitors [1]	Antibiotics	7.44	14.78	0.026
	Loop diuretics [1]	5.13	11.3	0.032
	Beta blockers [1]	11.03	19.13	0.034
	Proton pump inhibitors [1]	10.00	17.39	0.045
	Potassium spare diuretics [1]	1.03	4.35	0.049
Potassium spare diuretics [1]	Acetylsalicylic acid	0.77	4.35	0.023
	Adrenergic inhalatives	0.51	3.48	0.037
Loop diuretics [1]	Opioids [1]	2.82	7.83	0.032
Vitamin K antagonists [1]	Thyroid	0.51	3.48	0.037
NSAID	Other analgesics	10.26	3.48	0.038
Beta blockers [1]	Acetylsalicylic acid	10.77	18.26	0.048

[1] Drug subgroups that were associated with death or severe COVID-19 by Iloanusi et al. and McKeigue et al. [29,30].

Additionally, non-steroidal anti-inflammatory drugs (NSAIDs) were more often taken by patients with non-severe COVID-19, whereas the opposite was true for opioids (but only borderline significant).

Considering all patients, there are differences in combinations of drugs from anatomical/pharmacological group, drug group combinations, and drug subgroup combinations, but the weight of these edges (percentage of patients) is relatively low in most cases (<15%) (Table 3).

However, the disease-specific analysis revealed that the combination of *anti-hyperglycemics* and *anti-coagulants* was more common in non-severe COVID-19 in patients with cardiac conditions or cardiac conditions and diabetes. In the latter cohort, the combination of *anti-hyperglycemics* and *statins* had a higher percentage in non-severe COVID-19 (see Supplements, Table S4).

3.3. TDSI Network

The main molecular targets and their relative frequency per cohort are shown in the Supplements, Figure S1. Molecular targets with highly significant ($p < 0.001$) differences are given in the Supplements, Figure S2.

Differences in molecular targets can be divided into two groups. The first group comprises targets which interact with only one specific group of drugs, e.g., antithrombotic agents mostly interact with *coagulation factor X, P-selection*, and *antithrombin-III*, whereas diuretics may target members of the *solute carrier family 12*. The second group includes targets that cannot be assigned to just one indication or drug group. *Beta adrenergic receptors* are targets for anti-depressants, anti-hypertensives, and anti-arrhythmics. There are over 2690 significantly different edges in the molecular target network. In the Supplements, we included the 30 most common edges in the network (Figure S3) and the highly significant edges ($p < 0.001$) (Figure S2).

In Figure 3, we present a filtered version of molecular target networks of both severity cohorts, where only nodes with three or more edges are shown.

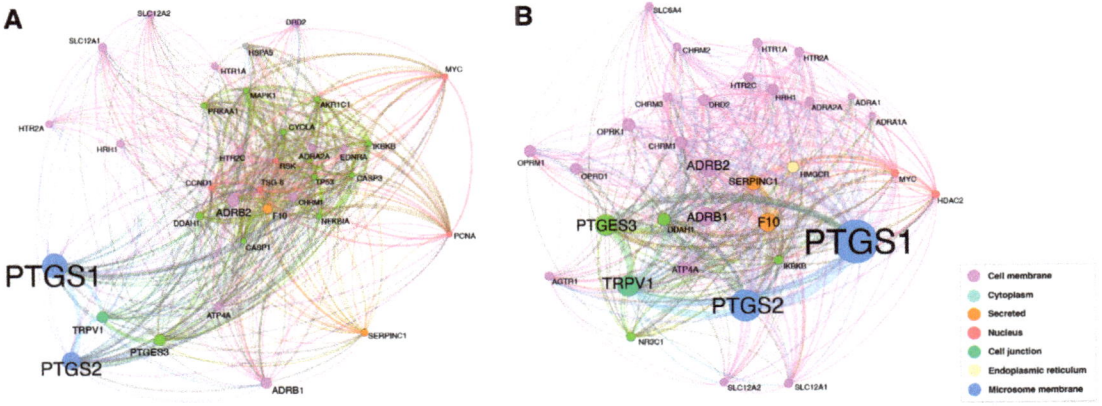

Figure 3. Molecular target networks for severe (**A**) and non-severe (**B**) COVID-19 (only nodes with three or more edges are shown); *ADRA1A/2A*: Alpha-1A/2A adrenergic receptor; *ADRB1/2*: Beta-1/2 adrenergic receptor; *AGTR1*: Type-1 angiotensin II receptor; *AKR1C1*: Aldo-keto reductase family 1 member C1; *ATP4A*: Potassium-transporting ATPase alpha chain 1; *CASP1/3*: Caspase-1/3; *CCND1*: G1/S-specific cyclin-D1; *CHRM1/M2/M3*: Muscarinic acetylcholine receptor M1/M2/M3; *CYCLA*: Cyclin A; *DDAH1*: N(G),N(G)-dimethylarginine dimethylaminohydrolase 1; *DRD2*: Dopamine D2 receptor; *EDNRA*: Endothelin-1 receptor; F10: Coagulation factor X; *HDAC2*: Histone deacetylase 2; *HMGCR*: 3-hydroxy-3-methylglutaryl-coenzyme A reductase; *HRH1*: Histamine H1 receptor; *HSPA5*: 78 kDa glucose-regulated protein; *HTR1A/2A/2C*: 5-hydroxytryptamine receptor 1A/2A/2C; *IKBKB*: Inhibitor of nuclear factor kappa-B kinase subunit beta; *MAPK1*: Mitogen-activated protein kinase 1; MYC: Myc proto-oncogene protein; *NFKBIA*: NF-kappa-B inhibitor alpha; *NR3C1*: Glucocorticoid receptor; *OPRD1*: Delta-type opioid receptor; *OPRK1*: Kappa-type opioid receptor; *OPRM1*: Mu-type opioid receptor; *PCNA*: Proliferating cell nuclear antigen; *PRKAA1*: 5'-AMP-activated protein kinase; *PTGES3*: Prostaglandin E synthase 3; *PTGS1/2*: Prostaglandin G/H synthase 1/2; *RSK*: Ribosomal protein S6 kinase alpha-3; *SERPINC1*: Antithrombin-III; *SLC12A1/2*: Solute carrier family 12 member 1/2; *SLC6A4*: Sodium-dependent serotonin transporter; *TP53*: Cellular tumor antigen p53; *TRPV1*: Transient receptor potential cation channel subfamily V member 1; *TSG-6*: Tumor necrosis factor-inducible gene 6 protein.

The color of the nodes indicates the location of the molecular target within the cell. In the non-severe cohort, more molecular targets are located within the cell membrane, whereas in the severe cohort more targets are located within the cytoplasm.

4. Discussion

The network analysis of drugs and their molecular targets revealed differences between the severity cohorts of COVID-19. Except for one edge, the main nodes (hubs) and edges are identical, however the weights were often slightly higher in the severe cohort. This suggests that the most important drugs and drug combinations are the same between the cohorts, but still, slightly more drugs and drug combinations are taken by the severe cohort. This may be indicative of a subpopulation with more co-morbidities. The larger diameter of the severe network indicates that the drugs and drug combinations are more heterogeneous in this cohort. This is supported by the generally lower betweenness of most nodes in this cohort in absolute values, but also in comparison to the non-severe cohort.

However, co-morbidities and co-medications did not always result in a more severe course. Noteworthy here is the higher percentage of patients with cardiac conditions, or cardiac conditions and diabetes, using anti-hyperglycemics, especially DPP4 inhibitors, and to a lower degree SGLT2 inhibitors in the non-severe COVID-19 cohort. These patients had at least two co-morbidities, which are considered risk factors for a severe course [15,42,43], but had a more favorable outcome under these treatment regimens. DPP4 inhibitors have been shown to be reno- and cardio-protective through the suppression of oxidative stress, inflammation, and improvement of endothelial function [44]. Furthermore, there is evidence that SARS-CoV-2, like MERS-CoV (Middle East respiratory syndrome-related coronavirus), also uses the membrane-bound DPP4 enzyme for viral entry. An inhibition of this enzyme is speculated to reduce viral entry and replication [45,46]. In SARS-CoV-2, a functional network analysis revealed that DPP4 is required in viral processes for viral entry and infection. Furthermore, protein-chemical interaction networks revealed important interactions between DPP4 and the DPP4 inhibitor sitagliptin [47]. Additionally, in animal experiments, DPP4 inhibition resulted in a rise of soluble DPP4 [48,49] which could bind to plasma SARS-CoV-2, reducing the amount of virus able to infect cells [50]. Mutations in DPP4 genes, leading to reduced levels for soluble DPP4, were identified as risk factors for increased susceptibility for MERS-CoV [51]. Within an infected cell, sitagliptin inhibited the SARS-CoV-2 papain-like proteases (PLpro) in an in-cell protease assay [52]. Clinical literature on DPP4 inhibitors in COVID-19 is ambiguous; several studies and meta-analyses have showed favorable effects [53–56], while some have not [57–59]. A review of clinical trials with the DPP4 inhibitor sitagliptin found that most studies showed a favorable effect on COVID-19 progression [50]. Several potential modes of action are discussed apart from the above-mentioned decrease in viral entry, increase in soluble DPP4, or inhibition of viral proteases. It is hypothesized that DPP4 inhibitors might attenuate COVID-19-related cardiovascular injury including arrhythmia, acute coronary syndrome and heart failure [60]. In addition, DPP4 inhibition has anti-inflammatory and immunomodulatory properties by decreasing activation of nuclear factor kappa beta (NF-κB) activation and expression of inflammatory cytokines [61,62]. These factors could also influence the progression.

A benefit of SGLT2 inhibitors is supported on pathophysiological grounds. SGLT2 inhibitors have been shown to downregulate systemic and adipose tissue inflammation by decreasing the expression of pro-inflammatory cytokines, lessen oxidative stress, and reduce sympathetic activity [63]. Furthermore, treatment with a SGLT2 inhibitors alleviated myocardial and renal fibrosis in mice [64]. In a large randomized trial with COVID-19 patients, treatment with dapagliflozin, a SGLT2 inhibitors, did not result in a statistically significant risk reduction in organ dysfunction and death, or speedier recovery [65].

Considering all patients, regardless of the diagnosed co-morbidities, there are some noteworthy differences in the drugs (nodes of the network, Table 2) used within the cohorts. Despite doubts early in the pandemic regarding the use of NSAIDs during COVID-19 [66], a systematic review and meta-analysis was not able to confirm this theoretical risk [67]. In human cell cultures and mice, NSAIDs reduced pro-inflammatory cytokines, and dampened the humoral immune response to SARS-CoV-2 [68]. This protective effect might be explained by reversing the progressive inflammation in different organs [69]. Even though this study included only few patients on NSAIDs, they were still more common in non-severe patients and thus corroborated earlier studies. Comparisons to other antipyretics with no anti-inflammatory action (e.g., acetaminophen) are necessary.

Some drugs with significant differences between cohorts might be more indicative of the severity of the underlying condition and not interact with COVID-19 prognosis directly. Loop diuretics, for instance are used in more advanced stages of renal failure [70]. As poor renal function is indicative of severe COVID-19 [71,72], this correlation might be due to the severity of the pre-existing condition, not the drug itself. Beta blockers were more often used in the severe cohort, but this might be explained by the higher prevalence of cardiovascular co-morbidities in this cohort. However, loop diuretics, beta blockers, and opioids are also associated with death or severe COVID-19 in a polypharmacy setting [29,30].

Overall, a relatively small percentage of patients received antipsychotic drugs, and the difference between cohorts was not significant (8% and 13% in the non-severe and severe cohorts, respectively). However, combinations with other drugs such as loop diuretics, opioids, beta-blockers, or proton pump inhibitors were more often seen in patients in the severe cohort. The influence of antipsychotic drugs on COVID-19 infection risk and prognosis is currently under discussion. A retrospective study in 698 patients using antipsychotic drugs revealed a lower infection risk and a better prognosis compared to non-users [73]. Comparable results were also reported from a study in patients with a pre-existing diagnosis of schizophrenia, schizoaffective disorder, or bipolar disorder [74]. On the other hand, a systematic review and meta-analysis showed a correlation between antipsychotics and COVID-19 mortality [75]. However, the reviewed studies included patients on antipsychotics independently of diagnoses, considered antipsychotics as a single homogenous pharmacological group, and did not test for adherence [76]. Our results suggest that not the use of a specific drugs per se, but the combination with other drugs influences the risk for severe COVID-19. Therefore, a detailed analysis of the most significantly different drug combinations (edges of the network, Table 3) was performed. Most drug combinations were taken by less than 15% of the patients, which makes a detailed analysis of cause and effect difficult, but trends are visible. In all cases but one (NSAIDs/other analgesics) a greater proportion was seen in the severe cohort. However, this difference is not due to general polypharmacy, which is known to influence disease severity in COVID-19 [29,30], as the number of drugs on admission was not significantly different in both cohorts. Not only polypharmacy, but also specific drug classes influence severity in COVID-19 [29,30]. Drug classes with an increased risk for severe COVID-19 are highlighted in red in Table 3. In seven and in eleven drug combinations, one or both drugs, respectively, were considered high risk. All these combinations were more prevalent in the severe cohort. Only in one combination (NSAIDs/other analgesics), neither drug was considered high risk. Interestingly, a higher proportion of non-severe patients took that combination.

In proton pump inhibitors (PPIs), the effect of combination with other drugs can be seen. PPIs are taken to the same extent by the non-severe and severe cohort (32.6% and 33.9%, respectively, $p = 0.88$, data not shown). However, combinations of PPIs with antipsychotics or platelet inhibitors were more prevalent in severe patients. Several review articles evaluating the effects of PPIs on COVID-19 progression and mortality revealed high heterogeneity in the outcomes [77–80]. However, those studies did not control for co-medication, except for one which looked at NSAIDs [80]. In summary, studies on drug effects should also consider including and ideally control for co-medication.

In the molecular target network of the non-severe cohort, there are more targets located in the cell membrane. Several hypotheses could help explain this finding. One hypothesis is that interaction of drugs with cell membrane receptors might interfere with viral entry into the cell. The host protein angiotensin-converting enzyme 2 (ACE2) is considered the main entry receptor for SARS-CoV-2 and the transmembrane serine protease 2 (TMPRSS2) an important priming enzyme required during this process [81,82]. In addition, other cell membrane receptors may be involved in cellular entry of SARS-CoV-2 [81,83,84], like neurophilin-I [85,86], or DPP4 [45,46]. Interference may be direct if a drug targets a protein, which is also important for viral entry. Studies on SARS-CoV-2–human protein-protein interaction revealed hundreds of further possible targets [87–90], however there is only minimal overlap with the target we identified. However, interference may also be indirect due to changes in membrane organization that negatively impact any part of the viral replication cycle. Functionally organized micro-domains (lipid rafts), characterized by highly ordered and tightly packed lipid molecules, within the cell membrane may play a pivotal role in different processes during the viral life-cycle, including coronaviruses [91]. Lipid raft involvement in viral entry was already shown for the murine hepatitis virus, a betacoronavirus such as SARS-CoV-2 [92]. A further study used SARS-CoV-2 pseudo viruses to demonstrate the importance of cholesterol-rich membrane lipid raft for infection [93]. Micro-domains may increase the efficiency of infection by clustering enzymes and receptors in certain membrane area, thus allowing multivalent binding of virus particles, but are not an absolute requirement for the entry process [94]. Several drugs acting on specific the cell membrane targets were shown to disrupt lipid rafts [95]. These included targets we identified in the non-severe cohort, such as alpha- and beta-adrenergic receptors, and opioid receptors. As the network visualizations only include nodes with three or more edges, one might conclude that the combination of several drugs, which interfere with the integrity of the lipid rafts, have an influence on COVID-19 progression.

Our study has some limitations. The severity cohorts had some significant differences in demographics and co-morbidities. The severe cohort was significantly older, had a higher BMI, and a higher share of male patients, all factors which are known risk factors for severe COVID-19 [5–12]. Even though the differences are significant, they are still rather small (median age difference three years, median BMI difference 1.68 points), so that a detailed analysis of these factors would require a larger sample size to obtain enough power with an unknown effect size. Additionally, more patients in the severe cohort suffered from arterial hypertension, chronic heart failure and/or coronary heart disease, again established risk factors in COVID-19 [16,17,22]. However, the presence and even the severity of co-morbidities were indirectly accounted for by the analysis of prescribed drugs. The number of drugs on admission was not significantly different between the cohorts. Even though we were able to include a total of 505 patients in our analysis, the number of patients receiving one specific drug was still relatively low, especially in the disease cohorts. Therefore, significant differences were in some cases only seen in the high-level pooled groups. For this reason, we also reported borderline significant results ($0.05 < p < 0.1$), which could be interpreted as a weak signal and should be investigated in further research. Furthermore, we were mainly able to consider hospitalized patients because of data availability issues. As the IHG is an important regional medical center, some patients were transferred from smaller hospitals. Drugs given in these smaller hospitals are recorded on the drugs on admission list.

The analysis only focused on dual combinations. While we did perform cluster analyses to find more complex combinations, the data available did not support this. Furthermore, even though there were significant differences between the severity cohort with regards to age and sex, we did not control for that.

5. Conclusions

In summary, the use of a network approach allowed for studying the impact of drugs from a novel vantage point. Most importantly, autonomic targets appear to be influential on the course of disease in COVID-19, mostly in the form of off-target effects, possibly by disrupting lipid rafts and impeding viral entry. This also holds for DPP4 inhibitors, which are known to interact with adrenergic receptors [96]. The impact of interference with autonomic receptors merits further study into potential future treatments for infection with SARS-CoV-2 and other viruses. Overall, our network analysis indicates that DPP4 inhibitors are related to a better prognosis for COVID-19 and thus represent potential repositioning drugs against SARS-CoV-2. Additionally, our study revealed (i) that drug-induced changes in cell membrane architecture might influence disease progression and (ii) that the influence of specific drugs on disease progression might be dependent on concurrent co-medication.

Supplementary Materials: The following supporting information can be downloaded at: https://www.mdpi.com/article/10.3390/pharmaceutics14091828/s1, Table S1: Assignment of ATC codes to the drug groups and subgroups; Table S2: Important network metrics of DDSI and TDSI network; Table S3: Significant nodes of the DDSI network, disease specific; Table S4: Significant edges of the DDSI network, disease specific; Figure S1: Main target nodes; Figure S2: Target nodes with significant differences; Figure S3: Main target edges; Figure S4: Target edges with highly significant differences ($p < 0.001$).

Author Contributions: V.S.: formal analysis, investigation, methodology, software, visualization, writing; F.H.: conceptualization, formal analysis, methodology, software, supervision, visualization, writing. All authors have read and agreed to the published version of the manuscript.

Funding: This research received no external funding.

Institutional Review Board Statement: The study was approved by the Cantonal Ethics Committee of Bern (Project-ID 2020-00973).

Informed Consent Statement: Participants either agreed to a general research consent or, for participants with no registered general research consent status (neither agreement nor rejection), a waiver of consent was granted by the ethics committee.

Data Availability Statement: The source code is available on GitHub: https://github.com/cptbern/Covid19-network-analysis.

Acknowledgments: We thank Noel Frey, Myoori Wijayasingham, and the Insel Data Science Center for database and infrastructure support.

Conflicts of Interest: The authors declare no conflict of interest.

References

1. Gnädinger, M.; Herzig, L.; Ceschi, A.; Conen, D.; Staehelin, A.; Zoller, M.; Puhan, M.A. Chronic conditions and multimorbidity in a primary care population: A study in the Swiss Sentinel Surveillance Network (Sentinella). *Int. J. Public Health* **2018**, *63*, 1017–1026. [CrossRef] [PubMed]
2. Déruaz-Luyet, A.; Goran, A.A.; Senn, N.; Bodenmann, P.; Pasquier, J.; Widmer, D.; Tandjung, R.; Rosemann, T.; Frey, P.; Streit, S.; et al. Multimorbidity and patterns of chronic conditions in a primary care population in Switzerland: A cross-sectional study. *BMJ Open* **2017**, *7*, e013664. [CrossRef] [PubMed]
3. Lynch, S.S. Drug Interactions. Available online: https://www.msdmanuals.com/home/drugs/factors-affecting-response-to-drugs/drug-interactions (accessed on 14 September 2021).
4. Galan-Vasquez, E.; Perez-Rueda, E. A landscape for drug-target interactions based on network analysis. *PLoS ONE* **2021**, *16*, e0247018. [CrossRef] [PubMed]
5. Bencivenga, L.; Rengo, G.; Varricchi, G. Elderly at time of COronaVIrus disease 2019 (COVID-19): Possible role of immunosenescence and malnutrition. *GeroScience* **2020**, *42*, 1089–1092. [CrossRef]
6. Cunha, L.L.; Perazzio, S.F.; Azzi, J.; Cravedi, P.; Riella, L.V. Remodeling of the Immune Response with Aging: Immunosenescence and Its Potential Impact on COVID-19 Immune Response. *Front. Immunol.* **2020**, *11*, 1748. [CrossRef]
7. Peckham, H.; de Gruijter, N.M.; Raine, C.; Radziszewska, A.; Ciurtin, C.; Wedderburn, L.R.; Rosser, E.C.; Webb, K.; Deakin, C.T. Male sex identified by global COVID-19 meta-analysis as a risk factor for death and ITU admission. *Nat. Commun.* **2020**, *11*, 6317. [CrossRef]
8. Klein, S.L.; Dhakal, S.; Ursin, R.L.; Deshpande, S.; Sandberg, K.; Mauvais-Jarvis, F. Biological sex impacts COVID-19 outcomes. *PLoS Pathog.* **2020**, *16*, e1008570. [CrossRef]
9. Kang, Z.; Luo, S.; Gui, Y.; Zhou, H.; Zhang, Z.; Tian, C.; Zhou, Q.; Wang, Q.; Hu, Y.; Fan, H.; et al. Obesity is a potential risk factor contributing to clinical manifestations of COVID-19. *Int. J. Obes.* **2020**, *44*, 2479–2485. [CrossRef]
10. Kwok, S.; Adam, S.; Ho, J.H.; Iqbal, Z.; Turkington, P.; Razvi, S.; Le Roux, C.W.; Soran, H.; Syed, A.A. Obesity: A critical risk factor in the COVID-19 pandemic. *Clin. Obes.* **2020**, *10*, e12403. [CrossRef] [PubMed]

11. Foldi, M.; Farkas, N.; Kiss, S.; Zadori, N.; Vancsa, S.; Szako, L.; Dembrovszky, F.; Solymar, M.; Bartalis, E.; Szakacs, Z.; et al. Obesity is a risk factor for developing critical condition in COVID-19 patients: A systematic review and meta-analysis. *Obes. Rev.* **2020**, *21*, e13095. [CrossRef]
12. Sattar, N.; McInnes, I.B.; McMurray, J.J.V. Obesity Is a Risk Factor for Severe COVID-19 Infection: Multiple Potential Mechanisms. *Circulation* **2020**, *142*, 4–6. [CrossRef] [PubMed]
13. Zhu, L.; She, Z.-G.; Cheng, X.; Qin, J.-J.; Zhang, X.-J.; Cai, J.; Lei, F.; Wang, H.; Xie, J.; Wang, W.; et al. Association of Blood Glucose Control and Outcomes in Patients with COVID-19 and Pre-existing Type 2 Diabetes. *Cell Metab.* **2020**, *31*, 1068–1077.e3. [CrossRef] [PubMed]
14. Tadic, M.; Cuspidi, C. The influence of diabetes and hypertension on outcome in COVID-19 patients: Do we mix apples and oranges? *J. Clin. Hypertens.* **2020**, *23*, 235–237. [CrossRef] [PubMed]
15. Lim, S.; Bae, J.H.; Kwon, H.-S.; Nauck, M.A. COVID-19 and diabetes mellitus: From pathophysiology to clinical management. *Nat. Rev. Endocrinol.* **2021**, *17*, 11–30. [CrossRef] [PubMed]
16. Ssentongo, P.; Ssentongo, A.E.; Heilbrunn, E.S.; Ba, D.M.; Chinchilli, V.M. Association of cardiovascular disease and 10 other pre-existing comorbidities with COVID-19 mortality: A systematic review and meta-analysis. *PLoS ONE* **2020**, *15*, e0238215. [CrossRef]
17. Inciardi, R.M.; Adamo, M.; Lupi, L.; Cani, D.S.; Di Pasquale, M.; Tomasoni, D.; Italia, L.; Zaccone, G.; Tedino, C.; Fabbricatore, D.; et al. Characteristics and outcomes of patients hospitalized for COVID-19 and cardiac disease in Northern Italy. *Eur. Heart J.* **2020**, *41*, 1821–1829. [CrossRef]
18. Yang, J.; Zheng, Y.; Gou, X.; Pu, K.; Chen, Z.; Guo, Q.; Ji, R.; Wang, H.; Wang, Y.; Zhou, Y. Prevalence of comorbidities and its effects in patients infected with SARS-CoV-2: A systematic review and meta-analysis. *Int. J. Infect. Dis.* **2020**, *94*, 91–95. [CrossRef]
19. Olloquequi, J. COVID-19 Susceptibility in chronic obstructive pulmonary disease. *Eur. J. Clin. Investig.* **2020**, *50*, e13382. [CrossRef]
20. Wang, Q.; Davis, P.B.; Gurney, M.E.; Xu, R. COVID-19 and dementia: Analyses of risk, disparity, and outcomes from electronic health records in the US. *Alzheimer's Dement.* **2021**, *17*, 1297–1306. [CrossRef]
21. Chudasama, Y.V.; Zaccardi, F.; Gillies, C.L.; Razieh, C.; Yates, T.; Kloecker, D.E.; Rowlands, A.V.; Davies, M.J.; Islam, N.; Seidu, S.; et al. Patterns of multimorbidity and risk of severe SARS-CoV-2 infection: An observational study in the U.K. *BMC Infect. Dis.* **2021**, *21*, 908. [CrossRef]
22. Hu, J.; Zhang, X.; Zhang, X.; Zhao, H.; Lian, J.; Hao, S.; Jia, H.; Yang, M.; Lu, Y.; Xiang, D.; et al. COVID-19 is more severe in patients with hypertension; ACEI/ARB treatment does not influence clinical severity and outcome. *J. Infect.* **2020**, *81*, 979–997. [CrossRef] [PubMed]
23. Sato, K.; White, N.; Fanning, J.P.; Obonyo, N.; Yamashita, M.H.; Appadurai, V.; Ciullo, A.; May, M.; Worku, E.T.; Helms, L.; et al. Impact of renin–angiotensin–aldosterone system inhibition on mortality in critically ill COVID-19 patients with pre-existing hypertension: A prospective cohort study. *BMC Cardiovasc. Disord.* **2022**, *22*, 123. [CrossRef] [PubMed]
24. Park, J.; Lee, S.-H.; You, S.C.; Kim, J.; Yang, K. Effect of renin-angiotensin-aldosterone system inhibitors on COVID-19 patients in Korea. *PLoS ONE* **2021**, *16*, e0248058. [CrossRef]
25. Braude, P.; Carter, B.; Short, R.; Vilches-Moraga, A.; Verduri, A.; Pearce, L.; Price, A.; Quinn, T.J.; Stechman, M.; Collins, J.; et al. The influence of ACE inhibitors and ARBs on hospital length of stay and survival in people with COVID-19. *IJC Heart Vasc.* **2020**, *31*, 100660. [CrossRef]
26. Vila-Córcoles, A.; Ochoa-Gondar, O.; Satué-Gracia, E.M.; Torrente-Fraga, C.; Gomez-Bertomeu, F.; Vila-Rovira, A.; Hospital-Guardiola, I.; de Diego-Cabanes, C.; Bejarano-Romero, F.; Basora-Gallisà, J. Influence of prior comorbidities and chronic medications use on the risk of COVID-19 in adults: A population-based cohort study in Tarragona, Spain. *BMJ Open* **2020**, *10*, e041577. [CrossRef]
27. Holt, A.; Mizrak, I.; Lamberts, M.; Lav Madsen, P. Influence of inhibitors of the renin-angiotensin system on risk of acute respiratory distress syndrome in Danish hospitalized COVID-19 patients. *J. Hypertens.* **2020**, *38*, 1612–1613. [CrossRef]
28. Jia, N.; Zhang, G.; Sun, X.; Wang, Y.; Zhao, S.; Chi, W.; Dong, S.; Xia, J.; Zeng, P.; Liu, D. Influence of angiotensin converting enzyme inhibitors/angiotensin receptor blockers on the risk of all-cause mortality and other clinical outcomes in patients with confirmed COVID-19: A systemic review and meta-analysis. *J. Clin. Hypertens.* **2021**, *23*, 1651–1663. [CrossRef]
29. Iloanusi, S.; Mgbere, O.; Essien, E.J. Polypharmacy among COVID-19 patients: A systematic review. *J. Am. Pharm. Assoc.* **2021**, *61*, e14–e25. [CrossRef]
30. McKeigue, P.M.; Kennedy, S.; Weir, A.; Bishop, J.; McGurnaghan, S.J.; McAllister, D.; Robertson, C.; Wood, R.; Lone, N.; Murray, J.; et al. Relation of severe COVID-19 to polypharmacy and prescribing of psychotropic drugs: The REACT-SCOT case-control study. *BMC Med.* **2021**, *19*, 51. [CrossRef]
31. Newman, M.E.J. *Networks: An Introduction*; Oxford University Press: Oxford, UK; New York, NY, USA, 2010.
32. Casas, A.I.; Hassan, A.A.; Larsen, S.J.; Gomez-Rangel, V.; Elbatreek, M.; Kleikers, P.W.M.; Guney, E.; Egea, J.; López, M.G.; Baumbach, J.; et al. From single drug targets to synergistic network pharmacology in ischemic stroke. *Proc. Natl. Acad. Sci. USA* **2019**, *116*, 7129–7136. [CrossRef]
33. Azad, A.K.M.; Fatima, S.; Capraro, A.; Waters, S.A.; Vafaee, F. Integrative resource for network-based investigation of COVID-19 combinatorial drug repositioning and mechanism of action. *Patterns* **2021**, *2*, 100325. [CrossRef] [PubMed]

34. Morselli Gysi, D.; do Valle, Í.; Zitnik, M.; Ameli, A.; Gan, X.; Varol, O.; Ghiassian, S.D.; Patten, J.J.; Davey, R.A.; Loscalzo, J.; et al. Network medicine framework for identifying drug-repurposing opportunities for COVID-19. *Proc. Natl. Acad. Sci. USA* **2021**, *118*, e2025581118. [CrossRef] [PubMed]
35. Sibilio, P.; Bini, S.; Fiscon, G.; Sponziello, M.; Conte, F.; Pecce, V.; Durante, C.; Paci, P.; Falcone, R.; Norata, G.D.; et al. In silico drug repurposing in COVID-19: A network-based analysis. *Biomed. Pharmacother.* **2021**, *142*, 111954. [CrossRef]
36. Schöning, V.; Liakoni, E.; Drewe, J.; Hammann, F. Automatic identification of risk factors for SARS-CoV-2 positivity and severe clinical outcomes of COVID-19 using Data Mining and Natural Language Processing. *medRxiv* **2021**. [CrossRef]
37. WHO Collaborating Centre for Drug Statistics Methodology. *ATC Classification Index with DDDs*; WHO Collaborating Centre for Drug Statistics Methodology: Oslo, Norway, 2021.
38. Gu, S.X.; Tyagi, T.; Jain, K.; Gu, V.W.; Lee, S.H.; Hwa, J.M.; Kwan, J.M.; Krause, D.S.; Lee, A.I.; Halene, S.; et al. Thrombocytopathy and endotheliopathy: Crucial contributors to COVID-19 thromboinflammation. *Nat. Rev. Cardiol.* **2021**, *18*, 194–209. [CrossRef]
39. Wishart, D.S.; Knox, C.; Guo, A.C.; Shrivastava, S.; Hassanali, M.; Stothard, P.; Chang, Z.; Woolsey, J. DrugBank: A comprehensive resource for in silico drug discovery and exploration. *Nucleic Acids Res.* **2006**, *34*, D668–D672. [CrossRef] [PubMed]
40. Csárdi, G.; Nepusz, T. The Igraph Software Package for Complex Network Research. *InterJournal Complex Syst.* **2006**, *1695*, 1–9.
41. Bastian, M.; Heymann, S.; Jacomy, M. Gephi: An Open Source Software for Exploring and Manipulating Networks. In Proceedings of the International AAAI Conference on Web and Social Media, San Jose, CA, USA, 17–20 May 2009; Volume 3, pp. 361–362.
42. Wolff, D.; Nee, S.; Hickey, N.S.; Marschollek, M. Risk factors for COVID-19 severity and fatality: A structured literature review. *Infection* **2020**, *49*, 15–28. [CrossRef]
43. Singh, A.K.; Gupta, R.; Misra, A. Comorbidities in COVID-19: Outcomes in hypertensive cohort and controversies with renin angiotensin system blockers. *Diabetes Metab. Syndr.* **2020**, *14*, 283–287. [CrossRef]
44. Tomovic, K.; Lazarevic, J.; Kocic, G.; Deljanin-Ilic, M.; Anderluh, M.; Smelcerovic, A. Mechanisms and pathways of anti-inflammatory activity of DPP-4 inhibitors in cardiovascular and renal protection. *Med. Res. Rev.* **2019**, *39*, 404–422. [CrossRef]
45. Solerte, S.B.; Di Sabatino, A.; Galli, M.; Fiorina, P. Dipeptidyl peptidase-4 (DPP4) inhibition in COVID-19. *Acta Diabetol.* **2020**, *57*, 779–783. [CrossRef] [PubMed]
46. Bassendine, M.F.; Bridge, S.H.; McCaughan, G.W.; Gorrell, M.D. COVID-19 and comorbidities: A role for dipeptidyl peptidase 4 (DPP4) in disease severity? *J. Diabetes* **2020**, *12*, 649–658. [CrossRef] [PubMed]
47. Bardaweel, S.K.; Hajjo, R.; Sabbah, D.A. Sitagliptin: A potential drug for the treatment of COVID-19? *Acta Pharm.* **2021**, *71*, 175–184. [CrossRef]
48. Varin, E.M.; Mulvihill, E.E.; Beaudry, J.L.; Pujadas, G.; Fuchs, S.; Tanti, J.-F.; Fazio, S.; Kaur, K.; Cao, X.; Baggio, L.L.; et al. Circulating Levels of Soluble Dipeptidyl Peptidase-4 Are Dissociated from Inflammation and Induced by Enzymatic DPP4 Inhibition. *Cell Metab.* **2019**, *29*, 320–334.e5. [CrossRef]
49. Baggio, L.L.; Varin, E.M.; Koehler, J.A.; Cao, X.; Lokhnygina, Y.; Stevens, S.R.; Holman, R.R.; Drucker, D.J. Plasma levels of DPP4 activity and sDPP4 are dissociated from inflammation in mice and humans. *Nat. Commun.* **2020**, *11*, 3766. [CrossRef] [PubMed]
50. Mikhael, E.M.; Ong, S.C.; Sheikh Ghadzi, S.M. Efficacy and Safety of Sitagliptin in the Treatment of COVID-19. *J. Pharm. Pract.* **2022**, 8971900221102119. [CrossRef] [PubMed]
51. Alkharsah, K.R.; Aljaroodi, S.A.; Rahman, J.U.; Alnafie, A.N.; Al Dossary, R.; Aljindan, R.Y.; Alnimr, A.M.; Hussen, J. Low levels of soluble DPP4 among Saudis may have constituted a risk factor for MERS endemicity. *PLoS ONE* **2022**, *17*, e0266603. [CrossRef]
52. Narayanan, A.; Narwal, M.; Majowicz, S.A.; Varricchio, C.; Toner, S.A.; Ballatore, C.; Brancale, A.; Murakami, K.S.; Jose, J. Identification of SARS-CoV-2 inhibitors targeting Mpro and PLpro using in-cell-protease assay. *Commun. Biol.* **2022**, *5*, 169. [CrossRef]
53. Rhee, S.Y.; Lee, J.; Nam, H.; Kyoung, D.-S.; Shin, D.W.; Kim, D.J. Effects of a DPP-4 Inhibitor and RAS Blockade on Clinical Outcomes of Patients with Diabetes and COVID-19. *Diabetes Metab. J.* **2021**, *45*, 251–259. [CrossRef]
54. Rakhmat, I.I.; Kusmala, Y.Y.; Handayani, D.R.; Juliastuti, H.; Nawangsih, E.N.; Wibowo, A.; Lim, M.A.; Pranata, R. Dipeptidyl peptidase-4 (DPP-4) inhibitor and mortality in coronavirus disease 2019 (COVID-19)—A systematic review, meta-analysis, and meta-regression. *Diabetes Metab. Syndr.* **2021**, *15*, 777–782. [CrossRef]
55. Mirani, M.; Favacchio, G.; Carrone, F.; Betella, N.; Biamonte, E.; Morenghi, E.; Mazziotti, G.; Lania, A.G. Impact of Comorbidities and Glycemia at Admission and Dipeptidyl Peptidase 4 Inhibitors in Patients with Type 2 Diabetes With COVID-19: A Case Series From an Academic Hospital in Lombardy, Italy. *Diabetes Care* **2020**, *43*, 3042–3049. [CrossRef]
56. Pal, R.; Banerjee, M.; Mukherjee, S.; Bhogal, R.S.; Kaur, A.; Bhadada, S.K. Dipeptidyl peptidase-4 inhibitor use and mortality in COVID-19 patients with diabetes mellitus: An updated systematic review and meta-analysis. *Ther. Adv. Endocrinol. Metab.* **2021**, *12*, 2042018821996482. [CrossRef] [PubMed]
57. Fadini, G.P.; Morieri, M.L.; Longato, E.; Bonora, B.M.; Pinelli, S.; Selmin, E.; Voltan, G.; Falaguasta, D.; Tresso, S.; Costantini, G.; et al. Exposure to dipeptidyl-peptidase-4 inhibitors and COVID-19 among people with type 2 diabetes: A case-control study. *Diabetes Obes. Metab.* **2020**, *22*, 1946–1950. [CrossRef] [PubMed]
58. Zhou, J.-H.; Wu, B.; Wang, W.-X.; Lei, F.; Cheng, X.; Qin, J.-J.; Cai, J.-J.; Zhang, X.-J.; Zhou, F.; Liu, Y.-M.; et al. No significant association between dipeptidyl peptidase-4 inhibitors and adverse outcomes of COVID-19. *World J. Clin. Cases* **2020**, *8*, 5576–5588. [CrossRef]

59. Morieri, M.L.; Bonora, B.M.; Longato, E.; Di Camilo, B.; Sparacino, G.; Tramontan, L.; Avogaro, A.; Fadini, G.P. Exposure to dipeptidyl-peptidase 4 inhibitors and the risk of pneumonia among people with type 2 diabetes: Retrospective cohort study and meta-analysis. *Diabetes Obes. Metab.* **2020**, *22*, 1925–1934. [CrossRef] [PubMed]
60. Du, H.; Wang, D.W.; Chen, C. The potential effects of DPP-4 inhibitors on cardiovascular system in COVID-19 patients. *J. Cell. Mol. Med.* **2020**, *24*, 10274–10278. [CrossRef]
61. Dastan, F.; Abedini, A.; Shahabi, S.; Kiani, A.; Saffaei, A.; Zare, A. Sitagliptin Repositioning in SARS-CoV-2: Effects on ACE-2, CD-26, and Inflammatory Cytokine Storms in the Lung. *Iran. J. Allergy Asthma Immunol.* **2020**, *19*, 10–12. [CrossRef]
62. Mozafari, N.; Azadi, S.; Mehdi-Alamdarlou, S.; Ashrafi, H.; Azadi, A. Inflammation: A bridge between diabetes and COVID-19, and possible management with sitagliptin. *Med. Hypotheses* **2020**, *143*, 110111. [CrossRef] [PubMed]
63. Koufakis, T.; Pavlidis, A.N.; Metallidis, S.; Kotsa, K. Sodium-glucose co-transporter 2 inhibitors in COVID-19: Meeting at the crossroads between heart, diabetes and infectious diseases. *Int. J. Clin. Pharm.* **2021**, *43*, 764–767. [CrossRef]
64. Li, X.-T.; Zhang, M.-W.; Zhang, Z.-Z.; Cao, Y.-D.; Liu, X.-Y.; Miao, R.; Xu, Y.; Song, X.-F.; Song, J.-W.; Liu, Y.; et al. Abnormal apelin-ACE2 and SGLT2 signaling contribute to adverse cardiorenal injury in patients with COVID-19. *Int. J. Cardiol.* **2021**, *336*, 123–129. [CrossRef]
65. Kosiborod, M.N.; Esterline, R.; Furtado, R.H.M.; Oscarsson, J.; Gasparyan, S.B.; Koch, G.G.; Martinez, F.; Mukhtar, O.; Verma, S.; Chopra, V.; et al. Dapagliflozin in patients with cardiometabolic risk factors hospitalised with COVID-19 (DARE-19): A randomised, double-blind, placebo-controlled, phase 3 trial. *Lancet Diabetes Endocrinol.* **2021**, *9*, 586–594. [CrossRef]
66. European Medicines Agency. EMA/136850/2020: EMA Gives Advice on the Use of Non-Steroidal Anti Inflammatories for COVID-19. Available online: https://www.ema.europa.eu/en/documents/press-release/ema-gives-advice-use-non-steroidal-anti-inflammatories-COVID-19_en.pdf (accessed on 6 December 2021).
67. Moore, N.; Bosco-Levy, P.; Thurin, N.; Blin, P.; Droz-Perroteau, C. NSAIDs and COVID-19: A Systematic Review and Meta-analysis. *Drug Saf.* **2021**, *44*, 929–938. [CrossRef]
68. Chen Jennifer, S.; Alfajaro Mia, M.; Chow Ryan, D.; Wei, J.; Filler Renata, B.; Eisenbarth Stephanie, C.; Wilen Craig, B.; Gallagher, T. Nonsteroidal Anti-inflammatory Drugs Dampen the Cytokine and Antibody Response to SARS-CoV-2 Infection. *J. Virol.* **2021**, *95*, e00014-21. [CrossRef]
69. Kelleni, M.T. Early use of non-steroidal anti-inflammatory drugs in COVID-19 might reverse pathogenesis, prevent complications and improve clinical outcomes. *Biomed. Pharmacother.* **2021**, *133*, 110982. [CrossRef]
70. Oh, S.W.; Han, S.Y. Loop Diuretics in Clinical Practice. *Electrolytes Blood Press.* **2015**, *13*, 17–21. [CrossRef] [PubMed]
71. Podestà, M.A.; Valli, F.; Galassi, A.; Cassia, M.A.; Ciceri, P.; Barbieri, L.; Carugo, S.; Cozzolino, M. COVID-19 in Chronic Kidney Disease: The Impact of Old and Novel Cardiovascular Risk Factors. *Blood Purif.* **2021**, *50*, 740–749. [CrossRef]
72. Schöning, V.; Liakoni, E.; Baumgartner, C.; Exadaktylos, A.K.; Hautz, W.E.; Atkinson, A.; Hammann, F. Development and validation of a prognostic COVID-19 severity assessment (COSA) score and machine learning models for patient triage at a tertiary hospital. *J. Trans. Med.* **2021**, *19*, 56. [CrossRef]
73. Canal-Rivero, M.; Catalán-Barragán, R.; Rubio-García, A.; Garrido-Torres, N.; Crespo-Facorro, B.; Ruiz-Veguilla, M.; Group, I.T.P. Lower risk of SARS-CoV2 infection in individuals with severe mental disorders on antipsychotic treatment: A retrospective epidemiological study in a representative Spanish population. *Schizophr. Res.* **2021**, *229*, 53–54. [CrossRef] [PubMed]
74. Nemani, K.; Conderino, S.; Marx, J.; Thorpe, L.E.; Goff, D.C. Association Between Antipsychotic Use and COVID-19 Mortality Among People with Serious Mental Illness. *JAMA Psychiatry* **2021**, *78*, 1391–1393. [CrossRef] [PubMed]
75. Vai, B.; Mazza, M.G.; Delli Colli, C.; Foiselle, M.; Allen, B.; Benedetti, F.; Borsini, A.; Casanova Dias, M.; Tamouza, R.; Leboyer, M.; et al. Mental disorders and risk of COVID-19-related mortality, hospitalisation, and intensive care unit admission: A systematic review and meta-analysis. *Lancet Psychiatry* **2021**, *8*, 797–812. [CrossRef] [PubMed]
76. Boland, X.; Dratcu, L. Antipsychotics and COVID-19: The debate goes on. *Lancet Psychiatry* **2021**, *8*, 1030. [CrossRef]
77. Zippi, M.; Fiorino, S.; Budriesi, R.; Micucci, M.; Corazza, I.; Pica, R.; de Biase, D.; Gallo, C.G.; Hong, W. Paradoxical relationship between proton pump inhibitors and COVID-19: A systematic review and meta-analysis. *World J. Clin. Cases* **2021**, *9*, 2763–2777. [CrossRef]
78. Fatima, K.; Almas, T.; Lakhani, S.; Jahangir, A.; Ahmed, A.; Siddiqui, A.; Rahim, A.; Qureshi, S.A.; Arshad, Z.; Golani, S.; et al. The Use of Proton Pump Inhibitors and COVID-19: A Systematic Review and Meta-Analysis. *Trop. Med. Infect. Dis.* **2022**, *7*, 37. [CrossRef]
79. Toubasi, A.A.; AbuAnzeh, R.B.; Khraisat, B.R.; Al-Sayegh, T.N.; AlRyalat, S.A. Proton Pump Inhibitors: Current Use and the Risk of Coronavirus Infectious Disease 2019 Development and its Related Mortality. Meta-analysis. *Arch. Med. Res.* **2021**, *52*, 656–659. [CrossRef]
80. Pranata, R.; Huang, I.; Lawrensia, S.; Henrina, J.; Lim, M.A.; Lukito, A.A.; Kuswardhani, R.A.T.; Wibawa, I.D.N. Proton pump inhibitor on susceptibility to COVID-19 and its severity: A systematic review and meta-analysis. *Pharmacol. Rep.* **2021**, *73*, 1642–1649. [CrossRef]
81. Jackson, C.B.; Farzan, M.; Chen, B.; Choe, H. Mechanisms of SARS-CoV-2 entry into cells. *Nat. Rev. Mol. Cell Biol.* **2021**, *23*, 3–20. [CrossRef]
82. Peng, R.; Wu, L.-A.; Wang, Q.; Qi, J.; Gao, G.F. Cell entry by SARS-CoV-2. *Trends Biochem. Sci.* **2021**, *46*, 848–860. [CrossRef] [PubMed]

83. Trbojević-Akmačić, I.; Petrović, T.; Lauc, G. SARS-CoV-2 S glycoprotein binding to multiple host receptors enables cell entry and infection. *Glycoconj. J.* **2021**, *38*, 611–623. [CrossRef] [PubMed]
84. Pruimboom, L. SARS-CoV 2; Possible alternative virus receptors and pathophysiological determinants. *Med. Hypotheses* **2021**, *146*, 110368. [CrossRef] [PubMed]
85. Daly James, L.; Simonetti, B.; Klein, K.; Chen, K.-E.; Williamson Maia, K.; Antón-Plágaro, C.; Shoemark Deborah, K.; Simón-Gracia, L.; Bauer, M.; Hollandi, R.; et al. Neuropilin-1 is a host factor for SARS-CoV-2 infection. *Science* **2020**, *370*, 861–865. [CrossRef] [PubMed]
86. Cantuti-Castelvetri, L.; Ojha, R.; Pedro Liliana, D.; Djannatian, M.; Franz, J.; Kuivanen, S.; van der Meer, F.; Kallio, K.; Kaya, T.; Anastasina, M.; et al. Neuropilin-1 facilitates SARS-CoV-2 cell entry and infectivity. *Science* **2020**, *370*, 856–860. [CrossRef]
87. Gordon, D.E.; Jang, G.M.; Bouhaddou, M.; Xu, J.; Obernier, K.; White, K.M.; O'Meara, M.J.; Rezelj, V.V.; Guo, J.Z.; Swaney, D.L.; et al. A SARS-CoV-2 protein interaction map reveals targets for drug repurposing. *Nature* **2020**, *583*, 459–468. [CrossRef]
88. Terracciano, R.; Preianò, M.; Fregola, A.; Pelaia, C.; Montalcini, T.; Savino, R. Mapping the SARS-CoV-2–Host Protein–Protein Interactome by Affinity Purification Mass Spectrometry and Proximity-Dependent Biotin Labeling: A Rational and Straightforward Route to Discover Host-Directed Anti-SARS-CoV-2 Therapeutics. *Int. J. Mol. Sci.* **2021**, *22*, 532. [CrossRef]
89. Kruse, T.; Benz, C.; Garvanska, D.H.; Lindqvist, R.; Mihalic, F.; Coscia, F.; Inturi, R.; Sayadi, A.; Simonetti, L.; Nilsson, E.; et al. Large scale discovery of coronavirus-host factor protein interaction motifs reveals SARS-CoV-2 specific mechanisms and vulnerabilities. *Nat. Commun.* **2021**, *12*, 6761. [CrossRef] [PubMed]
90. Khorsand, B.; Savadi, A.; Naghibzadeh, M. SARS-CoV-2-human protein-protein interaction network. *Inform. Med. Unlocked* **2020**, *20*, 100413. [CrossRef] [PubMed]
91. Helenius, A. Virus Entry: Looking Back and Moving Forward. *J. Mol. Biol.* **2018**, *430*, 1853–1862. [CrossRef] [PubMed]
92. Choi Keum, S.; Aizaki, H.; Lai Michael, M.C. Murine Coronavirus Requires Lipid Rafts for Virus Entry and Cell-Cell Fusion but Not for Virus Release. *J. Virol.* **2005**, *79*, 9862–9871. [CrossRef]
93. Li, X.; Zhu, W.; Fan, M.; Zhang, J.; Peng, Y.; Huang, F.; Wang, N.; He, L.; Zhang, L.; Holmdahl, R.; et al. Dependence of SARS-CoV-2 infection on cholesterol-rich lipid raft and endosomal acidification. *Comput. Struct. Biotechnol. J.* **2021**, *19*, 1933–1943. [CrossRef]
94. Sorice, M.; Misasi, R.; Riitano, G.; Manganelli, V.; Martellucci, S.; Longo, A.; Garofalo, T.; Mattei, V. Targeting Lipid Rafts as a Strategy Against Coronavirus. *Front. Cell Dev. Biol.* **2021**, *8*, 618296. [CrossRef]
95. Tsuchiya, H.; Mizogami, M. Interaction of drugs with lipid raft membrane domains as a possible target. *Drug Target Insights* **2020**, *14*, 34–47. [CrossRef]
96. Packer, M. Do DPP-4 Inhibitors Cause Heart Failure Events by Promoting Adrenergically Mediated Cardiotoxicity? *Circ. Res.* **2018**, *122*, 928–932. [CrossRef] [PubMed]

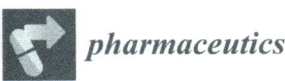

Systematic Review

Hidradenitis Suppurativa and Comorbid Disorder Biomarkers, Druggable Genes, New Drugs and Drug Repurposing—A Molecular Meta-Analysis

Viktor A. Zouboulis [1], Konstantin C. Zouboulis [2] and Christos C. Zouboulis [3,*]

1. Faculty of Medicine, Universitaetsklinikum Hamburg-Eppendorf (UKE), 20251 Hamburg, Germany; viktor.zouboulis@stud.uke.uni-hamburg.de
2. Department of Chemistry and Applied Biosciences, Swiss Federal Institute of Technology (ETH) Zurich, 8092 Zurich, Switzerland; zouboulk@ethz.ch
3. Departments of Dermatology, Venereology, Allergology and Immunology, Dessau Medical Center, Brandenburg Medical School Theodor Fontane and Faculty of Health Sciences Brandenburg, 06847 Dessau, Germany
* Correspondence: christos.zouboulis@mhb-fontane.de; Tel.: +49-340-5014000

Abstract: Chronic inflammation and dysregulated epithelial differentiation, especially of hair follicle keratinocytes, have been suggested as the major pathogenetic pathways of hidradenitis suppurativa/acne inversa (HS). On the other hand, obesity and metabolic syndrome have additionally been considered as an important risk factor. With adalimumab, a drug has already been approved and numerous other compounds are in advanced-stage clinical studies. A systematic review was conducted to detect and corroborate HS pathogenetic mechanisms at the molecular level and identify HS molecular markers. The obtained data were used to confirm studied and off-label administered drugs and to identify additional compounds for drug repurposing. A robust, strongly associated group of HS biomarkers was detected. The triad of HS pathogenesis, namely upregulated inflammation, altered epithelial differentiation and dysregulated metabolism/hormone signaling was confirmed, the molecular association of HS with certain comorbid disorders, such as inflammatory bowel disease, arthritis, type I diabetes mellitus and lipids/atherosclerosis/adipogenesis was verified and common biomarkers were identified. The molecular suitability of compounds in clinical studies was confirmed and 31 potential HS repurposing drugs, among them 10 drugs already launched for other disorders, were detected. This systematic review provides evidence for the importance of molecular studies to advance the knowledge regarding pathogenesis, future treatment and biomarker-supported clinical course follow-up in HS.

Keywords: hidradenitis suppurativa; acne inversa; transcriptome; proteome; comorbid disorder; biomarker; drug repurposing; signaling pathway; druggable gene

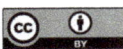

1. Introduction

Hidradenitis suppurativa/acne inversa (HS) is a chronic, inflammatory, recurrent, debilitating skin disease of the hair follicle that usually presents after puberty with painful, deep-seated, inflamed lesions in the apocrine gland-bearing areas of the body, most commonly at the axillae, inguinal and anogenital regions [1]. A consistent finding, regardless of disease duration, is follicular hyperkeratosis, leading to follicular rupture, inflammation and possible secondary bacterial colonization. The deep part of the follicle appears to be involved. HS is further associated with an initial lymphohistiocytic inflammation, granulomatous reaction, sinus tract formation and scarring [2].

Current own transcriptome and proteome studies highlighted a panel of immune-related drivers in HS, which induce an innate immunity response in epithelial skin cells in a targeted manner [3]. An inflammatory process coupled to impaired barrier function and bacterial activity were detected at the follicular and epidermal keratinocyte and at a minor grade at the skin-gland level. In addition, the adipose tissue was shown to be involved in HS at a real-world immune histochemical study [4].

Despite the beneficial therapeutic effectiveness of several compounds [5,6], treatment of HS is still challenging, since most patients only respond partially with subsequent recurrences. The large unmet need of new therapies requires the elucidation of disease-driving mechanisms and the recognition of the skin compartment initially involved [7,8]. This need can be covered by the development of novel therapeutic regimens for HS [9,10] or by drug repurposing through drug–gene interaction profiling [11,12].

New technology, including inverse virtual screening [13] and computational drug repurposing screening approaches [14], are widely engaged in identifying existing compounds as potential drugs for various diseases. The interaction level of disease and compound molecular profile patterns defines the probability of therapeutic activity of a certain drug. The aim of this study is to provide a wide and robust application of molecular pharmacology in HS through a systematic review of the relevant literature and identification of key molecular mediators in a real-world setting. Using the latter data, therapeutic agents that are currently available or under development for other indications are identified and potential paths for use in the medical management of HS are proposed.

2. Materials and Methods

2.1. Literature Search

This systematic review was conducted and narrated in accordance with the Preferred Reporting Items for Systematic Reviews and Meta-Analyses (PRISMA) [15] utilizing datasets from publicly available studies, as previously described [11]. A rigorous search of academic databases including PubMed, Web of Science and Ovid databases through August 2021 was conducted. A search strategy predefined and adapted for each aforementioned database included the following keywords: (transcriptome OR proteome OR biomarker(s) OR repurposing OR repositioning OR reprogramming) AND (hidradenitis suppurativa OR acne inversa OR Verneuil's disease). Additional records were obtained through the Gene Expression Omnibus, National Institutes of Health (Bethesda, MD, USA) [16] and the citation search of the bibliographic records obtained from the academic databases. There were no search filters pertaining to language or publication year.

2.2. Study Selection

First the duplicates among bibliographic records were removed. Titles and abstracts were then scrutinized by two reviewers (V.A.Z. and K.C.Z.) working independently according to predefined inclusion and exclusion criteria. This was followed by scrutiny of full texts of eligible studies. Discrepancies were resolved by discussion with the senior investigator (C.C.Z.). After eligible studies were identified, their bibliographies were screened for studies judged suitable for inclusion. Original investigations of HS molecular signatures and protein studies followed by the identification of molecular mediators were selected for further analysis.

2.3. Data Extraction

Data pertaining to characteristics of publications under study and quantitative data were extracted by two of the reviewers (V.A.Z. and K.C.Z.) working independently using a predetermined customized extraction form. Characteristics of publications included publication year and affiliation of corresponding authors. Molecular characteristics included transcriptome and/or proteome of HS, and drug repurposing/repositioning/reprogramming.

2.4. Data Analysis

Qualitative gene/protein data from the studies were pooled to detect HS signature pathways. Gene nomenclature was verified through the HUGO Gene Nomenclature Committee, European Bioinformatics Institute (Cambridge, UK) public domain [17]. Gene taxonomy was assessed through the biological DataBase network, National Cancer Institute (Frederick, MD, USA) [18]. The molecular pathways were assessed according to the g:Profiler, University of Tartu (Tartu, Estonia) [19], the Kyoto Encyclopedia of Genes and Genomes [KEGG, gene ontology (GO); Kyoto, Japan] [20], the Reactome (REAC), Ontario Institute for Cancer Research (Toronto, ON, Canada), New York University (New York, NY, USA), Oregon Health and Science University (Portland, OR, USA) and the European Molecular Biology Laboratory—European Bioinformatics Institute (Heidelberg, Germany) [21], the WikiPathways (WP) [22] and the Human Phenotype Ontology (HP; The Jackson Laboratory for Genomic Medicine, Farmington, CT, USA) [23] public domains. Random effects were applied throughout the analysis due to expected clinical heterogeneity encountered in different studies supported by g:Profiler [19]. This approach allows heterogeneity in the data to be addressed by considering that differences between studies are random.

2.5. Drug Repurposing Sources

For drug repurposing, the detected overall HS molecular signature was compared with the drugs' molecular signatures of The Drug Repurposing Hub public domain, Eli and Edy L. Broad Institute, MIT and Harvard University (Cambridge, MA, USA) [24] and the Gene Cards, Weizmann Institute of Science (Rehovot, Israel) [25] public domains.

2.6. Statistics

Statistics were automatically performed by the applied public domains used [19–23].

3. Results

3.1. Study Selection Process

A total of 123 bibliographic records were identified after electronic database searches, 36 through other sources and six through bibliographic record citation search. Among them, 61 records were removed as duplicates, leaving 104 titles and abstracts to be screened. After careful screening and manual search, six records were excluded based on title and abstract and 49 records due to inappropriate design and two records due to overlapping data sets with another record, resulting in 47 studies that were included in the quantitative synthesis [3,4,11,26–69] (Figure 1).

3.2. Differentially Expressed Genes and Proteins in HS

The comparison of lesional skin vs. non-lesional skin as well as of blood of patients vs. controls at the mRNA and protein levels (cumulatively reported as "targets") without restrictions revealed 386 differentially expressed genes (DEGs) in HS (Table S1).

3.3. HS Biomarkers

DEGs and differentially expressed proteins in blood and involved skin of HS patients in comparison to controls in at least two relevant articles or two targets were defined as HS biomarkers. Among the 109 detected genes/proteins out of the 386 genes/proteins detected without restrictions, which fulfilled this requirement, 43 DEGs (including the coding genes of detected differentially expressed proteins) have been described in 2/4 targets in two articles, seven in 3/4 targets (*CXCL10, IL6, IL17A, IL36A, IL36G, S100A8, S100A9*) and none in all four targets (Table 1). Additional 10 DEGs have been described in 2/4 targets, however, in a diversified direction (upregulated/downregulated). Among the 109 HS biomarkers, 65 are druggable.

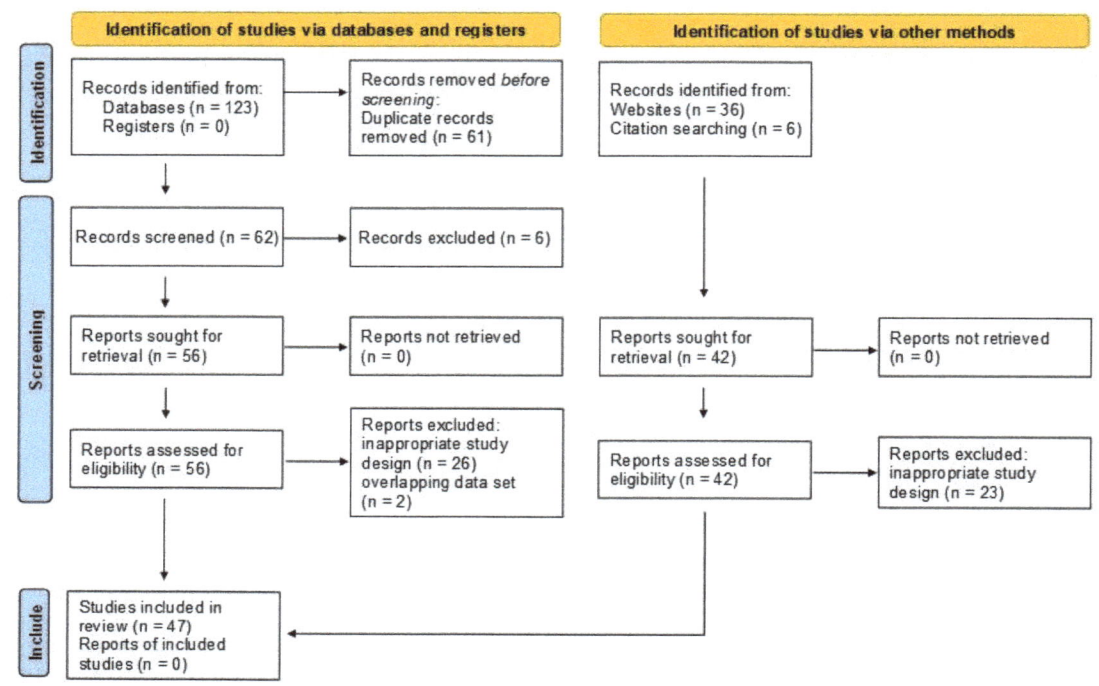

Figure 1. Preferred reporting items for systematic reviews and meta-analyses (PRISMA 2020 [15]) flow diagram.

Table 1. HS biomarkers resulting from the DEGs after transcriptomic profiling and protein expression studies between lesional HS and non-lesional skin biopsies and blood samples from HS patients and healthy controls, respectively and reported in at least two relevant articles. Bold letters indicate druggable genes. Background: white = similar results reported in one target (biological material) in at least two independent studies; orange = similar results reported in two targets in at least two independent studies; yellow = similar results reported in three targets in at least two independent studies. Gray = diversified result reported in at least two independent studies; + = upregulation; − = downregulation; +/− = diversified dysregulation in different studies; () = lower level of evidence.

Gene	Blood			Skin			Name	Other Skin Disorders	HS Comorbid Disorders	Drugs
	+/−	mRNA	Protein	+/−	mRNA	Protein				
ADAM12				+	[3,27]		ADAM Metal-lopeptidase Domain 12		Down syndrome	
ADIPOQ	−		[28]	−	[27]		Adiponectin		Glucose intolerance, metabolic syndrome	Piogitazone
AR				+	[3,33,34]	[35]	Androgen receptor	Polycystic ovary syndrome, alopecia	Androgen insensitivity syndrome	Cyproterone acetate, Flutamide, Nilutamide, Bicalutamide, 17α-Propionate, AZD3514
BTK				+/(−)	[3,27,33,34]		Betacellulin	Squamous cell carcinoma		Cetuximab
C3	−		[27]	+	[30]		Complement C3			Zinc, Zinc acetate

Table 1. Cont.

Gene	Blood +/−	Blood mRNA	Blood Protein	Skin +/−	Skin mRNA	Skin Protein	Name	Other Skin Disorders	HS Comorbid Disorders	Drugs
C5AR1				+	[3,30]		Complement C5a Receptor 1	Hypersensitivity reaction type III disease		Compstatin, PMX 205, PMX 53, W 54011
CASP1				+		[38,39]	Caspase 1	Schnitzler syndrome	Familial Mediterranean fever	Minocyclin
CCL18				+	[27,30]	[43]	C-C Motif Chemokine Ligand 18	Eczema		
CCL26	+		[41]	+	[30]		C-C Motif Chemokine Ligand 26			
CCR4	+	[45]		+	[30,45]		C-C Motif Chemokine Receptor 4	Mycosis fungoides, cutaneous T cell lymphoma, allergic contact dermatitis		
CD80				+	[30,38]		CD80 Molecule			Abatacept, Belatacept
CHI3L1	+		[49]	+		[50]	Chitinase 3-Like 1	Erysipelas		
CSF1				+	[3,33,34,40]		Colony-Stimulating Factor 1		Rheumatoid arthritis	
CXCL1				+	[27,40,42,44,45]	[40]	C-X-C Motif Chemokine Ligand 1	Kaposi sarcoma		Formic acid
CXCL8				+	[30,42,44]	[41]	C-X-C Motif Chemokine Ligand 8	Melanoma		Simvastatin
CXCL10	−		[41]	+	[30]	[41]	C-X-C Motif Chemokine Ligand 10			Eldelumab
CXCL13				+	[30,42,45]	[26]	C-X-C Motif Chemokine Ligand 13	T cell lymphoma		
CXCR5				+	[30]	[26]	C-X-C Motif Chemokine Receptor 5	T cell lymphoma		
DCD				−	[27,32,33]	[32]	Dermcidin	Netherton syndrome, tinea pedis		Basiliximab, Zinc sulfate
DEFB4A				+/(−)	[3,27,30,32,39,44–46]	[3,53]	Defensin β 4A	Tinea corporis, oral candidiasis		
DEFB103B				+	[46,52]		Defensin β 103B			
EGF				+	[3,33,34]		Epidermal Growth Factor			Cetuximab, AG 490, CGP 52411, Genistein, Zanubrutinib (receptor antagonist)
EPGN				+	[3,33,34]		Epithelial Mitogen	Seborrheic dermatitis		
ERBB4				−	[27,32]		Erb-B2 Receptor Tyrosine Kinase 4			Gefitinib, Afatinib, Fostamatinib, AG 490, CGP 52411, Genistein
EREG				+	[3,33,34]		Epiregulin			
GAS6				+/(−)	[3,33,34]		Growth Arrest Specific 6	Lupus erythematosus		
GDNF				+	[3,33,34]	[36]	Glial Cell Derived Neurotrophic Factor			Chondroitin sulphate
GJB2				+	[3]	[3]	Gap Junction Protein β2	Keratitis-Ichthyosis-Deafness Syndrome		Carbenoxolone disodium

Table 1. *Cont.*

Gene	Blood +/−	mRNA	Protein	+/−	Skin mRNA	Protein	Name	Other Skin Disorders	HS Comorbid Disorders	Drugs
HBEGF				+	[3,33,34]		Heparin Binding EGF-Like Growth Factor			
HGF				+	[3,33,34]		Hepatocyte Growth Factor			Dexamethasone, Neratinib, Erlotinib
HRG				+	[3,33,34]		Histidine-Rich Glycoprotein			Zinc sulfate
IFNA1				+	[3,26,30,33,34]		Interferon α1	Cryoblobulinemia		
IFNG				+	[3,26,30,33,34,40, 44–46]		Interferon γ			Oksalazine, Emapalumab, Glucosamine
IGF2				+	[3,33,34]		Insulin-Like Growth Factor 2			
IGHD				+	[27,30]		Immunoglobulin Heavy Constant δ			
IGHG3				+	[27,30]		Immunoglobulin Heavy Constant γ3 (G3m Marker)			
IGKV1D-13				+	[27,30]		Immunoglobulin κ Variable 1D-13			
IGLV				+	[27,30]		Immunoglobulin λ Variable Cluster			
IL1A				+	[3,26,30,33,34,40]	[39]	Interleukin 1α	Acne, Irritant dermatitis	Arthritis	Anakinra, Rinolacept, Olanzapine, Pirfenidone, Thalidomide, AMG-108
IL1B				+	[26,30,38,40,42,46]	[38,56]	Interleukin 1β	Gingivitis, Muckle–Wells syndrome, Toxic shock syndrome		Canakizumab, Anakinra (receptor antagonist), Rinolacept (receptor antagonist), Minocycline
IL2				+	[26,30]		Interleukin 2	Graft-versus-host disease, Leprosy		Suplatast tosylate, Daclizumab (receptor antagonist), Basiliximab (receptor antagonist), Rituxomab, Thalidomide, Cafazolin
IL2RA	+		[49,56]	+	[30]		Interleukin 2 Receptor Subunit α		Type 1 diabetes mellitus, Juvenile arthritis	Daclizumab, Basiliximab, Pirfenidone, Thalidomide
IL4				+	[3,30,33,34,40]		Interleukin 4	Atopy, Allergic rhinitis, Food allergy		Dupilumab (receptor antagonist), Calcitriol
IL6	+		[40]	+	[3,26,30,33,34,40, 42]	[40,58]	Interleukin 6			Siltuximab, Tocilizumab (receptor antagonist), Sarilumab (receptor antagonist), Satralizumab (receptor antagonist), Vitamin C, Vitamin E

Table 1. Cont.

Gene	Blood			Skin			Other Skin Disorders	HS Comorbid Disorders	Drugs
	+/−	mRNA	Protein	+/−	mRNA	Protein	Name		
IL10				+	[30,38,44,46]	[52,56]	Interleukin 10			Nicotinamide, Niacin, Cyclosporine A, Methotrexate, Mycofenolate mofetil
IL12A				+	[59]	[41]	Interleukin 12A	Adamantiades–Behçet's disease	Primary biliary cholangiitis	Mycophenolate mofetil, Ustekinumab (IL-12/23), Briakinumab (IL-12/23)
IL12B				+	[30]	[36]	Interleukin 12B	Psoriasis		Ustekinumab (IL-12/23), Briakinumab (IL-12/23)
IL13				+/(−)	[3,30,45]		Interleukin 13	Allergic rhinitis, Penicillin allergy		Suplatast tosylate, Montelukast, Omalizumab
IL16				+	[30]	[41]	Interleukin 16		Allergic asthma	
IL17A	+		[59]	+	[3,30,33,34,38–40,42,44,46,60]	[4,36,38,39,41]	Interleukin 17A	Allergic contact dermatitis	Arthritis	Secukizumab, Ixekizumab, Bimekizumab (IL-17A/F), Brodalumab (receptor antagonist), Vidofludimus
IL17F				+	[30,39,40,42,45]		Interleukin 17F	Candidiasis, Acute generalized exanthematous pustulosis, Mail diseases		Bimekizumab (IL-17A/F), Brodaluman (receptor antagonist)
IL17R				+	[3]	[4]	Interleukin 17 Receptor	Candidiasis	Arthritis	Brodalumab
IL18				+/−	[26,30]	[38]	Interleukin 18			IAP antagonist, Iboctadekin + Doxil
IL19				+	[3,30,40]		Interleukin 19	Psoriasis	Inflammatory bowel disease, Arthritis	
IL20				+/−	[30,46]	[46]	Interleukin 20	Psoriasis		
IL21				+	[30,39]		Interleukin 21		Dacryoadenitis, Inflammatory boel disease	
IL22				+/(−)	[3,30,40,42,46]	[46]	Interleukin 22	Candidiasis	Inflammatory bowel disease	
IL22RA1				−	[30]	[46]	Interleukin 22 Receptor Subunit α1		Spondyloarthropathy, rheumatoid arthritis, autoimmune uveitis	
IL23A				+	[30,40,61]		Interleukin 23 Subunit α	Autoimmune disease	Inflammatory bowel disease, Arthritis	Guselkumab, Risankinumab, Tildrakizumab, Ustekinumab (IL-12/23), Briakinumab (IL-12/23)
IL24				+	[30,42,46]		Interleukin 24	Melanoma, chronic spontaneous urticaria, psoriasis	Spondylarthropathy	
IL26				+	[42,46]		Interleukin 26	Psoriasis	Inflammatory bowel disease, Crohn's disease	
IL32				+	[30,40,61]		Interleukin 32	Cutaneous diphtheria		

Table 1. Cont.

Gene	Blood +/−	Blood mRNA	Blood Protein	Skin +/−	Skin mRNA	Skin Protein	Name	Other Skin Disorders	HS Comorbid Disorders	Drugs
IL36A	+		[62]	+	[30,40,42,45,61]	[39,61]	Interleukin 36α	Psoriasis		Spesolimab (receptor antagonist)
IL36B	+		[62]	+		[61]	Interleukin 36β		Periostitis	Spesolimab (receptor antagonist)
IL36G	+		[62]	+	[30,40,42,45]	[61]	Interleukin 36γ	Acute generalized exanthematous pustulosis, Psoriasis		Spesolimab (receptor antagonist)
IL37				−	[32,33,42]		Interleukin 37	Still's disease	Inflammatory bowel disease	Ustekinumab (IL-12/23)
JAK3				+	[3,30]		Janus Kinase 3		NK cell enteropathy	Decernatinib, Tofacitinib (JAK1/3), Ruxolitinib (JAK1/3), PF-06651600, AT-501, ATI-502, Cerdulatinib (JAK1/2/3, SYK), Delgocitinib (JAK1/2/3), Peficitinib (JAK1/2/3), Zanubrutinib (JAK3/ITR/EGFR), Cercosporamide JAK3/Mnk2)
KRT6A				+	[3,32]	[3]	Keratin 6A	Pachyonychia congenita, Lingua plicata, Cheilitis		Zinc, Zinc acetate
KRT16				+	[3,27,30,32]	[3]	Keratin 16	Pachyonychia congenita, palmoplantar keratoderma		
KRT77				−	[27,32,33]	[32]	Keratin 77	Epidermolytic palmoplantar keratoderma, Buschke-Ollendorff syndrome		
LCE3D				+	[32]	[32]	Late Cornified Envelope 3D	Psoriasis		
LGR5				−	[27,32]		Leucine Rich Repeat Containing G Protein-Coupled Receptor 5		Type II diabetes mellitus	
LTA4H	−		[27,65]	+	[31]		Leukotriene A4 Hydrolase			Captopril, Dexamethasone, Montelukast
MMP1				+	[3,30]	[3]	Matrix Metallopeptidase 1	Epidermolysis bullosa atrophica, Scleroderma		Zinc, Collagenase
MMP3				+	[40]	[40]	Matrix Metallopeptidase 3		Coronary heart disease, Arthritis	Pravastatin, Simvastatin, Prothalidone, Lisinopril
MMP9				+	[3,30,40]	[3]	Matrix Metallopeptidase 9			Minocycline, Caprovil, Simvastatin, Zinc, Zinc acetate
MMP12				+	[27,30]		Matrix Metallopeptidase 12	Dermatitis herpetiformis, Middermal elastolysis	Arthritis	Acetohydroxamic acid, Batimastat

Table 1. Cont.

Gene	Blood +/−	Blood mRNA	Blood Protein	Skin +/−	Skin mRNA	Skin Protein	Name	Other Skin Disorders	HS Comorbid Disorders	Drugs
NAMPT	+		[28,63]				Nicotinamide Phosphoribosyl transferase	Skin aging, pellagra, diabetes mellitus type 2, polycystic ovary syndrome		Nicotinamide, Niacin
NGF				+	[3,33,34]	[36]	Nerve Growth Factor			Clenbuterol
OSM				+	[3,26]	[36]	Oncostatin M	Kaposi sarcoma		
PI3				+	[3,27,32,33]	[3]	Peptidase Inhibitor 3	Pustular psoriasis, impetigo herpetiformis, erysipelas		
PIP				−	[27,32]		Prolactin Induced Protein			
PLIN1				+/−	[27,48]		Perilipin 1			Rosiglitazone
S100A7				+	[3,30,33,39,42,44,46]	[32]	S100 Calcium-Binding Protein A7	Psoriasis, Squamous cell carcinoma	Anal fistula	Ibuprofen, Dexibuprofen, Zinc, Zinc acetate, Zinc chloride
S100A7A				+	[3,27,32]	[3,32]	S100 Calcium-Binding Protein A7A	Psoriasis		
S100A8	+		[57]	+	[3,33,34,44]	[3,32]	S100 Calcium-Binding Protein A8			Zinc, Zinc acetate, Zinc chloride, Copper
S100A9	+		[57]	+	[3,27,32,33,42,44,46]	[3,32]	S100 Calcium-Binding Protein A9		Crohn's disease, Rheumatoid arthritis	Zinc, Zinc acetate, Zinc chloride, Calcium
S100A12				+	[3,30,32,42]	[3,41]	S100 Calcium-Binding Protein A12	Kawasaki disease	Psoriatic arthritis	Amlexanox, Olopatadine
SCGB1D2				−	[27,32]		Secretoglobin Family 1D Member 2			
SCGB2A2				−	[27,32,33]		Secretoglobin Family 2A Member 2			
SERPINB3				+	[3,27,30]	[3]	Serpin Family B Member 3	Squamous cell caecinoma		Phosphoserine
SERPINB4				+	[3,27,30]	[3]	Serpin Family B Member 4	Squamous cell carcinoma		
SLAMF7				+	[3,27]		SLAM Family Member 7	IgG4-related disease		Elotuzumab
SPRR2B				+	[32]	[32]	Small Proline Rich Protein 2B	Photosensitive trichothiodystrophy 1, Autosomal recessive congenital ichthyosis		
SPRR2C (pseudogene)				+	[32]	[32]	Small Proline Rich Protein 2C (Pseudogene)			
SPRR3				+	[3]	[3]	Small Proline Rich Protein 3	Genodermatoses		
STAT1				+	[3,26,30,44]	[36]	Signal Transducer and Activator of Transcription 1			Methimazole, Niclosamide, Nifuroxazide, Sulforaphane
TCN1				+	[3,27,45]	[3]	Transcobalamin 1			Hydroxycobalamin, Cyanocobalamin, Cobalt
TLR2				+	[3,68]		Toll-Like Receptor 2	Leprosy, Borreliosis	Colorectal cancer	Adapalene, Cyproterone acetate

Table 1. Cont.

Gene	Blood +/−	Blood mRNA	Blood Protein	Skin +/−	Skin mRNA	Skin Protein	Name	Other Skin Disorders	HS Comorbid Disorders	Drugs
TLR4				+/−	[26]	[53]	Toll-like Receptor 4			Paclitaxel, Tacrolimus, Cyclobenzaprine
TMPRSS1D				+	[3]	[3]	Transmembrane Serine Protease 11D			
TNF				+	[3,26,30,32,33,38,40]	[56]	Tumor Necrosis Factor	Psoriasis, Toxic shock syndrome	Inflammatory bowel diseases, Arthritis	Adalimumab, Infliximab, Golimumab, Etanercept (receptor antagonist), Certolizumab pegol, Thalidomide, Lenalidomide, Pomalidomide, Calcitriol, Bay 11-7821, (R)-DOI, Cannabidiol
TNFRSF4	+	[45]		+	[45]		TNF Receptor Superfamily Member 4	Kaposi sarcoma, Graft-versus-host disease, Drug reaction with eosinophilia		OX-40 ligand
TNFSF11				+	[30]	[36]	TNF Superfamily Member 11			Letrozole, Thiocolchicoside
TNFSF13 (APRIL)				+	[30]	[26]	TNF Superfamily Member 13	Autoimmune diseases	Rheumatoid arthritis	Pomalidomide, TACI-IG
TNFSF13B (BAFF)				+	[30]	[26]	TNF Superfamily Member 13b	Autoimmune diseases, Sialadenitis, Sjogren syndrome		Belimumab, Blisibimod, LY2127399, TACI-IG
TNFSF14				+	[30]	[36]	TNF Superfamily Member 14	Herpes simplex	Rheumatoid arthritis	
TNIP1				+/−	[26,30]		TNFAIP3 Interacting Protein 1	Systemic lupus erythematosus, Psoriatic arthritis	Rheumatoid arthritis, Arthritis	
WIF1				−	[27,32]		WNT Inhibitory Factor 1			

3.4. Enrichment Analysis of HS-Associated Genes

The 386 detected HS-associated DEGs and the 109 HS biomarkers were enriched into relevant signaling pathways, which were assessed according to the g:Profiler [19], the KEGG GO, [20], the REAC [21], the WP [22] and the HP [23] public domains in order to identify the major organismal and signal transduction pathways involved in HS. Gene clustering in chromosome 2 and 4 was detected.

Among the 386 HS-associated DEGs, 101 genes were enriched in the cytokine–cytokine (C–C) receptor interaction pathway ($-\log_{10} = 2.5 \times 10^{-74}$), 51 in the JAK-STAT signaling pathway (2.6×10^{-34}), 39 in the chemokine signaling pathway (2.7×10^{-18}), 32 in the IL-17 signaling pathway (1.8×10^{-22}), 31 in the Th17 cell differentiation pathway (2.6×10^{-18}), 28 in the Toll-like receptor (TLR) pathway (2.2×10^{-16}) and 26 in the inflammatory bowel disease pathway (3.6×10^{-26}) (Figure S1).

Furthermore, 45 HS biomarkers were enriched in the C–C receptor interaction pathway (5.6×10^{-43}, Figure 2, 19 in the IL-17 signaling pathway (8.8×10^{-19}, Figure 3), 19 in the JAK-STAT signaling pathway (6.0×10^{-14}, Figure 4), 18 in the inflammatory bowel disease pathway (1.1×10^{-20}), 18 in the rheumatoid arthritis pathway (1.2×10^{-17}), 13 in the Th17 cell differentiation pathway (1.5×10^{-9}), 13 in the lipid and atherosclerosis pathway (1.2×10^{-5}), 10 in the TLR pathway (4.3×10^{-6}), 9 in C-type leptin receptor signaling pathway (6.1×10^{-5}), 8 in the tumor necrosis factor (TNF) signaling pathway (1.1×10^{-3}) and 7 in the type I diabetes mellitus pathway (8.5×10^{-6}) (Figure 5).

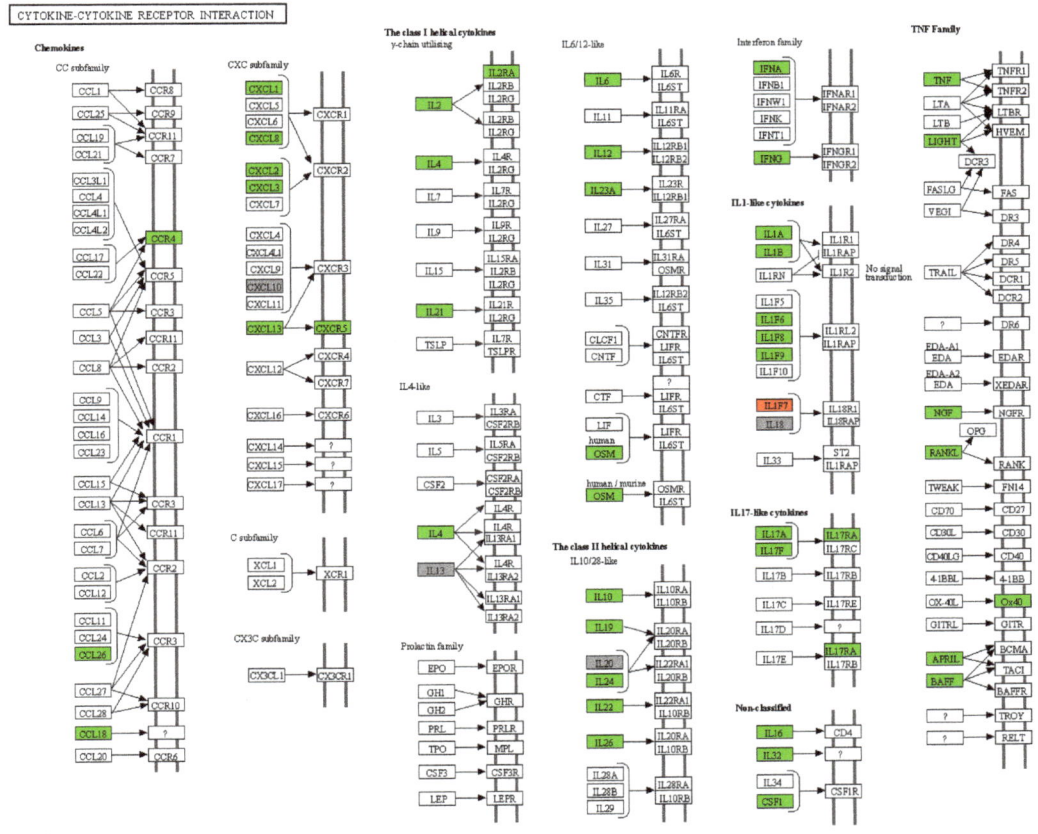

Figure 2. Hierarchical clustering of HS biomarkers in the KEGG GO C-C receptor interaction pathway. Genes which are positively regulated in HS are shown in green color, those downregulated with red color. Gray color corresponds to genes with a diversified reported regulation.

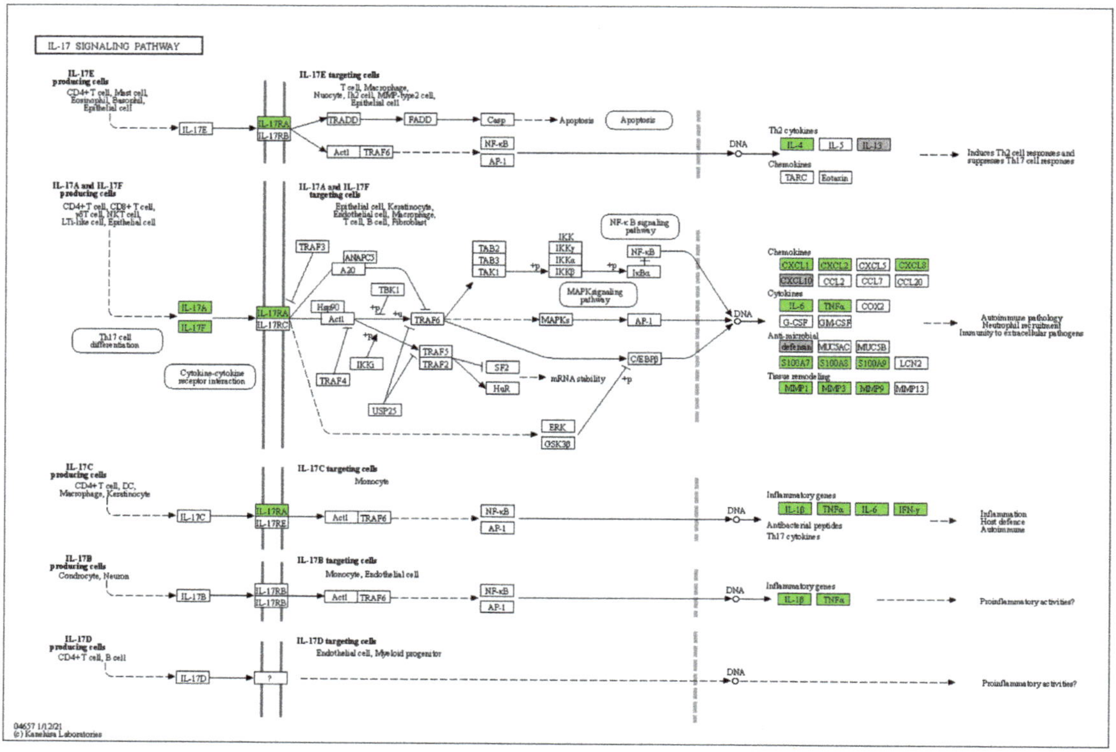

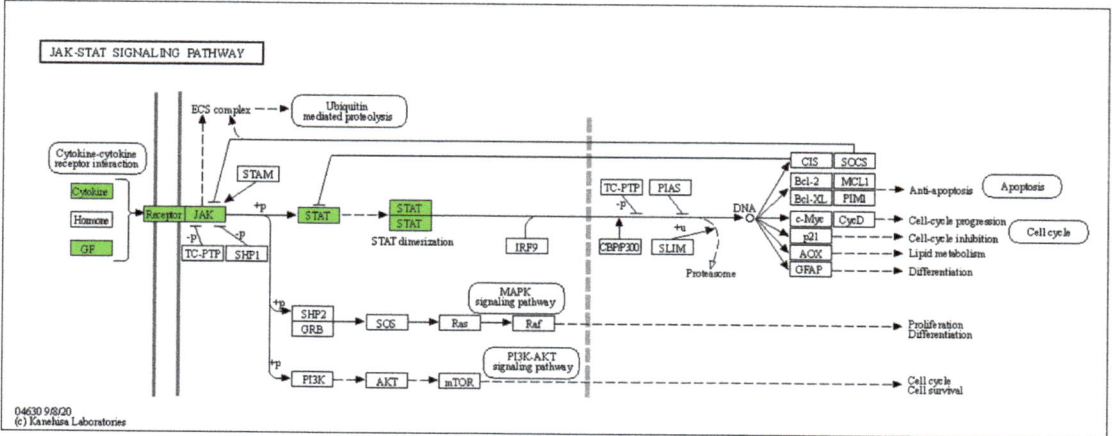

Figure 3. Hierarchical clustering of HS biomarkers in the KEGG GO IL-17 signaling pathway. Genes which are positively regulated in HS are shown in green color. Gray color corresponds to genes with a diversified reported regulation.

Figure 4. Hierarchical clustering of HS biomarkers in the KEGG GO JAK-STAT signaling pathway. Genes which are positively regulated in HS are shown in green color. Gray color corresponds to genes with a diversified reported regulation.

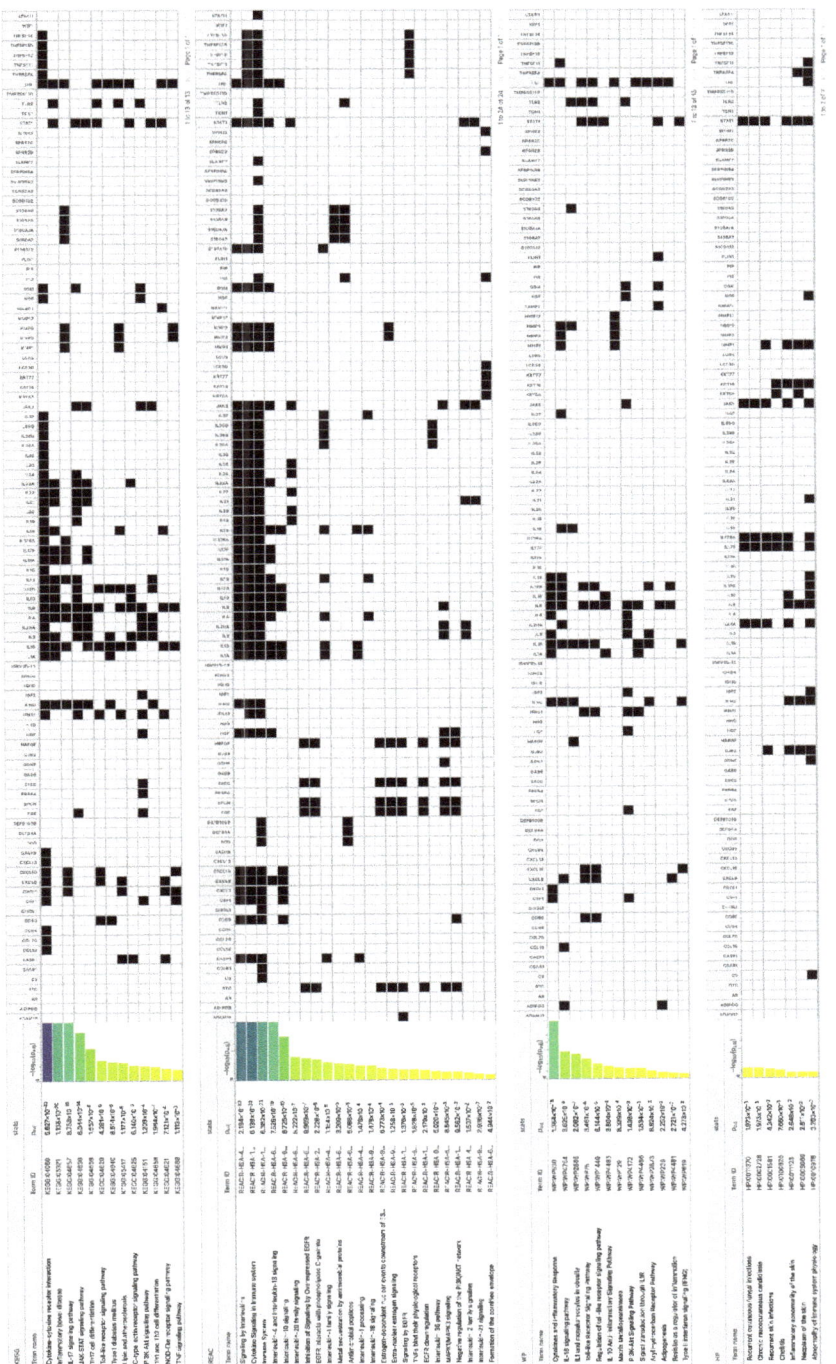

Figure 5. Enrichment of HS biomarkers resulting from the comparison of transcriptomic profiles and protein expression studies between lesional HS and non-lesional skin biopsies and blood samples from HS patients and healthy controls, respectively, in signaling pathways.

Concerning the individual cytokine signaling, IL-17, IL-4, IL-13, IL-10, IL-20 family, IL-1 family, IL-18, IL-36, IL-2 family, IL-21 and IL-12 family signaling included DEGs in HS (Figure 5).

Epithelial differentiation signaling dysregulation in HS was represented by the epidermal growth factor receptor (EGFR), IL-1, IL-1 receptor, formation of the cornified envelope, TLRs and antimicrobial peptides (Figure 5).

Metabolic/obesity-associated dysregulation in HS was detected through type I diabetes mellitus signaling, lipid and atherosclerosis, C-type leptin receptor signaling, estrogen-dependent nuclear events and extranuclear signaling, adipogenesis and resistin signaling (Figure 5).

Interestingly, infection-indicating signaling pathways did not exhibit any major involvement in our study (Figure 5).

At last, the REAC evaluation of globally involved pathways [70] revealed the innate immune system, the cytokine signaling in immune system (major pathways: regulation of *IFNG* signaling), signal transduction (nuclear receptor, *GPCR* and leptin pathways) and developmental biology (formation of the cornified envelope pathway) pathways as the mainly HS-associated ones (Figure S2).

The protein-based connectivity map occurring from an assumed gene biomarker translation (103 proteins our of 109 genes) resulted in 2465 interactions compared with the expected 531 interactions (4.64-fold; $p < 0.0001$), a result that indicates a robust strong protein–protein association in HS (Figure 6). On the other hand, the protein-based connectivity map occurring from the 386 HS-associated DEGs (372 proteins out of 386 genes) resulted in 19,823 interactions compared with the expected 6502 interactions (3.05-fold; $p < 0.0001$), indicating that the biomarker selection procedure increased the HS/protein association.

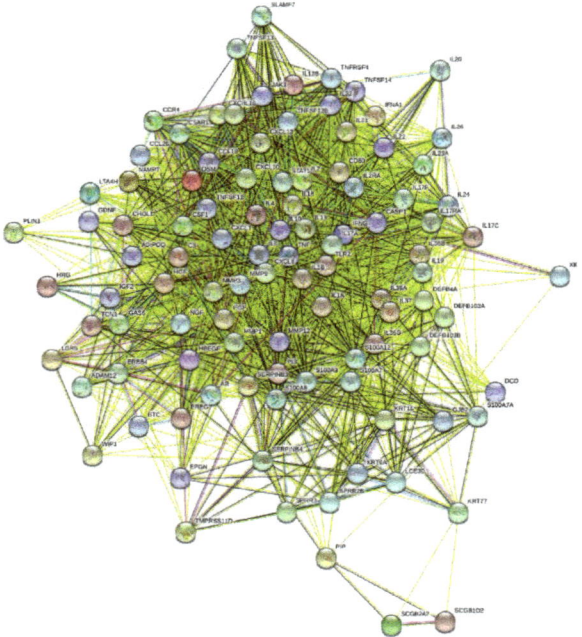

Figure 6. Biomarker-resulting protein-based connectivity map of HS.

3.5. Enrichment Analysis of HS Druggable Genes

Among the 386 HS-associated DEGs, 105 druggable genes were recognized. With the 11 additional druggable genes described by Zouboulis et al. [12], namely *ABAT, ADRA1A, CYP3A4, GRM4, HRH1, OPRD1, OPRM, PRKAB1, PTGS1, PTGS2* and *SLC6A4*, the overall detected druggable genes in HS are 116.

The 116 druggable genes were enriched in relevant signaling pathways according to the KEGG GO [20] and the Gene Cards [25] public domains to identify the major targeted organismal and signal transduction pathways (Figure S3). Twenty-two druggable genes were enriched in the lipid and atherosclerosis pathway (8.4×10^{-13}), 19 in the JAK-STAT signaling pathway (6.2×10^{-12}), 17 in the Th17 cell differentiation pathway (5.2×10^{-13}), 17 in the IL-17 signaling pathway (6.0×10^{-14}), 16 in the inflammatory bowel disease pathway (1.5×10^{-16}), 14 in the TLR signaling pathway (6.0×10^{-14}), 14 in the C-type leptin receptor signaling pathway (2.4×10^{-9}) and 13 in the TNF signaling pathway (8.4×10^{-8}).

3.6. Study Drugs and Drug Repurposing for HS

The majority of registered, studied or off-label administered drugs modify HS-associated DEGs. On the other hand, the evaluation of the detected 105 HS-associated druggable genes proposed 452 potentially therapeutic compounds, among them 120 launched drugs, 178 compounds in clinical studies and 154 in preclinical evaluation (Table S2). Among these potentially therapeutic compounds, the 31 drugs, which regulate three or more genes with all of them being HS-associated DEGs or at least four genes with 60% of them been DEGs were classified as probable repurposing drugs for HS (Table 2).

Table 2. Probable HS repurposing drugs * and molecular profile of drugs registered ** or off-label administered in HS.

Compound	Function	Gene Regulation	Development Phase
Probable repurposing HS drugs			
3,3′-Diindolylmethane	CHK inhibitor, cytochrome P450 activator, indoleamine 2,3-dioxygenase inhibitor	AR, HIF1A, **IFNG**, PI3	3
AG-490	EGFR inhibitor, JAK inhibitor	**EGFR, JAK2, JAK3**	preclinical
Andrographolide	tumor necrosis factor production inhibitor	**IL1B, IL6, NFKB1**, NFKB2, **TNF**	2
Apratastat	matrix metalloprotease inhibitor, tumor necrosis factor production inhibitor	ADAM17, **MMP1, MMP13, MMP9**	2
Atractylenolide-I	JAK inhibitor	**JAK1, JAK2, JAK3**	preclinical
AZD1480	JAK inhibitor	**JAK1, JAK2, JAK3**	1
Balsalazide	cyclooxygenase inhibitor	ALOX5, PPARG, **PTGS1, PTGS2**	launched
BMS-911543	JAK inhibitor	**JAK1, JAK2, JAK3**	1/2
Ciglitazone	PPARγ agonist	GPD1, PPARG, TBXA2R	2
Curcumol	JAK inhibitor	**JAK1, JAK2, JAK3**	1
Cyt387	JAK inhibitor	**JAK1, JAK2, JAK3**	3
Delgocitinib	JAK inhibitor	**JAK1, JAK2, JAK3**	2
Fedratinib	FLT3 inhibitor, JAK inhibitor	BRD4, **JAK1, JAK2, JAK3**, TYK2	launched
Filgotinib	JAK inhibitor	**JAK1, JAK2, JAK3**, TYK2	3
Ganoderic-acid-a	JAK inhibitor	**JAK1, JAK2, JAK3**	preclinical
JTE-607	cytokine production inhibitor	IL10, **IL1B, IL6, TNF**	2
Compound	Function	Gene Regulation	Development Phase
Latamoxef	Cephalosporine	DACB, MRCA, MRCB, PBPC	launched
LXR-623	Liver X receptor agonist	AR, NR1H2, NR1H3, NR1I2, NR3C1	1
NS-018	JAK inhibitor	**JAK1, JAK2, JAK3**, TYK2	1/2
Pacritinib	FLT3 inhibitor, JAK inhibitor	FLT3, **JAK1, JAK2, JAK3**	3
Paracetamol	cyclooxygenase inhibitor	FAAH, **PTGS1, PTGS2**, TRPV1	launched

Table 2. Cont.

Peficitinib	JAK inhibitor	**JAK1, JAK2, JAK3**	launched
PF-06651600	JAK inhibitor	**JAK1, JAK2, JAK3**	2/3
Plerixafor	CC chemokine receptor antagonist	ACKR3, **CCR4**, CXCR4, **MMP1, PI3**	launched
Ruxolitinib	JAK inhibitor	**JAK1, JAK2, JAK3**, TYK2	launched
Sirolimus	mTOR inhibitor	**CFD1, FKBP1A, GPD1, MMP1, MTOR, PI3, RPL38**	launched
Tofacitinib	JAK inhibitor	**JAK1, JAK2, JAK3**	launched
Trofinetide	cytokine production inhibitor	IFNG, IL6, TNFA	2
Upadacitinib	JAK inhibitor	**JAK1, JAK2, JAK3**	launched
WHI-P154	JAK inhibitor	EGFR, **JAK1, JAK2, JAK3**	preclinical
XL019	JAK inhibitor	**JAK1, JAK2, JAK3**	1
*Drugs with known molecular profile registered ** or off-label administered in HS*			
Acitretin	retinoid receptor agonist	**KRT16, PI3**, RARA, RARB, RARG, RBP1, RXRA, RXRB, RXRG, **STAT3**	launched
Adalimumab **	TNF-α inhibitor	TNF	launched
Anakinra	IL-1 receptor antagonist	IL1R1	launched
Avacopan	C5α receptor antagonist	C5AR1	2
Bimekizumab	IL-17A/F inhibitor	IL17A, IL17F	3
Brodalumab	IL-17 receptor inhibitor	IL17R, KRT6A, S100A7A, S100A8, S100A9	launched
Clindamycin	Protein synthesis inhibitor		launched
Cyproterone acetate	AR antagonist	ADORA1, **AR**	launched
Doxycycline	bacterial 30S ribosomal subunit inhibitor, metalloproteinase inhibitor	**MMP1, MMP8, PI3**	launched
Etanercept	TNF-α receptor antagonist	TNFRSF1A	launched
Golimumab	TNF inhibitor	TNF	launched
INCB 54707	JAK1 inhibitor	JAK1	2
Infliximab	TNF inhibitor	IL6, TNF	launched
Metformin	insulin sensitizer	ACACB, PRKAB1	launched
Rifampicin	RNA polymerase inhibitor	NR1I2, SLCO1A2, SLCO1B1, SLCO1B3	launched
Secukinumab	IL-17A inhibitor	IL17A	3
Spesolimab	IL-36R antagonist	IL36RN	2
Ustekinumab	IL12/IL23 inhibitor	FSH, HCG, LH, LTA4H	Launched
Vilobelimab	C5α inhibitor	C5	2

* The differentially regulated genes in HS are presented with bold letters.

4. Discussion

4.1. HS Pathogenesis

Inflammation doubtlessly plays a major role in the pathogenesis of HS [3,7,8]. Proteome studies provide evidence that the innate immunity system and both *IL-1* and *IL-17* signaling pathways are activated in HS lesions and circulating neutrophils [27,40,45,71–73], findings that have been confirmed in our systematic review. In addition, Th17 differentiation of CD4+ lymphocytes is activated in HS [57]. Among others, Kelly et al. [38] provided evidence that CD45+CD4+ T cells are responsible for IL-17 production and CD11c+CD1a-CD14+ dendritic cells are the main producers of IL-1β in lesional HS skin. The IL-17 cytokine family has been linked to the pathogenesis of diverse autoimmune and inflammatory diseases and also plays an essential role in host defense against extracellular microorganisms [2,74]. IL-17 has been shown to increase the expression of skin antimicrobial peptides, including human β-defensin 2, psoriasin (S100A7) and calprotectin (S100A8/9) in keratinocytes and of a number of cytokines attracting neutrophils [75]. Thus, IL-17 may contribute to inflammation by increasing the influx of neutrophils, dendritic cells and memory T cells into the lesions. On the other hand, the involvement of *IL-1* signaling pathway is also prominent in HS with upregulation of molecules causing immune cell infiltration and extracellular matrix degradation and could be reversed by application of IL-1 receptor antagonist [40,76]. *IL1B* signaling pathway-associated genes, such as *IL1R1, IL1RN*,

IFNG, *IL6*, *IL18*, *IL18R1*, *IL32*, *IL33*, *IL36A*, *IL36B*, *IL36G*, *IL36RN*, *IL37*, *TLR2*, *TLR3*, *TLR4*, *S100A7*, *S100A7A*, *S100A8*, *S100A9* and *S100A12* were HS-associated DEGs, as detected in our systemic review.

The inflammatory process in HS seems to be coupled with impaired barrier function, altered epidermal cell differentiation, formation of the cornified envelope, TLRs and antimicrobial peptides [3], the latter not being associated with any infection, as clearly shown in the present study. These events have been observed at the follicular and epidermal keratinocytes and at a minor grade at the skin glands [3]. Moreover, we could confirm a dysregulated expression pattern of serpins, small proline-rich proteins and certain keratins, which further support the involvement of the follicular infundibulum in the initiation of the lesions, especially at the anatomic area of communication with the apocrine gland duct and the ductus seboglandularis [3].

Although HS has well-documented associations with the metabolic syndrome, which is characterized by systemic inflammation identified at a molecular level [77], the role of adipose tissue in HS has barely been investigated. Obesity is currently shown to represent the primary risk factor in HS at the molecular level [4,28]. A chronic low-grade subclinical inflammatory response is strongly implicated in the pathogenesis of insulin resistance and metabolic syndrome. The clinically relevant peroxisome proliferator-activated receptor (PPAR) pathway was down-regulated in adipocytes of HS lesions [4]. In agreement with these data, reduced serum levels of adiponectin were currently found in non-diabetic patients with HS [28]. Since adiponectin inhibits the production of TNF-α, IL-6 and chemokines of human macrophages the upregulation of *ADIPOQ* and *PLIN1*, shown in this systematic review, might be beneficial in HS treatment. Indeed, thiazolidine derivatives act as PPARγ agonists and effectively increase the adiponectin concentration and adipogenic gene expression [28,78]. Unsaturated fatty acids, eicosanoids and non-steroidal anti-inflammatory drugs function in a similar manner [79]. Further metabolic pathways, e.g., the IGF transport and uptake of IGF-binding proteins pathway, type I diabetes mellitus signaling, lipid and atherosclerosis, C-type leptin receptor signaling, estrogen-dependent nuclear events and extranuclear signaling and *RETN* signaling, encoding resistin, are dysregulated in HS, as shown in the present review.

In conclusion, inflammatory signaling, mainly innate immunity signaling pathways, mostly that of IL-1 and IL-17, epithelial differentiation signaling pathways, primarily of follicular keratinocytes and skin gland duct cells and metabolic signaling pathways, especially that of obesity/adipogenesis, represent pathogenetic HS cascades, whose activity may be targeted by future therapeutic means.

4.2. HS Comorbid Disorders

HS has been associated with a variety of comorbid disorders, such as inflammatory bowel diseases, especially Crohn's disease, axial spondylarthritis without or with follicular occlusion, triad signs, genetic keratin disorders associated with follicular occlusion, such as pachyonychia congenita, steatocystoma multiplex, Dowling-Degos disease without and with arthritis, as well as other genetic disorders, such as keratitis–ichthyosis–deafness syndrome and Down syndrome [80]. Moreover, HS has been associated with reduced quality of life, metabolic syndrome, sexual dysfunction, working disability, depression and anxiety. Like in psoriasis, HS patients have higher prevalence of cardiovascular disease risk factors and suicide risk [81]. At last, the development of epithelial tumors on chronic HS lesions at the anogenital region may be considered as the consequence of chronic severe inflammatory skin disease. The current work has provided molecular evidence of HS association with inflammatory bowel disease pathway, rheumatoid arthritis pathway, type I diabetes mellitus signaling, lipid and atherosclerosis and adipogenesis signaling.

4.3. Study Drugs and Drug Repurposing for HS

In addition to the only registered drug in HS, namely adalimumab [9,82,83], the majority of studied and off-label administered drugs also regulate differentially expressed genes and their proteins in HS, as shown in the present review [10,65,76,81–95]. On the other hand, the 452 HS-associated druggable genes proposed can mostly be classified in receptor ligands, enzyme/protein inhibitors, JAK-STAT inhibitors, PI3K inhibitors, sodium/potassium/calcium channel activators and MMP inhibitors. Additionally, Gentamicin, Ibudilast, Spironolactone, Trastuzumab, Thalidomide, Apremilast, Glucosamine, Interferon-a-2b, Binimetinib and Midostaurin have previously been reported as repurposing drugs for HS [11]. The majority of the 31 probable repurposing drugs shown in Table 2 are JAK inhibitors, with cytokine inhibitors, such as anti-IL-17 compounds, tyrosine kinase receptor inhibitors, TNF inhibitors, cyclooxygenase inhibitors, EGF receptor inhibitors, MMP inhibitors and PPARγ ligands—among others—being represented. Ten of these drugs, which have not yet been administered in HS, are already launched for other indications and 17 are in clinical studies, not including HS.

5. Conclusions

The current review provides robust molecular evidence on the pathogenetic triads of HS, namely upregulated inflammation, dysregulated epithelial cell differentiation and obesity signaling/hormone involvement. In addition, evidence of the negligible role of infectious agents is included. Moreover, HS biomarkers with strong protein–protein connectivity in HS are presented. While adalimumab, the only currently registered drug in HS, and the majority of studied and off-label administered drugs regulate DEGs and their proteins in HS, numerous compounds are eligible for HS repurposing due to their molecular signaling. Among them, 31 compounds are designated probable, following our classification, with 10 of them already being launched for other indications.

Supplementary Materials: The following are available online at https://www.mdpi.com/article/10.3390/pharmaceutics14010044/s1: Figure S1: Enrichment of HS-associated DEGs in signaling pathways; Figure S2: Global REAC evaluation of possibly involved signaling pathways in HS; Figure S3: Enrichment of druggable HS-associated genes in signaling pathways; Table S1: DEGs resulting from the comparison of transcriptomic profiles and protein expression studies between lesional HS and non-lesional skin biopsies and blood samples from HS patients and healthy controls, respectively; Table S2. Drugs regulating HS-associated DEGs.

Author Contributions: Conceptualization, C.C.Z.; methodology, V.A.Z., K.C.Z. and C.C.Z.; software, V.A.Z. and K.C.Z.; validation, V.A.Z., K.C.Z. and C.C.Z.; formal analysis, V.A.Z. and K.C.Z.; investigation, V.A.Z. and K.C.Z.; resources, V.A.Z. and C.C.Z.; data curation, V.A.Z. and K.C.Z.; writing—original draft preparation, V.A.Z. and K.C.Z. and C.C.Z.; writing—review and editing, C.C.Z.; visualization, V.A.Z.; supervision, C.C.Z.; project administration, C.C.Z. All authors have read and agreed to the published version of the manuscript.

Funding: This research received no external funding.

Institutional Review Board Statement: Ethical review and approval were waived because the article reviews ethically approved published studies involving humans.

Informed Consent Statement: Patient consent was waived because the article reviews published studies involving humans. No patient can be identified.

Data Availability Statement: Data sets related to this article are hosted at the Gene Expression Omnibus (https://www.ncbi.nlm.nih.gov/geo/ (accessed on 21 November 2021)) data repositories GSE72702, GSE79150, GSE128637, GSE137141, GSE144801, GSE148027, GSE154773, GSE154775, GSE155176, GSE155850 and GSE175990.

Acknowledgments: The Departments of Dermatology, Venereology, Allergology and Immunology, Dessau Medical Center, Dessau, Germany are health care providers of the European Reference Network for Rare and Complex Skin Diseases (ERN Skin—ALLOCATE Skin group).

Conflicts of Interest: V.A.Z. and K.C.Z. declare no conflict of interest. C.C.Z. has received subject-relevant honoraria from AbbVie, Bayer Healthcare, Boehringer-Ingelheim, Idorsia, Incyte, Inflarx, Janssen, Novartis, Regeneron, UCB and Viatris, which were not associated with or have any influence on this study. His departments have received grants from AbbVie, AOTI, AstraZeneca, Celgene,

Galderma, Inflarx, NAOS-BIODERMA, Novartis, PPM and UCB for his participation as clinical investigator, which were not associated with this study.

References

1. Zouboulis, C.C.; Del Marmol, V.; Mrowietz, U.; Prens, E.P.; Tzellos, T.; Jemec, G.B.E. Hidradenitis suppurativa/acne inversa: Criteria for diagnosis, severity assessment, classification and disease evaluation. *Dermatology* **2015**, *231*, 184–190. [CrossRef] [PubMed]
2. Del Duca, E.; Morelli, P.; Bennardo, L.; Di Raimondo, C.; Nisticò, S.P. Cytokine pathways and investigational target therapies in hidradenitis suppurativa. *Int. J. Mol. Sci.* **2020**, *21*, 8436. [CrossRef]
3. Zouboulis, C.C.; Nogueira da Costa, A.; Makrantonaki, E.; Hou, X.X.; Almansouri, D.; Dudley, J.T.; Edwards, H.; Readhead, B.; Balthasar, O.; Jemec, G.B.E.; et al. Alterations in innate immunity and epithelial cell differentiation are the molecular pillars of hidradenitis suppurativa. *J. Eur. Acad. Dermatol. Venereol.* **2020**, *34*, 846–861. [CrossRef] [PubMed]
4. Kaleta, K.P.; Nikolakis, G.; Hossini, A.M.; Balthasar, O.; Almansouri, D.; Vaiopoulos, A.; Knolle, J.; Boguslawska, A.; Wojas-Pelc, A.; Zouboulis, C.C. Metabolic disorders/obesity is a primary risk factor in hidradenitis suppurativa: An immunohistochemical real-world approach. *Dermatology* **2021**. [CrossRef]
5. Zouboulis, C.C.; Desai, N.; Emtestam, L.; Hunger, R.E.; Ioannides, D.; Juhász, I.; Lapins, J.; Matusiak, L.; Prens, E.P.; Revuz, J.; et al. European S1 guideline for the treatment of hidradenitis suppurativa/acne inversa. *J Eur. Acad. Dermatol. Venereol.* **2015**, *29*, 619–644. [CrossRef]
6. Zouboulis, C.C.; Bechara, F.G.; Dickinson-Blok, J.L.; Gulliver, W.; Horváth, B.; Hughes, R.; Kimball, A.B.; Kirby, B.; Martorell, A.; Podda, M.; et al. Hidradenitis suppurativa/acne inversa: A practical framework for treatment optimization—Systematic review and recommendations from the HS ALLIANCE working group. *J. Eur. Acad. Dermatol. Venereol.* **2019**, *33*, 19–31. [CrossRef]
7. Zouboulis, C.C.; Benhadou, F.; Byrd, A.; Chandran, N.; Giamarellos-Bourboulis, E.; Fabbrocini, G.; Frew, J.; Fujita, H.; González-López, M.A.; Guillem, P.; et al. What causes hidradenitis suppurativa? 15 years after. *Exp. Dermatol.* **2020**, *29*, 1154–1170. [CrossRef]
8. Zouboulis, C.C.; Frew, J.W.; Giamarellos-Bourboulis, E.J.; Jemec, G.B.E.; del Marmol, V.; Marzano, A.V.; Nikolakis, G.; Sayed, C.J.; Tzellos, T.; Wolk, K.; et al. Target molecules for future hidradenitis suppurativa treatment. *Exp. Dermatol.* **2021**, *30* (Suppl. 1), 8–17. [CrossRef]
9. Kimball, A.B.; Okun, M.M.; Williams, D.A.; Gottlieb, A.B.; Papp, K.A.; Zouboulis, C.C.; Armstrong, A.W.; Kerdel, F.; Gold, M.H.; Forman, S.B.; et al. Two phase 3 trials of adalimumab treatment of hidradenitis suppurativa. *N. Engl. J. Med.* **2016**, *375*, 422–434. [CrossRef]
10. Glatt, S.; Jemec, G.B.; Forman, S.; Sayed, C.; Schmieder, G.; Weisman, J.; Rolleri, R.; Seegobin, S.; Baeten, D.; Ionescu, L.; et al. Bimekizumab in moderate-to-severe hidradenitis suppurativa: A phase 2, double-blind, placebo-controlled randomized clinical trial. *JAMA Dermatol.* **2021**, *157*, 1279–1288. [CrossRef] [PubMed]
11. Zouboulis, C.C.; Nogueira da Costa, A. Drug repurposing through drug-gene interaction profiles for hidradenitis suppurativa/acne inversa treatment. *J Eur Acad Dermatol Venereol.* **2021**, *35*, e251–e254. [CrossRef]
12. Zouboulis, C.C.; Readhead, B.; Dudley, J.T. An additional drug repurposing study for hidradenitis suppurativa/acne inversa. *Br. J. Dermatol.* **2021**, *184*, 748–750. [CrossRef]
13. Giordano, A.; Forte, G.; Massimo, L.; Riccio, R.; Bifulco, G.; Di Micco, S. Discovery of new erbB4 inhibitors: Repositioning an orphan chemical library by inverse virtual screening. *Eur. J. Med. Chem.* **2018**, *152*, 253–263. [CrossRef]
14. Yu, J.L.; Dai, Q.Q.; Li, G.B. Deep learning in target prediction and drug repositioning: Recent advances and challenges. *Drug Discov. Today* **2021**. [CrossRef] [PubMed]
15. Page, M.J.; McKenzie, J.E.; Bossuyt, P.M.; Boutron, I.; Hoffmann, T.C.; Mulrow, C.D.; Shamseer, L.; Tetzlaff, J.M.; Akl, E.A.; Brennan, S.E.; et al. The PRISMA 2020 statement: An updated guideline for reporting systematic reviews. *Bmj* **2021**, *372*, n71. [CrossRef]
16. Gene Expression Omnibus. Available online: https://www.ncbi.nlm.nih.gov/geo/ (accessed on 15 November 2021).
17. HUGO Gene Nomenclature Committee. Available online: https://www.genenames.org/tools/multi-symbol-checker/ (accessed on 15 November 2021).
18. Biological DataBase network. Available online: https://biodbnet-abcc.ncifcrf.gov/db/db2db.php (accessed on 15 November 2021).
19. g:Profiler. Available online: https://biit.cs.ut.ee/gprofiler/gost (accessed on 15 November 2021).
20. Kyoto Encyclopedia of Genes and Genomes. Available online: https://www.genome.jp/kegg/ (accessed on 15 November 2021).
21. Reactome. Available online: https://reactome.org/ (accessed on 15 November 2021).
22. WikiPathways. Available online: https://www.wikipathways.org/ (accessed on 15 November 2021).
23. Human Phenotype Ontology. Available online: https://hpo.jax.org/app/ (accessed on 15 November 2021).
24. The Drug Repurposing Hub. Available online: https://s3.amazonaws.com/data.clue.io/repurposing/downloads/repurposing_drugs_20200324.txt (accessed on 15 November 2021).
25. Gene Cards, The Human Gene Database. Available online: https://www.genecards.org/ (accessed on 15 November 2021).
26. Lowe, M.M.; Naik, H.B.; Clancy, S.; Pauli, M.; Smith, K.M.; Bi, Y.; Dunstan, R.; Gudjonsson, J.E.; Paul, M.; Harris, H.; et al. Immunopathogenesis of hidradenitis suppurativa and response to anti-TNF-alpha therapy. *JCI Insight* **2020**, *5*, e139932. [CrossRef]

27. Hoffman, L.K.; Tomalin, L.E.; Schultz, G.; Howell, M.D.; Anandasabapathy, D.; Alavi, A.; Suárez-Fariñas, M.; Lowes, M.A. Integrating the skin and blood transcriptomes and serum proteome in hidradenitis suppurativa reveals complement dysregulation and a plasma cell signature. *PLoS ONE* **2018**, *13*, e0203672. [CrossRef]
28. González-López, M.A.; Vilanova, I.; Ocejo-Viñals, G.; Arlegui, R.; Navarro, I.; Guiral, S.; Mata, C.; Pérez-Paredes, M.G.; Portilla, V.; Corrales, A.; et al. Circulating levels of adiponectin, leptin, resistin and visfatin in non-diabetics patients with hidradenitis suppurativa. *Arch. Dermatol. Res.* **2020**, *312*, 595–600. [CrossRef]
29. Hessam, S.; Sand, M.; Skrygan, M.; Bechara, F.G. The microRNA effector RNA-induced silencing complex in hidradenitis suppurativa: A significant dysregulation within active inflammatory lesions. *Arch. Dermatol. Res.* **2017**, *309*, 557–565. [CrossRef]
30. Rumberger, B.E.; Boarder, E.L.; Owens, S.L.; Howell, M.D. Transcriptomic analysis of hidradenitis suppurativa skin suggests roles for multiple inflammatory pathways in disease pathogenesis. *Inflamm. Res.* **2020**, *69*, 967–973. [CrossRef]
31. Penno, C.A.; Jäger, P.; Laguerre, C.; Hasler, F.; Hofmann, A.; Gass, S.K.; Wettstein-Ling, B.; Schaefer, D.J.; Avrameas, A.; Raulf, F.; et al. Lipidomics profiling of hidradenitis suppurativa skin lesions reveals lipoxygenase pathway dysregulation and accumulation of proinflammatory leukotriene B4. *J. Investig. Dermatol.* **2020**, *140*, 2421–2432. [CrossRef]
32. Coates, M.; Mariottoni, P.; Corcoran, D.L.; Kirshner, H.F.; Jaleel, T.; Brown, D.A.; Brooks, S.R.; Murray, J.; Morasso, M.I.; MacLeod, A.S. The skin transcriptome in hidradenitis suppurativa uncovers an antimicrobial and sweat gland gene signature which has distinct overlap with wounded skin. *PLoS ONE* **2019**, *14*, e0216249. [CrossRef]
33. Shanmugam, V.K.; Jones, D.; McNish, S.; Bendall, M.L.; Crandall, K.A. Transcriptome patterns in hidradenitis suppurativa: Support for the role of antimicrobial peptides and interferon pathways in disease pathogenesis. *Clin. Exp. Dermatol.* **2019**, *44*, 882–892. [CrossRef]
34. Blok, J.L.; Li, K.; Brodmerkel, C.; Jonkman, M.F.; Horváth, B. Gene expression profiling of skin and blood in hidradenitis suppurativa. *Br. J. Dermatol.* **2016**, *174*, 1392–1394. [CrossRef]
35. Buimer, M.G.; Wobbes, T.; Klinkenbijl, J.H.; Reijnen, M.M.; Blokx, W.A. Immunohistochemical analysis of steroid hormone receptors in hidradenitis suppurativa. *Am. J. Dermatopathol.* **2015**, *37*, 129–132. [CrossRef]
36. Vossen, A.; van der Zee, H.H.; Davelaar, N.; Mus, A.M.C.; van Doorn, M.B.A.; Prens, E.P. Apremilast for moderate hidradenitis suppurativa: No significant change in lesional skin inflammatory biomarkers. *J. Eur. Acad. Dermatol. Venereol.* **2019**, *33*, 761–765. [CrossRef]
37. Kanni, T.; Zenker, O.; Habel, M.; Riedemann, N.; Giamarellos-Bourboulis, E.J. Complement activation in hidradenitis suppurativa: A new pathway of pathogenesis? *Br. J. Dermatol.* **2018**, *179*, 413–419. [CrossRef]
38. Kelly, G.; Hughes, R.; McGarry, T.; van den Born, M.; Adamzik, K.; Fitzgerald, R.; Lawlor, C.; Tobin, A.M.; Sweeney, C.M.; Kirby, B. Dysregulated cytokine expression in lesional and nonlesional skin in hidradenitis suppurativa. *Br. J. Dermatol.* **2015**, *173*, 1431–1439. [CrossRef]
39. Vossen, A.; Stubbs, A.; van Doorn, M.; van Straalen, K.; van der Zee, H.; Prens, E. Profiling of the transcriptome in hidradenitis suppurativa: A case-control sample. *J. Investig. Dermatol.* **2016**, *136*, S193. [CrossRef]
40. Witte-Händel, E.; Wolk, K.; Tsaousi, A.; Irmer, M.L.; Mößner, R.; Shomroni, O.; Lingner, T.; Witte, K.; Kunkel, D.; Salinas, G.; et al. The IL-1 pathway is hyperactive in hidradenitis suppurativa and contributes to skin infiltration and destruction. *J. Investig. Dermatol.* **2019**, *139*, 1294–1305. [CrossRef]
41. Vossen, A.; van der Zee, H.H.; Tsoi, L.C.; Xing, X.; Devalaraja, M.; Gudjonsson, J.E.; Prens, E.P. Novel cytokine and chemokine markers of hidradenitis suppurativa reflect chronic inflammation and itch. *Allergy* **2019**, *74*, 631–634. [CrossRef]
42. Garcet, S.; Frew, J.W.; Navrazhina, K.; Krueger, J. Hidradenitis suppurativa RNA-seq skin transcriptome overlaps with psoriasis vulgaris and reveals a marked upregulation of multiple targetable cytokines. *J. Investig. Dermatol.* **2020**, *140*, S7. [CrossRef]
43. Byrd, A.S.; Kerns, M.L.; Williams, D.W.; Zarif, J.C.; Rosenberg, A.Z.; Delsante, M.; Liu, H.; Dillen, C.A.; Maynard, J.P.; Caffrey, J.A.; et al. Collagen deposition in chronic hidradenitis suppurativa: Potential role for CD163(+) macrophages. *Br. J. Dermatol.* **2018**, *179*, 792–794. [CrossRef]
44. Hotz, C.; Boniotto, M.; Guguin, A.; Surenaud, M.; Jean-Louis, F.; Tisserand, P.; Ortonne, N.; Hersant, B.; Bosc, R.; Poli, F.; et al. Intrinsic defect in keratinocyte function leads to inflammation in hidradenitis suppurativa. *J. Investig. Dermatol.* **2016**, *136*, 1768–1780. [CrossRef]
45. Gudjonsson, J.E.; Tsoi, L.C.; Ma, F.; Billi, A.C.; van Straalen, K.R.; Vossen, A.R.J.V.; van der Zee, H.H.; Harms, P.W.; Wasikowski, R.; Yee, C.M.; et al. Contribution of plasma cells and B cells to hidradenitis suppurativa pathogenesis. *JCI Insight* **2020**, *5*, e139930. [CrossRef] [PubMed]
46. Wolk, K.; Warszawska, K.; Hoeflich, C.; Witte, E.; Schneider-Burrus, S.; Witte, K.; Kunz, S.; Buss, A.; Roewert, H.J.; Krause, M.; et al. Deficiency of IL-22 contributes to a chronic inflammatory disease: Pathogenetic mechanisms in acne inversa. *J. Immunol.* **2011**, *186*, 1228–1239. [CrossRef]
47. Nelson, A.M.; Cong, Z.; Gettle, S.L.; Longenecker, A.L.; Kidacki, M.; Kirby, J.S.; Adams, D.R.; Stairs, D.B.; Danby, F.W. E-cadherin and p120ctn protein expression are lost in hidradenitis suppurativa lesions. *Exp. Dermatol.* **2019**, *28*, 867–871. [CrossRef] [PubMed]
48. Dany, M.; Elston, D. Gene expression of sphingolipid metabolism pathways is altered in hidradenitis suppurativa. *J. Am. Acad. Dermatol.* **2017**, *77*, 268–273. [CrossRef]
49. Matusiak, L.; Salomon, J.; Nowicka-Suszko, D.; Bieniek, A.; Szepietowski, J.C. Chitinase-3-like protein 1 (YKL-40): Novel biomarker of hidradenitis suppurativa disease activity? *Acta Dermatovenereol.* **2015**, *95*, 736–737. [CrossRef]

50. Salomon, J.; Piotrowska, A.; Matusiak, L.; Dziegiel, P.; Szepietowski, J.C. Chitinase-3-like protein 1 (YKL-40) Is expressed in lesional skin in hidradenitis suppurativa. *Vivo* **2019**, *33*, 141–143. [CrossRef]
51. Wolk, K.; Brembach, T.C.; Simaite, D.; Bartnik, E.; Cucinotta, S.; Pokrywka, A.; Irmer, M.L.; Triebus, J.; Witte-Handel, E.; Salinas, G.; et al. Activity and components of the granulocyte colony-stimulating factor pathway in hidradenitis suppurativa. *Br. J. Dermatol.* **2021**, *185*, 164–176. [CrossRef]
52. Hofmann, S.C.; Saborowski, V.; Lange, S.; Kern, W.V.; Bruckner-Tuderman, L.; Rieg, S. Expression of innate defense antimicrobial peptides in hidradenitis suppurativa. *J. Am. Acad. Dermatol.* **2012**, *66*, 966–974. [CrossRef]
53. Dréno, B.; Khammari, A.; Brocard, A.; Moyse, D.; Blouin, E.; Guillet, G.; Leonard, F.; Knol, A.C. Hidradenitis suppurativa: The role of deficient cutaneous innate immunity. *Arch. Dermatol.* **2012**, *148*, 182–186. [CrossRef]
54. Argyropoulou, M.; Grundhuber, M.; Kanni, T.; Tzanetakou, V.; Micha, S.; Stergianou, D.; Swiniarski, S.; Giamarellos-Bourboulis, E.J. A composite biomarker score for the diagnosis of hidradenitis suppurativa. *Exp. Dermatol.* **2019**, *28*, 18. [CrossRef]
55. Hessam, S.; Sand, M.; Skrygan, M.; Gambichler, T.; Bechara, F.G. Inflammation induced changes in the expression levels of components of the microRNA maturation machinery Drosha, Dicer, Drosha co-factor DGRC8 and Exportin-5 in inflammatory lesions of hidradenitis suppurativa patients. *J. Dermatol. Sci.* **2016**, *82*, 166–174. [CrossRef]
56. Van der Zee, H.H.; de Ruiter, L.; van den Broecke, D.G.; Dik, W.A.; Laman, J.D.; Prens, E.P. Elevated levels of tumour necrosis factor (TNF)-α, interleukin (IL)-1β and IL-10 in hidradenitis suppurativa skin: A rationale for targeting TNF-α and IL-1β. *Br. J. Dermatol.* **2011**, *164*, 1292–1298. [CrossRef]
57. Wieland, C.W.; Vogl, T.; Ordelman, A.; Vloedgraven, H.G.; Verwoolde, L.H.; Rensen, J.M.; Roth, J.; Boer, J.; Hessels, J. Myeloid marker S100A8/A9 and lymphocyte marker, soluble interleukin 2 receptor: Biomarkers of hidradenitis suppurativa disease activity? *Br. J. Dermatol.* **2013**, *168*, 1252–1258. [CrossRef]
58. Montaudié, H.; Seitz-Polski, B.; Cornille, A.; Benzaken, S.; Lacour, J.-P.; Passeron, T. Interleukin 6 and high-sensitivity C-reactive protein are potential predictive markers of response to infliximab in hidradenitis suppurativa. *J. Am. Acad. Dermatol.* **2017**, *76*, 156–158. [CrossRef]
59. Matusiak, L.; Szczech, J.; Bieniek, A.; Nowicka-Suszko, D.; Szepietowski, J.C. Increased interleukin (IL)-17 serum levels in patients with hidradenitis suppurativa: Implications for treatment with anti-IL-17 agents. *J. Am. Acad. Dermatol.* **2017**, *76*, 670–675. [CrossRef]
60. Schlapbach, C.; Hanni, T.; Yawalkar, N.; Hunger, R.E. Expression of the IL-23/Th17 pathway in lesions of hidradenitis suppurativa. *J. Am. Acad. Dermatol.* **2011**, *65*, 790–798. [CrossRef]
61. Thomi, R.; Kakeda, M.; Yawalkar, N.; Schlapbach, C.; Hunger, R.E. Increased expression of the interleukin-36 cytokines in lesions of hidradenitis suppurativa. *J. Eur. Acad. Dermatol. Venereol.* **2017**, *31*, 2091–2096. [CrossRef]
62. Hayran, Y.; Allı, N.; Yücel, Ç.; Akdoğan, N.; Turhan, T. Serum IL-36alpha, IL-36beta, and IL-36gamma levels in patients with hidradenitis suppurativa: Association with disease characteristics, smoking, obesity, and metabolic syndrome. *Arch. Dermatol. Res.* **2020**, *312*, 187–196. [CrossRef]
63. Akdogan, N.; Alli, N.; Uysal, P.I.; Topcuoglu, C.; Candar, T.; Turhan, T. Visfatin and insulin levels and cigarette smoking are independent risk factors for hidradenitis suppurativa: A case-control study. *Arch. Dermatol. Res.* **2018**, *310*, 785–793. [CrossRef] [PubMed]
64. Wolk, K.; Witte, E.; Tsaousi, A.; Witte, K.; Volk, H.; Sterry, W.; Wenzel, J.; Schneider-Burrus, S.; Sabat, R. Lipocalin-2 as a novel biomarker in acne inversa. *J. Investig. Dermatol.* **2016**, *136*, S235. [CrossRef]
65. Blok, J.L.; Li, K.; Brodmerkel, C.; Horvátovich, P.; Jonkman, M.F.; Horváth, B. Ustekinumab in hidradenitis suppurativa: Clin-ical results and a search for potential biomarkers in serum. *Br. J. Dermatol.* **2016**, *174*, 839–846. [CrossRef] [PubMed]
66. Tsaousi, A.; Witte, E.; Witte, K.; Rowert-Huber, H.J.; Volk, H.D.; Sterry, W.; Wolk, K.; Schneider-Burrus, S.; Sabat, R. MMP8 is increased in lesions and blood of acne inversa patients: A potential link to skin destruction and metabolic alterations. *Mediators Inflamm.* **2016**, *2016*, 4097574. [CrossRef]
67. Wang, B.; Yang, W.; Wen, W.; Sun, J.; Su, B.; Liu, B.; Ma, D.; Lv, D.; Wen, Y.; Qu, T.; et al. Gamma-secretase gene mutations in familial acne inversa. *Science* **2010**, *330*, 1065. [CrossRef]
68. Hunger, R.E.; Surovy, A.M.; Hassan, A.S.; Braathen, L.R.; Yawalkar, N. Toll-like receptor 2 is highly expressed in lesions of acne inversa and colocalizes with C-type lectin receptor. *Br. J. Dermatol.* **2008**, *158*, 691–697. [CrossRef]
69. Sartorius, K.; Emtestam, L.; Lapins, J.; Johansson, O. Cutaneous PGP 9.5 distribution patterns in hidradenitis suppurativa. *Arch. Dermatol. Res.* **2010**, *302*, 461–468. [CrossRef]
70. Fabregat, A.; Sidiropoulos, K.; Viteri, G.; Forner, O.; Marin-Garcia, P.; Arnau, V.; D'Eustachio, P.; Stein, L.; Hermjakob, H. Reactome pathway analysis: A high-performance in-memory approach. *BMC Bioinform.* **2017**, *18*, 142. [CrossRef]
71. Frew, J.W.; Hawkes, J.E.; Krueger, J.G. A systematic review and critical evaluation of immunohistochemical associations in hidradenitis suppurativa. *F1000Research* **2018**, *7*, 1923. [CrossRef] [PubMed]
72. Vossen, A.R.J.V.; van der Zee, H.H.; Prens, E.P. Hidradenitis suppurativa: A systematic review integrating inflammatory pathways into a cohesive pathogenic model. *Front. Immunol.* **2018**, *9*, 2965. [CrossRef]
73. Jenei, A.; Dajnoki, Z.; Medgyesi, B.; Gáspár, K.; Béke, G.; Kinyó, Á.; Méhes, G.; Hendrik, Z.; Dinya, T.; Törőcsik, D.; et al. Apocrine gland-rich skin has a non-inflammatory IL-17 related immune milieu, which turns to inflammatory IL-17 mediated disease in hidradenitis suppurativa. *J. Investig. Dermatol.* **2019**, *139*, 964–968. [CrossRef]
74. Bartlett, H.S.; Million, R.P. Targeting the IL-17-T(H)17 pathway. *Nat. Rev. Drug Discov.* **2015**, *14*, 11–12. [CrossRef]

75. Archer, N.K.; Adappa, N.D.; Palmer, J.N.; Cohen, N.A.; Harro, J.M.; Lee, S.K.; Miller, L.S.; Shirtliff, M.E. Interleukin-17A (IL-17A) and IL-17F are critical for antimicrobial peptide production and clearance of *Staphylococcus aureus* nasal colonization. *Infect. Immun.* **2016**, *84*, 3575–3583. [CrossRef] [PubMed]
76. Tzanetakou, V.; Kanni, T.; Giatrakou, S.; Katoulis, A.; Papadavid, E.; Netea, M.G.; Dinarello, C.A.; van der Meer, J.W.M.; Rigopoulos, D.; Giamarellos-Bourboulis, E.J. Safety and efficacy of anakinra in severe hidradenitis suppurativa: A randomized clinical trial. *JAMA Dermatol.* **2016**, *152*, 52–59. [CrossRef] [PubMed]
77. Mintoff, D.; Benhadou, F.; Pace, N.P.; Frew, J.W. Metabolic syndrome and hidradenitis suppurativa: Epidemiological, molecular, and therapeutic aspects. *Int. J. Dermatol.* **2021**. [CrossRef]
78. Salvator, H.; Grassin-Delyle, S.; Brollo, M.; Couderc, L.J.; Abrial, C.; Victoni, T.; Naline, E.; Devillier, P. Adiponectin inhibits the production of TNF-alpha, IL-6 and chemokines by human lung macrophages. *Front. Pharmacol.* **2021**, *12*, 718929. [CrossRef] [PubMed]
79. Zhang, J.; Li, Q.; Yan, Y.; Sun, B.; Wang, Y.; Tang, L.; Wang, E.; Yu, J.; Corpuz Nogoy, K.M.; Li, X.; et al. Effect of ciglitazone on adipogenic transdifferentiation of bovine skeletal muscle satellite cells. *J. Anim. Sci. Technol.* **2021**, *63*, 934–953. [CrossRef]
80. Fimmel, S.; Zouboulis, C.C. Comorbidities of hidradenitis suppurativa (acne inversa). *Derm.-Endocrinol.* **2010**, *2*, 9–16. [CrossRef] [PubMed]
81. Tzellos, T.; Zouboulis, C.C. Review of comorbidities of hidradenitis suppurativa: Implications for daily clinical practice. *Dermatol. Ther.* **2020**, *10*, 63–71. [CrossRef]
82. Zouboulis, C.C.; Okun, M.M.; Prens, E.P.; Gniadecki, R.; Foley, P.A.; Lynde, C.; Weisman, J.; Gu, Y.; Williams, D.A.; Jemec, G.B.E. Long-term adalimumab efficacy in patients with moderate-to-severe hidradenitis suppurativa/acne inversa: 3-year results of a phase 3 open-label extention study. *J. Am. Acad. Dermatol.* **2019**, *80*, 60–69. [CrossRef] [PubMed]
83. Zouboulis, C.C. Adalimumab for the treatment of hidradenitis suppurativa/acne inversa. *Expert Rev. Clin. Immunol.* **2016**, *12*, 1015–1026. [CrossRef]
84. Matusiak, L.; Bieniek, A.; Szepietowski, J.C. Acitretin treatment for hidradenitis suppurativa: A prospective series of 17 patients. *Br. J. Dermatol.* **2014**, *171*, 170–174. [CrossRef]
85. Frew, J.W.; Navrazhina, K.; Grand, D.; Sullivan-Whalen, M.; Gilleaudeau, P.; Garcet, S.; Ungar, J.; Krueger, J.G. The effect of subcutaneous brodalumab on clinical disease activity in hidradenitis suppurativa: An open-label cohort study. *J. Am. Acad. Dermatol.* **2020**, *83*, 1341–1348. [CrossRef]
86. Mortimer, P.S.; Dawber, R.P.; Gales, M.A.; Moore, R.A. A double-blind controlled cross-over trial of cyproterone acetate in females with hidradenitis suppurativa. *Br. J. Dermatol.* **1986**, *115*, 263–268. [CrossRef]
87. Nikolakis, G.; Kyrgidis, A.; Zouboulis, C.C. Is there a role for antiandrogen therapy for hidradenitis suppurativa? A systematic review of published data. *Am. J. Clin. Dermatol.* **2019**, *20*, 503–513. [CrossRef]
88. Van Straalen, K.R.; Tzellos, T.; Guillem, P.; Benhadou, F.; Cuenca-Barrales, C.; Daxhelet, M.; Daoud, M.; Efthymiou, O.; Giamarellos-Bourboulis, E.J.; Jemec, G.B.E.; et al. The efficacy and tolerability of tetracyclines and clindamycin plus rifampicin for the treatment of hidradenitis suppurativa: Results of a prospective European cohort study. *J. Am. Acad. Dermatol.* **2021**, *85*, 369–378. [CrossRef]
89. Lee, R.A.; Dommasch, E.; Treat, J.; Sciacca-Kirby, J.; Chachkin, S.; Williams, J.; Shin, D.B.; Leyden, J.J.; Vittorio, C.; Gelfand, J.M. A prospective clinical trial of open-label etanercept for the treatment of hidradenitis suppurativa. *J. Am. Acad. Dermatol.* **2009**, *60*, 565–573. [CrossRef] [PubMed]
90. Adams, D.R.; Yankura, J.A.; Fogelberg, A.C.; Anderson, B.E. Treatment of hidradenitis suppurativa with etanercept injection. *Arch. Dermatol.* **2010**, *146*, 501–504. [CrossRef] [PubMed]
91. Melendez-Gonzalez, M.D.M.; Hamad, J.; Sayed, C. Golimumab for the treatment of hidradenitis suppurativa in patients with previous TNF-alpha treatment failure. *J. Investig. Dermatol.* **2021**, *141*, 2975–2979. [CrossRef]
92. Grant, A.; Gonzalez, T.; Montgomery, M.O.; Cardenas, V.; Kerdel, F.A. Infliximab therapy for patients with moderate to severe hidradenitis suppurativa: A randomized, double-blind, placebo-controlled crossover trial. *J. Am. Acad. Dermatol.* **2010**, *62*, 205–217. [CrossRef] [PubMed]
93. Verdolini, R.; Clayton, N.; Smith, A.; Alwash, N.; Mannello, B. Metformin for the treatment of hidradenitis suppurativa: A little help along the way. *J. Eur. Acad. Dermatol. Venereol.* **2013**, *27*, 1101–1108. [CrossRef]
94. Prussick, L.; Rothstein, B.; Joshipura, D.; Saraiya, A.; Turkowski, Y.; Abdat, R.; Alomran, A.; Zancanaro, P.; Kachuk, C.; Dumont, N.; et al. Open-label, investigator-initiated, single-site exploratory trial evaluating secukinumab, an anti-interleukin-17A monoclonal antibody, for patients with moderate-to-severe hidradenitis suppurativa. *Br. J. Dermatol.* **2019**, *181*, 609–611. [CrossRef]
95. Giamarellos-Bourboulis, E.J.; Argyropoulou, M.; Kanni, T.; Spyridopoulos, T.; Otto, I.; Zenker, O.; Guo, R.; Riedemann, N.C. Clinical efficacy of complement C5a inhibition by IFX-1 in hidradenitis suppurativa: An open-label single-arm trial in patients not eligible for adalimumab. *Br. J. Dermatol.* **2020**, *183*, 176–178. [CrossRef]

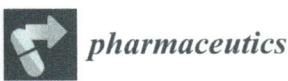

Review

Repurposing Drugs via Network Analysis: Opportunities for Psychiatric Disorders

Trang T. T. Truong [1], Bruna Panizzutti [1], Jee Hyun Kim [1,2] and Ken Walder [1,*]

1. IMPACT, The Institute for Mental and Physical Health and Clinical Translation, School of Medicine, Deakin University, Geelong 3220, Australia; truongtra@deakin.edu.au (T.T.T.T.); b.panizzuttiparry@deakin.edu.au (B.P.); jee.kim@deakin.edu.au (J.H.K.)
2. Mental Health Theme, The Florey Institute of Neuroscience and Mental Health, Parkville 3010, Australia
* Correspondence: ken.walder@deakin.edu.au

Abstract: Despite advances in pharmacology and neuroscience, the path to new medications for psychiatric disorders largely remains stagnated. Drug repurposing offers a more efficient pathway compared with de novo drug discovery with lower cost and less risk. Various computational approaches have been applied to mine the vast amount of biomedical data generated over recent decades. Among these methods, network-based drug repurposing stands out as a potent tool for the comprehension of multiple domains of knowledge considering the interactions or associations of various factors. Aligned well with the poly-pharmacology paradigm shift in drug discovery, network-based approaches offer great opportunities to discover repurposing candidates for complex psychiatric disorders. In this review, we present the potential of network-based drug repurposing in psychiatry focusing on the incentives for using network-centric repurposing, major network-based repurposing strategies and data resources, applications in psychiatry and challenges of network-based drug repurposing. This review aims to provide readers with an update on network-based drug repurposing in psychiatry. We expect the repurposing approach to become a pivotal tool in the coming years to battle debilitating psychiatric disorders.

Keywords: network analysis; drug repurposing; psychiatric disorders; medications; psychiatry; drug discovery; mental disorders

1. Challenges of Drug Research for Psychiatric Disorders

Psychiatric disorders are leading causes of disability, with an increasing burden and significant repercussions for health, society and the economy [1,2]. Despite some pharmacological advances, drug discovery for psychiatric disorders is particularly challenging and remains virtually stagnant. Out of 101 new drugs approved by the FDA in 2019 and 2020, only two were indicated for psychiatric disorders [3,4]. Such an outcome suggests that, compared with other diseases, drug development for psychiatric disorders has intrinsic bottlenecks that hinder the roadmap to new medications. In particular, there is a lack of understanding of the pathological mechanisms of neuropsychiatric disorders, largely due to their complex and ambiguous aetiology (genetics, environment, brain structure and function) [5,6]. Therefore, these disorders pose great challenges to the identification and characterization of biomarkers and molecular targets, as well as utilizing animal models adequately representing the disease.

Drug development is an inherently laborious, expensive, and time-consuming process, which becomes even more difficult for psychiatric disorders subserved by poorly understood mechanisms. Conventional drug discovery has long been considered a costly and risky journey (Figure 1a). The whole process usually takes approximately 13–15 years from initial discovery to final regulatory approval, and costs USD 2–3 billion [7]. The expenditure is predominated by failed candidates which are common given the low success rate of <10% [8].

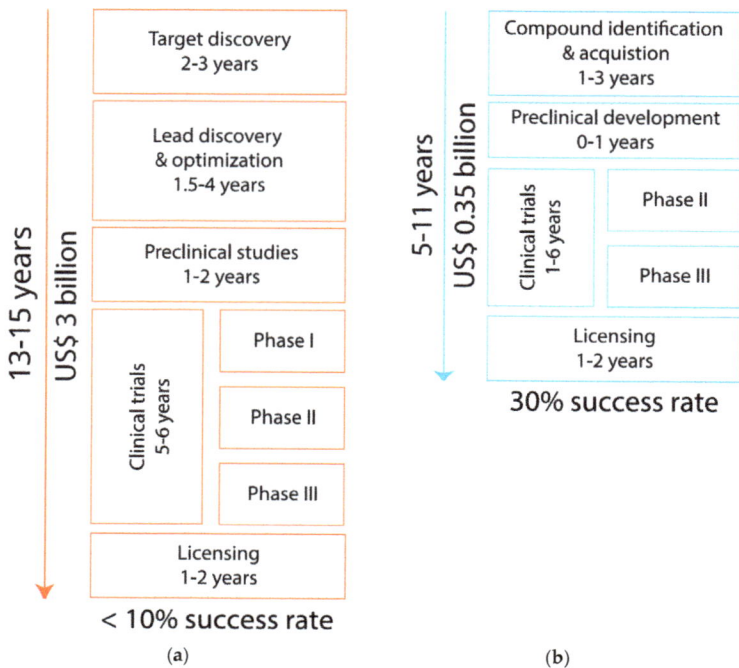

Figure 1. The comparison between (**a**) conventional drug discovery and (**b**) drug repurposing. (**a**) De novo drug discovery usually requires 13–15 years and may cost up to USD 3 billion from initial experiments to final marketing approval. Moreover, the overall success rate is only ~10%. (**b**) Drug repurposing typically bypasses several steps of the conventional approach, including not only early discovery and preclinical stages but also Phase I clinical trials. Hence, time and cost can be optimized to 5–11 years and USD 0.35 billion respectively, with an improved success rate of 30%.

In de novo drug discovery, a hypothesis related to the inhibition or activation of a protein/pathway would form the basis for the first step (target discovery—as shown in Figure 1a) [9]. However, psychiatric disorders are multi-faceted conditions, and it is still unknown whether targeting a key factor/pathway could lead to successful treatments [10]. The lack of experimental models not only poses further hurdles to answering that key mechanistic question but also prevents the next step of de novo drug discovery, i.e., lead discovery and optimisation (Figure 1a). This step is generally based on high-throughput compound screening or/and structure-based design but such approaches would require credible models to measure expected phenotypic traits [9]. Furthermore, novel compounds would undergo pharmacokinetics and pharmacodynamics testing including blood–brain barrier (BBB) penetration—another unique challenge of drugs targeting central nervous system (CNS) diseases such as psychiatric disorders [11].

2. Drug Repurposing—An Accelerated Framework for Psychiatric Drug Development

In recent years, drug repurposing or repositioning, i.e., finding new indications for drugs previously developed and/or marketed for a different disease, has become an attractive alternative to conventional drug discovery. Considering the high attrition rate of de novo drug discovery, a plethora of abandoned candidate drugs, including some that have passed safety assessment but failed due to lack of efficacy, can be recycled and utilized for new therapeutic purposes. Given the known safety profiles and bioavailability, as well as established manufacturing processes, drug repurposing can bypass some steps of conventional drug discovery and hence shorten the timeline from bench to bedside with lower cost and less risk (Figure 1b) [12–14]. Drug repurposing is playing an increasingly important role in the pharmaceutical industry. Out of 64 new drugs and biologics approved by the FDA in 2018, only 8 were first-in-class agents (i.e., novel drugs with a unique mechanism of action) [15]. As a shortcut to drug development, drug repurposing provides more feasible paradigms for organizations and institutions with limited resources, and potentially better financial incentives for companies to invest in rare, orphan diseases [16]. Importantly, governments and regulatory bodies are giving rigorous support including funding programs and drug repurposing public databases [17].

In the field of neuropharmacology, there have been a substantial number of repurposed drugs approved or in development. A review by Caban et al. in 2017 reported a total of 118 repurposed drugs for 203 cases in neurology and psychiatry (some drugs have been repurposed for more than one neuropsychiatric disease) [18]. Although most approved drug cases originated from the same discipline (i.e., neuropharmacology), the majority of developing cases are from outside the field [18]. For example, there are recent investigational candidates with positive results, such as tamoxifen repurposed from oncology for use as an antimanic agent (completed phase 3 clinical trials) [19], and quinidine which was repositioned from an anti-arrhythmia drug to an antipsychotic (currently entering phase 3 clinical trials) [20]. The early success of these candidates may be a glimpse of the vast untapped potential of recycling drugs from beyond the scope of neuropharmacology.

3. Why Networks Matter for Psychiatric Drug Research

Across the entire process of drug repurposing (Figure 1b), the first step of compound identification is critical. Such repurposing compounds could be recognized from empirical or even serendipitous observations, with the prominent examples of valproic acid for bipolar disorder and ketamine for major depression [21,22]. While these empirical findings have earned great success in psychiatric drug research, the advent of computational techniques as well as high-throughput data from "omics" technologies have enabled us to adopt a more systematic approach to discover new therapeutic agents. These approaches also require the design of methodologies that integrate the high-dimensional but noisy data efficiently to acquire useful insights for drug discovery, leading to the application of network science in medical research. Network science is the use of multiple layers of information to identify connections among biological components that are inherently and physiologically relevant [23].

The fusion of network science and drug research was first conceptualized by Andrew L. Hopkins based on the premise of poly-pharmacology—one drug, multiple targets [24]. This holistic view has been appreciated in psychiatry, in which many psychotropic drugs have been shown to exhibit promiscuity as an intrinsic feature of their therapeutic effects [25]. Antipsychotics are prominent examples. Each antipsychotic drug typically targets multiple receptors and they possess distinct pharmacological profiles [5]. Hence, poly-pharmacological profiles demand consideration of multiple factors (e.g., interactions with molecular targets, downstream affected pathways) to elucidate the mechanism(s) of action of known drugs as well as to discover new therapeutic agents for psychiatric disorders [6]. Network science enables the integration of various biological elements and simultaneous consideration of their relationships in complex systems, making it a powerful system for the poly-pharmacological paradigm.

Despite their pathological heterogeneity, psychiatric disorders have been suggested to share overlapping molecular mechanisms especially at the genetics level [26–29]. Comorbidity is the norm rather than the exception for psychiatric disorders [30–33]. While such commonality has posed challenges to the characterisation of distinct disorders, it also offers opportunities for the utilisation of existing drugs in multiple mechanistic-related disorders [34]. Therefore, network-based approaches can leverage the interconnection between different disorders to find potential latent connections suggesting the recycling of known targets of a disorder in another disorder.

4. Network-Based Drug Repurposing in Psychiatry

Previous publications have offered comprehensive reviews on network science theory [35] and capabilities in the context of medicine [36,37]. Herein, we will present major terminologies, repurposing strategies, main data resources and applications in psychiatric drug research.

Network-based interpretation comprises three major steps from understanding to predicting and possible manipulating biological systems: (1) network inference (reconstruction of network relationships from biomedical data, mostly from high-throughput assays), (2) network analysis (harnessing the topological relationships of networks), (3) network modelling (dynamic representations of time-course perturbations of network elements under different conditions) [38,39]. Most studies so far have utilised the first two steps for static networks, but very few have advanced to dynamic network modelling [36].

A network inference approach involves "simplifying" complex systems by describing them as a map of nodes connected by edges denoting their relationships or interactions [40] (Figure 2). While networks can represent a wide range of biological processes, in the context of drug discovery research, nodes are generally molecular targets (genes, proteins, compounds (drugs) or diseases, with their relationships inferred from structural interactions (e.g., protein–protein interactions), correlation (e.g., co-expression networks) or conditional dependences (e.g., Bayesian networks) [41]. Many real-world networks including biological networks, tend to exhibit scale-free properties, which means only a minority of nodes have a greater number of neighbours than average ("hubs"), while most nodes only have a few connections [42–44]. Selective targeting of hubs can therefore cause much greater impact on the function of the networks than those modulations on peripheral nodes, making hubs ideal drug targets [45].

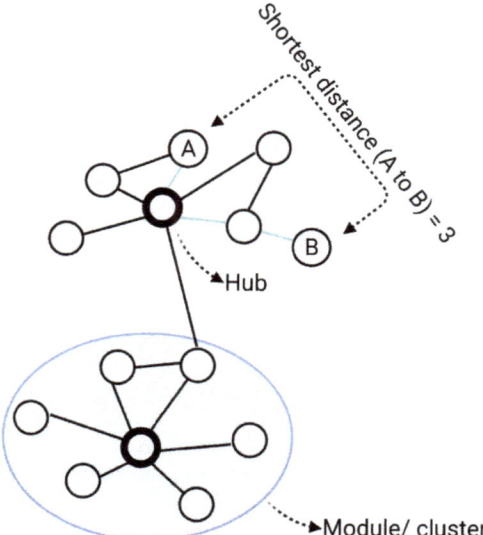

Figure 2. Main elements of a network. In the network, nodes (circles) are connected via edges (lines). For biological networks, nodes are usually biological entities (genes, proteins) and edges denote their relationships (interaction, association, similarity). From the networks, modules are clusters of closely connected nodes. Degree is the number of direct connections a node has to other nodes. Hubs are nodes with the highest degrees in the networks, meaning they have the highest number of connections. The shortest distance between node A and B is the path with the minimum number of edges from A to B. Created with BioRender.com (accessed on 2 June 2022).

Network-based drug repurposing efforts are generally based on Swanson's ABC model to retrieve unknown latent knowledge from multiple sources of data incorporated in the networks [46]. An assumption of this approach is that when term A is connected to term B, and term B is connected to term C, we can assume that terms A and C are also connected. For example, an indirect link between drug and disease can be inferred from a direct drug-target connection and a direct target-disease connection. In the ABC model, A and C must originate from different domains to yield new knowledge, and B can include multiple steps to abridge from A to C (A → B_1 → B_2 ... B_n → C) [47,48] (Figure 3).

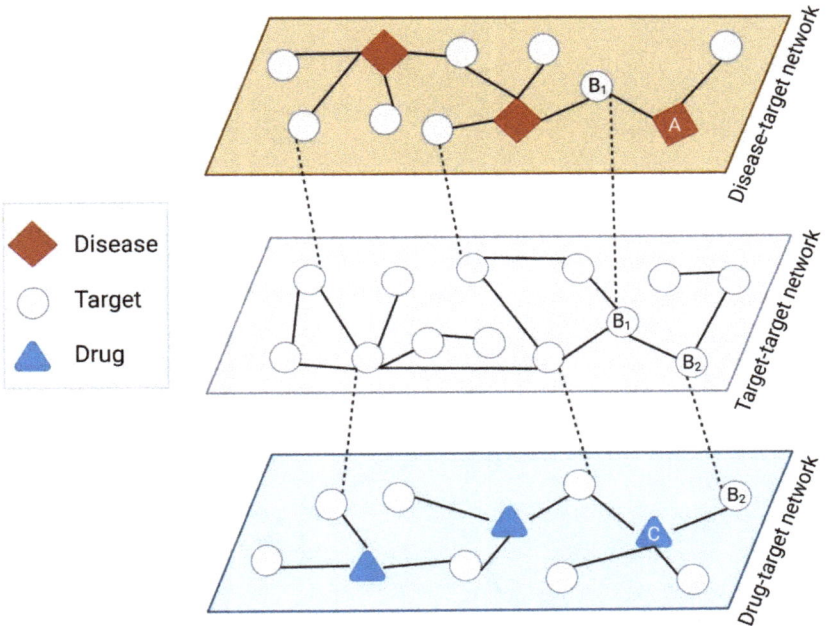

Figure 3. ABC model for network-based drug repurposing. Latent repurposing relationships can be inferred from multiple layers of network-based knowledge such as disease-target (diseasome), target–target (e.g., protein interactome), and drug–target interactions. As an example, disease A has target B_1 exhibiting direct interaction with target B_2 which in turn is targeted by drug C, suggesting drug C might be relevant for disease A (A → B_1 → B_2 → C). Created with BioRender.com (accessed on 2 June 2022).

Another common approach is "guilt-by-association" (GBA), which uses similarity measures to suggest new disease indications for drugs [49]. There are two main assumptions of GBA: (1) if two diseases share a significant number of characteristics (e.g., indications, medical descriptions, mechanisms), a drug known to treat one of them may also treat the other (Figure 4A); and (2) if a drug with unknown indications and another drug with known indications share similar properties (e.g., chemical structures, transcriptional effects), they may have the same indication profile (Figure 4B). The major challenge of this approach would be how to define the robust similarity metric between drugs or diseases that concurs with similarity in mechanisms of action.

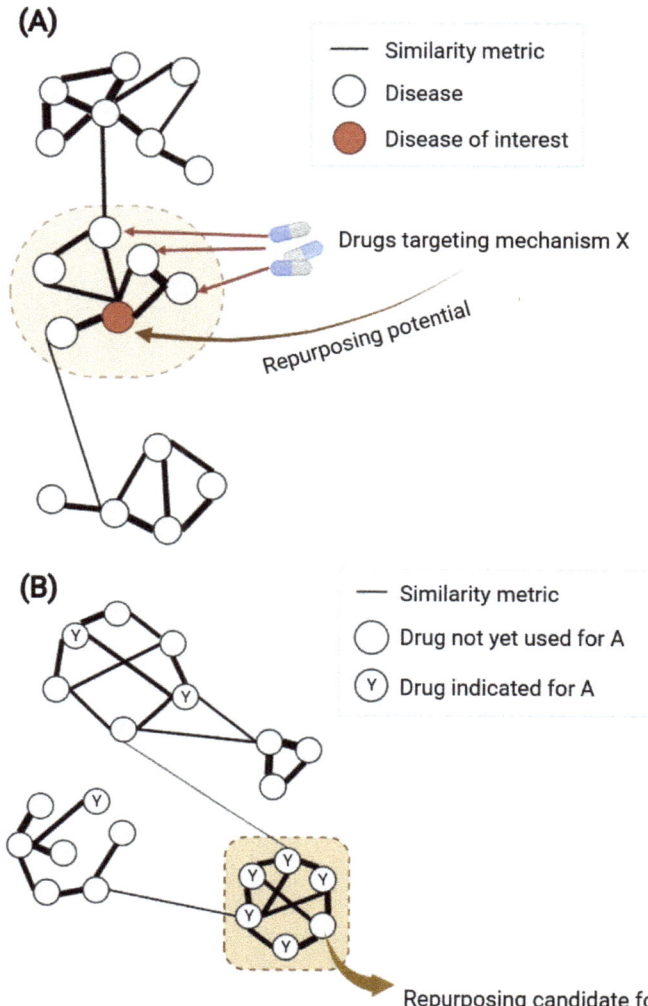

Figure 4. Guilt-by-association for network-based drug repurposing using (A) disease–disease or (B) drug–drug similarity. (A) Disease–disease similarity is generally inferred from one or several disease-related properties such as overlapping disease genes, symptoms or comorbidities. A weighted disease network (diseasome) can be built based on the similarity metric; herein, modules of similar nodes (diseases) can be identified. The module containing the disease of interest (highlighted in the brown dashed circle) might suggest potential shared mechanism(s) for repurposing drugs. Within this module, if multiple connected diseases have known drugs with similar mechanism X, such drugs might be repurposed for the disease of interest. (B) Drug–drug similarity can be calculated based on one or several properties such as chemical structures, targets, side effects or transcriptional profiles. Using the similarity metric as the weight of edges for network construction, ones can identify modules of highly similar nodes (drugs) suggesting similar mechanisms of action. When considering in the context of a certain disease A, it would be of interest to focus on the module containing multiple known drugs for disease A (highlighted as brown dashed square). Within such a module, a drug that has yet to be used for disease A might be a potential repurposing candidate due to its high similarity with other drugs used for disease A. Created with BioRender.com (accessed on 2 June 2022).

Data for network construction can be sourced from experimental data (e.g., high throughput screening), text mining or databases (e.g., phenotypic profiles, protein interactions). Text mining is also the main strategy of literature-based drug repurposing, which shares many integrative opportunities with network-centric approaches. Hence, readers can refer to previous reviews in this domain for an in-depth methodological presentation [50,51]. The advantage of network-based approaches is the possible integration of multiple data layers to complement the incompleteness of each domain's knowledge. Therefore, studies using network-based drug repurposing tend to utilise multiple data sources rather than one. There are various ways of data incorporation to find repurposing insights as shown in Figure 5. However, one should consider the relevance to the disease of interest (e.g., data yielded from brain tissue versus muscle tissue) and the robustness of the evidence supporting such a relationship (e.g., experimental evidence versus co-expression). Multi-omics integration has been playing a major role in the current biological interpretation and readers can refer to previous reviews of specific updates and recommendations for this approach [52]. Herein, we will focus on different types of biomedical database resources and their utility in the context of psychiatric drug discovery research (summarised in Table 1). A summary of studies using network-based drug repurposing in psychiatry is given in Table 2.

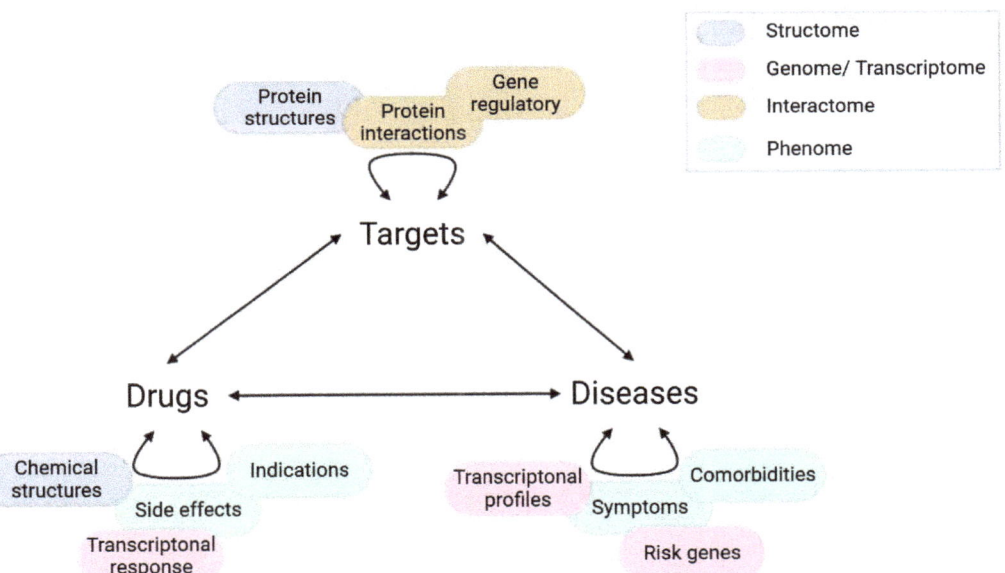

Figure 5. Different data sources for network-based drug repurposing. Curved arrows represent the associations of entities within one type (e.g., drug–drug). Multiple data sources (coloured correspondingly to their main domains such as transcriptome) can be applied to infer these associations, usually for the creation of similarity or interacting networks. Straight arrows represent the relationships between entities of different types (e.g., drug–target). For drug repurposing, the aim generally is to find a latent drug–disease connection, which can be achieved by taking the inference route from Drugs–Targets–Diseases (and vice-versa) as in the ABC model, or via Diseases–Diseases–Drugs (or Drugs–Drugs–Diseases) as in the GBA model. Created with BioRender.com (accessed on 2 June 2022).

Table 1. Summary of major data sources and their usage examples in psychiatry.

Type of Data	Description and Resource	Examples in Psychiatry
Structome	**Chemical structures:** ChemBL [53] ChemSpider [54] DrugBank [55] PubChem [56] **Macromolecular structures:** Protein Data Bank [57] AlphaFold Protein Structure Database [58]	Schizophrenia, sleep disorder [59]
Genome/Transcriptome	**GWAS (general):** GWAS ATLAS [60] NCBI Database of Genotypes and Phenotypes (dbGaP) [61] **GWAS (psychiatry):** NIMH Repository and Genomics Resource (NRGR) [62] Psychiatric Genomics Consortium (PGC) [63] Autism Sequencing Consortium (ASC) [64] Whole-Genome Sequencing Consortium for Psychiatric Disorders (WGSPD) [65] **Human brain resources:** PsychENCODE [66] Brain Somatic Mosaicism Network [67] CommonMind Consortium [68] Allen Brain Atlas [69] **Drug response:** Connectivity Map (CMap) [70] Library of Integrated Network-Based Cellular Signatures (LINCS) [71] Drug Gene Budger (DGB) [72]	Depression [73] Schizophrenia [74] Substance use disorder [75] Autism spectrum disorder [76]
Interactome	**Protein–protein interaction:** Search tool for retrieval of interacting genes/proteins (STRING) [77] Human Protein Reference Database (HPRD) [78] **Pathways:** Reactome [79] Kyoto Encyclopedia of Genes and Genomes (KEGG) [80] **Regulome:** The Human Transcription Factors [81] RegulomeDB [82] Catalog of inferred sequence binding preferences [83] JASPAR [84] UniPROBE [85] TRANSFAC [86] **Multiple collections:** OmniPath [87]	Schizophrenia [88,89] Bipolar disorder [90,91]
Phenome	**Side effects:** SIDER [92] **Drug targets:** DrugBank [55] PharmGKB [93] Drug–Gene Interaction Database (DGIdb) [94] DrugCentral [95] canSARblack [96] KEGG DRUG [97] IUPHAR/BPS Guide to PHARMACOLOGY (GtoPdb) [98] Search Tool for Interacting Chemicals (STITCH) [99,100] Therapeutic Target Database (TTD) [101] Drug Signatures Database (DSigDB) [102] Pharos [103] **Binding assay profiles:** Psychoactive Drug Screening Program (PDSP) [104] BindingDB [105] **Disease-associated targets:** Online Mendelian Inheritance in Man (OMIM) [106] ClinVar [107] MalaCards [108] DisGeNET [109] Human Phenotype Ontology (HPO) [110] Monarch [111] GPCards [112] **Disease symptoms:** Human symptoms–disease network [113] Human Phenotype Ontology (HPO) [110] DMPatternUMLS [114] **Clinical trials:** ClinicalTrials.gov [115]	Opioid use disorders [116] Schizophrenia [117] Schizophrenia, bipolar disorder, autism spectrum disorder [118]
Network-based drug discovery platforms	GRAND [119] PharmOmics [100] NeDRex [120] IBM Watson for Drug Discovery [121]	

Table 2. Summary of studies using network-based drug repurposing for psychiatric disorders. Abbreviations: ABC: ABC model; ASD: autism spectrum disorder; ADHD: attention-deficit/hyperactivity disorder; BD: bipolar disorder; GBA: guilt-by-association model; MDD: major depressive disorder; SCZ: schizophrenia; SUD: substance use disorder; TWAS: transcriptome-wide association study; ?: unclear mechanism.

Studies	Diseases	Databases Used	Inference Model and Network Type	Key Finding (Original Indication/Mechanism–Repurposed Indications)	Validation
[59]	Schizophrenia Sleep disorder	DrugBank PubChem	GBA: Drug–drug similarity	Raloxifene (estrogen receptor modulator → SCZ) Cyclobenzaprine (muscle relaxant → sleep disorder)	Literature-based (clinical trials, research articles), expert consultation
[73]	Depression	DGIdb ChEMBL PDSP Pharos PubChem DSigDB	ABC: Phenotype-informed drug-target network (http://drugtargetor.com/, accessed on 2 June 2022), i.e., an integration of drug-disease associations (GWAS pathway analysis p-values), target-disease associations (GWAS gene-wise analysis p-values, genetically predicted expression z-scores), and drug-target connections	Verapamil (calcium channel blocker → MDD) Pregabalin, Gabapentin and Nitrendipine (calcium channel modulators → MDD) Brompheniramine and Chlorphenamine (antihistamines → MDD) Lasofoxifene (estrogen receptor modulator → MDD) Levonorgestrel (sex hormones → MDD) Alizapride and Mesoridazine (D2 antagonists → MDD) Quinagolide (D2 agonist → MDD)	Literature-based (clinical trials, research articles)
[118]	Schizophrenia Bipolar Disorder Autism Spectrum Disorder	PubMed DrugBank Open Targets	ABC: Literature-mined disease–gene–drug association	AC-480, Mubritinib, CP724714, Trastuzumab, Ertumaxomab, and MM-302 (Target ERBB2 gene → SZ) SLC6A9 (glycine transporter → SZ) Bitopertin and PF-03463275 (? → SZ) Levetiracetam and Brivaracetam (anticonvulsant → SZ) CEACAM5 (? → BD) Lebrikizumab and Tralokinumab (act on IL3 →ASD)	Literature-based (clinical trials and research articles)
[74]	Schizophrenia	DGIdb	ABC: Brain co-expression network + TWAS predicted expression polygenic risk scores + drug-target interactions	Zonisamide (antiepileptic/ antiparkinsonian → SZ) Bevacizumab (antineoplastic agent → SZ) Fluticasone (cortisone analogue → SZ)	Literature-based (research articles)
[75]	Substance Use Disorder	DGIdb	ABC: Disease-related co-expression networks + drug-target interactions	MAOA inhibitors (antidepressants → SUD) Dextromethorphan (cough suppressant → SUB with suicide) Eglumegad and loxapine (? → non-suicidal SUD) Clozapine and olanzapine (antypsychotics SZ → non-suicidal SUD) Modafinil (sleep disorder → SUD)	Literature-based (research articles)
[76]	Autism Spectrum Disorder	STRING DrugBank Drug Targetor CMap	ABC: Disease-related co-expression networks + drug-gene interactome Mental disease and compounds knowledge graph (MCKG) based on literature mining for validation	Baclofen (GABA agonist for pain and muscle spasms → ASD) Sulpiride (D2 receptor antagonist, for SZ and ASD, confirmatory) Estradiol (steroid sex hormone → ASD) Entinostat (HDAC inhibitor → ASD) Everolimus (seizures → ASD) Fluvoxamine, Curcumin, Calcitriol, Metronidazole, and zinc (diverse mechanisms and uses → ASD)	Literature-based (research articles)

Table 2. Cont.

Studies	Diseases	Databases Used	Inference Model and Network Type	Key Finding (Original Indication/Mechanism–Repurposed Indications)	Validation
[116]	Opioid Use Disorders	STITCH SIDER STRING DrugBank	ABC: Drug side effect + protein interactome	Tramadol (pain → OUD) Olanzapine (SZ → OUD) Mirtazapine and Bupropion (MDD→OUD) Atomoxetine (ADHD → OUD)	Literature-based (clinical trials and research articles), clinical corroboration (retrospective case-control study of top candidates in population-level EHR data)
[117]	Schizophrenia	DrugBank MATADOR PDSP Ki Database BindingDB	GBA: SZ drug target–non-SZ drug interactome	264 SZ related drugs, 39 being investigated in clinical trials (Listed in Figure 3 of the corresponding publication)	Literature-based (clinical trials and research articles)
[122] repurposing based on network built by [88]	Schizophrenia	Psychiatric Genomics Consortium (PGC) HPRD Ensembl DrugBank	ABC: Disease risk gene–drug interactome	Sargramostin, Regorafenib, Theophylline (cancer and respiratory drugs → SZ) Cromoglicic acid (asthma prophylaxis → SZ) Acetazolamide (glaucoma, mountain sickness → SZ) Cinnarizine (Motion sickness, vertigo → SZ) Alfacalcidol (targets the VDR protein → SZ) Amiloride (on clinical trial for ADHD → SZ) Antazoline (targets ubiquitination and proteasome degradation → SZ) Danazol and Miconazole (target ESR1 and NOS3 associated with Alzheimer's Disease → SZ)	Literature-based (clinical trials and research articles)
[89]	Schizophrenia	Psychiatric Genomics Consortium (PGC) STRING DGIdb	ABC: Disease risk gene–untargeted neighbor gene interactome	19 drugs to repurpose, one major example: Galantamine (Alzheimer's disease → SZ)	Literature-based (research articles)
[91]	Bipolar Disorder	GEO CMap (via PharmacoGx package)	GBA: Transcription factor-target association	Chlorpromazine, Lavomepromazine, Perphenazine, Zuclopenthixol, Haloperidol, Promazine (antipsychotics → BD) Maprotiline, Desipramine, Mianserin (antidepressants → BD) Diflorasone (corticosteroid → BD) Meclofenamic acid, Ketorolac, Trolox c, and Acetylsalicylic acid (antiinflamatory/antirheumatic → BD)	Literature-based (research articles)

4.1. Structural Data (Structome)

Structural data from compounds and biological entities such as proteins and RNAs have been extensively utilized in structure-based drug repurposing [123]. The conventional structure-based approach usually requires a few predefined specific target molecules, which is not suitable for psychiatric disorders with complex pathology as mentioned in Section 3. However, network-centric approaches can incorporate the structome as a layer of information in a non-biased way to find new indications for drugs. Tan et al. used descriptions of 3D chemical structures from PubChem to calculate the similarity profiles of 965 drugs [59]. The Tanimoto-based 3D similarity scores were then combined with gene semantic similarity information and drug–target interactions to construct a drug similarity network. From this GBA approach, Tan et al. predicted new indications for 143 drugs and missing indications for 42 drugs without Anatomical Therapeutic Chemical (ATC) codes (indications not yet listed in ATC database) (Table 2). Psychotropic drugs suggested for repurposing from this study included raloxifene (from postmenopausal osteoporosis to schizophrenia) and cyclobenzaprine (from muscle spasms to sleep disorders) [59]. Raloxifene has passed a phase 4 clinical trial in participants with schizophrenia [124,125] while a phase 2 clinical trial of cyclobenzaprine was terminated prematurely due to inadequate recruitment [126].

4.2. Genome

Using the phenotype-to-genotype concept, multiple large-scale genome-wide association studies (GWAS) have identified thousands of genetic variants across the genome associated with psychiatric disorders [127,128]. Disease-associated genes located in risk loci can be inferred from GWAS data and are usually used in network analysis as a filtering layer to prioritise targets relevant to the disease. Ganapathiraju et al. used schizophrenia-associated genes in combination with protein–protein interactions to create a schizophrenia interactome [88]. Such a disease-specific network can be harnessed for target identification and testing of repurposed agents [122]. However, a major limitation of using GWAS data is the lack of directionality, making it difficult to determine whether a risk gene is up- or down-regulated in the disease phenotype. Gaspar et al. partially addressed this shortcoming via the incorporation of the GWAS summary statistics with gene expression to predict expression levels in different tissues, which were incorporated with drug–target interactions to build a bipartite tissue-specific drug–target network for major depression [73] (Table 2).

4.3. Transcriptome

Among the wealth of "omics" data, transcriptomic profiling has emerged as an efficient source for computational drug repurposing due to its standardized data format, multiple comprehensive public databases, and possible implementation with network biology approaches for complex diseases [12,129,130]. The expression patterns of gene products that are connected by signalling cascades or protein complexes are expected to be more similar than those of random gene products [40,131]. With this premise, co-expression networks built upon multi-dimensional data such as transcriptomics have aided in the identification of latent mechanistic patterns of psychiatric disorders and their medications, which could be missed by conventional differential expression analysis [131,132].

Psychiatric disease-related transcriptional profiles, generally from post-mortem brain samples, can be readily obtained from experiments, public databases, or psychiatric-centric consortiums such as PsychENCODE and CommonMind [66,68]. The transcriptomic data can be used on its own (gene expression levels) or incorporated with GWAS data to predict genetically regulated gene expression. As an example of the former, Cabrera-Mendoza et al. used transcriptional profiles from post-mortem brain samples of substance-use disorder individuals with and without suicidal behaviour to build gene co-expression networks associated with each phenotype (Table 2). The hub genes from these networks were then subjected to drug–gene interaction testing using the DGIdb database [94] to identify drug repurposing candidates [75]. Integration of transcriptomic profiles with GWAS data was adopted by Rodriguez-López et al. for finding druggable targets in schizophrenia. The authors estimated polygenic scores based on predicted expression and associated these scores with co-expression modules to find relevant hub target genes for early intervention [74]. Gaspar et al. also applied the genetically predicted gene expression approach [73].

Major sources of drug-induced transcriptional profiles are generated from cell lines after treatment exposure, utilising seminal reference databases for drug responses such as Connectivity Map (CMap) [133] and the Library of Integrated Network-based Cellular Signatures (LINCS) [134]. While transcriptional profiles have been used extensively in signature-based drug repurposing for the generation and comparison of selective genes representing the phenotype of interest [129,135], their network-centric drug repurposing application is still very limited in psychiatry. An emerging systems-level approach constructing gene-regulatory networks associated with each drug treatment-cell line pair using CMap expression data can offer a comprehensive characterisation of the mechanism of action of drugs. Such a systems-level approach includes information on complex interactions between multiple entities, beyond the reductionist consideration of several signature genes [119,136].

The major challenge of using drug-induced gene expression in psychiatry is the lack of biological and pathological representation of the treated model systems. Transcriptional perturbations are highly context-dependent; hence, the cancerous cells used commonly in CMap and LINCS might not recapitulate the tissue-specific effects in neuronal or glial cells. The advancement in stem cell technology has propelled the generation of patient-derived induced pluripotent stem cells (iPSC), leading to the genesis of the NeuroLINCS center of omics data generation for human iPSC response in neurological diseases [137]. Since iPSCs carry the genetic information of the patients, they recapitulate the disease-related mutations that would be more representative for diseases with significant genetic factors such as psychiatric disorders [138].

4.4. Interactome

Interactomes encompass the functional interactions of biological components, which might include physical contact between proteins (protein–protein interaction networks), metabolites (metabolic networks), transcription factors and putative regulatory elements (gene regulatory networks) or functional relationships only such as phenotypic profiling networks (phenome networks) [40]. The interactome might be placed in specific biological contexts such as signalling pathways or disease-related pathways [139]. The functional interactome based on phenotypic profiles have been broadly applied for drug discovery and will be discussed separately in the context of phenome-based networks. Interactome networks tend to possess small world property: nodes are well connected with only a few paths required for the shortest distance (Figure 2). This holds highly relevant for functionally associated nodes, ensuring a quick flow of regulatory information passing between them [140]. With the premise that risk genes tend to be more connected in the network than a set of random genes, Kauppi et al. utilised the protein interactome to map drug targets of antipsychotic drugs with networks of schizophrenia risk genes (Table 2). Using network topological analysis of shortest distance, they found risk genes were significantly localised into a distinct module and overlapped with antipsychotic drug targets. Kauppi et al. then evaluated druggable risk genes without direct links to known antipsychotic drug targets to find potential novel targets for schizophrenia such as nicotinic acetylcholine receptor genes [89].

Given the key contribution of transcription factors in the modulation of gene expression and driving phenotypic perturbations, the transcriptional regulome has been employed by De Bastiani et al. for drug repurposing in bipolar disorders [91]. Their study inferred transcription factors–targets interactions via a reverse-engineering prediction algorithm applied on human prefrontal cortex microarray data. The transcription factor-centric network comprised of modules of gene targeted by each transcription factor, called "regulons". Based on case-control transcriptomics data, gene set enrichment analysis (GSEA) was applied on the regulons to find enriched regulons in bipolar disorder. These regulons were used as gene expression signatures to query connectivity map for potential drug candidates reverting disease-related regulon signatures. Several compounds with known clinical relevance in bipolar disorders were identified such as antipsychotics (chlorpromazine, haloperidol) and antidepressants (maprotiline, mianserin, and desipramine). The study also found novel repurposing candidates including non-steroidal anti-inflammatory agents (meclofenamic acid, ketorolac, acetylsalicylsalicylic acid and diflorasone) and an antioxidant agent (trolox C) (Table 2) [91].

4.5. Phenome

The collection of phenotypic data collected from drug-induced (indications, side-effects) or disease-associated phenotypes (symptoms, disease genes) has been extensively used for drug repurposing with the availability of comprehensive public sources such as DrugBank and PharmGKB [55,93]. Zhou et al. built a drug side effect–gene system comprising two networks: drug phenotypic network of side effect profiles from SIDER [92] and protein interactome network from STRING [141]. The two networks were interconnected via drug-target associations from DrugBank [55]. Zhou et al. then applied this phenome-driven drug discovery system in finding repurposing agents for opioid use disorders. Rather than finding drugs targeting the pathological mechanism of the disorder, which is still mainly unknown, the system explored repurposing candidates sharing similar side effects or common targets with drugs causing or indicated for opioid use disorders. Using a network-based iterative algorithm, top-ranked repurposing candidates including tramadol, olanzapine, mirtazapine, bupropion and atomoxetine were identified with supporting clinical corroboration (Table 2) [116].

As presented in Section 3, psychiatric disorders tend to share mechanisms, such as pleiotropic genes associated with multiple disorders. By incorporating disease phenome and disease genome networks together, one can explore the common pathophysiology between diseases and infer potential reusable targets of one disease in a different disease. Such a disease-gene network was first proposed by Goh et al. as a "diseasome"—a bipartite graph including all known genetic disorders and disease genes connected by the association of genetic mutations to disorders [142]. Such a network can be interpreted for gene-gene similarity (connected if two genes share a disorder), or disease–disease similarity (linked if two disorders share a gene). While the specific application of diseasome in psychiatric disorders is still limited, Lüscher Dias et al. built a diseasome network considering multiple psychiatric and neurological disorders using text mining. They found several clusters shared by multiple disorders and their enriched functional annotations, e.g., depression with anxiety disorder (enriched for inflammatory response), bipolar disorder with schizophrenia (enriched for long-term potentiation and circadian entrainment). However, Lüscher Dias et al. did not consider common genes for their drug repurposing steps but focused on unique genes associated with each disorder as potential targets for the corresponding disorder (ABC model), shifting back to a single-disease context [118]. To our knowledge, there have been no cases using disease–disease similarity networks for drug repurposing in psychiatric disorders. An example outside of psychiatry from Langhauser et al. demonstrated how the repurposing hypothesis can be generated from a disease–disease similarity network of the diseasome, even from seemingly distinct diseases [143]. They built diseasome networks for 132 diseases based on four different relationships: shared genes, protein interactome, common symptoms and co-morbidity. From the diseasome, Langhauser et al. found the cGMP signalling pathway was associated with a cluster of disease phenotypes including neurological, cardiovascular, metabolic and respiratory diseases. This GBA approach suggested cGMP modulators as treatments for diseases belonging to this cluster. Based on this premise, the authors repurposed soluble guanylate cyclase (sGC) activators—cGMP generation facilitators—from their exclusive indications for cardiovascular diseases to neurological disorders and successfully validated their neuroprotection effects in vivo [143].

4.6. Network-Based Drug Repurposing Platforms

There are various approaches to yield network-based repurposing insights from biomedical data if one would like to build networks from the ground up, which has been comprehensively reviewed [36,37,41]. However, there are several platforms that can serve as a "one-stop shop" for network repurposing with the incorporation of multiple biological datasets, pre-constructed networks, pre-set analyses for easy access and queries of existing or user-generated data: for example, GRAND, a web-based database of gene regulatory networks specific for disease- or drug-related phenotypes inferred from prior experimental data such as protein–protein interactions, transcriptional profiles, transcriptional factor binding motifs and miRNAs predicted targets [119]. Using similarity scores based on properties of inferred regulatory networks, the CLUEreg tool of GRAND allows users to query a list of "high-targeted" and "low-targeted" genes or transcriptional factors of the disease to identify single or combinations of compounds that might "reverse" aberrant regulatory patterns [119]. Other examples of open-sourced platforms include PharmOmics and NeDRex; the former is a knowledgebase supporting gene-network-based drug repurposing and the latter allows heterogeneous network construction to mine disease modules for drug prioritization [100,120]. While these platforms would be easy to use with curated networks, users are limited by the scope of the current platforms, and how regularly they are updated. Reproducibility would be a challenge especially with commercial platforms such as IBM Watson for Drug Discovery where detailed analysing workflows are not publicly accessible [121]. Moreover, most datasets incorporated were yielded from different domains such as oncology, weakening the robustness of interpretations in psychiatry.

5. Challenges of Network-Based Drug Repurposing in Psychiatry

Despite its great potential, there are major obstacles preventing network-based drug repurposing from making substantial impact:

(1) While previous knowledge plays a major role in network construction, our current understanding of psychiatric disorders remains inadequate and biased towards well-studied mechanisms and biological entities. Even high-throughput screening data such as for protein interactions can only capture 20% of all potential interactions, leaving us an 80% incomplete interactome network with a great deal of missing gaps and fragmented clusters [144].

(2) Furthermore, the integration of heterogenous and high-dimensional datasets generally has to deal with disparate, incompatible or missing information [145]. To merge multiple datasets into a homogenous network would compromise accuracy due to the disregarding of biological and experimental variations affiliated with each dataset [146].

(3) Regardless of the scale of the network and data integrated, network representation in drug repurposing so far has only recapitulated static snapshots of the biological systems despite their dynamic nature. However, dynamic network modelling is still a major challenge due to the limited knowledge of interaction kinetics [147].

(4) Whilst phenotypic profiles are important data for network-based drug repurposing, similar phenotypes are not necessarily the result of similar modes of action. Genes, medication histories, and traits all play a significant role in the phenotypic outcomes of a drug's mode of action [148].

(5) Repurposing candidates have been implied from various network-based approaches, yet the preclinical validation of these candidates is limited. Even though biological follow-ups are the gold-standard, the lack of representative experimental models for psychiatric disorders has posed a great obstacle to in vitro and in vivo validation of drug efficacy [6]. Most studies in psychiatry resorted to in silico validation such as literature cross-referencing, domain expert consultation and electronic health records (EHR) [149]. The literature-based validation is undertaken by mining clinical trials or PubMed articles to find supportive evidence such as the work of Lüscher Dias et al. [118]. Expert consultation is employed for a more credible evaluation of results and literature support, as done by Tan et al. [59]. While these validations are dependent on the inference of prior knowledge,

the EHR-based validation can provide a more observational corroboration based on real-world clinical data. Zhou et al. employed EHR of nearly 73 million patients provided by the IBM Watson Health platform to validate repurposing candidates for opioid use disorders (OUD), using the odds of OUD remission as the outcome measure [116]. To validate repurposing drug X, they identified a cohort of OUD patients diagnosed with repurposing drug X's original indication (disease A). This group was then split into an exposure group (patients with OUD, disease A, using drug X) and a comparison group (patients with OUD, disease A, not using drug X). The odds ratios of remission rates between these groups were then measured. They reported patient cohorts using top-ranked repurposing candidates had higher odds of OUD remission than corresponding groups without these drugs, supporting their repurposing potential for OUD [116]. A list of EHR resources can be referred from the collection of Observational Medical Outcomes Partnership (OMOP) Common Data Model (CDM) compliance databases [150]. Most of this list are commercial and private databases whose utility is mostly hampered by the restrictive access policies. However, recent initiatives such as "All of Us" have been collecting large-scale EHR data and making data widely available for approved researchers, offering valuable resources for biomedical research [151].

6. Conclusions and Future Perspectives

Drug repurposing has emerged as a promising alternative for de novo drug discovery and has become a vital shift in the pharmaceutical industry. Taking advantage of the expanding accumulation of biomedical data, various computational drug repurposing approaches have been facilitating informed decisions for drug research. Among those, network-based approaches offer a unique opportunity to integrate various domains of biological knowledge to discover latent repurposing candidates for complex diseases such as psychiatric disorders. Given the virtually stagnant progress of drug discovery in psychiatry, we have presented the incentives for using network-based drug repurposing for psychiatric disorders: the efficiency of repurposing drugs with verified safety records and the compatibility of network science with the poly-pharmacology concept for complex disorders. We then summarised major concepts and main strategies for network-based drug repurposing, including the ABC model and GBA approaches. Data sources and current repurposing applications for psychiatric disorders were then summarised to offer readers an update with the progress of this approach in psychiatry. However, no methodology is without limitations; thus, we presented common challenges of using network-centric approaches for drug repurposing—mostly with the noisiness and insufficiency of data resources, lack of appropriate models for follow-up validation and the dynamic representation of complex systems.

Nevertheless, network-based repurposing holds great potential for expanding the knowledge of drug research, especially for complex disorders. Emerging techniques and resources will complement its capabilities for psychiatric research. Neuroimaging techniques such as functional magnetic resonance imaging (fMRI) offer the detection of the drug-induced perturbations of brain activity for predicting the efficacy of drug action [152]. A library of drug-related fMRI patterns might offer biomarker refences to compare the similarity between repurposing drugs with existing ones [153,154]. Its unique ability of non-evasively capturing functional differences at the brain systems level would be beneficial for psychiatric drug research given the complex nature of these diseases and inadequate experimental models. However, it is still an open challenge to incorporate the human connectome, i.e., the map of neural connections mapped via brain imaging, into the network-based drug repurposing given most biological data resources were measured at the molecular level. The emerging application of more pathological-representative preclinical models for psychiatric disorders such as iPSCs and organoids is also expected to provide more phenotypic-relevant datasets for drug repurposing and validation. A patient-derived stem cells library of drug response specifically for psychiatric disorders would offer a more accurate context-specific overview of drug action and therefore improve the robustness of network-based drug repurposing.

To address the incompleteness of data, computational approaches are being developed for the integration of multi-dimensional data with differences in statistical properties and biological objectives. It is challenging to represent relationships between multitudinous omics data solely with traditional linear modelling. Therefore, multi-omics tools employing multivariate statistics, machine learning (ML) and deep learning (DL) approaches have been proposed to extract and predict complex non-linear patterns [52,155]. While much development and optimization are needed to generalize ML/DL models for systems-level capture of dynamics and kinetics underlying phenotypes, ML/DL has been aiding network inference and improving network coverage via the prediction of missing connections with supervised and unsupervised analyses [52,156]. While data integration is a cornerstone of network-based inference, most aggregation results in a single network endeavoring to represent a population with a broad spectrum of phenotypic differences. Despite being informative in terms of finding shared characteristics of the inspected population, aggregated networks generally ignore population heterogeneity. Emerging attention for precision medicine has facilitated the development of personalized characterization of biological perturbations. Several efforts have been made in network medicine to account for individual-level estimations, e.g., via overlaying the sample-specific expression data on the known biological networks, or interpolation of aggregated networks with and without a sample to estimate network contribution of such sample [157,158].

Empowered by the ever-growing amount of biomedical data and new computational analyses, the network-centric approach will keep proving itself as a powerful tool for the comprehension of vast knowledge to shed light on new repurposing candidates for psychiatric disorders.

Author Contributions: Conceptualization: T.T.T.T., J.H.K. and K.W.; writing—original draft preparation, T.T.T.T. and B.P.; writing—review and editing, T.T.T.T., B.P., J.H.K. and K.W.; visualization, T.T.T.T.; supervision, J.H.K. and K.W.; funding acquisition, K.W. All authors have read and agreed to the published version of the manuscript.

Funding: This research was funded by National Health and Medical Research Council (NHMRC) Project Grant (1078928) and Centre of Research Excellence (1153607).

Institutional Review Board Statement: Not applicable.

Informed Consent Statement: Not applicable.

Data Availability Statement: Data sharing not applicable.

Conflicts of Interest: The authors declare no conflict of interest.

References

1. Vos, T.; Abajobir, A.A.; Abate, K.H.; Abbafati, C.; Abbas, K.M.; Abd-Allah, F.; Abdulkader, R.S.; Abdulle, A.M.; Abebo, T.A.; Abera, S.F. Global, regional, and national incidence, prevalence, and years lived with disability for 328 diseases and injuries for 195 countries, 1990–2016: A systematic analysis for the Global Burden of Disease Study 2016. *Lancet* **2017**, *390*, 1211–1259. [CrossRef]
2. Scott, K.M.; de Jonge, P.; Stein, D.J.; Kessler, R.C. *Mental Disorders around the World: Facts and Figures from the WHO World Mental Health Surveys*; Cambridge University Press: Cambridge, UK, 2018.
3. U.S. Food and Drug Administration. *New Molecular Entity (NME) Drug and New Biologic Approvals*; U.S. Food and Drug Administration: Silver Spring, MD, USA, 2019.
4. U.S. Food and Drug Administration. *New Molecular Entity (NME) Drug and New Biologic Approvals*; U.S. Food and Drug Administration: Silver Spring, MD, USA, 2020.
5. Stahl, S.M. *Stahl's Essential Psychopharmacology: Neuroscientific Basis and Practical Applications*; Cambridge University Press: Cambridge, UK, 2013.
6. Lee, H.-M.; Kim, Y. Drug Repurposing Is a New Opportunity for Developing Drugs against Neuropsychiatric Disorders. *Schizophr. Res. Treat.* **2016**, *2016*, 6378137. [CrossRef] [PubMed]
7. Scannell, J.W.; Blanckley, A.; Boldon, H.; Warrington, B. Diagnosing the decline in pharmaceutical R&D efficiency. *Nat. Rev. Drug Discov.* **2012**, *11*, 191–200. [CrossRef] [PubMed]

8. Akhondzadeh, S. The Importance of Clinical Trials in Drug Development. *Avicenna J. Med. Biotechnol.* **2016**, *8*, 151. [PubMed]
9. Hughes, J.P.; Rees, S.; Kalindjian, S.B.; Philpott, K.L. Principles of early drug discovery. *Br. J. Pharmacol.* **2011**, *162*, 1239–1249. [CrossRef]
10. Blokhin, I.O.; Khorkova, O.; Saveanu, R.V.; Wahlestedt, C. Molecular mechanisms of psychiatric diseases. *Neurobiol. Dis.* **2020**, *146*, 105136. [CrossRef]
11. Gribkoff, V.K.; Kaczmarek, L.K. The need for new approaches in CNS drug discovery: Why drugs have failed, and what can be done to improve outcomes. *Neuropharmacology* **2017**, *120*, 11–19. [CrossRef]
12. Pushpakom, S.; Iorio, F.; Eyers, P.A.; Escott, K.J.; Hopper, S.; Wells, A.; Doig, A.; Guilliams, T.; Latimer, J.; McNamee, C.; et al. Drug repurposing: Progress, challenges and recommendations. *Nat. Rev. Drug Discov.* **2019**, *18*, 41–58. [CrossRef]
13. Ashburn, T.T.; Thor, K.B. Drug repositioning: Identifying and developing new uses for existing drugs. *Nat. Rev. Drug Discov.* **2004**, *3*, 673–683. [CrossRef]
14. Ko, Y. Computational Drug Repositioning: Current Progress and Challenges. *Appl. Sci.* **2020**, *10*, 5076. [CrossRef]
15. Graul, A.I.; Pina, P.; Cruces, E.; Stringer, M. The year's new drugs and biologics 2018: Part I. *Drugs Today* **2019**, *55*, 35–87. [CrossRef] [PubMed]
16. Sardana, D.; Zhu, C.; Zhang, M.; Gudivada, R.C.; Yang, L.; Jegga, A.G. Drug repositioning for orphan diseases. *Brief. Bioinform.* **2011**, *12*, 346–356. [CrossRef] [PubMed]
17. Power, A.; Berger, A.C.; Ginsburg, G.S. Genomics-enabled drug repositioning and repurposing: Insights from an IOM Roundtable activity. *JAMA* **2014**, *311*, 2063–2064. [CrossRef] [PubMed]
18. Caban, A.; Pisarczyk, K.; Kopacz, K.; Kapuśniak, A.; Toumi, M.; Rémuzat, C.; Kornfeld, A. Filling the gap in CNS drug development: Evaluation of the role of drug repurposing. *J. Mark Access Health Policy* **2017**, *5*, 1299833. [CrossRef] [PubMed]
19. Yildiz, A.; Aydin, B.; Gökmen, N.; Yurt, A.; Cohen, B.; Keskinoglu, P.; Öngür, D.; Renshaw, P. Antimanic Treatment With Tamoxifen Affects Brain Chemistry: A Double-Blind, Placebo-Controlled Proton Magnetic Resonance Spectroscopy Study. *Biol. Psychiatry Cogn. Neurosci. Neuroimaging* **2016**, *1*, 125–131. [CrossRef]
20. Pharmaceuticals, A. A Multicenter, Randomized, Double-blind, Placebo-Controlled, Parallel-Arm Study to Assess the Efficacy, Safety, and Tolerability of AVP-786 (Deudextromethorphan Hydrobromide [d6-DM]/Quinidine Sulfate [Q]) for the Treatment of Negative Symptoms of Schizophrenia. Available online: https://www.clinicaltrials.gov/ct2/show/study/NCT03896945 (accessed on 16 May 2022).
21. Bowden, C. The effectiveness of divalproate in all forms of mania and the broader bipolar spectrum: Many questions, few answers. *J. Affect. Disord.* **2004**, *79*, 9–14. [CrossRef]
22. Schwartz, J.; Murrough, J.W.; Iosifescu, D.V. Ketamine for treatment-resistant depression: Recent developments and clinical applications. *Evid. Based Ment. Health* **2016**, *19*, 35. [CrossRef]
23. Maron, B.A.; Altucci, L.; Balligand, J.-L.; Baumbach, J.; Ferdinandy, P.; Filetti, S.; Parini, P.; Petrillo, E.; Silverman, E.K.; Barabási, A.-L.; et al. A global network for network medicine. *NPJ Syst. Biol. Appl.* **2020**, *6*, 29. [CrossRef] [PubMed]
24. Hopkins, A.L. Network pharmacology: The next paradigm in drug discovery. *Nat. Chem. Biol.* **2008**, *4*, 682–690. [CrossRef]
25. Bianchi, M.T.; Botzolakis, E.J. Targeting ligand-gated ion channels in neurology and psychiatry: Is pharmacological promiscuity an obstacle or an opportunity? *BMC Pharmacol.* **2010**, *10*, 3. [CrossRef]
26. Cross-Disorder Group of the Psychiatric Genomics Consortium. Identification of risk loci with shared effects on five major psychiatric disorders: A genome-wide analysis. *Lancet* **2013**, *381*, 1371–1379. [CrossRef]
27. Anttila, V.; Bulik-Sullivan, B.; Finucane, H.K.; Walters, R.K.; Bras, J.; Duncan, L.; Escott-Price, V.; Falcone, G.J.; Gormley, P.; Malik, R.; et al. Analysis of shared heritability in common disorders of the brain. *Science* **2018**, *360*, eaap875. [CrossRef]
28. Gandal Michael, J.; Haney Jillian, R.; Parikshak Neelroop, N.; Leppa, V.; Ramaswami, G.; Hartl, C.; Schork Andrew, J.; Appadurai, V.; Buil, A.; Werge Thomas, M.; et al. Shared molecular neuropathology across major psychiatric disorders parallels polygenic overlap. *Science* **2018**, *359*, 693–697. [CrossRef]
29. Gandal, M.J.; Zhang, P.; Hadjimichael, E.; Walker, R.L.; Chen, C.; Liu, S.; Won, H.; van Bakel, H.; Varghese, M.; Wang, Y.; et al. Transcriptome-wide isoform-level dysregulation in ASD, schizophrenia, and bipolar disorder. *Science* **2018**, *362*, eaat8127. [CrossRef] [PubMed]
30. Jacobi, F.; Wittchen, H.U.; HÖLting, C.; Höfler, M.; Pfister, H.; Müller, N.; Lieb, R. Prevalence, co-morbidity and correlates of mental disorders in the general population: Results from the German Health Interview and Examination Survey (GHS). *Psychol. Med.* **2004**, *34*, 597–611. [CrossRef]
31. Andrews, G.; Henderson, S.; Hall, W. Prevalence, comorbidity, disability and service utilisation: Overview of the Australian National Mental Health Survey. *Br. J. Psychiatry* **2001**, *178*, 145–153. [CrossRef]
32. Kessler, R.C.; McGonagle, K.A.; Zhao, S.; Nelson, C.B.; Hughes, M.; Eshleman, S.; Wittchen, H.-U.; Kendler, K.S. Lifetime and 12-Month Prevalence of DSM-III-R Psychiatric Disorders in the United States: Results From the National Comorbidity Survey. *Arch. Gen. Psychiatry* **1994**, *51*, 8–19. [CrossRef]
33. Merikangas, K.R.; Angst, J.; Eaton, W.; Canino, G.; Rubio-Stipec, M.; Wacker, H.; Wittchen, H.U.; Andrade, L.; Essau, C.; Whitaker, A.; et al. Comorbidity and boundaries of affective disorders with anxiety disorders and substance misuse: Results of an international task force. *Br. J. Psychiatry Suppl.* **1996**, *168*, 58–67. [CrossRef]
34. Qu, X.A.; Gudivada, R.C.; Jegga, A.G.; Neumann, E.K.; Aronow, B.J. Inferring novel disease indications for known drugs by semantically linking drug action and disease mechanism relationships. *BMC Bioinform.* **2009**, *10* (Suppl. S5), S4. [CrossRef]

35. Barabási, A.-L. *Network Science*; Cambridge University Press: Cambridge, UK, 2016.
36. Recanatini, M.; Cabrelle, C. Drug Research Meets Network Science: Where Are We? *J. Med. Chem.* **2020**, *63*, 8653–8666. [CrossRef]
37. Csermely, P.; Korcsmáros, T.; Kiss, H.J.M.; London, G.; Nussinov, R. Structure and dynamics of molecular networks: A novel paradigm of drug discovery: A comprehensive review. *Pharmacol. Ther.* **2013**, *138*, 333–408. [CrossRef] [PubMed]
38. Albert, R.K. Network Inference, Analysis, and Modeling in Systems Biology. *Plant Cell* **2007**, *19*, 3327–3338. [CrossRef]
39. Kitano, H. Systems Biology: A Brief Overview. *Science* **2002**, *295*, 1662–1664. [CrossRef] [PubMed]
40. Vidal, M.; Cusick, M.E.; Barabási, A.-L. Interactome Networks and Human Disease. *Cell* **2011**, *144*, 986–998. [CrossRef] [PubMed]
41. *Network Medicine: Complex Systems in Human Disease and Therapeutics*; Harvard University Press: Cambridge, MA, USA, 2017.
42. Barabási, A.-L.; Albert, R. Emergence of Scaling in Random Networks. *Science* **1999**, *286*, 509–512. [CrossRef]
43. Seebacher, J.; Gavin, A.C. SnapShot: Protein-protein interaction networks. *Cell* **2011**, *144*, 1000. [CrossRef]
44. Barabási, A.-L.; Oltvai, Z.N. Network biology: Understanding the cell's functional organization. *Nat. Rev. Genet.* **2004**, *5*, 101–113. [CrossRef]
45. Penrod, N.M.; Cowper-Sal-lari, R.; Moore, J.H. Systems genetics for drug target discovery. *Trends Pharmacol. Sci.* **2011**, *32*, 623–630. [CrossRef]
46. Swanson, D.R. Fish oil, Raynaud's syndrome, and undiscovered public knowledge. *Perspect. Biol. Med.* **1986**, *30*, 7–18. [CrossRef]
47. Baek, S.H.; Lee, D.; Kim, M.; Lee, J.H.; Song, M. Enriching plausible new hypothesis generation in PubMed. *PLoS ONE* **2017**, *12*, e0180539. [CrossRef]
48. Weeber, M.; Klein, H.; de Jong-van den Berg, L.T.W.; Vos, R. Using concepts in literature-based discovery: Simulating Swanson's Raynaud–fish oil and migraine–magnesium discoveries. *J. Am. Soc. Inf. Sci. Technol.* **2001**, *52*, 548–557. [CrossRef]
49. Chiang, A.P.; Butte, A.J. Systematic evaluation of drug-disease relationships to identify leads for novel drug uses. *Clin. Pharm.* **2009**, *86*, 507–510. [CrossRef] [PubMed]
50. Andronis, C.; Sharma, A.; Virvilis, V.; Deftereos, S.; Persidis, A. Literature mining, ontologies and information visualization for drug repurposing. *Brief. Bioinform.* **2011**, *12*, 357–368. [CrossRef] [PubMed]
51. Lekka, E.; Deftereos, S.N.; Persidis, A.; Persidis, A.; Andronis, C. Literature analysis for systematic drug repurposing: A case study from Biovista. *Drug Discov. Today Ther. Strateg.* **2011**, *8*, 103–108. [CrossRef]
52. Krassowski, M.; Das, V.; Sahu, S.K.; Misra, B.B. State of the Field in Multi-Omics Research: From Computational Needs to Data Mining and Sharing. *Front. Genet.* **2020**, *11*, 610798. [CrossRef]
53. Mendez, D.; Gaulton, A.; Bento, A.P.; Chambers, J.; De Veij, M.; Félix, E.; Magariños, M.P.; Mosquera, J.F.; Mutowo, P.; Nowotka, M.; et al. ChEMBL: Towards direct deposition of bioassay data. *Nucleic Acids Res.* **2019**, *47*, D930–D940. [CrossRef]
54. Pence, H.E.; Williams, A. ChemSpider: An Online Chemical Information Resource. *J. Chem. Educ.* **2010**, *87*, 1123–1124. [CrossRef]
55. Wishart, D.S.; Feunang, Y.D.; Guo, A.C.; Lo, E.J.; Marcu, A.; Grant, J.R.; Sajed, T.; Johnson, D.; Li, C.; Sayeeda, Z.; et al. DrugBank 5.0: A major update to the DrugBank database for 2018. *Nucleic Acids Res.* **2018**, *46*, D1074–D1082. [CrossRef]
56. Kim, S.; Chen, J.; Cheng, T.; Gindulyte, A.; He, J.; He, S.; Li, Q.; Shoemaker, B.A.; Thiessen, P.A.; Yu, B.; et al. PubChem 2019 update: Improved access to chemical data. *Nucleic Acids Res.* **2019**, *47*, D1102–D1109. [CrossRef]
57. Burley, S.K.; Bhikadiya, C.; Bi, C.; Bittrich, S.; Chen, L.; Crichlow, G.V.; Christie, C.H.; Dalenberg, K.; Di Costanzo, L.; Duarte, J.M.; et al. RCSB Protein Data Bank: Powerful new tools for exploring 3D structures of biological macromolecules for basic and applied research and education in fundamental biology, biomedicine, biotechnology, bioengineering and energy sciences. *Nucleic Acids Res.* **2021**, *49*, D437–D451. [CrossRef]
58. Jumper, J.; Evans, R.; Pritzel, A.; Green, T.; Figurnov, M.; Ronneberger, O.; Tunyasuvunakool, K.; Bates, R.; Žídek, A.; Potapenko, A.; et al. Highly accurate protein structure prediction with AlphaFold. *Nature* **2021**, *596*, 583–589. [CrossRef] [PubMed]
59. Tan, F.; Yang, R.; Xu, X.; Chen, X.; Wang, Y.; Ma, H.; Liu, X.; Wu, X.; Chen, Y.; Liu, L.; et al. Drug repositioning by applying 'expression profiles' generated by integrating chemical structure similarity and gene semantic similarity. *Mol. Biosyst.* **2014**, *10*, 1126–1138. [CrossRef]
60. Watanabe, K.; Stringer, S.; Frei, O.; Umićević Mirkov, M.; de Leeuw, C.; Polderman, T.J.C.; van der Sluis, S.; Andreassen, O.A.; Neale, B.M.; Posthuma, D. A global overview of pleiotropy and genetic architecture in complex traits. *Nat. Genet.* **2019**, *51*, 1339–1348. [CrossRef] [PubMed]
61. Tryka, K.A.; Hao, L.; Sturcke, A.; Jin, Y.; Wang, Z.Y.; Ziyabari, L.; Lee, M.; Popova, N.; Sharopova, N.; Kimura, M.; et al. NCBI's Database of Genotypes and Phenotypes: dbGaP. *Nucleic Acids Res.* **2014**, *42*, D975–D979. [CrossRef] [PubMed]
62. Home | NRGR. NIMH Repository and Genomics Resource. Available online: https://www.nimhgenetics.org/ (accessed on 1 June 2022).
63. The Psychiatric, G.C.S.C. A framework for interpreting genome-wide association studies of psychiatric disorders. *Mol. Psychiatry* **2009**, *14*, 10–17. [CrossRef]
64. Buxbaum, J.D.; Daly, M.J.; Devlin, B.; Lehner, T.; Roeder, K.; State, M.W. The autism sequencing consortium: Large-scale, high-throughput sequencing in autism spectrum disorders. *Neuron* **2012**, *76*, 1052–1056. [CrossRef]
65. Sanders, S.J.; Neale, B.M.; Huang, H.; Werling, D.M.; An, J.-Y.; Dong, S.; Abecasis, G.; Arguello, P.A.; Blangero, J.; Boehnke, M.; et al. Whole genome sequencing in psychiatric disorders: The WGSPD consortium. *Nat. Neurosci.* **2017**, *20*, 1661–1668. [CrossRef]
66. Akbarian, S.; Liu, C.; Knowles, J.A.; Vaccarino, F.M.; Farnham, P.J.; Crawford, G.E.; Jaffe, A.E.; Pinto, D.; Dracheva, S.; Geschwind, D.H.; et al. The PsychENCODE project. *Nat. Neurosci.* **2015**, *18*, 1707–1712. [CrossRef]

67. McConnell, M.J.; Moran, J.V.; Abyzov, A.; Akbarian, S.; Bae, T.; Cortes-Ciriano, I.; Erwin, J.A.; Fasching, L.; Flasch, D.A.; Freed, D.; et al. Intersection of diverse neuronal genomes and neuropsychiatric disease: The Brain Somatic Mosaicism Network. *Science* **2017**, *356*, eaal1641. [CrossRef]
68. Hoffman, G.E.; Bendl, J.; Voloudakis, G.; Montgomery, K.S.; Sloofman, L.; Wang, Y.-C.; Shah, H.R.; Hauberg, M.E.; Johnson, J.S.; Girdhar, K.; et al. CommonMind Consortium provides transcriptomic and epigenomic data for Schizophrenia and Bipolar Disorder. *Sci. Data* **2019**, *6*, 180. [CrossRef]
69. Sunkin, S.M.; Ng, L.; Lau, C.; Dolbeare, T.; Gilbert, T.L.; Thompson, C.L.; Hawrylycz, M.; Dang, C. Allen Brain Atlas: An integrated spatio-temporal portal for exploring the central nervous system. *Nucleic Acids Res.* **2013**, *41*, D996–D1008. [CrossRef] [PubMed]
70. Lamb, J. The Connectivity Map: A new tool for biomedical research. *Nat. Rev. Cancer* **2007**, *7*, 54–60. [CrossRef]
71. Subramanian, A.; Narayan, R.; Corsello, S.M.; Peck, D.D.; Natoli, T.E.; Lu, X.; Gould, J.; Davis, J.F.; Tubelli, A.A.; Asiedu, J.K.; et al. A Next Generation Connectivity Map: L1000 Platform and the First 1,000,000 Profiles. *Cell* **2017**, *171*, 1437–1452.e1417. [CrossRef] [PubMed]
72. Wang, Z.; He, E.; Sani, K.; Jagodnik, K.M.; Silverstein, M.C.; Ma'ayan, A. Drug Gene Budger (DGB): An application for ranking drugs to modulate a specific gene based on transcriptomic signatures. *Bioinformatics* **2019**, *35*, 1247–1248. [CrossRef] [PubMed]
73. Gaspar, H.A.; Gerring, Z.; Hübel, C.; Middeldorp, C.M.; Derks, E.M.; Breen, G.; Major Depressive Disorder Working Group of the Psychiatric Genomics Consortium. Using genetic drug-target networks to develop new drug hypotheses for major depressive disorder. *Transl. Psychiatry* **2019**, *9*, 117. [CrossRef]
74. Rodriguez-López, J.; Arrojo, M.; Paz, E.; Páramo, M.; Costas, J. Identification of relevant hub genes for early intervention at gene coexpression modules with altered predicted expression in schizophrenia. *Prog. Neuro-Psychopharmacol. Biol. Psychiatry* **2020**, *98*, 109815. [CrossRef]
75. Cabrera-Mendoza, B.; Martínez-Magaña, J.J.; Monroy-Jaramillo, N.; Genis-Mendoza, A.D.; Fresno, C.; Fries, G.R.; Walss-Bass, C.; López Armenta, M.; García-Dolores, F.; Díaz-Otañez, C.E.; et al. Candidate pharmacological treatments for substance use disorder and suicide identified by gene co-expression network-based drug repositioning. *Am. J. Med. Genet. Part B Neuropsychiatr. Genet.* **2021**, *186*, 193–206. [CrossRef]
76. Gao, H.; Ni, Y.; Mo, X.; Li, D.; Teng, S.; Huang, Q.; Huang, S.; Liu, G.; Zhang, S.; Tang, Y.; et al. Drug repositioning based on network-specific core genes identifies potential drugs for the treatment of autism spectrum disorder in children. *Comput. Struct. Biotechnol. J.* **2021**, *19*, 3908–3921. [CrossRef]
77. Szklarczyk, D.; Gable, A.L.; Nastou, K.C.; Lyon, D.; Kirsch, R.; Pyysalo, S.; Doncheva, N.T.; Legeay, M.; Fang, T.; Bork, P.; et al. The STRING database in 2021: Customizable protein–protein networks, and functional characterization of user-uploaded gene/measurement sets. *Nucleic Acids Res.* **2021**, *49*, D605–D612. [CrossRef]
78. Peri, S.; Navarro, J.D.; Kristiansen, T.Z.; Amanchy, R.; Surendranath, V.; Muthusamy, B.; Gandhi, T.K.B.; Chandrika, K.N.; Deshpande, N.; Suresh, S.; et al. Human protein reference database as a discovery resource for proteomics. *Nucleic Acids Res.* **2004**, *32*, D497–D501. [CrossRef]
79. Croft, D.; O'Kelly, G.; Wu, G.; Haw, R.; Gillespie, M.; Matthews, L.; Caudy, M.; Garapati, P.; Gopinath, G.; Jassal, B.; et al. Reactome: A database of reactions, pathways and biological processes. *Nucleic Acids Res.* **2011**, *39*, D691–D697. [CrossRef] [PubMed]
80. Kanehisa, M.; Goto, S. KEGG: Kyoto Encyclopedia of Genes and Genomes. *Nucleic Acids Res.* **2000**, *28*, 27–30. [CrossRef] [PubMed]
81. Lambert, S.A.; Jolma, A.; Campitelli, L.F.; Das, P.K.; Yin, Y.; Albu, M.; Chen, X.; Taipale, J.; Hughes, T.R.; Weirauch, M.T. The Human Transcription Factors. *Cell* **2018**, *172*, 650–665. [CrossRef]
82. Boyle, A.P.; Hong, E.L.; Hariharan, M.; Cheng, Y.; Schaub, M.A.; Kasowski, M.; Karczewski, K.J.; Park, J.; Hitz, B.C.; Weng, S.; et al. Annotation of functional variation in personal genomes using RegulomeDB. *Genome Res.* **2012**, *22*, 1790–1797. [CrossRef] [PubMed]
83. Weirauch, M.T.; Yang, A.; Albu, M.; Cote, A.G.; Montenegro-Montero, A.; Drewe, P.; Najafabadi, H.S.; Lambert, S.A.; Mann, I.; Cook, K.; et al. Determination and inference of eukaryotic transcription factor sequence specificity. *Cell* **2014**, *158*, 1431–1443. [CrossRef] [PubMed]
84. Castro-Mondragon, J.A.; Riudavets-Puig, R.; Rauluseviciute, I.; Berhanu Lemma, R.; Turchi, L.; Blanc-Mathieu, R.; Lucas, J.; Boddie, P.; Khan, A.; Manosalva Pérez, N.; et al. JASPAR 2022: The 9th release of the open-access database of transcription factor binding profiles. *Nucleic Acids Res.* **2022**, *50*, D165–D173. [CrossRef] [PubMed]
85. Hume, M.A.; Barrera, L.A.; Gisselbrecht, S.S.; Bulyk, M.L. UniPROBE, update 2015: New tools and content for the online database of protein-binding microarray data on protein-DNA interactions. *Nucleic Acids Res.* **2015**, *43*, D117–D122. [CrossRef] [PubMed]
86. Matys, V.; Kel-Margoulis, O.V.; Fricke, E.; Liebich, I.; Land, S.; Barre-Dirrie, A.; Reuter, I.; Chekmenev, D.; Krull, M.; Hornischer, K.; et al. TRANSFAC and its module TRANSCompel: Transcriptional gene regulation in eukaryotes. *Nucleic Acids Res.* **2006**, *34*, D108–D110. [CrossRef]
87. Türei, D.; Korcsmáros, T.; Saez-Rodriguez, J. OmniPath: Guidelines and gateway for literature-curated signaling pathway resources. *Nat. Methods* **2016**, *13*, 966–967. [CrossRef]
88. Ganapathiraju, M.K.; Thahir, M.; Handen, A.; Sarkar, S.N.; Sweet, R.A.; Nimgaonkar, V.L.; Loscher, C.E.; Bauer, E.M.; Chaparala, S. Schizophrenia interactome with 504 novel protein–protein interactions. *NPJ Schizophr.* **2016**, *2*, 16012. [CrossRef]

89. Kauppi, K.; Rosenthal, S.B.; Lo, M.-T.; Sanyal, N.; Jiang, M.; Abagyan, R.; McEvoy, L.K.; Andreassen, O.A.; Chen, C.-H. Revisiting Antipsychotic Drug Actions Through Gene Networks Associated With Schizophrenia. *Am. J. Psychiatry* **2018**, *175*, 674–682. [CrossRef] [PubMed]
90. Li, H.; Zhou, D.-S.; Chang, H.; Wang, L.; Liu, W.; Dai, S.-X.; Zhang, C.; Cai, J.; Liu, W.; Li, X.; et al. Interactome Analyses implicated CAMK2A in the genetic predisposition and pharmacological mechanism of Bipolar Disorder. *J. Psychiatr. Res.* **2019**, *115*, 165–175. [CrossRef] [PubMed]
91. De Bastiani, M.A.; Pfaffenseller, B.; Klamt, F. Master Regulators Connectivity Map: A Transcription Factors-Centered Approach to Drug Repositioning. *Front. Pharmacol.* **2018**, *9*, 697. [CrossRef]
92. Kuhn, M.; Campillos, M.; Letunic, I.; Jensen, L.J.; Bork, P. A side effect resource to capture phenotypic effects of drugs. *Mol. Syst. Biol.* **2010**, *6*, 343. [CrossRef] [PubMed]
93. Whirl-Carrillo, M.; Huddart, R.; Gong, L.; Sangkuhl, K.; Thorn, C.F.; Whaley, R.; Klein, T.E. An Evidence-Based Framework for Evaluating Pharmacogenomics Knowledge for Personalized Medicine. *Clin Pharm.* **2021**, *110*, 563–572. [CrossRef]
94. Freshour, S.L.; Kiwala, S.; Cotto, K.C.; Coffman, A.C.; McMichael, J.F.; Song, J.J.; Griffith, M.; Griffith, O.L.; Wagner, A.H. Integration of the Drug–Gene Interaction Database (DGIdb 4.0) with open crowdsource efforts. *Nucleic Acids Res.* **2021**, *49*, D1144–D1151. [CrossRef]
95. Avram, S.; Bologa, C.G.; Holmes, J.; Bocci, G.; Wilson, T.B.; Nguyen, D.-T.; Curpan, R.; Halip, L.; Bora, A.; Yang, J.J.; et al. DrugCentral 2021 supports drug discovery and repositioning. *Nucleic Acids Res.* **2021**, *49*, D1160–D1169. [CrossRef]
96. Mitsopoulos, C.; Di Micco, P.; Fernandez, E.V.; Dolciami, D.; Holt, E.; Mica, I.L.; Coker, E.A.; Tym, J.E.; Campbell, J.; Che, K.H.; et al. canSAR: Update to the cancer translational research and drug discovery knowledgebase. *Nucleic Acids Res.* **2021**, *49*, D1074–D1082. [CrossRef]
97. Kanehisa, M.; Furumichi, M.; Tanabe, M.; Sato, Y.; Morishima, K. KEGG: New perspectives on genomes, pathways, diseases and drugs. *Nucleic Acids Res.* **2017**, *45*, D353–D361. [CrossRef]
98. Harding, S.D.; Armstrong, J.F.; Faccenda, E.; Southan, C.; Alexander, S.P.H.; Davenport, A.P.; Pawson, A.J.; Spedding, M.; Davies, J.A.; Nc, I. The IUPHAR/BPS guide to pharmacology in 2022: Curating pharmacology for COVID-19, malaria and antibacterials. *Nucleic Acids Res.* **2022**, *50*, D1282–D1294. [CrossRef]
99. Szklarczyk, D.; Santos, A.; von Mering, C.; Jensen, L.J.; Bork, P.; Kuhn, M. STITCH 5: Augmenting protein–chemical interaction networks with tissue and affinity data. *Nucleic Acids Res.* **2016**, *44*, D380–D384. [CrossRef] [PubMed]
100. Chen, Y.-W.; Diamante, G.; Ding, J.; Nghiem, T.X.; Yang, J.; Ha, S.-M.; Cohn, P.; Arneson, D.; Blencowe, M.; Garcia, J.; et al. PharmOmics: A species- and tissue-specific drug signature database and gene-network-based drug repositioning tool. *iScience* **2022**, *25*, 104052. [CrossRef] [PubMed]
101. Zhou, Y.; Zhang, Y.; Lian, X.; Li, F.; Wang, C.; Zhu, F.; Qiu, Y.; Chen, Y. Therapeutic target database update 2022: Facilitating drug discovery with enriched comparative data of targeted agents. *Nucleic Acids Res.* **2022**, *50*, D1398–D1407. [CrossRef] [PubMed]
102. Yoo, M.; Shin, J.; Kim, J.; Ryall, K.A.; Lee, K.; Lee, S.; Jeon, M.; Kang, J.; Tan, A.C. DSigDB: Drug signatures database for gene set analysis. *Bioinformatics* **2015**, *31*, 3069–3071. [CrossRef] [PubMed]
103. Nguyen, D.-T.; Mathias, S.; Bologa, C.; Brunak, S.; Fernandez, N.; Gaulton, A.; Hersey, A.; Holmes, J.; Jensen, L.J.; Karlsson, A.; et al. Pharos: Collating protein information to shed light on the druggable genome. *Nucleic Acids Res.* **2017**, *45*, D995–D1002. [CrossRef] [PubMed]
104. Jensen, H.N.; Roth, L.B. Massively Parallel Screening of the Receptorome. *Comb. Chem. High Throughput Screen.* **2008**, *11*, 420–426. [CrossRef] [PubMed]
105. Gilson, M.K.; Liu, T.; Baitaluk, M.; Nicola, G.; Hwang, L.; Chong, J. BindingDB in 2015: A public database for medicinal chemistry, computational chemistry and systems pharmacology. *Nucleic Acids Res.* **2016**, *44*, D1045–D1053. [CrossRef]
106. Amberger, J.S.; Bocchini, C.A.; Scott, A.F.; Hamosh, A. OMIM.org: Leveraging knowledge across phenotype–gene relationships. *Nucleic Acids Res.* **2019**, *47*, D1038–D1043. [CrossRef]
107. Landrum, M.J.; Chitipiralla, S.; Brown, G.R.; Chen, C.; Gu, B.; Hart, J.; Hoffman, D.; Jang, W.; Kaur, K.; Liu, C.; et al. ClinVar: Improvements to accessing data. *Nucleic Acids Res.* **2020**, *48*, D835–D844. [CrossRef]
108. Rappaport, N.; Twik, M.; Plaschkes, I.; Nudel, R.; Iny Stein, T.; Levitt, J.; Gershoni, M.; Morrey, C.P.; Safran, M.; Lancet, D. MalaCards: An amalgamated human disease compendium with diverse clinical and genetic annotation and structured search. *Nucleic Acids Res.* **2017**, *45*, D877–D887. [CrossRef]
109. Piñero, J.; Ramírez-Anguita, J.M.; Saüch-Pitarch, J.; Ronzano, F.; Centeno, E.; Sanz, F.; Furlong, L.I. The DisGeNET knowledge platform for disease genomics: 2019 update. *Nucleic Acids Res.* **2020**, *48*, D845–D855. [CrossRef] [PubMed]
110. Köhler, S.; Carmody, L.; Vasilevsky, N.; Jacobsen, J.O.B.; Danis, D.; Gourdine, J.-P.; Gargano, M.; Harris, N.L.; Matentzoglu, N.; McMurry, J.A.; et al. Expansion of the Human Phenotype Ontology (HPO) knowledge base and resources. *Nucleic Acids Res.* **2019**, *47*, D1018–D1027. [CrossRef] [PubMed]
111. Shefchek, K.A.; Harris, N.L.; Gargano, M.; Matentzoglu, N.; Unni, D.; Brush, M.; Keith, D.; Conlin, T.; Vasilevsky, N.; Zhang, X.A.; et al. The Monarch Initiative in 2019: An integrative data and analytic platform connecting phenotypes to genotypes across species. *Nucleic Acids Res.* **2020**, *48*, D704–D715. [CrossRef] [PubMed]
112. Li, B.; Wang, Z.; Chen, Q.; Li, K.; Wang, X.; Wang, Y.; Zeng, Q.; Han, Y.; Lu, B.; Zhao, Y.; et al. GPCards: An integrated database of genotype–phenotype correlations in human genetic diseases. *Comput. Struct. Biotechnol. J.* **2021**, *19*, 1603–1611. [CrossRef]
113. Zhou, X.; Menche, J.; Barabási, A.-L.; Sharma, A. Human symptoms–disease network. *Nat. Commun.* **2014**, *5*, 4212. [CrossRef]

114. Xu, R.; Li, L.; Wang, Q. Towards building a disease-phenotype knowledge base: Extracting disease-manifestation relationship from literature. *Bioinformatics* **2013**, *29*, 2186–2194. [CrossRef]
115. Gillen, J.E.; Tse, T.; Ide, N.C.; McCray, A.T. Design, implementation and management of a web-based data entry system for ClinicalTrials.gov. *Stud. Health Technol. Inform.* **2004**, *107*, 1466–1470.
116. Zhou, M.; Wang, Q.; Zheng, C.; John Rush, A.; Volkow, N.D.; Xu, R. Drug repurposing for opioid use disorders: Integration of computational prediction, clinical corroboration, and mechanism of action analyses. *Mol. Psychiatry* **2021**, *26*, 5286–5296. [CrossRef]
117. Huang, L.-C.; Soysal, E.; Zheng, W.J.; Zhao, Z.; Xu, H.; Sun, J. A weighted and integrated drug-target interactome: Drug repurposing for schizophrenia as a use case. *BMC Syst. Biol.* **2015**, *9*, S2. [CrossRef]
118. Lüscher Dias, T.; Schuch, V.; Beltrão-Braga, P.C.B.; Martins-de-Souza, D.; Brentani, H.P.; Franco, G.R.; Nakaya, H.I. Drug repositioning for psychiatric and neurological disorders through a network medicine approach. *Transl. Psychiatry* **2020**, *10*, 141. [CrossRef]
119. Ben Guebila, M.; Lopes-Ramos, C.M.; Weighill, D.; Sonawane, A.R.; Burkholz, R.; Shamsaei, B.; Platig, J.; Glass, K.; Kuijjer, M.L.; Quackenbush, J. GRAND: A database of gene regulatory network models across human conditions. *Nucleic Acids Res.* **2022**, *50*, D610–D621. [CrossRef] [PubMed]
120. Sadegh, S.; Skelton, J.; Anastasi, E.; Bernett, J.; Blumenthal, D.B.; Galindez, G.; Salgado-Albarrán, M.; Lazareva, O.; Flanagan, K.; Cockell, S.; et al. Network medicine for disease module identification and drug repurposing with the NeDRex platform. *Nat. Commun.* **2021**, *12*, 6848. [CrossRef] [PubMed]
121. Chen, Y.; Elenee Argentinis, J.D.; Weber, G. IBM Watson: How Cognitive Computing Can Be Applied to Big Data Challenges in Life Sciences Research. *Clin. Ther.* **2016**, *38*, 688–701. [CrossRef] [PubMed]
122. Karunakaran, K.B.; Chaparala, S.; Ganapathiraju, M.K. Potentially repurposable drugs for schizophrenia identified from its interactome. *Sci. Rep.* **2019**, *9*, 12682. [CrossRef] [PubMed]
123. Batool, M.; Ahmad, B.; Choi, S. A Structure-Based Drug Discovery Paradigm. *Int. J. Mol. Sci.* **2019**, *20*, 2783. [CrossRef]
124. Kulkarni, J. Selective Estrogen Receptor Modulators-A Potential Treatment for Psychotic Symptoms of Schizophrenia? NCT00361543. Available online: https://clinicaltrials.gov/ct2/show/NCT00361543 (accessed on 28 January 2015).
125. Kulkarni, J.; Gavrilidis, E.; Gwini, S.M.; Worsley, R.; Grigg, J.; Warren, A.; Gurvich, C.; Gilbert, H.; Berk, M.; Davis, S.R. Effect of Adjunctive Raloxifene Therapy on Severity of Refractory Schizophrenia in Women: A Randomized Clinical Trial. *JAMA Psychiatry* **2016**, *73*, 947–954. [CrossRef]
126. Henry, L. UMCC 2013.051: Prospective Pilot Study Evaluating the Use of Cyclobenzaprine for Treatment of Sleep Disturbance, Fatigue, and Musculoskeletal Symptoms in Aromatase Inhibitor-Treated Breast Cancer Patients. NCT01921296. Available online: https://clinicaltrials.gov/ct2/show/NCT01921296 (accessed on 21 March 2016).
127. Hebbring, S.J. The challenges, advantages and future of phenome-wide association studies. *Immunology* **2014**, *141*, 157–165. [CrossRef]
128. Senthil, G.; Dutka, T.; Bingaman, L.; Lehner, T. Genomic resources for the study of neuropsychiatric disorders. *Mol. Psychiatry* **2017**, *22*, 1659–1663. [CrossRef]
129. Shukla, R.; Henkel, N.D.; Alganem, K.; Hamoud, A.-R.; Reigle, J.; Alnafisah, R.S.; Eby, H.M.; Imami, A.S.; Creeden, J.F.; Miruzzi, S.A.; et al. Signature-based approaches for informed drug repurposing: Targeting CNS disorders. *Neuropsychopharmacology* **2020**, *46*, 116–130. [CrossRef]
130. Iorio, F.; Rittman, T.; Ge, H.; Menden, M.; Saez-Rodriguez, J. Transcriptional data: A new gateway to drug repositioning? *Drug Discov. Today* **2013**, *18*, 350–357. [CrossRef]
131. Gaiteri, C.; Ding, Y.; French, B.; Tseng, G.C.; Sibille, E. Beyond modules and hubs: The potential of gene coexpression networks for investigating molecular mechanisms of complex brain disorders. *Genes Brain Behav.* **2014**, *13*, 13–24. [CrossRef] [PubMed]
132. Truong, T.T.; Bortolasci, C.C.; Spolding, B.; Panizzutti, B.; Liu, Z.S.; Kidnapillai, S.; Richardson, M.; Gray, L.; Smith, C.M.; Dean, O.M.; et al. Co-Expression Networks Unveiled Long Non-Coding RNAs as Molecular Targets of Drugs Used to Treat Bipolar Disorder. *Front. Pharmacol.* **2022**, *13*, 873271. [CrossRef] [PubMed]
133. Lamb, J.; Crawford, E.D.; Peck, D.; Modell, J.W.; Blat, I.C.; Wrobel, M.J.; Lerner, J.; Brunet, J.-P.; Subramanian, A.; Ross, K.N.; et al. The Connectivity Map: Using Gene-Expression Signatures to Connect Small Molecules, Genes, and Disease. *Science* **2006**, *313*, 1929–1935. [CrossRef] [PubMed]
134. Vidović, D.; Koleti, A.; Schürer, S.C. Large-scale integration of small molecule-induced genome-wide transcriptional responses, Kinome-wide binding affinities and cell-growth inhibition profiles reveal global trends characterizing systems-level drug action. *Front. Genet.* **2014**, *5*, 342. [CrossRef]
135. Kidnapillai, S.; Bortolasci, C.C.; Udawela, M.; Panizzutti, B.; Spolding, B.; Connor, T.; Sanigorski, A.; Dean, O.M.; Crowley, T.; Jamain, S.; et al. The use of a gene expression signature and connectivity map to repurpose drugs for bipolar disorder. *World J. Biol. Psychiatry* **2020**, *21*, 775–783. [CrossRef]
136. Liu, W.; Tu, W.; Li, L.; Liu, Y.; Wang, S.; Li, L.; Tao, H.; He, H. Revisiting Connectivity Map from a gene co-expression network analysis. *Exp. Med.* **2018**, *16*, 493–500. [CrossRef]
137. Keenan, A.B.; Jenkins, S.L.; Jagodnik, K.M.; Koplev, S.; He, E.; Torre, D.; Wang, Z.; Dohlman, A.B.; Silverstein, M.C.; Lachmann, A.; et al. The Library of Integrated Network-Based Cellular Signatures NIH Program: System-Level Cataloging of Human Cells Response to Perturbations. *Cell Syst.* **2018**, *6*, 13–24. [CrossRef]

138. Dolmetsch, R.; Geschwind, D.H. The human brain in a dish: The promise of iPSC-derived neurons. *Cell* **2011**, *145*, 831–834. [CrossRef]
139. Huang, J.K.; Carlin, D.E.; Yu, M.K.; Zhang, W.; Kreisberg, J.F.; Tamayo, P.; Ideker, T. Systematic Evaluation of Molecular Networks for Discovery of Disease Genes. *Cell Syst.* **2018**, *6*, 484–495.e485. [CrossRef]
140. Zhang, Z.; Zhang, J. A Big World Inside Small-World Networks. *PLoS ONE* **2009**, *4*, e5686. [CrossRef]
141. Szklarczyk, D.; Morris, J.H.; Cook, H.; Kuhn, M.; Wyder, S.; Simonovic, M.; Santos, A.; Doncheva, N.T.; Roth, A.; Bork, P.; et al. The STRING database in 2017: Quality-controlled protein–protein association networks, made broadly accessible. *Nucleic Acids Res.* **2017**, *45*, D362–D368. [CrossRef] [PubMed]
142. Goh, K.-I.; Cusick Michael, E.; Valle, D.; Childs, B.; Vidal, M.; Barabási, A.-L. The human disease network. *Proc. Natl. Acad. Sci. USA* **2007**, *104*, 8685–8690. [CrossRef] [PubMed]
143. Langhauser, F.; Casas, A.I.; Dao, V.-T.-V.; Guney, E.; Menche, J.; Geuss, E.; Kleikers, P.W.M.; López, M.G.; Barabási, A.-L.; Kleinschnitz, C.; et al. A diseasome cluster-based drug repurposing of soluble guanylate cyclase activators from smooth muscle relaxation to direct neuroprotection. *NPJ Syst. Biol. Appl.* **2018**, *4*, 8. [CrossRef]
144. Menche, J.; Sharma, A.; Kitsak, M.; Ghiassian, S.D.; Vidal, M.; Loscalzo, J.; Barabási, A.-L. Disease networks. Uncovering disease-disease relationships through the incomplete interactome. *Science* **2015**, *347*, 1257601. [CrossRef] [PubMed]
145. Palsson, B.; Zengler, K. The challenges of integrating multi-omic data sets. *Nat. Chem. Biol.* **2010**, *6*, 787–789. [CrossRef]
146. Guo, M.G.; Sosa, D.N.; Altman, R.B. Challenges and opportunities in network-based solutions for biological questions. *Brief. Bioinform.* **2022**, *23*, bbab437. [CrossRef] [PubMed]
147. Dai, Y.-F.; Zhao, X.-M. A Survey on the Computational Approaches to Identify Drug Targets in the Postgenomic Era. *BioMed Res. Int.* **2015**, *2015*, 239654. [CrossRef]
148. Arrell, D.K.; Terzic, A. Network systems biology for drug discovery. *Clin. Pharm.* **2010**, *88*, 120–125. [CrossRef]
149. Jarada, T.N.; Rokne, J.G.; Alhajj, R. A review of computational drug repositioning: Strategies, approaches, opportunities, challenges, and directions. *J. Cheminform.* **2020**, *12*, 46. [CrossRef]
150. List of Databases Converted to the OMOP CDM. Available online: https://www.ohdsi.org/web/wiki/doku.php?id=resources:2020_data_network (accessed on 16 May 2022).
151. The All of Us Research Program Investigators. The "All of Us" Research Program. *N. Engl. J. Med.* **2019**, *381*, 668–676. [CrossRef]
152. Agid, Y.; Buzsáki, G.; Diamond, D.M.; Frackowiak, R.; Giedd, J.; Girault, J.-A.; Grace, A.; Lambert, J.J.; Manji, H.; Mayberg, H.; et al. How can drug discovery for psychiatric disorders be improved? *Nat. Rev. Drug Discov.* **2007**, *6*, 189–201. [CrossRef] [PubMed]
153. Wager, T.D.; Woo, C.W. fMRI in analgesic drug discovery. *Sci. Transl. Med.* **2015**, *7*, 274fs276. [CrossRef] [PubMed]
154. Duff, E.P.; Vennart, W.; Wise, R.G.; Howard, M.A.; Harris, R.E.; Lee, M.; Wartolowska, K.; Wanigasekera, V.; Wilson, F.J.; Whitlock, M.; et al. Learning to identify CNS drug action and efficacy using multistudy fMRI data. *Sci. Transl. Med.* **2015**, *7*, 274ra216. [CrossRef] [PubMed]
155. Subramanian, I.; Verma, S.; Kumar, S.; Jere, A.; Anamika, K. Multi-omics Data Integration, Interpretation, and Its Application. *Bioinform. Biol. Insights* **2020**, *14*, 1177932219899051. [CrossRef]
156. Mirza, B.; Wang, W.; Wang, J.; Choi, H.; Chung, N.C.; Ping, P. Machine Learning and Integrative Analysis of Biomedical Big Data. *Genes* **2019**, *10*, 87. [CrossRef]
157. Kuijjer, M.L.; Tung, M.G.; Yuan, G.; Quackenbush, J.; Glass, K. Estimating Sample-Specific Regulatory Networks. *iScience* **2019**, *14*, 226–240. [CrossRef]
158. Liu, C.; Louhimo, R.; Laakso, M.; Lehtonen, R.; Hautaniemi, S. Identification of sample-specific regulations using integrative network level analysis. *BMC Cancer* **2015**, *15*, 319. [CrossRef]

MDPI
St. Alban-Anlage 66
4052 Basel
Switzerland
Tel. +41 61 683 77 34
Fax +41 61 302 89 18
www.mdpi.com

Pharmaceutics Editorial Office
E-mail: pharmaceutics@mdpi.com
www.mdpi.com/journal/pharmaceutics

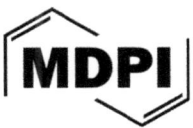